Barcode No: 12003760

WW
100
DEN.

D0492393

OXFORD MEDICAL PUBLICATIONS

Oxford Handbook of
Ophthalmology

Published and forthcoming Oxford Handbooks

Oxford Handbook of
Ophthalmology

Third edition

Alastair K.O. Denniston
Consultant Ophthalmologist
& Honorary Senior Lecturer
Queen Elizabeth Hospital Birmingham
University Hospitals Birmingham NHSFT
& University of Birmingham, UK

Philip I. Murray
Professor of Ophthalmology
& Honorary Consultant Ophthalmologist
University of Birmingham
& Birmingham & Midland Eye Centre
Sandwell & West Birmingham Hospitals NHS Trust, UK

OXFORD
UNIVERSITY PRESS

OXFORD
UNIVERSITY PRESS

Great Clarendon Street, Oxford, OX2 6DP,
United Kingdom

Oxford University Press is a department of the University of Oxford.
It furthers the University's objective of excellence in research, scholarship,
and education by publishing worldwide. Oxford is a registered trade mark of
Oxford University Press in the UK and in certain other countries

© Oxford University Press 2014

The moral rights of the authors have been asserted

First edition published 2006
Second edition published 2009
This edition published 2014

Impression: 1

Published in the United States of America by Oxford University Press
198 Madison Avenue, New York, NY 10016, United States of America

British Library Cataloguing in Publication Data
Data available

Library of Congress Control Number: 2014930096

ISBN 978–0–19–967998–0

Printed and bound in China by
C&C Offset Printing Co., Ltd.

Foreword

It is my great pleasure to write the foreword for this third edition of the *Oxford Handbook of Ophthalmology* by Alastair Denniston and Phil Murray. From the outset, the handbook has been closely aligned to the needs of trainees who have delighted in its ubiquitous support in clinic, theatre, and casualty, and for its help in preparing for postgraduate exams. It has also become popular with senior ophthalmologists who want a portable 'vade mecum' for those times when they have to stray outside their subspecialty. Although small in dimensions, it is quite remarkable how much is contained within it. With its standardized format and pithy style of writing, information is easily navigated, accessed, and remembered.

This new edition is completely revised and updated to reflect the exciting advances in knowledge and treatments of the last few years. In addition, as subspecialization continues to grow, so has the authorship team. Alastair Denniston and Phil Murray have assembled an excellent team across all specialties, comprising established clinical leaders, balanced by senior trainees, to ensure that the text is up to the minute and relevant. The scope of the book continues to impress, with advances in medical retina and refractive surgery rubbing shoulders with new sections on patient-reported outcome measures and Bayesian statistics. New trainees may also be particularly pleased to welcome a new chapter 'Theatre notes' which will help them navigate theatre with greater confidence, correctly identifying surgical instruments and understanding issues around sterilization and so on.

I hope this new edition of the handbook will continue to help you to improve the care of your patients. The patient remains at the heart of all we do. Lists are more than just a way to pass examinations—they help to make us think around diagnoses and management, and they will help to ensure we do not miss something that may be sight- or even life-threatening to our patients. The *Oxford Handbook of Ophthalmology* continues to demonstrate its essential place among the books that help us all learn, enjoy, and deliver the wonderful specialty that is ophthalmology.

Sir Peng Tee Khaw
Professor & Consultant Ophthalmic Surgeon,
Director, National Institute for Health Research Biomedical Research
Centre at Moorfields Eye Hospital and UCL Institute of Ophthalmology,
London 2014

Preface to the third edition

This is surely the most exciting time to be involved in the care of patients with eye disease. Our understanding of ocular pathology is increasing exponentially; our treatment options are multiplying faster than ever before, and the sophistication and specificity of some investigative tools and treatments are quite breathtaking. Now is also a period of great hope for our patients, as they continue to benefit from the success stories of the last decade (such as anti-VEGF therapies for neovascular age-related macular degeneration and other retinal diseases) and become increasingly aware of the dawn of gene therapy, cell-based therapies, and personalized medicine.

There are, however, two occasions when an ophthalmologist may have cause to regret this explosion of knowledge: first, in their youth as they have to hurdle an apparently never-ending succession of exams; and second, in their old(er) age when they have the equally challenging task of distilling all that knowledge into a single lucid volume of text. It is our great privilege—on behalf of a wonderful team of authors—to present to you this third edition of the best-selling *Oxford Handbook of Ophthalmology*. We trust that this edition will continue to provide you with knowledge—that essential information you need in an easily accessible format—but also that it may inspire you as you care for patients suffering from ophthalmic disease.

AKOD, PIM
2014

Preface to the first edition

Welcome to the first edition of the *Oxford Handbook of Ophthalmology*.

The aspiration of the *OHO* is to be your portable repository of knowledge, accessible in emergencies and easily dipped in and out of between examining patients. It provides immediate access to the detailed clinical information you need—in casualty, clinic, theatre, and on the wards. It is also highly suitable for revision for postgraduate examinations. It is not exhaustive, and we would expect it to complement, rather than replace, your collection of desktop ophthalmology heavyweights.

The core of the book comprises a systematic synopsis of ophthalmic disease directed towards diagnosis, interim assessment, and ongoing management. Assessment boxes for common clinical conditions and algorithms for important clinical presentations illustrate this practical approach. The information is easily accessed, being presented in standard format with areas of importance being highlighted. Key sections for the trainee include: clinical skills, aids to diagnosis, and investigations and their interpretation. Basic perioperative care and advanced life support protocols are included, since specialists often find their general medical knowledge somewhat hazy at times of crisis.

Primarily intended for ophthalmologists, this handbook is a valuable resource for anyone working with ophthalmic patients, whether optometrists, orthoptists, ophthalmic nurses, or other health professionals in ophthalmology. Whilst the earlier pages may be thumbed mainly by the trainee, it is envisaged that even the experienced consultant will find the *OHO* useful. We have tried to include information that you would not easily find elsewhere: vision in context (low vision, registration and benefits, driving requirements), management of systemic disease (diabetes, thyroid disorders, systemic immunosuppression), a glossary of eponymous syndromes, and NICE and RCOphth guidelines.

Although we have endeavoured to provide up-to-date, accurate, evidence-based information, any comments would be gratefully received so that we can make future editions even better. Point your web browser to: ✆ http://www.oup.co.uk/academic/medicine/handbooks, where you will be able to have your say and to download any updates.

We hope the *OHO* will be an essential addition to your personal library of ophthalmology textbooks and be an invaluable companion to you in your practice of ophthalmology.

Alastair K.O. Denniston, Philip I. Murray
2006

Acknowledgements

As authors and editors of this book, we are privileged to coordinate a wonderful team of ophthalmologists, orthoptists, optometrists, visual scientists, ophthalmic technicians, and other professionals who care for people with eye disease. These people are not only experts in their fields but are passionate about ensuring that this wisdom is passed on to the rest of us. These authors continue to distil the complexities of their subspecialties in a way that is concise, clear, memorable, and easily applied in clinic, theatre, or eye casualty. We are deeply indebted to them, and the junior authors who assisted them, for all their hard work.

There are also many senior ophthalmologists who, like us, can measure the passage of the years by their contributions to successive editions of this handbook. Significant contributors to previous editions include: Miss Susan Mollan, Mr Arun Reginald, Mr Geraint Williams, Mr Paul Tomlins, Mr Anil Arilakatti, Miss Rosemary Robinson, Mr Paul Chell, Miss Monique Hope-Ross, Mr Graham Kirkby, Miss Fiona Dean, Prof Sunil Shah, Mrs Waheeda Illahi, Mr Mike Burdon, Sonal Rughani, Mr Vijay Savant, Mr Sumit Dhingra, Mr Rajen Gupta, Mr Joseph Abbott, Mr James iDOC Cameron, Mr James Flint, Mr Tahir Masoud, and Mr David Lockington. We also thank Rizwana Siddiqui, Musarrat Allie, and Dr Peter Good for images. We are grateful to Angela Luck for yet more beautiful anatomical illustrations and her ongoing appreciation of the artistic merits of the slit-lamp. Additionally, new for this edition, we thank Altomed and John Weiss for kindly giving us permission to include images of their surgical instruments, and to Paul Sims of Action for Blind People for his valuable input to the 'Vision in context' chapter.

It has been a great pleasure to work with the staff of OUP throughout. We thank Kate Smith, Elizabeth Reeve, Michael Hawkes, Beth Womack, and Anna Winstanley for their enthusiasm and practical assistance.

AD wishes to thank his wife (Sarah) and his two boys (Arran and Ewan) for their critical assessment of this work and allowing the evolving manuscript to join us for almost all of our holidays. He also wishes to thank his clinical mentors (Marie Tsaloumas, Andrew Dick, Phil Murray) for their ongoing advice and encouragement.

PIM wishes to thank his family (Tricia, Hannah, Ella) for trying to keep out of his way while attempting to write this book. He is grateful to Out of the Blue Jazz Orchestra and The Soul Providers for almost keeping him sane and thanks his local garage who keeps his 1997 Porsche 993 Targa (which he may have reluctantly sold by the time this edition hits the shelves) on the road—except in the snow and ice. He also thanks Birmingham public transport and all the colleagues who have given him lifts to and from work. He does not wish to thank Brentford FC who seem only capable of scoring or letting in goals in the 95th minute and their abject failure in taking penalties.

AKOD, PIM, 2014

Additional acknowledgements

We are indebted to a number of colleagues from across the UK and the rest of the world who have given us invaluable feedback which has helped direct the development of successive editions. We thank: Mr Ajay Tyagi, Mr Sam Elsherbiny, Mr Sam Mirza, Mr Velota Sung, Dr Zakaria, Dr Hannah Baker, Mr Maged Nessim, Dr Imran Khan, Dr Anna Gao, Miss Lei Liu, Mr Nachiketa Acharya, Mr James Denniston, Dr Estelle Manson-Whitton, Mr Ali Bell, Dr Ed Moran, Miss Vaneeta Sood, Miss Anne Williams, Miss Katya Tambe, Dr Liz Justice, Mr Imran Masood, Mr Pravin Pandey, Miss Dipti Trivedi, and Mr Richard Lee.

Contents

Chapter authors

Clinical skills
Mr Alastair K.O. Denniston
Prof James Wolffsohn
Ms Rosie Auld
Prof Philip I. Murray

Investigations and their interpretation
Miss Susan P. Mollan
Mr Antonio Calcagni
Dr Steve Colley
Mr Pearse A. Keane

Ocular trauma
Wg Cdr Malcolm Woodcock
Mr Matthew Edmunds
Mr Omar Durrani
Miss Saaeha Rauz

Lids
Miss Julia Hale
Miss Saaeha Rauz
Mr Aidan Murray

Lacrimal
Miss Julia Hale
Mr Aidan Murray

Conjunctiva
Miss Saaeha Rauz

Cornea
Miss Saaeha Rauz
Mr Sai Kolli

Sclera
Mr Alastair K.O. Denniston
Mr Carlos E. Pavesio
Prof Philip I. Murray

Lens
Mr Vijay Savant
Mr Sai Kolli

Glaucoma
Miss Freda Sii
Mr Mark Chiang
Prof Peter Shah

Uveitis
Mr Alastair K.O. Denniston
Prof Philip I. Murray

Vitreoretinal
Mr Kwesi Amissah-Arthur
Mr Ash Sharma

Medical retina
Mr Pearse A. Keane
Mr Michel Michaelides
Mr Alastair K.O. Denniston
Mr Adnan Tufail

Orbit
Mr Matthew Edmunds
Mr Omar Durrani

Intraocular tumours
Dr Hibba Quhill
Mr Manoj V. Parulekar
Prof Ian G. Rennie

Neuro-ophthalmology
Miss Susan P. Mollan
Lt Col Andrew S. Jacks

Strabismus
Mr Joseph Abbott
Mr Tim D. Matthews

Paediatric ophthalmology
Mr Thomas Jackson
Miss Lucilla Butler

Refractive ophthalmology
Mr Sai Kolli
Prof James S. Wolffsohn

Aids to diagnosis
Mr Alastair K.O. Denniston
Mr Mike A. Burdon
Prof Philip I. Murray

Vision in context
Mr Alastair K.O. Denniston
Prof Philip I. Murray

Ophthalmic surgery: anaesthetics and perioperative care

Dr Shashi Vohra
Mr Alastair K.O. Denniston
Prof Philip I. Murray

Ophthalmic surgery: theatre notes

Dr Priscilla Mathewson
Mr Alastair K.O. Denniston
Prof Philip I. Murray

Laser

Mr Samer Elsherbiny
Mr Alastair K.O Denniston

Therapeutics

Miss Vaneeta Sood
Mrs Lucy C. Titcomb
Prof Philip I. Murray
Mr Alastair K.O. Denniston

Evidence-based ophthalmology

Mr Alastair K.O. Denniston
Dr Merrick Moseley
Prof Philip I. Murray

Resources

Mr Andrej Kidess
Mr Alastair K.O. Denniston
Prof Philip I. Murray

Author affiliations

Mr Joseph Abbott

FRCOphth
Consultant Ophthalmologist
Birmingham Children's Hospital
NHSFT

Mr Kwesi Amissah-Arthur

FRCOphth
Specialist Trainee (Ophthalmology)
West Midlands Deanery

Ms Rosie Auld

CBE
Head of Orthoptic Services
Birmingham & Midland Eye Centre,
Sandwell & West Birmingham
Hospitals NHS Trust

Mr Mike A. Burdon

MRCP FRCOphth
Consultant Ophthalmologist
University Hospitals Birmingham
NHSFT
Birmingham & Midland Eye Centre,
Sandwell & West Birmingham
Hospitals NHS Trust

Miss Lucilla Butler

MA FRCSEd (Ophth) FRCOphth
Consultant Ophthalmologist &
Hon. Senior Lecturer
Birmingham & Midland Eye Centre,
Sandwell & West Birmingham
Hospitals NHS Trust
Birmingham Women's NHSFT
Royal Wolverhampton NHS Trust
University of Birmingham

Dr Antonio Calcagni

MD MRCOphth
Clinician Scientist
University of Aston

Mr Mark Chiang

MBBS MPhil FRANZCO
Consultant Ophthalmologist
Queensland Eye Institute
City Eye Centre
Brisbane, Australia

Dr Steve Colley

FRCR
Consultant Radiologist
University Hospitals Birmingham
NHSFT

Mr Alastair K.O. Denniston

PhD MRCP FRCOphth
Consultant Ophthalmologist &
Hon. Senior Lecturer
University Hospitals Birmingham
NHSFT
Birmingham & Midland Eye Centre,
Sandwell & West Birmingham
Hospitals NHS Trust
Bristol Eye Hospital, University
Hospitals Bristol NHSFT
Moorfields Eye Hospital NHSFT
University of Birmingham

Mr Omar M. Durrani

FRCOphth
Consultant Ophthalmologist &
Hon. Senior Lecturer
Birmingham & Midland Eye Centre,
Sandwell & West Birmingham
Hospitals NHS Trust
University of Birmingham

Mr Matthew Edmunds

MRCP MRCOphth
Wellcome Trust Clinical Research
Fellow
University of Birmingham
West Midlands Deanery

Mr Samer Elsherbiny
FRCS(Ed) FRCOphth
Consultant Ophthalmologist &
Hon. Senior Lecturer
Birmingham & Midland Eye Centre,
Sandwell & West Birmingham
Hospitals NHS Trust
University of Birmingham

Miss Julia Hale
FRCOphth
Consultant Ophthalmologist
Royal Cornwall Hospitals NHS
Trust

Lt Col Andrew S. Jacks
OStJ FRCOphth
Consultant Ophthalmologist
University Hospitals Birmingham
NHSFT
Royal Centre for Defence Medicine
Birmingham & Midland Eye Centre,
Sandwell & West Birmingham
Hospitals NHS Trust

Mr Thomas Jackson
FRCOphth
Specialist Trainee (Ophthalmology)
West Midlands Deanery

Mr Pearse A. Keane
MD FRCOphth
NIHR Clinical Lecturer
NIHR Biomedical Research Centre
at Moorfields Eye Hospital and
UCL, Institute of Ophthalmology
Moorfields Eye Hospital NHSFT

Mr Andrej Kidess
MD
Senior Fellow
University Hospitals Birmingham
NHSFT

Mr Sai Kolli
MA PhD FRCOphth
Consultant Ophthalmologist
University Hospitals Birmingham
NHSFT

Dr Priscilla Mathewson
MA MBBChir
Specialist Trainee (Ophthalmology)
West Midlands Deanery

Mr Tim D. Matthews
BSc DO FRCS FRCOphth
Consultant Ophthalmologist
University Hospitals Birmingham
NHSFT
Birmingham & Midland Eye Centre,
Sandwell & West Birmingham
Hospitals NHS Trust

Mr Michel Michaelides
BSc MD(Res) FRCOphth FACS
Consultant Ophthalmologist &
Clinical Senior Lecturer
Moorfields Eye Hospital NHSFT
NIHR Biomedical Research Centre
at Moorfields Eye Hospital and
UCL Institute of Ophthalmology

Miss Susan P. Mollan
FRCOphth
Consultant Ophthalmologist
University Hospitals Birmingham
NHSFT

Prof Philip I. Murray
PhD FRCP FRCS FRCOphth
Professor of Ophthalmology &
Hon. Consultant Ophthalmologist
University of Birmingham
Birmingham & Midland Eye Centre,
Sandwell & West Birmingham
Hospitals NHS Trust

Mr Aidan Murray
FRCOphth
Consultant Ophthalmologist
University Hospitals Birmingham
NHSFT
Birmingham & Midland Eye Centre,
Sandwell & West Birmingham
Hospitals NHS Trust

Mr Manoj V. Parulekar
MS FRCS
Consultant Ophthalmologist
Birmingham Children's Hospital
NHSFT

Mr Carlos E. Pavesio
MD FRCOphth
Consultant Ophthalmologist &
Hon. Senior Lecturer
Moorfields Eye Hospital NHSFT
NIHR Biomedical Research Centre
at Moorfields Eye Hospital and
UCL Institute of Ophthalmology

Mrs Hibba Quhill
MRCOphth
Specialist Trainee
(Ophthalmology)
Yorkshire and the Humber
Deanery

Miss Saaeha Rauz
PhD FRCOphth
Clinical Senior Lecturer
in Ophthalmology & Hon.
Consultant Ophthalmologist
University of Birmingham
Birmingham & Midland Eye Centre,
Sandwell & West Birmingham
Hospitals NHS Trust

Prof Ian G. Rennie
MBChB FRCS FRCOphth
Professor of Ophthalmology
University of Sheffield
Royal Hallamshire Hospitals
NHSFT

Mr Vijay Savant
FRCOphth
Consultant Ophthalmologist
University Hospitals Leicester
NHSFT

Prof Peter Shah
BSc(Hons) MBChB FRCOphth
FRCP Edin
Consultant Ophthalmologist &
Hon. Professor of Glaucoma
University Hospitals Birmingham
NHSFT
NIHR Biomedical Research Centre
at Moorfields Eye Hospital and
UCL Institute of Ophthalmology
University of Wolverhampton

Mr Ash Sharma
FRCOphth
Consultant Ophthalmologist
Birmingham & Midland Eye Centre,
Sandwell & West Birmingham
Hospitals NHS Trust

Miss Freda Sii
MBBS
Senior Glaucoma Fellow
University Hospitals Birmingham
NHSFT
NIHR Biomedical Research Centre
at Moorfields Eye Hospital and
UCL Institute of Ophthalmology

Miss Vaneeta Sood
FRCOphth
Specialist Trainee (Ophthalmology)
West Midlands Deanery

Mrs Lucy C. Titcomb
BSc FRPharmS MCPP
Lead Ophthalmic Pharmacist
Birmingham & Midland Eye Centre,
Sandwell & West Birmingham
Hospitals NHS Trust

Mr Adnan Tufail
MD FRCOphth
Consultant Ophthalmologist &
Hon. Senior Lecturer
Moorfields Eye Hospital NHSFT
NIHR Biomedical Research Centre
at Moorfields Eye Hospital and
UCL Institute of Ophthalmology

Dr Shashi B. Vohra
FRCA
Consultant Anaesthetist
Birmingham & Midland Eye Centre,
Sandwell & West Birmingham
Hospitals NHS Trust

Wg Cdr Malcolm Woodcock
MSc MRCOphth FRCS (Ed)
Consultant Ophthalmologist
Worcestershire Acute Hospitals
NHS Trust
Royal Centre for Defence Medicine

Prof James S. Wolffsohn
MBA PhD FCOptom
Deputy Dean
Life and Health Sciences
Aston University

Symbols and abbreviations

↑	increased
↓	decreased
→	leading to
Δ	prism dioptre
➔	book reference
♀	female
♂	male
1°	primary
2°	secondary
±	plus/minus
~	approximately
>	more than
<	less than
≥	equal to or greater than
≤	equal to or less than
°	degree
+ve	positive
−ve	negative
IIn	optic nerve
IIIn	oculomotor nerve
IVn	trochlear nerve
Vn	trigeminal nerve
Va, b, c	ophthalmic, maxillary, and mandibular divisions of Vn
VIn	abducens nerve
VIIn	facial nerve
AA	attendance allowance
AACG	acute angle closure glaucoma
AAPOX	adult-onset asthma and periocular xanthogranuloma
AAU	acute anterior uveitis
AC	anterior chamber
ACCORD	Action to Control Cardiovascular Risk in Diabetes
ACE	angiotensin-converting enzyme
ACh	acetylcholine
ACIOL	anterior chamber intraocular lens
AD	autosomal dominant
A&E	accident and emergency

AF	atrial fibrillation
AIDS	acquired immune deficiency syndrome
AIIR	angiotensin II receptor
AION	anterior ischaemic optic neuropathy
AK	arcuate keratotomy
ALPI	argon laser peripheral iridoplasty
ALT	argon laser trabeculoplasty; alanine aminotransferase
AM	amniotic membrane
AMD	age-related macular degeneration
AMG	amniotic membrane graft
ANA	antinuclear antibody
ANCA	antineutrophil cytoplasmic antibody
AOA	American Optometric Association
AOX	adult-onset xanthogranuloma
APAC	acute primary angle closure
APMPPE	acute posterior multifocal placoid pigment epitheliopathy
APTT	activated partial thromboplastin time
AR	autosomal recessive
ARC	abnormal retinal correspondence
AREDS	Age-Related Eye Disease Study
ARN	acute retinal necrosis
ARR	absolute risk reduction
ASA	American Society of Anesthesiologists
asb	apostilb
ASD	atrial septal defect
ASFA	anterior segment fluorescein angiography
AST	aspartate aminotransferase
AV	arteriovenous
AVM	arteriovenous malformation
AVMD	adult vitelliform macular dystrophy
BC	base curve
BCC	basal cell carcinoma
BCG	bacille Calmette–Guérin
BCL	bandage contact lens
bd	twice daily
BDUMP	bilateral diffuse uveal melanocytic proliferation
BE	base excess
BHL	bihilar lymphadenopathy
BM	basement membrane
BMI	body mass index

BNF	*British National Formulary*
BP	blood pressure; bullous pemphigoid
BRAO	branch retinal artery occlusion
BRVO	branch retinal vein occlusion
BSA	body surface area
BSS	balanced salt solution
BSV	binocular single vision
BVD	back vertex distance
Bx	biopsy
Ca^{2+}	calcium ion
CAA	Civil Aviation Authority
CAS	clinical activity score
CCP	cyclic citrullinated peptide
cCSNB	complete congenital stationary night blindness
CCT	central corneal thickness
CCTV	closed circuit television
C/D	cup:disc ratio
CDC	Centers for Disease Control and Prevention
CDI	colour Doppler imaging
C3F8	perfluoropropane
cf.	compare with
CF	counting fingers
CFEOM	congenital fibrosis of extraocular muscles
cGMP	cyclic guanosine monophosphate
CHED	congenital hereditary endothelial dystrophy
Chr	chromosome
CHRPE	congenital hypertrophy of retinal pigment epithelium
CK	conductive keratoplasty
Cl^-	chloride ion
CL	contact lens
cmH_2O	centimetre of water
CMO	cystoid macular oedema
CMV	cytomegalovirus
CNS	central nervous system
CNV	choroidal neovascularization
COMS	Collaborative Ocular Melanoma Study
COPD	chronic obstructive pulmonary disease
COSA	chronic obstructive sleep apnoea
COX	cyclo-oxygenase
CPEO	chronic progressive external ophthalmoplegia

CPR	cardiopulmonary resuscitation
CRAO	central retinal artery occlusion
CRP	C-reactive protein
CRVO	central retinal vein occlusion
cs	centistoke
CSF	cerebrospinal fluid
CSNB	congenital stationary night blindness
CSR	central serous retinopathy
CT	computerized tomography
CTA	computerized tomography angiography
CTV	computerized tomography venography
CVA	cerebrovascular accident
CVI	Certificate of Vision Impairment
CVS	cardiovascular system
CVST	cerebral venous sinus thrombosis
CWS	cotton wool spot
CXR	chest X-ray
d	day
D	dioptre
Da	dalton
DA	dark adaptation/adaptometry
DALK	deep anterior lamellar keratoplasty
dB	decibel
DC	dioptre cylinder
DCCT	Diabetes Control and Complications Trial
DCG	dacryocystogram
DCR	dacryocystorhinostomy
DD	disc diameter
DHA	docosahexaenoic acid
DIC	disseminated intravascular coagulopathy
DLA	disability living allowance
DMO	diabetic macular oedema
DMPK	dystrophica myotonica protein kinase
DNA	deoxyribonucleic acid
dsDNA	double-stranded deoxyribonucleic acid
DS	dioptre sphere
DSG	dacryoscintigraphy
DUSN	diffuse unilateral subacute neuroretinitis
DVD	dissociated vertical deviation
DVLA	Driver and Vehicle Licensing Agency

DVT	deep vein thrombosis
Dx	drug history
DXA	dual X-ray absorptiometry
EBV	Epstein–Barr virus
ECCE	extracapsular cataract extraction
ECD	Erdheim–Chester disease
ECG	electrocardiogram
ECP	endoscopic cyclophotocoagulation; endodiode laser photocoagulation
EDI	enhanced depth imaging
EDT	electrodiagnostic test
eGFR	estimated glomerular filtration rate
ELISA	enzyme-linked immunosorbent assay
ELM	external limiting membrane
EMG	electromyogram
EMGT	Early Manifest Glaucoma Trial
ENT	ear, nose, and throat specialty (otorhinolaryngology)
EOG	electro-oculogram
EOM	extraocular muscle
EPA	eicosapentaenoic acid
ERD	exudative retinal detachment
ERG	electroretinogram
ERM	epiretinal membrane
ESR	erythrocyte sedimentation rate
ETDRS	Early Treatment of Diabetic Retinopathy Study
EUA	examination under anaesthesia
E-W	Edinger–Westphal (nucleus)
FAF	fundus autofluorescence
FB	foreign body
FBC	full blood count
FDA	Food and Drug Administration
FEF	frontal eye fields
FEVR	familial exudative vitreoretinopathy
FFA	fundus fluorescein angiography
FH	family history
FHU	Fuchs' heterochromic uveitis
FNA	fine-needle aspiration
FSH	follicle-stimulating hormone
FSL	femtosecond laser
ft	foot

FTA-ABS	fluorescent treponemal antibody absorption
5-FU	5-fluorouracil
g	gram; drop (*guttae*)
G	gauge
GA	general anaesthesia
GAT	Goldmann applanation tonometry
GCA	giant cell arteritis
GCS	Glasgow coma scale
γGT	gamma glutamyl transferase
GI	gastrointestinal system
Glu	glucose
GP	general practitioner
GPA	granulomatosis with polyangiitis
GU	genitourinary
GVHD	graft-versus-host disease
Gy	gray
h	hour
HAART	highly active antiretroviral therapy
Hb	haemoglobin
HCV	hepatitis C virus
HES	hospital eye service
HHV8	human herpesvirus 8
HIV	human immune deficiency virus
HLA	human leucocyte antigen
HM	hand movements
HPC	history of presenting complaint
HPV	human papillomavirus
HR	hazard ratio
HRCT	high-resolution computerized tomography
HRT	Heidelberg Retinal Tomography; hormone replacement therapy
HRVO	hemiretinal vein occlusion
HSV	herpes simplex virus
HTLV-1	human T-cell lymphotropic virus type 1
Hx	history
Hz	hertz
HZO	herpes zoster ophthalmicus
IBD	inflammatory bowel disease
ICA	internal carotid artery
ICD	implantable cardioverter defibrillator

ICE	iridocorneal endothelial (syndrome)
ICG	indocyanine green (angiography)
ICP	intracranial pressure
ICRS	intracorneal ring segment
iCSNB	incomplete congenital stationary night blindness
IGRA	interferon γ release assay
IGT	impaired glucose tolerance
IHD	ischaemic heart disease
IHS	International Headache Society
IIH	idiopathic intracranial hypertension
ILAR	International League of Associations of Rheumatologists
ILM	internal limiting membrane
IM	intramuscular
in	inch
INO	internuclear ophthalmoplegia
INR	international normalized ratio
IO	inferior oblique
IOFB	intraocular foreign body
IOL	intraocular lens
IOOA	inferior oblique overaction
IOP	intraocular pressure
IPCV	idiopathic polypoidal choroidal vasculopathy
IPD	interpupillary distance
IQ	intelligence quotient
IR	inferior rectus
IRMA	intraretinal microvascular abnormality
ISCEV	International Society for Clinical Electrophysiology of Vision
IS-OS	inner segment-outer segment
ITC	iridotrabecular contact
ITU	intensive therapy unit
IUSG	International Uveitis Study Group
IV	intravenous
IVC	inferior vena cava
IVMP	intravenous methylprednisolone
Ix	investigation
J	joule
JIA	juvenile idiopathic arthritis
K^+	potassium ion
KCS	keratoconjunctivitis sicca
kDa	kilodalton

kHz	kilohertz
KP	keratic precipitate
kPa	kilopascal
L	litre
LA	linolenic acid
LASEK	laser-assisted subepithelial keratomileusis
LASIK	laser stromal *in situ* keratomileusis
LCA	Leber's congenital amaurosis
LCT	lateral canthal tendon
LE	left eye
LEMS	Lambert–Eaton myasthenic syndrome
LESC	limbal epithelial stem cell
LFT	liver function tests
LGN	lateral geniculate nucleus
LH	luteinizing hormone
LHON	Leber's hereditary optic neuropathy
LN	lymph node; latent nystagmus
LOC	loss of consciousness
logMAR	logarithm of the minimum angle of resolution
LP	lumbar puncture
LPA	laser protection advisor
LPS	levator palpebrae superioris
LR	lateral rectus
LRI	limbal relaxing incision
LTK	laser thermokeratoplasty
LTS	lateral tarsal strip
LVL	Low Vision Leaflet
MALT	mucosa-associated lymphoid tissue
MBq	mega becquerel
MCP	multifocal choroiditis with panuveitis
MC&S	microscopy, culture, and sensitivity
MD	mean deviation
MEWDS	multiple evanescent white dot syndrome
mfERG	multifocal electroretinogram
MG	Meibomian gland; myasthenia gravis
MGD	Meibomian gland dysfunction
MHz	mega hertz
MI	myocardial infarction
MIGS	minimally invasive glaucoma surgery
min	minute

mJ	millijoule
mL	millilitre
MLF	medial longitudinal fasciculus
MMC	mitomycin C
mmHg	millimetre of mercury
mmol	millimole
MMP	mucous membrane pemphigoid; matrix metalloproteinase
mo	month
mol	mole
MPS	mucopolysaccharidosis
MR	medial rectus
MRA	magnetic resonance angiography
MRI	magnetic resonance imaging
MRSA	meticillin-resistant *Staphylococcus aureus*
MRV	magnetic resonance venography
ms	millisecond
MS	multiple sclerosis
MSICS	manual small incision cataract surgery
mTOR	mammalian target of rapamycin
mW	milliwatt
n.	nerve
Na^+	sodium ion
NAA	National Assistance Act
NaCl	sodium chloride
NBX	necrobiotic xanthogranuloma
Nd-YAG	neodymium-yttrium-aluminium-garnet laser
NEI VFQ-25	National Eye Institute Visual Functioning Questionnaire-25
NF	neurofibromatosis
NHS	National Health Service
NIBP	non-invasive blood pressure
NICE	National Institute for Health and Care Excellence
nm	nanometre
NMO	neuromyelitis optica
NNT	number needed to treat
norA	noradrenaline
NPDR	non-proliferative diabetic retinopathy
NPGS	non-penetrating glaucoma surgery
NPL	no perception of light
NPV	negative predictive value
NRR	neuroretinal rim

ns	nanosecond
NSAID	non-steroidal anti-inflammatory drug
NTG	normal-tension glaucoma
NVA	neovascularization of the angle
NVD	new vessels on the optic disc
NVE	new vessels elsewhere
NVG	neovascular glaucoma
NVI	neovascularization of the iris
oc	ocular
Oc	ointment
OcMMP	ocular mucous membrane pemphigoid
OCT	optical coherence tomography
od	once daily
O/E	on examination
OHT	ocular hypertension
OHTS	Ocular Hypertension Treatment Study
OIS	ocular ischaemic syndrome
OKN	optokinetic
ONTT	Optic Neuritis Treatment Trial
OTC	over the counter
OVD	ophthalmic viscosurgical device
p	probability
PAC	primary angle closure
PACG	primary angle-closure glaucoma
PAM	primary acquired melanosis
PAN	polyarteritis nodosa
PAS	periodic acid–Schiff; peripheral anterior synechiae
PC	presenting complaint
PCG	primary congenital glaucoma
PCIOL	posterior chamber intraocular lens
PCO	posterior capsular opacification
PCR	polymerase chain reaction
PCV	polypoidal choroidal vasculopathy
PDR	proliferative diabetic retinopathy
PDS	pigment dispersion syndrome
PDT	photodynamic therapy
PE	pulmonary embolism
PED	pigment epithelium detachment
PEP	post-exposure prophylaxis
PERG	pattern electroretinogram

PET	positron emission tomography
PF	preservative-free
pg	picogram
PHMB	polyhexamethylene biguanide
PI	peripheral iridotomy
PIC	punctate inner choroidopathy
PION	posterior ischaemic optic neuropathy
PIP	personal independence payment
PK	penetrating keratoplasty
PL	perception of light
Plt	platelets
PMH	past medical history
PMMA	polymethylmethacrylate
pmol	picomole
PNS	peripheral nervous system
PO	*per os* (by mouth)
POAG	primary open-angle glaucoma
POH	past ophthalmic history
POHS	presumed ocular histoplasmosis syndrome
PORN	progressive outer retinal necrosis
PPA	peripapillary atrophy
PPCD	posterior polymorphous corneal dystrophy
PPD	posterior polymorphous dystrophy
ppm	part per million
PPRF	paramedian pontine reticular formation
PPV	positive predictive value
PRK	photorefractive keratectomy
prn	as required
PRO	patient-reported outcome
PROM	patient-reported outcome measure
PRP	pan-retinal photocoagulation
PR-VEP	pattern reversal visual evoked potential
PS	posterior synechiae
PSP	progressive supranuclear palsy
PTK	phototherapeutic keratectomy
PTT	prothrombin time
PUK	peripheral ulcerative keratitis
PVD	posterior vitreous detachment
PVR	proliferative vitreoretinopathy
PVRL	primary vitreoretinal lymphoma

PXE	pseudoxanthoma elasticum
PXF	pseudoexfoliation (syndrome)
q	every (e.g. q 1h = every 1h)
QALY	quality-adjusted life year
QFT-G	QuantiFERON-TB Gold
RA	rheumatoid arthritis
rAAV	recombinant adeno-associated virus
RAP	retinal angiomatous proliferation
RAPD	relative afferent pupillary defect
RCES	recurrent corneal erosion syndrome
RCOphth	Royal College of Ophthalmologists
RCT	randomized controlled trial
RE	right eye
RF	rheumatoid factor
RGP	rigid gas permeable (of contact lenses)
RK	radial keratotomy
RLE	refractive lens exchange
RNA	ribonucleic acid
RNFL	retinal nerve fibre layer
ROP	retinopathy of prematurity
RP	retinitis pigmentosa
RPE	retinal pigment epithelium
RPR	rapid plasma reagin
RRD	rhegmatogenous retinal detachment
RRMS	relapsing/remitting multiple sclerosis
RS	respiratory system
RT-PCR	reverse transcriptase polymerase chain reaction
RVO	retinal vein occlusion
s	second
SBS	shaken baby syndrome
SC	subcutaneous
SCC	squamous cell carcinoma
SD	standard deviation
SF	short-term fluctuation
SF-36	Short Form-36
SH	social history
Si	silicone (of oil)
SIGN	Scottish Intercollegiate Network
SITA	Swedish interactive threshold algorithm
SJS	Stevens–Johnson syndrome

SLE	systemic lupus erythematosus
SLO	scanning laser ophthalmoscopy
SLT	selective laser trabeculoplasty
SO	superior oblique
SOM	Special Order Manufacturers
SpO_2	oxygen saturation
spp.	species
SR	superior rectus
SRF	subretinal fluid
SSPE	subacute sclerosing panencephalitis
SUN	Standardization of Uveitis Nomenclature
SVC	superior vena cava
SVP	spontaneous venous pulsation
T4	thyroxine
TAB	temporal artery biopsy
TAP	Treatment of AMD with Photodynamic therapy
TASS	toxic anterior segment syndrome
TB	tuberculosis
tds	three times daily
TED	thyroid eye disease
TEN	toxic epidermal necrolysis
TFBUT	tear film break-up time
TFT	thyroid function tests
Th2	T helper 2
TIA	transient ischaemic attack
TIBC	total iron binding capacity
TINU	tubulointerstitial nephritis with uveitis
TNF	tumour necrosis factor
TPC	tenacious proximal convergence
TPHA	treponema pallidum haemagglutination assay
TRD	tractional retinal detachment
TSE	transmissible spongiform encephalitis
TSH	thyroid-stimulating hormone
TST	tuberculin skin test
U	unit
UC	ulcerative colitis
U+E	urea and electrolytes
UGH	uveitis-glaucoma–hyphaema (syndrome)
UKPDS	UK Prospective Diabetic Study
URTI	upper respiratory tract infection

US	ultrasound
USP	United States Pharmacopeia
UV	ultraviolet
UVA	ultraviolet A
UVB	ultraviolet B
UVC	ultraviolet C
VA	visual acuity
VCM1	Vision Core Module 1
VDRL	venereal disease research laboratory
VDU	visual display unit
VEGF	vascular endothelial growth factor
VEP	visual evoked potential
VF	visual field
VHL	von Hippel–Lindau
VKC	vernal keratoconjunctivitis
VKH	Vogt–Koyanagi–Harada (syndrome)
VOR	vestibulo-ocular reflex
VR	vitreoretinal
vs	versus
VSD	ventricular septal defect
VZV	varicella-zoster virus
WBC	white blood cell
WHO	World Health Organization
wk	week
WNV	West Nile virus
XD	X-linked dominant
XL	X-linked
XLRS	X-linked retinoschisis
XR	X-linked recessive
y	year

Orthoptic abbreviations

ACS	alternating convergent strabismus
ADS	alternating divergent strabismus
AHP	abnormal head posture
ARC	abnormal retinal correspondence
BD	base down (of prism)
BI	base in (of prism)
BO	base out (of prism)
BU	base up (of prism)
BSV	binocular single vision
CC	Cardiff cards
CI	convergence insufficiency
Conv XS	convergence excess
CSM	central steady maintained (of fixation)
CT	cover test
DVD	dissociated vertical deviation
DVM	delayed visual maturation
Ecc fix	eccentric fixation
EP	esophoria
ET	esotropia
E(T)	intermittent esotropia
FCPL	forced choice preferential looking
FL/FLE	fixing with left eye
FR/FRE	fixing with right eye
HP	hyperphoria
HT	hypertropia
Hypo	hypophoria
HypoT	hypotropia
KP	Kay's pictures
LCS	left convergent strabismus
LDS	left divergent strabismus
MLN	manifest latent nystagmus
MR	Maddox rod
MW	Maddox wing
NPA	near point of accommodation
NPC	near point of convergence
NRC	normal retinal correspondence

o/a	overaction
Obj	objection
Occ	occlusion
OKN	optokinetic nystagmus
PCT	prism cover test
PFR	prism fusion range
PRT	prism reflection test
RCS	right convergent strabismus
RDS	right divergent strabismus
Rec	recovery
SG	Sheridan Gardiner test
Sn	Snellen chart
SP	simultaneous perception
Supp	suppression
u/a	underaction
VOR	vestibulo-ocular reflex
XP	exophoria
XT	exotropia
X(T)	intermittent exotropia

More complex variations for intermittent strabismus include:
R(E)T, intermittent right esotropia predominantly controlled
RE(T), intermittent right esotropia predominantly manifest.

Adjust according to whether:
R (right), L (left), or A (alternating)
ET (esotropia), XT (exotropia), HT (hypertropia), or hypoT (hypotropia).

These abbreviations are in common usage and are approved by the British and Irish Orthoptic Society.

Chapter 1

Clinical skills

Taking an ophthalmic history

One of the first and most vital skills acquired by those involved in eye care is the accurate and efficient taking of an ophthalmic history. In ophthalmology, clinical examination is very rewarding, probably more so than in any other medical specialty. This should, however, supplement, rather than replace, the clinical history. In addition to the information gained, a rapport is established which should help the patient tolerate the relatively 'invasive' ophthalmic examination. The patient is also more likely to accept any subsequent explanation of diagnosis and ongoing management if they know they have been heard.

Presenting complaint (PC)

Why are they here? Have they got a problem at all?

Routine optometric review has a valuable role in screening for asymptomatic disease (notably glaucoma) but may generate unnecessary referrals for benign variants (e.g. anomalous discs, early lens opacities). Consider who has the problem—the patient or the referring practitioner? Also consider what anxieties and expectations they bring with them.

History of presenting complaint (HPC)

The analysis of most ophthalmic complaints centre on general questions regarding onset, precipitants, associated features (e.g. pain, redness, discharge, photophobia, etc.), duration, relieving factors, recovery, and specific questions directed by the presentation. Even after clinical examination, further information may be needed to 'rule in' or 'rule out' diagnoses. Although some of these processes can be formalized as algorithms, their limitations should be recognized—they cannot emulate the multivariate processing, recognition of exceptions, and calculation of diagnostic probabilities subconsciously practised by an experienced clinician (see Box 1.1).

Past ophthalmic history (POH)

The background for each presentation is important. Ask about previous surgery/trauma, previous/concurrent eye disease, and refractive error. The differential diagnosis of an acute red eye will be affected by knowing that they had complicated cataract surgery 2d previously, or that they have a 10y history of recurrent acute anterior uveitis, or even that they wear contact lenses (CL).

Past medical history (PMH)

Similarly, consider the whole patient. Ask generally about any medical problems. In addition, ask specifically about relevant conditions that they may have omitted to mention. The patient presenting with recurrently itchy eyes may not mention that they have eczema or asthma. Similarly, if presenting with a vascular event, ask specifically about diabetes, hypertension, and hypercholesterolaemia.

Family history (FH)

This is relevant both to diseases with a significant genetic component (e.g. retinitis pigmentosa (RP), glaucoma, some corneal dystrophies; there may be consanguinity) and to infective conditions (e.g. conjunctivitis, tuberculosis (TB), etc.).

Social history (SH)

Ask about smoking, alcohol intake, if relevant to the ophthalmic disease (e.g. vascular event or unexplained optic neuropathy, respectively). Consider the social context of the patient. Will they manage hourly drops? Can they even get the top off the bottle?

Drugs and allergies

Ask about concurrent medication and any allergies to previous medications (e.g. drops), since these may limit your therapeutic options. In addition to actual allergies, consider contraindications (e.g. asthma/chronic obstructive pulmonary disease (COPD) and β-blockers). Make it clear to the patient that you want to know about all their medication—not just their eye drops.

Box 1.1 Taking the HPC—an example

Patient presenting with loss of vision

Did it happen suddenly or gradually? Sudden loss of vision is commonly due to a vascular occlusion (e.g. anterior ischaemic optic neuropathy (AION), central retinal artery occlusion (CRAO), central retinal vein occlusion (CRVO)) or bleed (e.g. vitreous haemorrhage, 'wet' macular degeneration). Gradual loss of vision is coammonly associated with degenerations/depositions (e.g. cataract, macular dystrophies or 'dry' macular degeneration, corneal dystrophies).

Is it painful? Painful blurring of vision is most commonly associated with anterior ocular processes (e.g. keratitis, anterior uveitis), although orbital disease, optic neuritis, and giant cell arteritis (GCA) may also cause painful loss of vision.

Is the problem transient or persistent? Transient loss of vision is commonly due to temporary/subcritical vascular insufficiency (e.g. GCA, amaurosis fugax, vertebrobasilar artery insufficiency), whereas persistent loss of vision suggests structural or irreversible damage (e.g. vitreous haemorrhage, macular degeneration).

Does it affect one or both eyes? Unilateral disease may suggest a local (or ipsilateral) cause. Bilateral disease may suggest a more widespread or systemic process.

Is the vision blurred, dimmed, or distorted? Blurring or dimming may arise due to pathology anywhere in the visual pathway, from cornea to cortex; common problems include refractive error, cataract, and macular disease. Distortion is commonly associated with macular pathology but may arise due to high refractive error (high ametropia/astigmatism) or other ocular disease.

Where is the problem with their vision? A superior or inferior hemispheric field loss suggests a corresponding inferior or superior vascular event involving the retina (e.g. retinal vein occlusion (RVO)) or disc (e.g. segmental AION). Peripheral field loss may indicate retinal detachment (usually rapidly evolving from far periphery), optic nerve disease, chiasmal compression (typically bitemporal loss), or cortical pathology (homonymous hemianopic defects). Central blurring of vision suggests disease of the macula (positive scotoma: a 'seen' spot) or optic nerve (negative scotoma: an unseen defect).

When is there a problem? For example, glare from headlights or bright sunlight is commonly due to posterior subcapsular lens opacities.

Assessment of vision: acuity

Measuring visual acuity (VA) (See Box 1.2)

Box 1.2 An approach to measuring VA

Select (and document) appropriate test (see Table 1.1)	Consider age, language, literacy, general faculties of patient
Check distance acuity (for each eye)	Unaided With distance prescription With pinhole (if <0.2 LogMAR, <6/9.5)
Check near acuity (for each eye) (where appropriate)	Unaided With near prescription

Selecting the appropriate clinical test

Table 1.1 Tests of VA

Patient	Distance	Near
Adult: literate	Snellen LogMAR	Test type N chart LogMAR
Adult: illiterate	Keeler logMAR (crowded/uncrowded)* Sheridan Gardiner (single optotype)* Kay picture test (crowded/uncrowded)*	Reduced Sheridan Gardiner*
Children: age ≥3y	LogMAR Keeler logMAR (crowded/uncrowded)† Kay picture test (crowded/uncrowded)†	
Children: age ≥2y	Kay picture test (single optotype)* Cardiff Cards	Reduced Kay picture test*
Babies/infants	Preferential looking tests: Keeler, Teller, Cardiff cards Clinical tests: fixing and following, objection to occlusion, picking up fine objects Electrodiagnostic tests (EDTs): visual evoked potential (VEP) response to alternating chequerboard of varying frequency	

* Use with matching cards;

† Use with or without matching cards, as needed

Distance acuity

Snellen charts

The optotypes (letters) subtend 5min of arc if read at the distance ascribed to that line, with each component of the letter subtending just 1min. This is the denominator. The actual distance at which it is used (usually 6m; 20ft in the USA) is the numerator. Thus, if the top (60m) line can only be read at 2m, the Snellen acuity is 2/60. Normal VA in the young eye is at least is 1min of arc or 6/6, although Vernier acuity may be up to 5s of arc. A change of two lines should be regarded as significant. Decimal acuity is the numerator divided by the denominator (see Fig. 1.1).

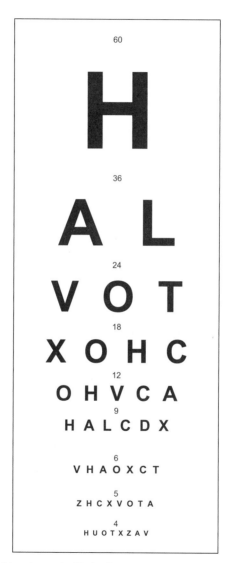

Fig. 1.1 Schematic example of Snellen chart.

LogMAR charts

This records the logarithm of the minimum angle of resolution. Based on the Bailey–Lovie logMAR chart, the actual chart in common usage is the Ferris modification, known as the 'ETDRS' chart (see Fig. 1.2). LogMAR testing has marked advantages over Snellen, notably that: (1) all letters are equally legible, (2) it controls the crowding phenomenon with five letters on each line and appropriate separation, (3) there is a logical geometric progression of resolution. Starting with the logMAR 1.0 line (Snellen 6/60), each letter is read and scored. The chart is usually positioned at a working distance of 4m, although it can be scaled to any distance. Each correct line (worth 0.1U) or each correct letter (worth 0.02U) is subtracted from 1.0 to give the final score (see Table 1.2).

Table 1.2 Distance acuity scoring systems

Snellen (UK; in m)	LogMAR	Decimal	Snellen (USA; in ft)
6/60	1.0	0.1	20/200
6/24	0.6	0.25	20/80
6/12	0.3	0.5	20/40
6/6	0.0	1.0	20/20
6/3	−0.3	2.0	20/10

Crowding is a phenomenon by which neighbouring targets interfere as proximity increases. Amblyopic patients are particularly susceptible and may score better with single optotype tests (e.g. Sheridan Gardiner) than on a multiple test (e.g. Snellen). This has led to the use of multiple optotype forms of letter matching or picture tests. Although other tests may approximate to a Snellen acuity reading, they are not exactly equivalent. It is therefore important to document which test has been used.

Pinhole acuity

A pinhole (stenopaeic aperture, typically 1.2mm diameter) can neutralize up to 3DS of refractive error, due to resulting increased depth of focus.

Near (reading) acuity

Various charts are available. Most have paragraphs of text that are read by the patient at their usual reading distance (typically around 30–40cm). N notation corresponds to the point size of the text being read, with a range from about N5 to N48. M notation is more common in the USA, with 1M corresponding to N8. Note these are sizes and not acuities without a working distance. N5 read at 30cm is equivalent to about 6/12.

Testing low VA

If the vision is <6/60, walk the patient, metre by metre, to the chart (or chart to patient). If <1/60, try counting fingers (scores CF), then hand movements (HM). If less than this, light perception (PL) is tested with a bright light. If PL is present, try all four quadrants, and ask the patient to point to which quadrant the light is perceived as arising from (accurate projection).

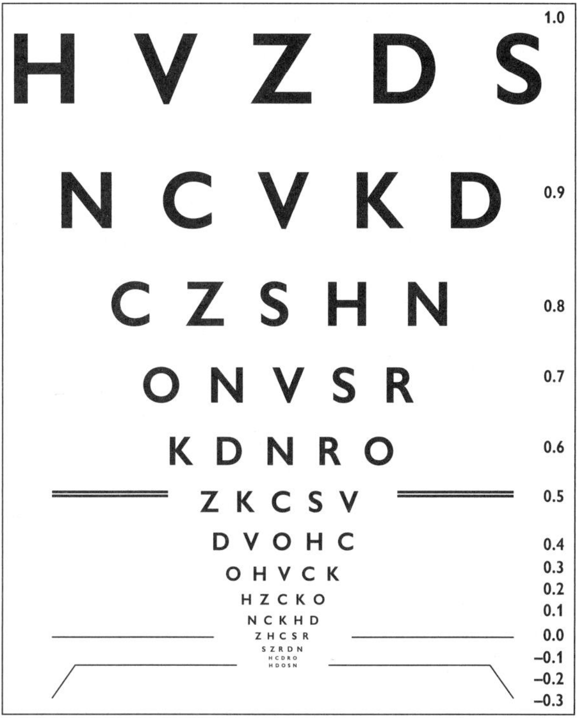

Fig. 1.2 Schematic example of LogMAR chart.

Assessment of vision: clinical tests in children and tests of binocular status

Behavioural tests for babies/infants

Fixing and following

From 3mo of age, a baby should be able to fix and follow a target. Note whether fixation is central, steady, and maintained when the target is moved. The use of different size targets can give an estimation of acuity.

Further information can be gained by observation of behaviour. Do they respond to fine stimuli ('hundreds and thousands test')? Do they object to occlusion of one eye more than the other?

Preferential looking tests

These tests depend on the normal preference to look at the more visually interesting target, i.e. patterned, rather than blank.

- *Keeler and Teller acuity cards*: comprise a series of cards, each of which has a black and white grating on a grey background of matching luminance. The spatial frequency of the grating (i.e. the thinness of the lines) approximates to different acuity levels. The cards are presented so that the observer has to decide which direction the child has looked before knowing whether this corresponds to the position of the grating, i.e. it is 'forced choice'.
- *Cardiff acuity cards*: have 'vanishing optotypes'. These are a series of pictures with increasingly fine outlines which are correspondingly difficult to see. These can either be used as a preferential looking test or as a picture test (if verbal).

Recognition tests for older children

Picture tests

These include Cardiff acuity cards, Kay picture cards (single picture opto-types; optotypes vary in size), and multiple picture cards (similar but multiple optotypes on each card). The patient then selects the matching optotype on a handheld card or identifies the object verbally.

Keeler LogMAR tests

The Keeler LogMAR tests (uncrowded and crowded) are performed at 3m. The optotypes are presented on a single line in a booklet format. The uncrowded test presents two optotypes of each size on each page, from 0.8 to 0.0. The crowded test presents four optotypes of each size within a rec-tangular outline. Both tests can be used with a matching card (see Fig. 1.3).

Sheridan Gardiner test

This test has five booklets with single letter optotypes which are presented at 6m (or, if necessary, 3m); intended for use with a matching card.

Sonsken–Silver test

This is similar to the Sheridan Gardiner test but is a crowded test (multiple optotypes); intended for use with a matching card.

Tests of binocular status

Binocular vision may be graded from simultaneous perception to fusion, and finally to stereopsis (a 'three-dimensional' perception).

- Simultaneous perception and fusion are assessed, using the Worth's Lights or Bagolini Glasses tests, when dissimilar images are presented to each eye, and the patient is asked to report what they see. The tests determine whether the patient can fuse the dissimilar images.
- Prisms can be used to assess the range of motor fusion when the patient is instructed to maintain a single image with the introduction of increasing prism power.
- Stereoacuity is measured, using a range of three-dimensional tests, based on disparity of images and or colour dissociation. Stereoacuity is measured in seconds of arc. Normal disparity perceived is 60s of arc but may be up to 15s.

The synoptophore is rarely used now. It is an instrument which allows the simultaneous presentation of separate images to each eye. Depending on the images presented and the degree of binocular vision, the patient might report: simultaneous perception of two images, fusion of two images, or perception of depth in a fused image (see Table 1.3).

Table 1.3 Tests of binocular status

Test	Icon	Mechanism	Monocular clues	Disparity
Titmus		Polaroid glasses	Yes	40–3,000s of arc
TNO		Red-green glasses	No	15–480s of arc
Lang	☆	Intrinsic cylinder lenses	Yes, if not held perpendicular	550–1,200s of arc
Frisby		Intrinsic plate thickness	Yes, if not held perpendicular	15–600s of arc
Synoptophore		Separate eyepieces	No	90–720s of arc

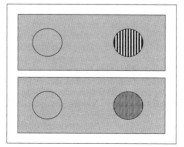

Fig. 1.3 Schematic example of Keeler acuity cards.

Assessment of vision: contrast and colour

Contrast sensitivity

Whilst VA charts (e.g. Snellen) test high contrast (black letters on a white background), most daily visual tasks require resolution of low/medium contrast. Contrast sensitivity may be reduced, even when high contrast testing (such as Snellen acuity) is normal. It may be measured by a number of charts, all of which score the minimum contrast detectable for a specified target size. The *Vistech chart* employs rows of broken circles which decrease in contrast across the row and diminish in size from row to row. Identification of target orientation is plotted on a template to give a graph of contrast vs spatial frequency. Charts are available for use at 45cm and 3m. Alternative charts maintaining a constant target size include the *Pelli–Robson* chart (triplets of capital letters, usually read at 1m, read until two or three mistakes in one triplet) (see Fig. 1.4), or *Cambridge chart* (square wave gratings, usually read at 6m, forced choice as to which of two luminance-matched pages the grating is on).

Colour vision

- *Red desaturation*: compare the perception of 'redness' (e.g. of a red pin) between eyes, occluding one at a time. This can be done for both central vision (reduced in an optic neuropathy) or peripheral field (bitemporally reduced in a chiasmal lesion). An approximate score can be assigned by the patient to the 'washed-out' image in relation to the normal image, e.g. 5/10.
- *Ishihara pseudo-isochromatic plates*: use at 2/3m under good illumination in patients with VA ≥6/18. The first test plate (seen even by achromats with sufficient acuity) is followed by a series of plates testing red-green confusion. Some of the plates differentiate whether the defect is of the protan (red) or deutan (green) system. It does not test the tritan (blue) system. Patients with congenital red-green colour blindness (protanopia, deuteranopia) tend to make predictable mistakes; in acquired disease (optic neuropathy), the mistakes do not follow a specific pattern.
- *Hardy–Rand–Rittler plates*: less commonly used but has the advantage of testing tritan as well as protan and deutan discrimination.
- *Holmes Wright lantern*: a test of binary choice of two or three coloured spots of light viewed at 6m. Colours are red, green, and white. This is a more practical assessment that aims to predict red-green discrimination in a work situation, e.g. distinguishing red and green lights on a runway. Used in conjunction with Ishihara plates for testing colour vision in military personnel.
- *Farnsworth-D15 test*: a colour tile ordering test of confusion, giving limited information on the protan, deutan, and tritan systems. It may be used as a screening test of colour vision.
- *Farnsworth–Munsell 100-Hue test*: a more time-consuming colour tile ordering test of discrimination where the patient attempts to order 85 coloured caps by hue. When this is plotted onto a dedicated chart, it provides detailed information on protan, deutan, and tritan systems. This test is often used as the final arbitrator for colour vision-requiring professions.

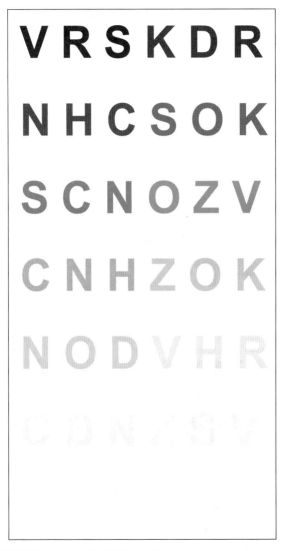

Fig. 1.4 Schematic example of Pelli–Robson chart.

Biomicroscopy: slit-lamp overview

The slit-lamp (biomicroscope) provides excellent visualization of both the anterior segment and, with the help of additional lenses, the posterior segment of the eye. Advantages of the slit-lamp view are that it is magnified (typically 6–40×) and stereoscopic. Although basic slit-lamp skills are quickly gained, mastering its finer points enables one to use it to its full potential. Careful preparation of slit-lamp and patient is essential to optimize both quality of view and patient/clinician comfort.

Optical and mechanical features

The slit lamp consists of a binocular compound microscope and an adjustable illumination system. Since it has a fixed focal plane, objects are brought into focus by moving the slit-lamp forward or back. Movement of the slit-lamp laterally (adjusted with the joystick) and vertically (a dial often attached to the joystick) permits visualization of eye and adnexae without having to adjust patient position.

Magnification

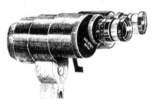

Fig. 1.5 Eyepieces.

Most conventional slit-lamps have two objective settings (1× and 1.6×) and two eyepiece options (10× and 16×). The total magnification thus ranges from 10× to 25× (see Fig. 1.5).

Others have a series of Galilean telescopes which can be dialled into position to give magnifications ranging from 6.3× to 40×. Less commonly, a zoom system is used.

Illumination: filters

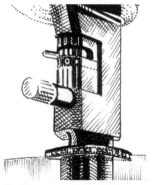

Fig. 1.6 Illumination filters.

The illumination can be adjusted by a series of filters (see Fig. 1.6). Options are typically unfiltered, heat-absorbing filter, 10% grey filter, red-free filter, and blue filter (traditionally cobalt blue, but optionally with a 495nm peak). In practice, the heat-absorbing filter is generally used for high illumination and the grey filter for lower illumination. The red-free filter increases visualization of the vitreous and retinal nerve fibre layer/vasculature. The blue illumination filter is best combined with a yellow enhancement observational filter to maximize visualization of fluorescein; the blue filter may also assist detection of iron lines.

The beam height and width are adjusted by apertures; the beam height is incremented in mm and may be useful in measurement (e.g. disc size, corneal ulcer, etc.).

Illumination: orientation and angulation

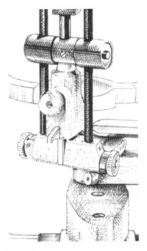

Fig. 1.7 Illumination arm.

(Note Haag-Streit type illumination column illustrated.) The orientation of the beam may be adjusted from vertical to horizontal (or any other angle) by swinging the superior aspect of the illumination arm to left or right (useful for gonioscopy or in measuring lesions). Angulation of the beam is achieved by swinging the whole illumination arm to the side (horizontal) or tilting the illumination arm upward (vertical) (see Fig. 1.7). The alternative techniques of direct illumination, retroillumination, scleral scatter, specular reflection (see ➔ Additional techniques for anterior segment examination, p. 17) require different angulations of the illumination arm, and some require the illumination arm to be 'uncoupled' to displace the beam from the centre of the field of view. Tilting the beam vertically may reduce troublesome reflections when using handheld lenses.

Illumination: mirrors

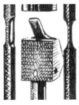

Fig. 1.8 Mirror.

In certain situations, such as when using small angulations (3–10°), the standard long mirror may partially obscure the view. If this is troublesome, it can be replaced by the short mirror (see Fig. 1.8).

Fixation lamp

Many slit-lamps have a fixation target, either a standard fixation lamp or an annular target with a focusing range of –15 to +10D. This can be adjusted to the patient's refractive error, enabling them to see the target clearly.

Stereovariator

Some slit-lamps have a stereovariator which changes the angle of convergence from 13° to 4.5°. The conventional 13° provides better stereopsis, but the 4.5° provides a larger binocular field of view and thus improved acuity (binocular acuity > monocular acuity). This means that the 4.5° setting may be advantageous for detailed examination of certain ocular surfaces (e.g. corneal endothelium).

Biomicroscopy: use of the slit-lamp

Outline of slit-lamp examination (See Fig. 1.9)

Set-up

For each clinic

- Adjust the eyepieces. Set the eyepieces to their maximum plus. Place the focusing rod in the centre column (remove the tonometer plate, if present), with the flat surface of the rod facing you. Adjust the slit-lamp beam to minimal thickness and maximum brightness to optimize detection of defocus. For each eyepiece, in turn, viewing through the respective eye reduce the amount of plus until the slit first becomes clear. This prevents stimulating the accommodation system.
- Adjust the interpupillary distance (IPD).

For each patient

- Adjust patient chair, slit-lamp, and your chair so that you can both be comfortable during the examination.
- Adjust chin-rest until patient's eyes are at level of the marker (on the side of the head rest).

Examination

- Start examination with lowest magnification and low illumination. Rather than inadvertently dazzling your patient first, test the brightness, e.g. on your hand.
- Start examination with direct illumination (usually fairly thin beam, angled 30–60°).
- Examine in a methodical manner from 'outside in', i.e. orbit/adnexae, lids, anterior segment (see ➔ Anterior segment examination, p. 16), posterior segment (see ➔ Posterior segment examination, p. 22).
- Throughout examination: (1) adjust illumination: adjust filter, orientation and angulation, and illumination technique (direct illumination, retroillumination, scleral scatter, specular reflection) to optimize visualization; (2) adjust magnification: to optimize visualization (e.g. of cells in the anterior chamber (AC)).
- At the end of the examination, do not leave your patient stranded on the slit-lamp. Switch the slit-lamp off (for the sake of the patient and the bulb), and encourage the patient to sit back.

Additional techniques

- *Tonometry*: Goldmann tonometer used with fluorescein and blue light.
- *Gonioscopy and indirect fundoscopy*: performed with appropriate handheld lenses.

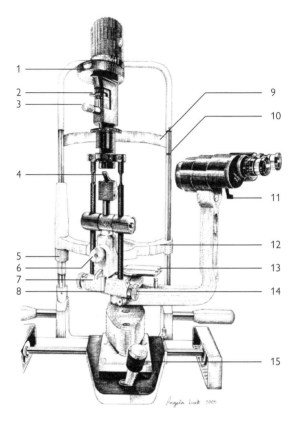

1	Indicator for beam height	9	Head band
2	Lever for selecting filters	10	Height marker (patient eye level)
3	Control for beam height	11	Lever for selecting magnification
4	Mirror	12	Chin rest
5	Control for chin rest height	13	Tonometer plate
6	Centring screw	14	Control for beam width
7	5° stops	15	Joystick
8	Latch for vertically tilting beam		

Fig. 1.9 Slit-lamp (Haag-Streit type) with key features identified.

Anterior segment examination (1)

See Table 1.4 for examination of the anterior segment.

Table 1.4 An approach to examining the anterior segment

Observe	Habitus, face, orbits
Examine *lashes*	Loss, colour, position, crusting
Examine *lid margins*	Position, contour, skinfolds, defects, inflammation, lumps
Examine *palpebral conjunctiva* • *Explain, then gently evert the lids*	Papillae, follicles, exudate, membrane, pseudomembrane
Examine *fornices*	Loss of fornices, symblepharon, ankyloblepharon
Examine bulbar *conjunctiva/episclera*	Hyperaemia, haemorrhage, lumps, degenerations, foreign bodies (FBs)/deposits
Examine *sclera*	Hyperaemia, thinning, perforation
Examine *cornea* • *Use diffuse/direct illumination/scleral scatter/specular reflection, as required*	Diameter, thickness, shape; pre-corneal tear film, epithelium, Bowman's layer, stroma, Descemet's membrane, endothelium
Examine *AC*	*Grade* flare/cells/depth; fibrin, pigment, level
Examine *iris* • *Use direct/retroillumination*	Colour, structure, movement, transillumination defects
Examine *lens* • *Use direct/retroillumination*	Opacity (pattern and maturity), size, shape, position, stability, capsule (anterior and posterior)
Examine *anterior vitreous*	Cells, flare, lens–vitreous interface, degenerations
Stain cornea • *Use fluorescein ± Lissamine green*	Tear film break-up time (TFBUT), Seidel's test
Check corneal sensation • *Use topical anaesthetic*	
Perform applanation *tonometry*	

Additional techniques for anterior segment examination

Illumination techniques

Although *direct illumination* is most commonly used, additional pathology may be revealed by the following techniques:

- *Sclerotic scatter*: uncouple the light source so that the slit beam can be displaced laterally to fall on the limbus while the microscope remains focused on the central cornea. Total internal reflection results in a generalized glow around the limbus and the highlighting of subtle opacities within the cornea, e.g. early oedema, deposits, etc.
- *Retroillumination*: direct the light source at a relatively posterior reflecting surface (e.g. iris or retina), and focus on the structure of interest (e.g. cornea, or iris and lens). View undilated for iris transillumination defects, dilated for lens opacities.
- *Specular reflection*: focus on the area of interest, and change the angle of illumination until you get a bright reflection (Purkinje image: I=tear film, II=endothelium, III=anterior lens) when the angle of incidence equals the angle of reflection, to highlight discontinuities in an otherwise smooth reflecting surface, e.g. examining the endothelium for guttata.

TFBUT

Place a drop of fluorescein into the lower fornix. Ask the patient to blink once and then not to blink (or hold lids open, if necessary). Observe with the blue light and yellow observational filter the time taken until the tear film breaks up (dark areas appear). A result <10s is usually considered abnormal (less in Asian eyes).

Seidel's test

Place a drop of 2% fluorescein over the area of concern, and observe with the blue light and yellow observational filter. The test is positive if there is a luminous green flow of aqueous. This results from local dilution of the stain by aqueous leaking from a surgical wound, penetrating injury, or bleb.

Schirmer's test

Whatman test paper is folded, 5mm from the end, and inserted in the temporal fornix of both lower lids. After 5min, the strips are removed and the length wetted is measured. This result is an indication of basic and reflex tearing. It is normal if >10mm, borderline 5–10mm, and abnormal if <5mm. Repeating the test after the addition of a topical anaesthetic gives an indication of basal secretion alone.

Applanation tonometry

Place a drop of local anaesthetic and fluorescein into the lower fornix. Rotate the tonometer dial, and record the pressure at which the inner aspect of the two luminous green circles just touch. Usually the white line on the prism is aligned with the horizontal meridian; however, in high astigmatism, the red line should be aligned with the minor axis. This is also affected by corneal thickness (see ➲ Ocular hypertension, p. 352).

- *Tonometer checks and calibration*: Goldmann tonometers may be checked by using the metal bar and control weight supplied. With the weight exactly midway along the bar (central stop), the tonometer should read 0mmHg. The next two stops correspond to 20 and 60mmHg, respectively. Significant deviation from this indicates a need for formal recalibration by the supplier.

Anterior segment examination (2)

AC depth measurement

Peripheral AC depth can be estimated using the Van Herick method; set the slit beam at 60° and directed just anterior to the limbus. If the AC depth is less than one-quarter of the corneal thickness, the angle is narrow and should be assessed on gonioscopy. A more central AC depth can be measured with a pachymeter. Alternatively, use a horizontal beam set at 60° to the viewing arm, and measure the length of beam at which the image on the cornea just abuts the image on the iris. Multiply this by 1.4 to get the depth in mm.

AC activity

The AC is initially assessed by using an angled thin ('conic') beam; the AC should appear dark in the absence of inflammation or hyphaema. In the presence of AC inflammation, grade both the flare (visible as haze illuminated by the slit-lamp beam) and cells (seen as particles slowly moving through the beam). This is important both in detecting intraocular inflammation and in monitoring response to treatment. A 1mm × 1mm slit is required for assessing cellular activity, according to the Standardization of Uveitis Nomenclature (SUN) standards.[1] (See Table 1.5 for grading of AC flare and Table 1.6 for grading of AC cells.)

Table 1.5 Grading of AC flare*

Flare grade	Description
0	None
1+	Faint
2+	Moderate (iris + lens clear)
3+	Marked (iris + lens hazy)
4+	Intense (fibrin or plastic aqueous)

* Jabs DA et al. Standardization of Uveitis Nomenclature (SUN) for reporting clinical data. Am J Ophthalmol 2005;**140**:509–16.

Table 1.6 Grading of AC cells[*]

Cell grade	Number of cells counted with 1mm × 1mm slit
0	<1
0.5+	1–5
1+	6–15
2+	16–25
3+	26–50
4+	>50

* Jabs DA *et al.* Standardization of Uveitis Nomenclature (SUN) for reporting clinical data. *Am J Ophthalmol* 2005;**140**:509–16.

1. Jabs DA *et al.* Standardization of Uveitis Nomenclature (SUN) for reporting clinical data. *Am J Ophthalmol* 2005;**140**:509–16.

Gonioscopy

Use an indirect (Goldmann, Zeiss) or direct (Koeppe) goniolens to assess the iridocorneal angle, including the iris insertion, the iris curvature, and the angle approach. If angle is closed, indent (with a Zeiss lens) to see if it can be opened ('appositional closure') or zipped shut ('synechial closure'). Describe according to Shaffer (see Table 1.7) or Spaeth (see Table 1.8), and record which classification used or a limited key (e.g. '4 = wide open', if using Shaffer) (see Fig. 1.10).

Shaffer classification

The Shaffer classification is outlined in Table 1.7.

Table 1.7 Shaffer classification

Shaffer grade	Grade 4	Grade 3	Grade 2	Grade 1	Grade 0
Angular approach	40°	30°	20°	10°	0
Most posterior structure clearly visualized	Ciliary body	Scleral spur	Trabeculum	Schwalbe's line	Cornea
Risk of closure	Closure not possible	Closure not possible	Closure possible	Closure probable	Closed
Summary	Wide open	Moderately open	Moderately narrow	Very narrow	Closed

Spaeth classification

Categorize according to iris insertion, angular approach, and iris curvature. e.g. D40R (see Table 1.8).

Table 1.8 Spaeth classification

Iris insertion	A	B	C	D	E
	Above Schwalbe's line	Below Schwalbe's line	Below scleral spur	Deep	Extremely deep
Angular approach	°				
	Estimate in °				
Iris curvature	R	S		Q	
	Regular convex	Steep convex		Queer, i.e. concave	

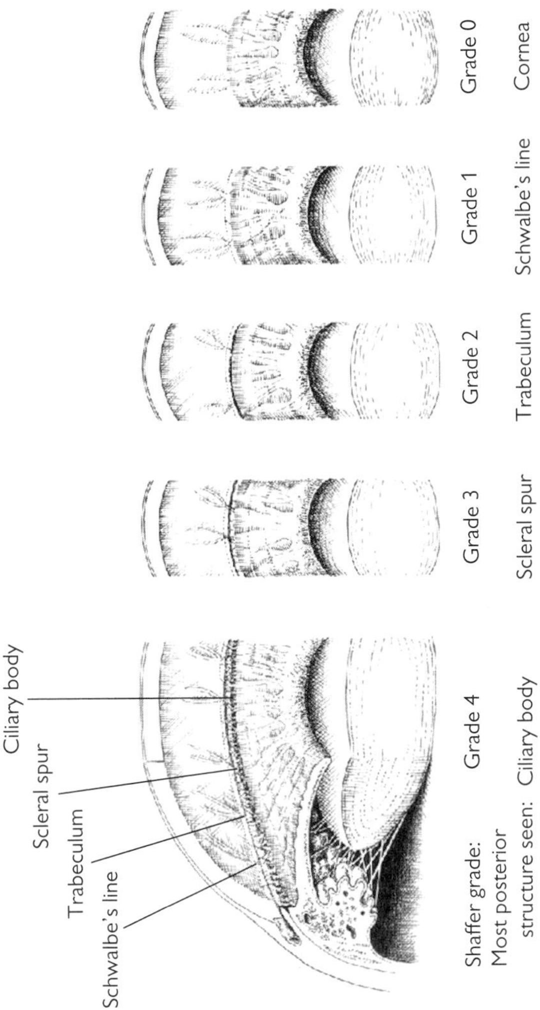

Fig. 1.10 AC angle with gonioscopic views. See Shaffer classification.

Shaffer grade:	Grade 4	Grade 3	Grade 2	Grade 1	Grade 0
Most posterior structure seen:	Ciliary body	Scleral spur	Trabeculum	Schwalbe's line	Cornea

Ciliary body
Scleral spur
Trabeculum
Schwalbe's line

Posterior segment examination

Table 1.9 An approach to examining the posterior segment

Pre-dilation perform RAPD, consider:	Amsler testing
Observe	Habitus, face, orbits
Examine *iris*	Adequate dilation, aniridia, albinism
Examine *lens*	Clarity, position, a-/pseudophakia
Examine *vitreous* • *Use conventional/red-free illumination*	Cells, flare, pigment, haemorrhage, opacities, posterior vitreous detachment (PVD), optical emptiness
Examine *disc*	Size, vertical cup:disc (C/D) ratio, colour, flat/elevated/tilted, neuroretinal rim (NRR) (e.g. contour, notches, haemorrhages), pits/colobomata
Examine *disc margin*	Oedema, capillaries, drusen
Examine *disc vessels*	Baring, bayonetting, anomalous vasculature, presence of spontaneous venous pulsation (SVP)
Examine *peripapillary area* • *Use conventional/red-free illumination*	Haemorrhages, atrophy, pigmentation, retinal nerve fibre layer (RNFL) defects
Examine *macula*	Position, flat/elevated, fluid/haemorrhage/exudate, drusen/atrophy/gliosis, angioid streaks/lacquer cracks, retinal striae/choroidal folds, cherry-red spot
Examine *retinal vessels*	Attenuation/dilation, tortuosity, sheathing, emboli, IRMA/neovascularization/telangiectasia/shunt vessels
Examine *peripheral fundus*	Degenerations/breaks/retinal detachments/dialysis/retinoschisis fluid/haemorrhage/exudate pigmentary retinopathy, chorioretinal scars, tumours, laser/cryotherapy/buckles

At the *slit-lamp*, consider: choice of lens, Watzke–Allen test.

With the *indirect ophthalmoscope*, consider choice of lens, scleral indentation.

Instruments used in posterior segment examination

Slit-lamp

Most ophthalmologists examining the posterior segment use the slit-lamp with a handheld lens (e.g. 90D or equivalent) (see Table 1.9).

- *Optical features*: the choice of lens balances the advantages of greater magnification (e.g. 66D lens) against wider field of view (e.g. 90D lens). Some (e.g. superfield/super 66) attempt to combine both these qualities. CL provide the highest clarity and may be useful in assessing detail (e.g. area centralis for macular pathology) or where the view is poor (e.g. media opacities). The retinal view using these lenses is inverted. Three-mirror CL (e.g. Goldmann) facilitate examination of the periphery; the views are mirror-image, rather than fully inverted.
- *Method*: ideally, the patient is dilated; the fundal view obtained without dilation is usually limited both in extent and in stereopsis. Adjust the slit-lamp so that it is coaxial and focused on the centre of the cornea. Interpose the lens 1cm in front of the eye, and draw the slit-lamp back until a clear fundal view is obtained. To view the peripheral retina, ask the patient to look in the direction of the area you wish to examine (i.e. down to view inferior retina). Troublesome reflections can be reduced by moving the illumination beam slightly off axis.

Indirect ophthalmoscope and scleral indenter

The indirect ophthalmoscope (assisted by scleral indentation) is the instrument of choice for examination of the peripheral fundus (see Table 1.9).

- *Optical features*: the choice of lens depends on the need for greater magnification (e.g. 3-fold with 20D lens but smaller field of view) vs wider field of view (e.g. larger field of view with 28D lens but only 2-fold magnification). The retinal view is inverted.
- *Method*: ensure patient is well dilated, positioned flat, and looking straight up at the ceiling. Have lens, indenter, and retinal chart/paper (for recording findings) available. Align eyepieces and illumination by viewing your outstretched thumb. Ensure that the headband is sufficiently tight that the ophthalmoscope will remain secure as you move around. Illumination brightness is adjusted according to quality of view and patient comfort.

View from above, with the ophthalmoscope directed downwards towards the pupil and with the lens held directly in the line of illumination. Resting this hand lightly against the patient's face helps steady the lens at an appropriate focal distance for a clear fundal view. To view the peripheral retina, change the angulation by asking the patient to look in the direction of the area to be examined (i.e. down to view inferior retina), whilst angling your head and lens in the opposite direction.

- *Scleral indentation*: to view, e.g. the inferior ora, ask the patient to look straight up, and place the indenter on the outside of the lower lid, resting tangentially against the area to be indented; then ask the patient to look straight down, moving the indenter with the globe. Observe the area of interest, whilst gently exerting pressure over it. Continue for 360°. Warn the patient that the procedure may be uncomfortable.

Direct ophthalmoscope

For those who see ophthalmic patients in the community, this may be the only option available for fundal examination. Ophthalmologists may also choose to use it where access to a slit-lamp is not possible (e.g. on ITU).

- *Optical features*: there is high magnification (15×) but only a small field of view. The retinal view is not inverted.
- *Method*: optimize your view with adequate dilation, dimmed room, and a fully charged ophthalmoscope. The field of view should be maximized by coming as close as possible to the eye. Optimal view of the optic disc is achieved by approaching from 15 to 20° temporally, while on the same horizontal level as the patient.

Additional examination techniques

Amsler grid

View at 1/3m. Ask the patient to fixate one eye at a time on the central dot and comment on whether any of the small squares are missing or distorted. There are seven charts, of which chart 1 is suitable for most patients. It consists of a 20 × 20 grid of 5mm squares, each representing 1° of central field (if viewed at 1/3m) (see Table 1.10).

Table 1.10 Amsler charts

Chart	Design	Colour	Use
1	Standard grid	White on black	Most patients
2	Standard grid with diagonals	White on black	Helps fixation
3	Standard grid	Red on black	Tests colour scotoma, e.g. optic neuropathy
4	Random dots	White on black	Tests scotoma only (no lines to become distorted)
5	Horizontal lines	White on black	Tests in one meridian (standard horizontal lines)
6	Horizontal lines	Black on white	Tests in one meridian (standard/fine horizontal lines)
7	Standard/fine central grid	White on black	High sensitivity for central lesions

Watzke–Allen test

Whilst using the slit lamp and handheld lens to view the macula, project a thin strip of light across the fovea. Ask the patient whether the line they see is broken, narrowed, or complete. A clear gap (Watzke–Allen positive) suggests a full-thickness macular defect/hole.

Goldmann three-mirror lens

This CL is used with the slit-lamp to examine the central and peripheral fundus. Note that this is a mirror image, rather than a rotated image of the peripheral fundus (cf. standard indirect ophthalmoscopy). It comprises four parts: central (view central 30°), equatorial mirror (largest; views 30° to equator), peripheral mirror (intermediate; views equator to ora), and gonioscopic mirror (smallest; views ora, pars plana, and angle).

Retinal charts

One standardized representation of vitreoretinal pathology uses the code in Table 1.11. See Table 1.12 for optical properties of lenses.

Table 1.11 Retinal chart key

Structure	Colour
Detached retina	Blue
Flat retina	Red
Retinal veins	Blue
Retinal breaks	Red within a blue outline
Retinal thinning	Red hatching within a blue outline
Lattice degeneration	Blue hatching within a blue outline
Pigment	Black
Exudate	Yellow
Vitreous opacities	Green

Table 1.12 Optical properties of commonly used lenses

Lens	Field of view	Magnification of image	Magnification of laser spot
With indirect ophthalmoscope			
20D	46°/60°	3.1	0.3
28D	53°/69°	2.3	0.4
Non-CL with slit-lamp			
60D	81°	1.2	0.9
Super 66	96°	1.0	1.0
78D	73°/97°	0.9	1.1
90D	69°/89°	0.8	1.3
Superfield NC	116°	0.8	1.3
Super vitreofundus	124°	0.6	1.8
CL with slit-lamp			
Area centralis	84°	1.1	0.9
Three-mirror		0.9	1.1
Transequator	132°	0.7	1.4
QuadrAspheric	144°	0.5	2.0

When using lenses with the slit-lamp, the overall magnification seen = lens magnification (listed above) × slit-lamp magnification (varies from 10 to 25×).

Pupils examination

Clinical examination
(See Box 1.3.)

> **Box 1.3 An approach to examining the pupils**
>
> Observe   Check lids, iris colour
>
> *Ask patient to look at a distant target*
>
> Measure pupil diameters in ambient *bright* light
>
> Measure pupil diameters in ambient *dim* light
>
> Check *direct* and *consensual* pupillary response for each side
>
> Check for relative afferent pupillary defect *(RAPD)*
>
> *Ask patient to look at a near target*   Check near
>   response

For an approach to diagnosing anisocoria, see ➔ Anisocoria, p. 708.

Anatomy and physiology

Parasympathetic pathway (light response) (See Fig. 1.11)

| IIn → | Pretectal nucleus | → | E-W nuclei (bilateral) | → | IIIn (inf) | → | Ciliary ganglion | → | Short ciliary n. | → | CONSTRICT |

Fig. 1.11 Light response of parasympathetic pathway. Known synapses are marked in bold.

Parasympathetic pathway (near response) (See Fig. 1.12)

VACx (area 19)	→	FEF	→	III/E-W nuclei	→	Ciliary ganglion	→	Short ciliary n.	→	CONSTRICT ACCOMMODATE
				↓						
				→ Medial rectus				→			CONVERGE

Fig. 1.12 Near response of parasympathetic pathway.

- *Light-near dissociation*: this is where dorsal midbrain pathology selectively reduces the response to light whilst preserving the response to near. This is thought to be due to the fact that the near pathway is placed ventral to the more dorsal pretectal nucleus serving the light pathway.

Sympathetic pathway (See Fig. 1.13)

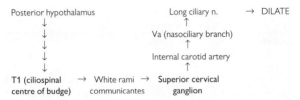

Fig. 1.13 Sympathetic pathway.

Pharmacological testing

The diagnosis of anisocoria (see ➡ Anisocoria, p. 708) may, in some cases, be assisted by pharmacological testing. These tests depend on comparing the response of the abnormal and the normal pupils, thus the agent should be instilled in both eyes and the response measured.

Diagnostic agents for an abnormally large pupil

(e.g. for diagnosing Adie's pupil)

Pharmacology

- *Pilocarpine*: is a direct muscarinic agonist. A normal pupil will constrict in response to 1% pilocarpine. A response to 0.125% indicates denervation hypersensitivity as occurs in an Adie's pupil.

Method

- Administer a drop of 0.125% pilocarpine to both eyes. At 0 and 30min, measure pupil size when fixing on a distant target in identical dim lighting conditions. In Adie's, the affected eye shows a significantly greater response.

Diagnostic agents for an abnormally small pupil

(e.g. for diagnosing Horner's pupil)

Pharmacology

- *Apraclonidine*: has weak alpha1-agonist activity, with little effect on the normal pupil. In a Horner's syndrome the abnormal pupil will dilate in response to apraclonidine; there may also be reversal of the associated ptosis.
- *Cocaine*: inhibits noradrenaline (NorA) reuptake at the neuromuscular junction of the dilator pupillae so increasing sympathetic tone. In the presence of a normal sympathetic pathway, cocaine results in dilation. In a Horner's syndrome, the abnormal pupil does not dilate.
- *Hydroxyamfetamine*: stimulates release of preformed NorA. In a 1st or 2nd order Horner's, the post-ganglionic neurone is intact, and thus the pupil will dilate in response to hydroxyamfetamine. In a 3rd order Horner's, the pupil will not dilate.

Method

See ➡ Anisocoria: sympathetic chain, p. 710.

Ocular motility examination

Table 1.13 An approach to examining ocular motility

Note VA	
Observe head posture	Face turn, head tilt, chin up/down
Hirschberg test	Manifest deviation
Cover/uncover + alternate cover test • With/without glassesTargets: near (1/3m), distance (6m), non-accommodative	Manifest or latent deviation
Examine *ductions* and *versions* into nine positions of gaze • Ask patient to follow target (usually a pen-torch) • Perform cover test in each position • Ask patient to report any diplopia in 1° position or during test	Any abnormality: Under-/overaction Paresis/restriction alphabet patterns Lid/head movements
Examine horizontal and vertical *saccades* • Ask patient to look rapidly between targets positioned at 30° on either side of the midline	Normal/slow Hypo-/hypermetric
Examine *convergence* • Assess to both an accommodative and non-accommodative target	Normal/reduced
Examine horizontal/vertical *doll's head movements*	Normal/absent
Examine horizontal/vertical *optokinetic (OKN) nystagmus* • Slowly rotate an OKN drum in horizontal and vertical direction	Normal/absent/convergence retraction nystagmus

Baseline tests should include tests which allow quantitative assessment of the ocular deviation (such as the prism cover test and Krimsky test).
Consider: caloric tests.

General approach

See Table 1.13 and ➲ Strabismus: outline, p. 744. Once a deviation has been detected, try to identify it as:
• Manifest or latent.
• Concomitant (constant in all positions of gaze) or incomitant (varying).

For incomitant deviations, identify:
• Direction of maximum separation of diplopic images.
• Pattern typical of neurogenic (see ➲ Neurogenic strabismus, p. 752), mechanical (see ➲ Mechanical strabismus, p. 752), or other (supranuclear, see ➲ Supranuclear eye movement disorders, p. 696; myasthenic, see ➲ Myasthenia gravis, p. 722; myopathic, see ➲ Myopathies p. 726, etc.) pathology.

It is common practice to use a pen-torch as a target when examining versions and vergences, since the positions of the eyes are highlighted by the corneal reflexes and it is a non-accommodative target. However, try to ensure that the pen-torch is not too bright, since dazzling the patient is counterproductive.

Corneal reflection tests

Hirschberg test

To detect/estimate the size of a manifest deviation. Ask the patient to fix on a pen-torch at 1/3m, and note the corneal reflections. The normal position is just nasal to the centre of the cornea. Every 1mm deviation represents $7°$ or 15Δ. If the reflection is deflected nasally, the eye is divergent (i.e. exotropic); if deflected temporally, the eye is convergent (i.e. esotropic).

Krimsky test

In the Krimsky test, this deviation is measured by placing a prism bar in front of the deviating eye and finding the prism strength at which the corneal reflexes are symmetrical. The prism should be orientated to 'point' in the direction of deviation, i.e. base-out for an esotropia, base-in for an exotropia.

Cover tests

Cover–uncover test

The cover test reveals a manifest deviation. Ask the patient to fix on a target (near, distance, non-accommodative, and sometimes far distance). Occlude each eye in turn (starting with the fixing eye), and observe any movement of the uncovered eye. For example, inward movement indicates that the eye was previously divergent (i.e. exotropic) and downward movement that it was previously elevated (i.e. hypertropic).

The uncover test may reveal a latent deviation. Occlude the first eye again for a few seconds. Look for any movement of the covered eye as the occluder is removed. Repeat for the other eye. For example, inward movement indicates that the occluded eye has drifted out (i.e. exophoric).

Perform the cover test in the nine positions of gaze to: (1) identify the direction of maximum separation of diplopia (indicates the direction of paretic muscle's action/maximum restriction) and (2) compare ductions and versions.

Alternate cover test

This detects the total deviation (latent + manifest) by causing dissociation of binocular single vision (BSV). Ask the patient to fix on a target (near/distance/non-accommodative). Repeatedly cover each eye in turn for 2–3s, so that one eye is always covered. Note the direction and amplitude of any deviation elicited. Once BSV is broken down, remove the occluder and note the speed of recovery of each eye in turn. Also look for dissociated vertical deviation (DVD) and manifest latent nystagmus (MLN) which are common in infantile esotropia.

Prism cover test

This measures the angle of deviation. Repeat the alternate cover test, but with a prism bar placed in front of one eye, adjusting the prism strength until first neutralization and then reversal of the corrective movement occurs. The prism should be orientated to 'point' in the direction of deviation, i.e. base-out for an esotropia.

Maddox tests

In these dissociative tests, different images are presented to each eye. They are generally used for assessing symptomatic phorias: whether for distance (Maddox rod), for near (Maddox wing), or torsional (two Maddox rods).

Maddox rod

For distance, a single Maddox rod (series of red cylinders) is placed horizontally in front of the right eye, and the patient (with distance correction) fixates on a distant spot of white light. The patient will see a vertical red line and a white spot. If there is no phoria, the line will pass straight through the spot. If the image is crossed (i.e. the line is to the left of the light), there is an exophoria; if the line is to the right, there is an esophoria. The phoria is then quantified by finding the prism required to neutralize it. The Maddox rod is then orientated vertically and the procedure repeated to identify any vertical phoria. If the line appears below the light, there is a right hyperphoria; if below, there is a left hyperphoria. This is again quantified by neutralizing with prisms.

Maddox wing

For near, a Maddox wing is used. The patient (wearing their usual reading correction) looks through the apertures to view a vertical and horizontal arrow (with the right eye) and corresponding vertical and horizontal scales (with the left eye). The numbers indicated by the arrows (as seen by the patient) indicates the direction and size of the near phoria.

Double Maddox rod test

For torsion, a horizontally orientated Maddox rod is placed in front of each eye (one red, one white). The colour of the tilted line is identified by the patient. The corresponding Maddox rod is rotated until the patient reports that it is vertical. The rotation required indicates the size of torsion. The two lines will fuse if there is no residual non-torsional deviation.

Parks–Bielschowsky 3-step test

This is used to identify a single underacting muscle in vertical/torsional deviations. It is particularly useful in superior oblique (SO) palsies.
- *Step 1*: perform cover test in 1° position; identify higher eye.
- *Step 2*: perform cover test with gaze to right, then left; identify where separation (and diplopia) is greatest.
  - This stage is based on the eye position where greatest vertical action occurs; for the obliques, this is when the eye is adducted, whereas, for the vertical recti, this is when the eye is abducted.
- *Step 3*: perform cover test with head tilt to right, then left shoulder; identify where separation (and diplopia) is greatest.
  - This stage is based on the fact that the superior muscles intort the eyes, whereas the inferior muscles extort.

See Fig. 1.14 and Table 1.14.

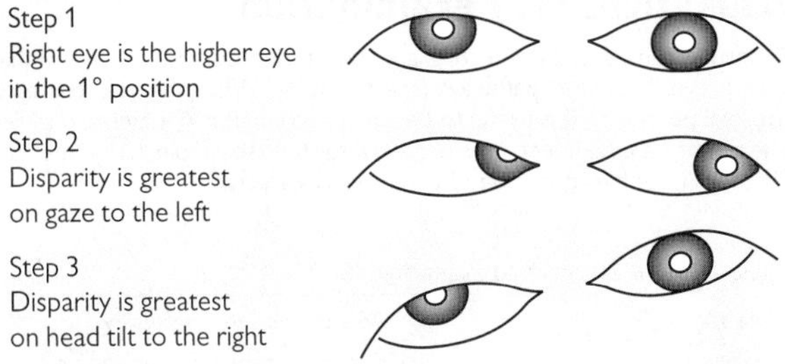

Step 1
Right eye is the higher eye
in the 1° position

Step 2
Disparity is greatest
on gaze to the left

Step 3
Disparity is greatest
on head tilt to the right

Fig. 1.14 Parks–Bielschowsky 3-step test: example of right SO underaction.

Table 1.14 Parks–Bielschowksy 3-step test

Step 1	Step 2	Step 3	Conclusion
Higher eye	Worst with gaze to	Worst with head tilt to	Underaction
Right eye	Right	Left	RIR
		Right	LIO
	Left	Left	LSR
		Right	RSO
Left eye	Right	Left	LSO
		Right	RSR
	Left	Left	RIO
		Right	LIR

LIR, left inferior rectus; RIR, right inferior rectus; LIO, left inferior oblique; RIO, right inferior oblique; LSR, left superior rectus; RSR, right superior rectus; LSO, left superior oblique; RSO, right superior oblique.

Caloric tests

This tests the vestibular/nuclear/infranuclear pathways and can be useful in patients with decreased consciousness. Ideally position the patient, with the head inclined backwards at 60°. Water placed in either ear causes nystagmus, with fast phase as follows: cold—opposite, warm—same (COWS).

Visual field (VF) examination

VF testing can assist in detecting and monitoring diseases of the retina, optic nerve, and visual pathways (see Fig. 1.14). While the gold standard is formal perimetry, it is useful to be able to screen for VF defects in clinics where time or equipment does not allow for this (see Table 1.15). See also Chapter 20 for interpretation of common VF defects.

Table 1.15 An approach to examining VF

Note VA	Adjust target size, if necessary
Observe	Features of stroke, acromegaly, etc.
• *Patient with both eyes open and looking at the bridge of your nose*	Gross homonymous defects
Ask if any part of your face appears to be missing	
• *Patient with non-testing eye occluded:*	Peripheral defects
Check they can see a white pin head against a dark background	
Map out right/left VF with the white pin (coming from unseen to seen, asking the patient to identify when they first see the pin)	
Repeat with the red pin to map right/ left central 30° (asking the patient to identify when the pin appears red)	Central defects
Use red pin to map out right/left *physiological blind spots*	Enlarged/ part of centrocaecal scotoma

Any VF abnormality should be confirmed on formal perimetry (see ➲ Visual field testing: general, p. 48; ➲ Goldmann perimetry, p. 56).

Consider:

- Simultaneous presentation of gross targets to elicit inattention (this may occur in the context of stroke syndromes).
- Simultaneous presentation of red targets across vertical and horizontal midlines (e.g. present across the vertical midline to elicit the temporal depression of red perception of early chiasmal disease—ask patient to report any difference in red colour between targets).

Additional clinical examinations may include pupils, discs, ocular motility, cranial nerves, peripheral nervous system (PNS).

Lids/ptosis examination

See Table 1.16 for an approach to examination.

Table 1.16 An approach to examining the lids (with particular regard to ptosis)

Shake hands	Check for myotonia (note slow release of grip)
Observe	
• Face	Any asymmetry, lesions
• Brow	Any frontalis overaction
• Globes	Position, asymmetry
• Lids	Position, asymmetry, scars
• Pupils	Anisocoria, hypochromia
Measure *palpebral aperture*	
Measure *upper margin reflex distance*	
Measure *position of upper lid crease*	
Measure *levator function*	
• *Inhibit frontalis by placing a thumb on the brow*	
Measure any *lagophthalmos*	
• *Ask patient to close eyes, gently at first, and then to squeeze eyes shut*	
Assess *orbicularis function* and *Bell's phenomenon*	
• *Try to open patient's eyes against resistance*	
Assess *fatiguability* over 1min	Any worsening of ptosis
• *Ask patient to keep looking upward at a target held superiorly*	
Examine for *Cogan's twitch*	Any overshoot
• *Ask patient to look rapidly from downgaze to a target held in 1° position*	
Assess for *jaw-winking*	Any change in ptosis
• *Ask patient to simulate chewing and to move jaw from side to side*	
Biomicroscope examination of *lid* and *subtarsal* conjunctiva	Inflammation/masses/scars
Check *corneal sensation*	Implications for surgery
Examine *ocular motility*	Motility abnormality, change in ptosis
Examine *pupils*	Anisocoria (in response to light and near)

Consider: ice-pack test (see ➲ Investigations p. 722), full VIIn assessment, full cranial n. assessment, examination of fundus, systemic review (myopathy, fatiguability).

Special tests

Fatiguability

The ability to sustain lid elevation is assessed in upgaze. Hold a target superiorly, and ask the patient to maintain fixation on it for a minute. Note if either lid drifts down over that time, and reassess palpebral aperture in the 1° position at the end of this period. If fatiguability is demonstrated, examine for associated fatiguability of ocular motility and general musculature. This is usually a sign of myasthenia (see ⮕ Myasthenia gravis, p. 722); consider the ice-pack test (see ⮕ Investigations, p. 722) and further investigation.

Cogan's twitch

Cogan's twitch is an overshoot of the eyelid which occurs on rapid elevation of the eyes from downgaze to the 1° position. Ask the patient to look down and then to look at a target held directly in front of them. Cogan's twitch may be seen in myasthenia.

Jaw-winking

Synkinesis ('miswiring') may result in a ptosis which varies with use of other facial muscles (pterygoids). This may be seen as jaw-winking where the lid can be elevated by movement of the jaw (e.g. chewing, side-to-side movement of the jaw) (see ⮕ Ptosis: congenital, p. 162).

Normal lid measurements

See Table 1.17.

Table 1.17 Normal lid measurements

Palpebral aperture	8–11mm (♀ > ♂)
Upper margin reflex distance	4–5mm
Upper lid excursion (levator function)	13–16mm
Upper lid crease position	8–10mm from margin (♀ > ♂)

Orbital examination

See Table 1.18 for an approach to examination.

Table 1.18 An approach to examining the orbit

Vision	VA, colour
Observe	Behaviour, habitus, face, lids
Observe from above	Globe position
Palpate orbital margins	Notches, instability, soft tissue signs; check for lacrimal gland
Palpate globe (gentle *retropulsion*)	Pulsation, resistance, pain
Check *infraorbital sensation*	Hypoaesthesia
Perform *exophthalmometry* • *Document which model used (e.g. Hertel, Rodenstock)*	Globe position
If proptosis, assess whether axial or non-axial • *Use two clear rulers, one horizontally over the bridge of the nose and one vertically to detect whether axial or non-axial*	
Auscultate the globe/temporal region • *Use stethoscope bell*	Bruit
Assess any effect of the *Valsalva* manoeuvre	Increased proptosis
Check *corneal sensation*	Hypoaesthesia
Proceed to *full ophthalmic examination*, including:	
Pupils	RAPD, anisocoria
VF	
Ocular motility (± forced duction test)	Restriction, paresis
Cranial nerves	
Conjunctiva	Chemosis, injection
Cornea/sclera	Vessels, integrity
Tonometry	Change in upgaze, wide pulse pressure
Optic disc	Oedema, pallor, abnormal vessels
Fundus	Choroidal folds
Consider: refraction, neurological, and general systemic examination, as indicated.	

Special tests

Exophthalmometry

A number of exophthalmometers are available, and there is some variation in technique used, even with the common Hertel device. The following is one approach:

- Using the Hertel exophthalmometer, place it level with the orbits, and adjust the separation so that the foot plates rest on the lateral orbital rims at the level of the lateral canthi. Close your right eye, and ask the patient to fix on your open (left) eye, while you align the parallax markers (usually red), and read off where the patient's right corneal apex appears on the scale. Repeat with your right eye and the patient's left eye.
- Measurements >20mm or a difference of >2mm between globes is suggestive of proptosis. Beware of patient variables (racial differences, lateral orbitotomy), instrument variability (try to use the same exophthalmometer each time), and operator inconsistency.
- The consistency of serial measurements may be improved by ensuring that the intercanthal distance is kept the same.

Two-ruler test

Horizontal and vertical displacement of the globe may be demonstrated by using two clear plastic rulers. One is placed horizontally over the bridge of the nose at the level of the lateral canthi. Look for horizontal displacement by comparing the distance from the centre of the nasal bridge to equivalent points on the globe (e.g. nasal limbus). Look for vertical displacement by measuring vertically (second ruler) to compare the distance from the horizontal meridian (i.e. the first ruler) to equivalent points on the globe (e.g. the inferior limbus).

Nasolacrimal system examination

See Table 1.19 for an approach to examination.

Table 1.19 An approach to examining the nasolacrimal system

Observe face	Asymmetry, scars, nasal bridge
Observe/palpate *lacrimal sac*	Mass, inflammation
• Check for regurgitation from canaliculi on pressing sac	
Observe *lids*	Contour, position, chronic lid disease
• Assess with eyes open and closed	
Assess lid laxity	
• Draw lid laterally, medially, and anteriorly	
Examine *puncta*	Position, calibre, discharge
• Assess with eyes open and closed	
Examine *conjunctiva/cornea*	Inflammation
Measure *tear meniscus*	
• Instil 2% fluorescein in lower fornix	
Assess *dye disappearance*	
Check *dye recovery* from nose	
• Use nasendoscope or cotton bud	
Cannulate and probe *puncta/canaliculi*	Patency of puncta, hard or soft stop
• Use lacrimal cannula attached to a syringe of saline (+ fluorescein)	
Irrigate with saline to estimate flow/ regurgitation	Upper/lower systems
Consider: nasendoscopy, formal Jones testing.	

Dye disappearance test

Instil a drop of fluorescein 2% into each lower fornix. Reassess at 2min, by which time (almost) complete clearance should have occurred. Prolonged retention indicates inadequate drainage.

Probing

Under topical anaesthesia, insert a straight lacrimal cannula into the lower canaliculus, and guide it towards the medial wall of the lacrimal sac whilst exerting gentle lateral traction on the lower lid (see Table 1.20 for interpretation of tests). Assess whether there is a:

• *Hard (abrupt) stop*: indicates a patent system as far as the lacrimal sac, or a
• *Soft (spongy) stop*: indicates a canalicular block.

Irrigation

Under topical anaesthesia, insert a lacrimal cannula into the lower canaliculus, and place a finger against the lacrimal sac. Irrigate with saline, and assess:

- *Flow*: estimate flow (e.g. in %) conducted (i.e. down nose/back of the throat) vs regurgitated; if regurgitated, note from which canaliculus.
- *Quality of regurgitated fluid*: clear or purulent
- *Lacrimal sac distension* (see Table 1.20 for interpretation of tests).

Table 1.20 Interpretation of probing and irrigation tests

Level of block	Probing	Irrigation
Punctum	Cannot cannulate	Not possible
Canaliculus (upper/lower)	Soft stop	Regurgitates through same canaliculus only (high pressure)
Common canaliculus	Soft stop	May regurgitate through either canaliculus
Nasolacrimal duct	Hard stop	Lacrimal sac dilates; may regurgitate (± mucus) through either canaliculus

Jones testing

This may be considered in cases of partial obstruction to ascertain the level of block (see Table 1.21 for interpretation).

- *1° test*: instil fluorescein 2% into the lower fornix. After 5min, assess for dye recovery with a cotton bud (can be moistened with 4% cocaine) placed at the nasolacrimal duct opening (below the inferior turbinate) or with a nasendoscope; an alternative way of looking for dye recovery is to ask the patient to blow one nostril at a time onto a tissue.
- *2° test*: wash out the fluorescein from the lower fornix. Under topical anaesthesia, insert a lacrimal cannula into the lower canaliculus and irrigate. Assess dye recovery from the nose as before.

Table 1.21 Interpretation of Jones test

	Result	Interpretation
1° test		
Dye recovered	Positive	Normal patency
Dye not recovered	Negative	Partial obstruction or lacrimal pump failure
2° test		
Dye recovered	Positive	Partial obstruction of nasolacrimal duct
Dye not recovered	Negative	Partial obstruction above the lacrimal sac

Refraction: outline (1)

History

Essential history
- Reason for visit/rationale for refraction such as symptoms.
- Demographics, including age.
- Visual requirement such as occupation, VDU use, driving, and hobbies.
- POH, including previous surgery, allergies, and use of refractive corrections such as spectacles and CL.
- Family ophthalmic history.
- PMH.

Examination

Preparation
Focimetry on current spectacles (see ➔ Focimetry, p. 44)

ROOM LIGHTS ON
- VA—unaided + with current prescription + with pinhole if <6/9.
- Cover/uncover test at distance and near.
- Motility and pupil examination (if not already conducted).
- Measure IPD (distance) → set up trial frame.

Retinoscopy

ROOM LIGHTS OFF
- Ask patient to look at a non-accommodative target distance (e.g. green duochrome).
- Estimate refractive error from previous prescription and VA (1.0D of blur reduces VA by about 4 logMAR lines if no accommodation exerted), and start with this lens compensated for your working distance (e.g. if you work at 2/3m, add +1.5D DS).
- Fog fellow eye with a high plus powered lens to prevent accommodation.
- Aim to be as close to the patient's visual axis without obscuring their fixation target. If your head gets in the way, they are likely to look at it and start accommodating. Ask the patient to tell you if this happens.
- Check retinoscopy reflex:
  - Identify axis of astigmatism from movement of retinoscopy light as sweep across eye.
  - Neutralize reflex in one meridian with DS lenses.
  - If reflex is 'with', then add PLUS; if 'against', then add MINUS.
  - When point of reversal is reached in one meridian, add cylindrical lenses to neutralize in the other meridian.

Plus or minus cylinders

Be consistent; either work with *plus* or with *minus* cylindrical lenses.

- If using *plus* cylindrical lenses, you will wish to correct the most *minus* meridian first. This is identified by:
  - If both reflexes are *against*, then it is the *slower* reflex.
  - If one is *with* and one *against*, then it is the *against* reflex.
  - If both reflexes are *with*, then it is the *faster* reflex.
- If using *minus* cylindrical lenses, you will wish to correct the most *plus* meridian first. This is identified similarly:
  - If both reflexes are *against*, then it is the *faster* reflex.
  - If one is *with* and one *against*, then it is the *with* reflex.
  - If both reflexes are *with*, then it is the *slower* reflex.

Poor reflex

- *Consider media opacity*: optimize illumination; check that they are not accommodating on your head.
- *Consider high refractive error*: use large steps, e.g. ± 5DS or ±10DS.
- *Consider keratoconus*: if swirling reflex or oil drop sign.

Refraction: outline (2)

Subjective refraction

Remove 'working distance' lenses   ROOM LIGHTS ON
Occlude eye not being tested
Check VA

Verify sphere
- Ask patient to look at the smallest line that they can see clearly.
- Verify sphere by offering ± DS (usually ± 0.25DS to fine-tune but may need ± 0.5DS if poor VA).
- Ask, 'Is the line clearer and easier to read with lens 1 or 2?'
- Do not make the prescription more minus if the lens does not improve the number of letters than can be read and just makes the letter look 'darker'. Put higher power lenses at back of trial frame.
- Measure and document back vertex distance (BVD), especially if >4.0DS.

Verify cylinder axis
- Ask patient to look at a round target/easily readable such as 'O' or dots.
- Use cross-cylinder (± 0.25D cross-cylinder, or ± 0.50 or ± 1.00D if VA poor).
- Align handle with axis of trial cylinder.
- Ask, 'Is the circle rounder and clearer with lens 1 or 2?'
- Rotate trial cylinder towards the preferred cross-cylinder position respecting its sign, i.e. a plus trial cylinder is rotated towards the plus sign of the cross-cylinder. Try not to remove the cross-cylinder from in front of the eyes as you rotate the axis; explain to the patient it will be clearer without this lens.

Verify cylinder power
- Once there is no difference between the two positions with the cross-cylinder handle along the axis of the cross-cylinder, repeat the procedure but with the handle at 45° to axis of trial cylinder. This will in effect offer ± 0.25D cyl (if using the 0.50 cross-cylinder).
- Add the sign of the cylinder preferred in 0.25D steps until there is a reversal.
- Add 0.25DS for every 0.5DC lost.

Refine best sphere
- Plus 1 blur test (should reduce a VA of 6/5 or 6/6 to about 6/12—if not, add more plus).
- Duochrome test (monocular and binocular; aim for no preference/slight red preference).

Measure and record BVD; most important if >4DS.

Check near requirement—at usual reading/working distance. If presbyopic (typically over age 45y), add a near addition suitable for the patient's age (see Table 1.22), and refine for the patient's preferred working distance and working range. The residual accommodation remaining can be determined with the RAF rule (perform 3× for each test) or rule and near target, determining the closest distance the text can be moved towards the eyes before the letters blur and cannot be made clear with effort.

Table 1.22 Estimated near corrections

Age 45–50y	+1.0DS
Age 50–55y	+1.5DS
Age 55–60y	+2.0DS
Age >60y or pseudophake	+2.5DS

Muscle balance, accommodation, and convergence

A measure of the oculomotor balance between the eyes is required, with the prescription determined in place. This could be a cover test or fixation disparity at distance and near, or dissociative tests (no fusional lock) such as Maddox rod and Wing (see ⟳ Maddox tests, p. 30). Do not prescribe prisms unless symptomatic, and first consider whether further investigation (including orthoptic referral) is necessary.

Causes of spectacle intolerance

The following may lead to asthenopia (refractive discomfort or 'eye strain'):
- Significant change in axis or size of cylinder.
- Change of lens form.
- Overcorrection, especially of myopes who will end up permanently accommodating.
- Excessive near correction resulting in an uncomfortably near and narrow reading distance.
- Unsuitable bifocal or progressive lenses—consider occupation, requirements, and general faculties of the patient.

Focimetry

The focimeter or lensometer measures the axis and power of spectacles and CL. The instrument can also be used to find the optical centre and the power and base direction of any prism in unknown lenses (see Fig. 1.15).

Manual focimetry

The vertex power of the lens is measured by taking the inverse of the focal length of the unknown lens. Green light is used to eliminate chromatic aberration.

Components
- Moveable illumination target.
- Viewing telescope.
- Fixed collimating lens (renders light parallel).

Method
- Ensure the eyepiece is focused and target seen sharply focused.
- Insert unknown lens (spectacles mounted with the back surface of the lens against the rest to measure back vertex power).

For simple spherical lenses
Dial (this moves the target backwards or forwards) until the graticules are sharp, and read off the power.

For cylindrical power
The target is rotated as well as dialled until one set of lines is sharp. The reading is noted. The target is then dialled again until the other lines are sharp. The difference in these two readings is the cylindrical power. The axis of the cylinder is then read from the dialling wheel.

Bifocal addition
Turn the spectacles around to measure the front vertex power. The difference between the front vertex power of the distance and near portions is the bifocal add.

Automated focimetry

In principle, four parallel beams of light pass through the unknown lens and strike a photosensitive surface. The deflection of the beams from their original path is measured and used to compute the lens power.

There is a support frame for the spectacles; changing the lever on the unit above the support frame will automatically read either the right or the left lens, as required.

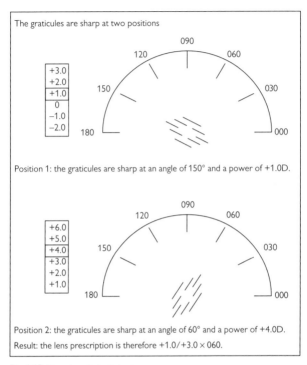

The graticules are sharp at two positions

Position 1: the graticules are sharp at an angle of 150° and a power of +1.0D.

Position 2: the graticules are sharp at an angle of 60° and a power of +4.0D.

Result: the lens prescription is therefore +1.0/+3.0 × 060.

Fig. 1.15 View through the focimeter.

Chapter 2

Investigations and their interpretation

Visual field testing: general

The VF is 'an island of vision surrounded by a sea of darkness' (Traquair's analogy). It is a three-dimensional hill, the peak of the hill being the fovea, and, at ground level, it extends ~50° superiorly, 60° nasally, 70° inferiorly, and 90° temporally.

Indications

Aids diagnosis and monitors certain ophthalmic (e.g. glaucoma) and neurological disease.

Definitions

- A *scotoma* is an area of visual loss or depression surrounded by an area of normal or less depressed vision. An absolute scotoma represents a total loss of vision where no light can be perceived. A relative scotoma is an area of partial visual loss where bright lights or larger targets are seen, whereas smaller and dimmer ones cannot be seen.
- *Homonymous*: this is where the defects are in the corresponding region of the VF in both eyes. For example, in a right homonymous hemianopia, there is a defect to the right of the midline in both VFs.
- *Congruousness*: describes the degree to which the field defects match between the two eyes. Generally, the more congruous the field defect, the more posterior along the visual pathway the lesion is located.
- *Isopter*: this is a threshold line joining points of equal sensitivity on a VF chart.

Caution

Interpretation problems of all VFs can include refractive status (overcorrection by 1D will cause a reduction in sensitivity of 3.6dB). To compare serial VFs, background luminance, stimulus size, intensity, and exposure times need to be standardized.

Confrontational VFs

This is a simple qualitative method for gross detection of defects in the peripheral VF (see ➔ Visual field (VF) examination, p. 32). The use of hat pins (white and red) enables more subtle defects to be plotted. Results should be recorded the way the patient sees them; however, there can be inter-examiner variability.

Amsler grid

This assesses the central 10° of the VF. Easy to perform and portable, it is used to detect central and paracentral scotomas. Held at a testing distance of 33cm, each square subtends 1° of VF (see ➔ Posterior segment examination, p. 22).

Kinetic perimetry

This presents a moving stimulus of known luminance from a non-seeing area to a seeing area. The target is then presented at various points around the clock and marked when recognized; these points are then joined, producing a line of equal threshold sensitivity, which is named the isopter.

Tangent screen

The tangent screen (Bjerrum screen) is not commonly used in clinical practice.

Indication

Examining the central 30° of VF, usually at 2m, although a 1m chart is available.

Method

Patient sits 2m (2,000mm) away from the screen, wears corrective lens for distance, if required. The non-tested eye is occluded in turn. The patient fixates at a central spot and informs the operator when they see the target. White (w) or red (r) disc targets are used, either 1 or 2mm in diameter.

Results

The results are plotted on charts as the patient sees them. The target size and colour is the numerator (1w, 2w, 1r, or 2r), and the denominator is the distance (mm) of the patient from the chart (e.g. 1r/2,000).

Goldmann perimetry

This is the commonest type of kinetic perimetry in clinical practice (see ➋ Goldmann perimetry, p. 56). Both automated (Haag-Streit) and manual machines are in clinical use.

Static perimetry

Most automated perimetry is based on static on–off stimuli of variable luminance presented throughout the potential field (see ➋ Static automated perimetry: performance and interpretation, p. 50).

Static automated perimetry: performance and interpretation

In static perimetry, the stimulus is stationary but changes its intensity until the sensitivity of the eye at that point is found. It is measured at preselected locations in the VF. Program selection includes the central 30°, 24°, 10°, or full field.

- *Suprathreshold* tests are quickest to perform and are screening tests. They calculate the threshold adjusted for age by testing a few predefined spots using a 4–6dB step. They may miss subtle variations in the scotoma's contour, as they do not go on to map defects. They should not be used to monitor glaucoma.
- *Threshold* testing steps of 4dB are used until detected, then retested at this point in 2dB steps. This is the gold standard for monitoring glaucoma and requires patient cooperation and concentration. There is an appreciable subject learning curve seen in the first few tests.

Humphrey perimetry

- Sensitive and reproducible but difficult to perform.
- Fixation monitoring (by tracking gaze and retesting the blind spot).

Method

The machine automatically calibrates itself on start-up. Selection of programs includes:

- Threshold (full threshold or SITA central 30-2, 24-2, 10-2).
- Suprathreshold testing (screening central 76 point, full field 120 point, and Esterman (Driver and Vehicle Licensing Agency (DVLA) visual driving standard test)).
- Coloured stimuli can also be used.

Interpretation of Humphrey perimetry

See Table 2.1 and Table 2.2.

When analysing the results of automated perimetry, consider reliability indices, absolute retinal thresholds, comparison with age-matched controls, and overall performance indices (global indices).

Table 2.1 Reliability indices (subject reliability)

Fixation losses	Fixation plotted, if patient moves and the machine retests and patient sees spot, then a fixation loss is recorded. Fixation losses above 20% may significantly compromise the test
False positives	Patient responds to the normal whirr of the computer noise when it sounds, as if it is about to present a light but does not. A high false positive occurs in 'trigger happy' patients
False negatives	A brighter light is presented in an area in which the threshold has already been determined and the patient does not see it. A high false negative score occurs in fatigued or inattentive patients

Table 2.2 Common VF abnormalities

Altitudinal field defects	Ischaemic optic neuropathy
	Hemibranch retinal artery or vein occlusion
	Glaucoma
	Optic nerve or chiasmal lesions
	Optic nerve coloboma
Arcuate scotoma	Glaucoma
	Ischaemic optic neuropathy
	Optic disc drusen
Binasal field defect	Glaucoma
	Bitemporal retinal disease (e.g. RP)
	Bilateral occipital disease
	Compressive lesion of both optic nerves or chiasm
	Functional visual loss
Bitemporal hemianopia	Chiasmal lesions
	Titled optic discs
	Sectoral RP
Central scotoma	Macular lesions
	Optic neuritis
	Optic atrophy
	Occipital cortex lesions
Homonymous hemianopia	Optic tract or lateral geniculate lesions
	Temporal, parietal, or occipital lobe lesions
Constriction of peripheral fields	Glaucoma
	Retinal disease (e.g. RP)
	Bilateral pan-retinal photocoagulation (PRP)
	CRAO
	Bilateral occipital lobe lesions with macular sparing
	Papilloedema
	Functional visual loss (spiral VFs)
Blind spot enlargement	Papilloedema
	Glaucoma
	Optic nerve drusen
	Optic nerve coloboma
	Myelinated nerve fibres
	Myopic discs
Pie in the sky	Temporal lobe lesion
Pie on the floor	Parietal lobe lesion

Probability values (p)

Indicate the significance of the defect <5%, <2%, <1%, and <0.5%. The lower the *p* value, the greater its clinical significance and the lesser the likelihood of the defect having occurred by chance (see Table 2.3 and Table 2.4 and Fig. 2.1).

Table 2.3 Global indices (a summary of the results as a single number used to monitor change)

Mean deviation (MD)	A measure of overall field loss
Pattern standard deviation (PSD)	Measure of focal loss or variability within the field, taking into account any generalized depression. An increased PSD is more indicative of glaucomatous field loss than MD
Short-term fluctuation (SF)	An indication of the consistency of responses. It is assessed by measuring threshold twice at ten preselected points and calculated on the difference between the 1st and 2nd measurements
Corrected PSD	A measure of variability within the field after correcting for SF (intra-test variability)

Table 2.4 Typical graphical results from automated perimetry

The grey scale	Decreasing sensitivity is represented by the darker tones. Grey scale tones correspond to 5dB change in threshold
Numerical display	Gives the threshold for all points checked (in dB). Bracketed results show the initial test if the sensitivity was 5dB less sensitive than expected
Total deviation	Calculated by comparing the patient's measurements with age-matched controls. Upper chart is in dB, and lower is in grey scale
Pattern deviation	Adjusted for any generalized depression in the overall field. This highlights focal depressions in the field, which might be masked by generalized depressions in sensitivity (e.g. cataract and corneal opacities)

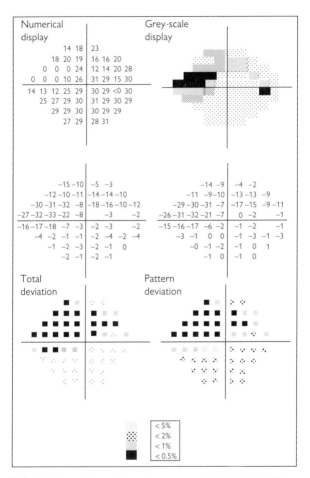

Fig. 2.1 Typical graphical results from automated perimetry of the right eye of a patient with glaucoma, demonstrating nasal step and developing superior arcuate field defect.

Automated perimetry: protocols

Swedish interactive threshold algorithm (SITA; fast or standard)

SITA strategies were created to take 50% less time than conventional algorithms to perform, thus increasing reliability. They are carried out by using prior information and establishing threshold values more quickly.

Esterman grid

Different grids are available for the central field, whole field, and binocular field. Subjects are tested, and a percentage score of functional field is given. The binocular field test is used by the DVLA as a measure of visual disability for drivers. It is not necessary for the subject to see all the points, but to see points within the UK's current driving standard protocols (see ➜ Driving standards, p. 916).

Short wavelength automated perimetry

Short wavelength automated perimetry uses standard static threshold testing strategies with a blue test object on a yellow background (red and green cones are desensitized by adapting the eye to yellow light). Results suggest that this is more sensitive than conventional white on white perimetry to early glaucomatous damage.[1]

Caution
- Increased total test time.
- Difficulty to set up test.
- High SF.
- Data affected by lens opacities.

Frequency doubling perimetry

This measures the function of a subset of specialized retinal ganglion cells (the large magnocellular (M-cell) pathway fibres) by rapid reversal of broad black and white bars, creating a doubling frequency illusion. These M-fibres are thought to be lost early in glaucoma.

Owing to its high sensitivity and specificity, frequency doubling perimetry may be useful in glaucoma screening. It is a small portable unit that is not sensitive to background illumination levels. It is reported to work independently of refractive errors up to ± 7D.

---

1. Johnson CA *et al.* Progression of early glaucomatous visual field loss as detected by blue on yellow and standard white on white automated perimetry. *Arch Ophthalmol* 1993;**111**:651–6.

Glaucoma progression analysis

Identifying VF progression, using serial printout of stored field tests (as single charts) in consecutive order, allows subjective comparison of charts to show change over time. Trend and event analyses allow quantitative assessment of progression in a VF series.

Trend analysis

Measures rate of change of the VF and the statistical significance. Can be measured point by point (point-wise linear regression) or on a cluster basis. Examples: PROGRESSOR software (Institute of Ophthalmology, London) and PeriData.

Event analysis

Designed to highlight any VF changes from baseline that are larger than typical clinical variability. Examples include: the Glaucoma Progression Analysis for the Humphrey Field Analyser.

Glaucoma progression analysis

Glaucoma progression analysis is simple to interpret and corrects for media opacities (such as progressive cataracts that cause a generalized depression).

It defines visual progression according to the Early Manifest Glaucoma Trial (EMGT) criteria:[2] any patient who lost three or more test points in the same location on three consecutive field tests. The EMGT criteria has been shown to identify progression earlier and more often than the Advanced Glaucoma Intervention Study (AGIS) or the Collaborative Initial Glaucoma Treatment Study (CIGTS) criteria.[3]

Results

Glaucoma progression analysis can calculate the variability then adjusts for this to calculate the probability that a change at a specific point is indeed true change or not. The probability plot progression symbol key:

- *Open triangles*: when a point is a statistically significant from baseline fields at that location.
- *Half-black triangle*: if a point has changed on two consecutive fields (indicates possible progression).
- *Black triangle*: if three consecutive fields show change at that particular location (indicates likely progression).

Glaucoma Progression Analysis Alert™

- Three half-black triangles in one analysis indicate 'possible progression'.
- Three black triangles in one analysis indicate 'likely progression'.

Caution

Full threshold strategy fields can only be used as baseline and not as follow-up tests (SITA, standard or fast, must be used).

2. Heijl A *et al.* Reduction of IOP and glaucoma progression: results from the Early Manifest Glaucoma Trial. *Arch Ophthalmol* 2002;**120**:1268–79.

3. Heijl A *et al.* A comparison of visual field progression criteria of 3 major glaucoma trials in early manifest glaucoma trial patients. *Ophthalmology* 2008;**115**:1557–65.

Goldmann perimetry

Basic principles
- Usually kinetic (static perimetry is used for the central field).
- Skilled operators are required for the manual Goldmann Perimeter.
- Newer software packages on automated machines simulate full field Goldmann kinetic perimetry (e.g. OCTOPUS 900™).
- Useful for neuro-ophthalmic patients and those needing significant supervision to produce a VF.

Method

The Goldmann Perimeter should be calibrated at the start of each session. Distance and near add with wide aperture lenses should be used (to prevent ring scotoma). Aphakic eyes should, where possible, be corrected with CL. Seat patient, with chin on chin-rest and forehead against rest; occlude non-test eye; ask patient to fix on central target and to press the buzzer whenever they see the light stimulus.

From the opposite side of the Goldmann, the examiner directs the stimulus to map out their field of vision to successive stimuli (isopters). Move the stimulus slowly and steadily from unseen to seen, i.e. inward for periphery and outward for mapping the blind spot/central scotomas. To move the stimulus arm from one side to the other, it must be swung around the bottom of the chart. Once the peripheral isopters are plotted, the central area is examined for scotoma. The examiner should monitor patient fixation via the viewing telescope. The central 20° with an extension to the nasal 30° is appropriate to pick up early glaucomatous scotomas. Points either side of the vertical meridian are explored in suspected chiasmal and post-chiasmal disease. The physiological blind spot should be mapped (see Fig. 2.2).

Results

Isopters are contours of visual sensitivity. Common isopters plotted are:
- I-4e (0.25mm², 1000asb stimulus).
- I-2e (0.25mm², 100asb stimulus).
- II-4e (1.0mm², 1000asb stimulus).
- IV-4e if smaller targets not seen (16mm², 1000asb stimulus).

Interpretation

The target sizes are indicated by Roman numerals (0–V), representing the size of the target in square millimetres, each successive number being equivalent to a 4-fold increase in area.

The intensity of the light is represented by an Arabic numeral (1–4), each successive number being 3.15 times brighter (0.5 log unit steps). It is measured in apostilb (asb).

A lower-case letter indicates additional minor filters, progressing from 'a', the darkest, to 'e' being the brightest. Each progressive letter is an increase of 0.1 log unit.

Caution

Potential sources of error/artefact include miosis, media opacities, uncorrected refractive error, rim of the trial frame, ptosis or dermatochalasis, incomprehension of the test, tremor, or inadequate retinal adaptation.

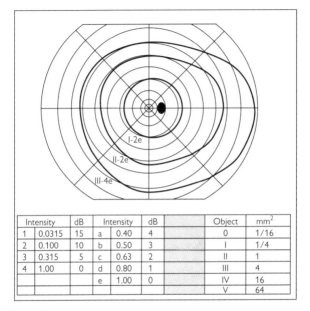

Intensity		dB	Intensity		dB		Object	mm²
1	0.0315	15	a	0.40	4		0	1/16
2	0.100	10	b	0.50	3		I	1/4
3	0.315	5	c	0.63	2		II	1
4	1.00	0	d	0.80	1		III	4
			e	1.00	0		IV	16
							V	64

Fig. 2.2 Normal Goldmann VF of the right eye.

Anterior segment imaging (1)

Keratometry

Basic principles

Keratometry is measurement of the anterior surface curvature of the central cornea (~3mm diameter). It is used to assess the axis and magnitude of astigmatism and is typically expressed as two corneal curvature values, 90° apart (i.e. max and min 'k' values in dioptres and axis readings).

Technology

Traditionally performed manually, using either a Helmholtz (e.g. Bausch & Lomb) or Javal Schiotz keratometer, where the cornea is assumed to be spherical and a skilled operator is required. Automated keratometry devices provide these readings, in addition to other functions, e.g autorefractors that measure refraction, corneal topographers that map the corneal surface, and the IOLMaster that provides intraocular lens (IOL) calculations for cataract surgery (see ➔ Cataract surgery: perioperative, p. 312).

Indications

- CL fitting.
- Ocular biometry.
- Assessment of changes in corneal curvature post-surgery.

Caution

Keratometry provides no information about points central or peripheral to the points measured.

Corneal topography

Basic principles

This is mapping of curvature across the entire corneal surface.

Technology

Traditionally performed using Placido-based systems, analysing multiple concentric rings of light reflected off the anterior corneal surface, and thus indirectly measuring corneal curvature ('video keratoscopy'). Now direct measurements of corneal curvature are possible, using scanning slit technology (Orbscan™, Bausch & Lomb) or Scheimpflug imaging (Pentacam™, Oculus), These systems allow evaluation of the posterior corneal surface, corneal thickness maps, and greater coverage of the peripheral cornea.

Indications

- Assess the corneal curvature (post-operative changes and prior to laser refractive procedures).
- Detection of macro-irregularities such as astigmatism, keratoconus, and pellucid marginal degeneration.
- Assessment of CL fit and monitoring of warpage.
- Measurement of corneal thickness.

Interpretation

Curvature is expressed as radii of curvature in mm or in keratometric dioptres. A colour scale is used, representing the range of values. Curvature maps are constructed by either comparing the data with themselves (relative or normalized scales) or to set ranges (absolute scale). Consequently, different colour maps cannot be directly compared and must be interpreted, based on their actual numerical values. Normal corneas are usually classified as: (1) round, (2) oval, (3) symmetric bow tie, (4) asymmetric bow tie, and (5) irregular. The average adult cornea is steeper in the vertical meridian, compared with the horizontal (i.e. has 'with-the-rule' astigmatism).

Scanning slit videokeratography

Basic principles

In scanning slit videokeratography, a high-resolution video camera is used to capture reflections from multiple slits of light projected through the cornea at 45°. Software then calculates the corneal thickness and posterior corneal surface by direct triangulation. Precise calculation of the anterior corneal surface is provided by the addition of Placido-ring based measurements.

Technology

The Orbscan™ (Bausch & Lomb) provides accurate and repeatable measurements under optimal conditions, in the range of 4 microns for the central cornea and 7 microns for the peripheral cornea. The software calculates elevation, i.e. the points per half slit from both the anterior and posterior surfaces. It then indirectly calculates the corneal thickness.

Caution

Inability to detect interfaces (e.g. post-LASIK flap).

Scheimpflug imaging

Indications

- Corneal topography with high resolution of the entire cornea and ability to measure corneas with severe irregularities.
- Corneal wavefront analysis for measurement of higher-order aberrations.
- Measurement of corneal thickness from limbus to limbus.
- Measurement of AC depth and angle estimation.

Basic principles

Scheimpflug imaging differs from conventional techniques in that the object plane, lens plane, and image plane are not parallel to each other but intersect in a common straight line. This allows generation of optical sections with a wide depth of focus. A three-dimensional mathematical model of the anterior segment is generated from 50 slit images, evaluating 500 measured points from each image, in 2s taken with the non-contact rotating Scheimpflug camera.

Technology

The Pentacam™ (Oculus) is commonly used in clinical practice.

Anterior segment imaging (2)

In vivo **confocal microscopy**

Non-invasive technique that images the cornea and conjunctiva *in vivo*.

Indications
- Diagnosis of infectious keratitis (e.g. fungal elements and *Acanthamoeba* cysts).
- Detection of corneal pathology, including dystrophies, degenerations, deposits, and infections (e.g. fungi elements and *Acanthamoeba*).
- Post-surgical analysis (e.g. refractive surgery, collagen cross-linking, filtering blebs post-trabeculectomy).

Basic principles
In conventional light microscopy, a light source is used to evenly flood-illuminate a tissue of interest. All parts of the tissue in the optical path are thus illuminated. Therefore, light is reflected and scattered from images outside the focal plane, leading to image degradation. In confocal microscopy, pinhole apertures are used to both focus a point source of light on the tissue and to collect light waves reflected specifically from this point (as these apertures are conjugate to the focal plane, the term 'confocal' microscopy is adopted).

An array of apertures is then used to examine many points simultaneously, and this array is scanned rapidly across the field to create a two-dimensional corneal image. The device can then scan down through the cornea, creating a series of *en face* optical sections, allowing visualization of corneal microstructure at various depths.

Technology
In the HRT Rostock Cornea Module™ (Heidelberg), a laser scanning (670nm) confocal microscope is used to obtain high-quality, high-resolution images of the cornea (lateral resolution and depth of field reported as 1 micron and 4 microns, respectively).

Anterior segment optical coherence tomography (OCT)

Indications
- Direct visualization of the AC angle for assessment of patient with glaucoma, especially angle-closure glaucoma and plateau iris configuration.
- Measurement of relative corneal epithelial thickness and depth of anterior stromal scars.
- Post-operative assessment of lamellar corneal graft positioning and thickness.
- Assessment of post-LASIK flap thickness.
- Measurement of AC depth prior to insertion of phakic IOLs.
- Imaging of glaucoma filtering blebs.

Basic principles

OCT uses interferometry to provide cross-sectional images of the cornea and anterior segment (see ➍ Optical coherence tomography, p. 72). Anterior segment OCT is similar to posterior segment OCT, although longer wavelengths light sources are commonly used, typically 1,310nm vs 800nm.

Technology

- Time domain OCT devices are commonly used, e.g. Visante™ (Zeiss).
- Spectral domain OCT devices with anterior segment modules (e.g. RTVue™, Optovue™, and Spectralis™) provide greatly increased image acquisition speed for greater coverage of the corneal surface and improved resolution.
- Slit-lamp adapted OCT devices include the SL SCAN-1™ (Topcon) and SL-OCT™ (Heidelberg).

Posterior segment imaging

Colour fundus photography

Indications

- Screening for posterior segment disease (e.g. diabetic retinopathy screening).
- Diagnosis and monitoring of posterior segment disease.
- Assessment of anatomic end-points in clinical trials (e.g. Early Treatment Diabetic Retinopathy Study (ETDRS)).
- Evaluation of disease risk factors in epidemiological studies (e.g. Beaver Dam Eye Study).

Basic principles

Specially modified cameras may be used to acquire photographs of the ocular fundus. In such devices, a bright ring of white light is used to illuminate the ocular fundus—the light reflected is then captured on the pixel array of a charge-coupled device (CCD) and a digital image generated. Commercial fundus cameras have undergone substantial refinement since their introduction, including optimization for non-mydriatic and stereoscopic image acquisition and transition from analogue to digital image capture.

Technology

Commonly used fundus cameras include the Topcon TRC-50DX™ (Topcon) and the Zeiss FF450plus™ (Zeiss). At present, retinal cameras are typically described by their optical field of view, with an angle of 30° or 35° most commonly used.

Ultra-widefield imaging

Conventional fundus imaging (30° or 35° field of view) allows optimal visualization of the posterior pole; however, the peripheral retina is not captured. Recent advances in optics have greatly extended the field of view in so-called 'ultra-widefield' imaging.

Technology

The Optos 200 Tx system (Optos) is non-contact and uses scanning laser ophthalmoscopy (SLO) (see ➔ SLO, p. 68), in combination with a large ellipsoid mirror, to obtain fundal images with a 200° field of view through an undilated pupil. ~80% of the total retinal surface area is visualized. The use of appropriate light filters allows ultra-widefield autofluorescence and angiographic imaging.

Indications

- Assessment of peripheral non-perfusion in retinal vascular diseases (e.g., diabetic retinopathy).
- Assessment of patients with uveitis demonstrating scattering inflammatory foci.
- Assessment of patients with posterior segment pathology (e.g. vitreous detachment, retinal tears, and retinal detachments).

Fundus autofluorescence (FAF)

Many structures in the posterior segment of the eye possess innate fluorescent properties—'FAF'; when stimulated by light of a specific wavelength, they emit light of a longer wavelength, even in the absence of any fluorescent contrast agent.

Indications

- Diagnosis and monitoring of geographic atrophy progression in patients with age-related macular degeneration (AMD).
- Assessment of patients with inherited retinal degenerative disease.
- Screening and assessment of patients with toxic retinopathies.

Basic principles

Incorporating appropriate light filters, FAF images can be obtained with either fundus cameras or SLO devices. FAF properties are dependent on the wavelengths of light used:

- Blue or green light highlights lipofuscin, a by-product of photoreceptor outer segment degradation that accumulates in retinal pigment epithelium (RPE) cells.
- Near-infrared light highlights melanin.

Technology

- FAF imaging with a fundus camera and longer wavelength filters are used to reduce the effects of lens autofluorescence (Spaide Autofluorescence Filters, Topcon; excitation: 535–580nm).
- The SLO device most commonly used for FAF imaging is the HRA-2, 'Bluepeak' autofluorescence system (Heidelberg Engineering), with an excitation wavelength of 488nm.

Monochromatic imaging

Indications

- Near-infrared reflectance imaging for assessment of drusen subtypes in patients with AMD.
- Blue light reflectance imaging for assessment of RNFL defects in glaucoma, epiretinal membranes (ERM), capillary non-perfusion in retinal vascular disease, and abnormally increased reflectance in macular telangiectasia.
- Red-free imaging for assessment of preretinal, intraretinal, and subretinal haemorrhage.

Basic principles

Uses monochromatic light filters. Longer wavelengths of light (near infrared) penetrate more deeply for visualization of subretinal and choroidal structures. Shorter wavelengths (blue light) allow imaging of superficial retinal structures.

Technology

SLO devices (see ➲ SLO, p. 68) typically employ laser light sources at fixed wavelengths which allow monochromatic acquisition.

Fundus fluorescein angiography (FFA)

In FFA, a rapid series of fundus images are acquired following IV injection of a fluorescent contrast agent sodium fluorescein ($C_{20}H_{10}O_5Na_2$). This organic, water-soluble dye aids visualization of the choroidal and retinal vasculature. Fluorescein is stimulated by blue light (490nm) and emits green light (530nm). Therefore, FFA images are acquired, using fundus cameras or SLO devices incorporating spectrally appropriate blue excitation and yellow–green barrier filters. Sodium fluorescein (weight 376Da) is 70–85% bound to plasma albumin, metabolized by the liver, and excreted by the kidneys in 24h. Good visualization requires clear media and dilated pupils.

Indications

- Diagnosis of chorioretinal vascular disease (e.g. diabetic retinopathy, neovascular AMD).
- Diagnosis of macular disease (e.g. central serous chorioretinopathy).
- Assessment of intermediate and posterior uveitis.
- Planning of retinal laser procedures.

Relative contraindications

- A previous history of severe reactions to fluorescein.
- Pregnancy.
- Lower doses of fluorescein are advisable for patients with renal impairment.

Side effects

- Transient skin and urine discoloration.
- Extravasation of dye at injection site with local irritation/thrombophlebitis.
- Nausea and vomiting.
- Pruritis.
- Vasovagal syncope (1 in 340).
- Severe anaphylaxis (1 in 1,900).
- Fatal anaphylaxis (1 in 220,000).

Method

- *Prepare patient*: explain procedure, risks, and benefits, and take formal consent; dilate; check BP; cannulate (medium-/large-bore vein); ensure resuscitation facilities (including 'crash' trolley) are readily available.
- Seat patient at camera, and adjust height for patient comfort and camera alignment. Ask patient to fix on the fixation target.
- Take colour and 'red-free' fundal photographs.
- Inject fluorescein (5mL 10% IV), and take early rapid sequence photographs (at about 1s intervals for 25–30s). Continue less frequent shots, alternating between eyes for up to 5–10min. Late images may be taken at 10–20min.
- *The early shots are critical*: it is generally only possible to get a good series of early shots from one eye due to the time it takes to move between eyes. It is therefore important that the photographer is informed which eye takes priority.

Interpretation (See Box 2.1)

Box 2.1 Reporting an FFA

1. Report the red-free photo.
2. Specify the phase.
3. Note hyper- and hypofluorescence and any delay in filling (see Table 2.5).
4. Note distinctive features (petalloid, smoke stack, etc.).
5. Note any change in area, intensity, or the fluorescence over time.

FFAs should be read sequentially, according to their phases: choroidal (pre-arterial), arterial, capillary, venous, and late. This test should be reported in conjunction with patient history and examination (see Table 2.5).

Table 2.5 Morphological analysis of FFA features

Feature	Common causes
Hyperfluorescence	
Window defect	RPE defect (e.g. RPE atrophy, macular hole)
Leakage of dye	*At macula*: cystoid macular oedema (CMO) (petalloid appearance), other macular oedema
	At disc: papilloedema, ischaemic optic neuropathy, inflammation
	Elsewhere: new retinal vessels, vasculitis, choroidal neovascularization (CNV)
Pooling of dye	Detachment of the neural retina or RPE (e.g. central serous retinopathy (CSR), AMD)
Staining of dye	Drusen, disc, disciform scars sclera (seen if overlying chorioretinal atrophy/thinning)
Abnormal vessels	Tumours (haemangiomas, melanomas, etc.)
Autofluorescence (visible without dye)	Disc drusen, large lipofuscin deposits
Hypofluorescence	
Transmission defect	*Preretinal* (blocks view of retinal and choroidal circulations): media opacity, especially vitreous opacities (inflammation, haemorrhage, degenerative), preretinal haemorrhage
	Inner retinal (blocks view of capillary circulation, but larger retinal vessels seen): dot and blot haemorrhages (e.g. vein occlusion), intraretinal lipid (e.g. diabetic retinopathy)
	Prechoroidal (blocks view of choroidal circulation, but retinal circulation seen): subretinal haemorrhage, pigment (e.g. choroidal naevi, congenital hypertrophy of the retinal pigment epithelium (CHRPE), melanoma, lipid, lipofuscin
Filling defects (circulation abnormalities)	Retinal arteriolar non-perfusion (e.g. arterial occlusion)
	Retinal capillary non-perfusion (e.g. ischaemia 2° to diabetes, vein occlusion)
	Choroidal non-perfusion (e.g. infarcts 2° to accelerated hypertension, etc.)
	Disc non-perfusion (e.g. ischaemic optic neuropathy)

Indocyanine green (ICG) angiography and other vascular assessments

ICG angiography

ICG angiography is usually performed in association with FFA (see ➲ Fundus fluorescein angiography (FFA), p. 64) and used to study the choroidal circulation. ICG is 98% bound to serum proteins that do not pass through choriocapillaris vessel fenestrations; the larger choroidal vessels are not obscured by early leakage of dye from this layer. With an excitation peak at 810nm and emission of 830nm, the dye is excited by infrared radiation. The use of this long wavelength light enhances depth penetration, especially in cases of retinal haemorrhage.

Indications

- Diagnosis of CNV not clearly visualized on FFA (e.g. extensive submacular haemorrhage or serous RPE detachments).
- Identification of idiopathic polypoidal choroidal vasculopathy (IPCV), particularly in patients with neovascular AMD appearing 'refractory' to conventional treatment.
- Assessment of choroidal tumours and ocular inflammatory disease.

Method

- ICG powder is mixed with aqueous solvent to make a solution of 40mg in 2mL. A red-free photo is taken, and the bolus IV injection is given. Frequent images are taken over the first 3min and then later images at, e.g. 5, 10, 15, 20, and 30min.

Contraindications

- Pregnancy.
- Iodine allergy (ICG contains 5% iodine).

Side effects

- Nausea and vomiting.
- Sneezing and pruritus.
- Backache.
- Staining of stool.
- Vasovagal syncope.
- Severe anaphylaxis (1 in 1,900).

Interpretation

- *Early phase (2–60s)*: prominent filling of choroidal arteries, which appear tortuous.
- *Early mid-phase (1–3min)*: increased prominence of choroidal veins, which appear straight and drain towards the vortex vein in each quadrant.
- *Late mid-phase (3–15min)*: diffuse hyperfluorescence due to diffusion of dye from the choriocapillaris).
- *Late phase (15–30min)*: dye may remain in neovascular tissue after it has left the choroidal and retinal circulations.

See Table 2.6.

Table 2.6 Morphological analysis of ICG features

Feature	Common causes
Hyperfluorescence	
Window defect	RPE defect
Leakage of dye	CNV
	IPCV: polyps and branching vascular network
Abnormal blood vessels	Choroidal haemangioma
Hypofluorescence	
Transmission defect	RPE detachment (hypofluorescent centrally); blood, pigment and exudate cause less blockage than in FFA
Filling defects (circulation abnormalities)	Choroidal infarcts 2° to accelerated hypertension, SLE, etc.
	Choroidal atrophy (e.g. atrophic AMD, some chorioretinal scars, choroideraemia)

Quantification of retinal and choroidal blood flow

Measurement of retinal and choroidal blood flow is also possible, using quantitative angiography, based on dye dilution techniques where the concentration of fluorescein at a particular point is graphed over time.

Measurement of the Doppler effect can also be used for calculation of ocular blood flow velocities. If the diameter of the blood vessel is known, then absolute values for blood flow volume may also be determined. Laser Doppler devices have been developed for this purpose (e.g. the Canon Laser Blood Flowmeter and the Heidelberg Retina Flowmeter).

Retinal oximetry

In spectral imaging, measurement of light reflected from the retina at multiple wavelengths is used to assess retinal oxygen saturation. A multispectral imaging device (Oxymap T1, Iceland) is available for research purposes, and hyperspectral devices are in development; however, detailed validation and reproducibility assessments are required prior to future routine clinical usage.

Imaging the retinal nerve fibre layer

SLO

Indications
- Similar indications as for colour fundus photography, but enhanced capabilities for evaluation of patients with medical retina pathology.

Basic principles

SLO devices employ a confocal ('pinhole') aperture, generating a single point of laser light at a specific wavelength that is scanned across the retina in a raster pattern (i.e. series of parallel horizontal lines). As only a small area of the fundus is illuminated at any time, the effects of light scatter are reduced and higher contrast images are generated.

Technology

The Heidelberg Retina Angiograph-2™ (HRA-2) (Heidelberg Engineering) and the Nidek F-10™ (Nidek) are in common use.

Caution

Fundus cameras typically have higher temporal and spatial resolution.

Scanning laser tomography

Indications
- To distinguish normal optic disc anatomy from glaucomatous optic neuropathy.
- To monitor longitudinal or progressive change of glaucomatous optic neuropathy.

Basic principles

The confocal aperture used in SLO devices allows acquisition of images at different focal planes within a tissue of interest (i.e. generation of a 'stack' of *en face* images). Three-dimensional reconstruction of the images then allows tomographic (cross-sectional) visualization of the fundus.

Technology

The Heidelberg Retina Tomograph-3 (HRT-3) (Heidelberg Engineering) is an SLO that allows for three-dimensional reconstruction of the optic nerve head.

Interpretation

After acquisition, the stack of confocal images is aligned and their reflectivities summed, generating a false-colour topographic image. Software then calculates detailed measurements of optic nerve head morphology (e.g. disc and cup area). These stereometric parameters are compared with a normative database and risk of glaucoma assessed using a regression model (Moorfields Regression Analysis). The topographic image is then divided into six sectors; a green tick indicates within normal limits, a yellow exclamation mark borderline, and a red cross outside normal limits.

Caution

This technology is lower resolution than OCT. Media opacities and the ability of patient to fixate can all affect the quality and variability of the results. Measurements are also influenced by acute changes in intraocular pressure (IOP) and possibly the cardiac cycle.

Scanning laser polarimetry

Indications

- To distinguish normal optic disc anatomy from glaucomatous optic neuropathy.
- To monitor progression of glaucomatous optic neuropathy.

Basic principles

Due to the parallel arrangement of its axons, the RNFL is birefringent (a ray of light entering a birefringent substance is broken into two rays). Polarized light reflected from the RNFL undergoes a phase shift, dependent on the amount of birefringent material present. Scanning of polarized light across a region centred on the optic nerve head can therefore be used to assess phase shifts in this region and estimate RNFL thickness.

Technology

The GDx (Zeiss) is the only commercially available scanning laser polarimeter. Newer models compensate for corneal birefringence to improve the accuracy of results (variable and enhanced corneal compensation (VCC and ECC, respectively)).

Interpretation

Nerve fibre thickness maps are presented in a colour-coded spectrum from blue to red. Deviation maps are used to show the magnitude and location of RNFL defects using colour-coded squares. TSNIT graphs compare the RNFL thickness to a normative database.

The nerve fibre indicator (NFI) is a global value, based on the entire thickness map, used for discriminating normal vs glaucomatous eyes: normal 1–30, borderline 31–50, and abnormal 51–100.

The advanced serial analysis provides trend analysis over time from baseline.

Caution

Measurements may be erroneous in areas of peripapillary atrophy (PPA) or chorioretinal scarring.

NB Mild to moderate cataracts do not degrade the result.

Adaptive optics

Indications
- Evaluation of photoreceptor loss in inherited retinal degenerations.
- Assessment of geographic atrophy and drusen progression in patients with AMD.
- Assessment of anatomical outcomes in clinical trials of photoreceptor and RPE stem cell therapies.

Basic principles
The transverse optical resolution of fundus cameras (see ➲ Fundus fluorescein angiography, p. 64) and SLO devices (see ➲ SLO, p. 68) is limited by the presence of defects or aberrations in the optical system of the eye (i.e. the cornea and lens). Real-time measurement of these aberrations is possible using a Hartman Shack wavefront sensor. Once measured, highly deformable mirrors (mirrors with large numbers of small, electronically controlled actuators on their rear surface that can push and pull them to adopt any desired configuration) can be used to compensate for these aberrations. By incorporating wavefront sensing and correction into existing optical imaging platforms—'adaptive optics'—it is possible to acquire images of the retina with cellular level resolution in a non-invasive fashion.

Cone photoreceptors are the dominant feature seen with adaptive optics systems. Rods are smaller and less easily seen (the smallest cones at the foveal centre are also often difficult to visualize).

Technology
Adaptive optics has been incorporated into both fundus cameras and SLO systems. Adaptive optics 'flood-illuminated' fundus cameras are commercially available and approved for use in clinical settings (e.g. 'rtx1 Adaptive Optics Retinal Camera', Imagine Eyes).

Caution
Adaptive optic devices offer greatly improved transverse resolution; however, their field of view is still limited (e.g. 4° × 4°).

Optical coherence tomography

OCT provides high-resolution images of the neurosensory retina in a non-invasive manner. OCT is analogous to ultrasonography but measures light waves, rather than sound waves.

Basic principles

OCT measurements are achieved indirectly using interferometry. In this technique, the combination of light reflected from a tissue of interest and light reflected from a reference path produces characteristic interference patterns, dependent on the mismatch between the reflected waves. Since the time delay and amplitude of one of the waves (i.e. the reference path) are known, the time delay and intensity of light returning from the sample tissue may be determined. The resulting plot of light intensity vs time delay is known as an A-scan and describes the anatomy of the eye tissue at a specific point. A-scans are then repeated at multiple transverse locations and mapped to a grey or false-colour scale, giving rise to two-dimensional cross-sectional (tomographic) images (termed B-scans).

Indications

- Monitoring of response to treatment and/or disease activity in patients with chorioretinal vascular and inflammatory diseases (e.g. neovascular AMD, diabetic retinopathy, RVO, CMO).
- Diagnosis of clinically occult macular pathology (e.g. subtle abnormalities of the vitreoretinal interface).
- Detection of glaucomatous damage to the RNFL and/or optic nerve head.
- Assessment and longitudinal monitoring of disc volume in disc swelling and papilloedema.

Examples of the use of OCT in common macular conditions are provided in Figs. 2.4–2.10.

Interpretation

On OCT false-colour B-scans, highly reflective tissue is reddish white in colour, while hyporeflective tissue is blue–black in colour. Alternatively, images can be shown in 256 shades of grey, corresponding to different optical reflectivities (see Fig. 2.3). The inner and outer nuclear layers and ganglion cell layer are typically hyporeflective, while the inner and outer plexiform layers and nerve fibre layer are hyperreflective. Larger retinal vessels are seen on OCT as circular hyperreflective foci located in the inner retina, with underlying 'shadowing'. A number of hyperreflective bands may be seen in the outer retina, typically consisting of the external limiting membrane, photoreceptor inner segment-outer segment (IS-OS) junction (or ellipsoid zone), and RPE. Using specialized scanning protocols ('enhanced depth imaging'), the choroid and choroidal–scleral junction may also be seen.

Technology

Time domain OCT using the Stratus OCT (Carl Zeiss Meditec) acquires images at 400 axial scans/s, with an axial resolution of 10 microns.

Spectral (or Fourier) domain OCT using the Spectralis HRA/OCT (Heidelberg Engineering) or Cirrus HD-OCT (Carl Zeiss Meditec) scan at a rate of at least 20,000 axial scans/s, with an axial resolution typically between 3 and 8 microns.

Quantitative image analysis

Each OCT device incorporates image analysis software that provides measurement of retinal thickness via automated detection ('segmentation') of the inner and outer retinal boundaries. Using these techniques, it is possible to measure retinal thickness at multiple locations and to construct retinal thickness maps corresponding to the ETDRS subfields.

Newer OCT systems also allow for automated quantitative assessment of drusen and geographic atrophy in patients with AMD.

In patients with glaucoma, specialized circular OCT scanning protocols are employed—a single circular B-scan, centred on the optic disc and 3.4mm in diameter, is obtained. Segmentation of the inner and outer boundaries of the RNFL then allows assessment of peripapillary RNFL thickness. The presence of glaucomatous RNFL thinning can then be determined by comparison with normative databases.

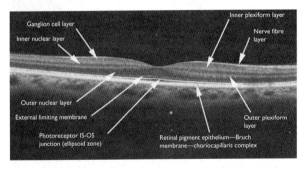

Fig. 2.3 Imaging of the healthy neurosensory retina produced using spectral domain OCT.

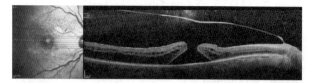

Fig. 2.4 SD-OCT of full-thickness macular hole (stage 3).

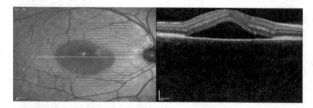

Fig. 2.5 SD-OCT of central serous chorioretinopathy.

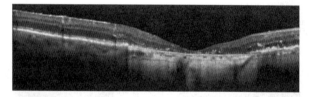

Fig. 2.6 SD-OCT of geographic atrophy.

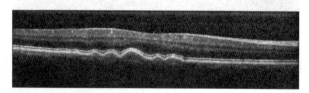

Fig. 2.7 SD-OCT of soft drusen.

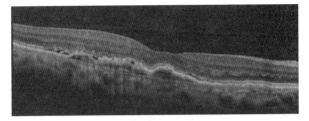

Fig. 2.8 SD-OCT of fibrovascular pigment epithelial detachment (PED).

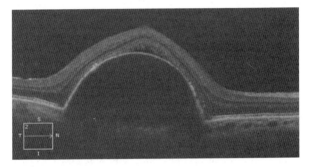

Fig. 2.9 SD-OCT of serous PED.

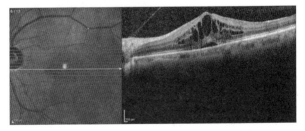

Fig. 2.10 SD-OCT of CMO.

Ophthalmic ultrasonography (1)

Diagnostic ultrasonography

Basic pinciples

'Ultrasound' (US) describes sound waves with frequency above the upper limit audible to humans (i.e. >20kHz). In medical ultrasonography, these high-frequency sound waves (ocular 8–10MHz; orbital 4–5MHz; anterior segment 50–100MHz) are focused on a tissue of interest and the 'echoes' of reflected sound waves measured.

Ultrasonic probes contain a piezoelectric crystal for both sound wave generation and echo measurement. A piezoelectric material is one that expands or contracts at high frequency when an electrical voltage is applied across it and that produces an electrical current when sound waves are applied across it. Once captured, the reflected signal is amplified; the 'gain' control can be used to adjust this amplification. The resulting plot of amplitude vs time delay is known as an A-scan and describes tissue structure at a specific point. By multiplying the time delay from any reflective interface by the speed of sound in the tissue, A-scans can be used to obtain accurate measurements of ocular structures (corrections are required for different media, such as silicone oil, within the eye due to their effects on the speed of sound). A-scans can be repeated at multiple transverse locations and mapped to a grey scale, producing two-dimensional cross-sectional images termed B-scans. Examples are shown in Figs. 2.11–16.

Ocular US

Basic principles

Ocular ultrasonography can be performed with medical ultrasonography devices that accept 8–10MHz transducers, or with dedicated ophthalmic devices. The axial resolution is typically 150 microns, while the transverse resolution is typically 450 microns.

Indications (A-scan)

- Measurement of axial length (biometry).
- Measurement of AC depth or other intraocular distances.
- Measurement of intraocular mass thickness and characterization of acoustic properties.

Indications (B-scan)

- Identification of posterior segment pathology in the presence of media opacity preventing fundal view, e.g. identifying retinal break/detachment obscured by vitreous haemorrhage.
- Characterization of intraocular masses.
- Location of intraocular FBs.
- Detection of calcification in retinoblastomas and optic disc drusen.

Method

- Topical anaesthetic drops are applied.
- Coupling agent (e.g. methylcellulose) is applied to the tip of the probe or to the closed eyelids.
- The patient is reclined or placed in a supine position.

- A marker on the US probe is used for orientation. When the marker is lined horizontally with the lids, the image displayed is in a horizontal plane. Vertical placement (marker pointing to eyebrows) generates an image in the vertical plane.
- Scans are captured with the patient's eye in 1° position and then sequentially in all four quadrants, horizontally, and vertically. **NB** If the probe is moved temporally from the 1° position, the scan shows the nasal retina. If the patient moves their left eye nasally, while probe is moved temporally, the nasal retina anterior to the equator can be scanned.
- Scanning during eye movements can help differentiate between PVDs and retinal detachments (dynamic scanning).

Caution (A-scan)

This is a one-dimensional time–amplitude display. Corrections need to be made for different mediums, such as silicone oil, in the eye, as the speed of sound varies in different media (slower in oil, compared with vitreous media). Artefactually, low axial lengths may occur in conditions, such as ateroid hyalosis, and with inappropriate application.

Orbital US

Basic principles

A lower frequency ultrasonic transducer is used (3–5MHz), allowing enhanced depth penetration.

Indications

- Assessment of orbital tumours.
- Assessment of orbital disease (thyroid eye disease (TED), measurement of muscles).

Corneal ultrasonic pachymetry

Basic principles

Simple measurements of corneal thickness can be obtained using a 20MHz ultrasonic probe. Average central corneal thickness (CCT) is 490–560 microns.

Indications

- Prior to laser refractive surgery (e.g. LASIK), to assess risk of postoperative ectasia.
- In patients with suspected glaucoma, to estimate accuracy of applanation tonometry (in thick corneas, IOP may be overestimated, while, in thin corneas, IOP may be underestimated).

Method

- Topical anaesthetic is applied.
- No coupling agent is required.
- The ultrasonic probe is held in direct contact with, and at 90° to, the corneal surface.

NB Inaccurate positioning of the probe may result in erroneous results.

Ophthalmic ultrasonography (2)

Ultrasound biomicroscopy (UBM)

Basic principles

Use of a higher frequency transducer (35–50MHz) allows generation of images with much higher resolution (typically 30 microns axial and 60 microns transverse resolution), but with less depth penetration. UBM is suitable for imaging of anterior segment structures (see Fig. 2.17 and Fig. 2.18).

Indications

- Corneal biometry.
- Glaucoma (e.g. pupil block, plateau iris, malignant glaucoma, pigment dispersion).
- Evaluation of unexplained hypotony (e.g. due to cyclitic membranes and cyclodialysis clefts).
- Anterior segment tumours (e.g. 1° and 2° cysts, iris and ciliary body melanomas).
- Assessment of crystalline lens and/or implant position, including phakic and piggyback implants.
- Assessment of the anterior segment in cases of corneal opacification (e.g. Peter's anomaly and sclerocornea).

Method

- Topical anaesthetic is applied.
- Eyelids open with an immersion bath (water or methylcellulose) used as coupling agent.
- High-frequency scans are taken, radial and parallel to the limbus, at various predetermined positions.

Colour Doppler imaging (CDI)

Basic principles

CDI is a duplex US technique that combines conventional B-scan grey scale imaging, with Doppler-based assessment of blood flow. Blood flow is detected, using the frequency shift of sound waves reflected from moving blood columns. Colour is then added to represent the motion of blood through the vessels. Colour varies in proportion to flow velocity and is colour-coded, according to its direction to or from the probe.

Using the resulting image, the operator can identify a vessel of interest and place the sampling window for pulsed Doppler measurements.

Indications

- Assessment of blood flow in central retinal artery, posterior ciliary arteries, ophthalmic artery, and central retinal vein.
- 1° evaluation and follow-up of orbital vascular lesions (e.g. varices, arteriovenous malformations (AVMs), and carotid–cavernous sinus fistulas).
- Semi-quantitative assessment of perfusion in retinal and choroidal vascular disease (e.g. ocular ischaemic syndrome (OIS)).

Interpretation
- CDI describes blood flow in terms of parameters, including: (1) peak systolic velocity, (2) end-diastolic velocity, and (3) resistance index. It does not provide absolute measurements of blood flow (no quantitative information on vessel diameter is obtained).
- With a 7.5MHz probe, CDI is able to resolve structures 0.2mm (200 microns) or larger but can also be used to measure Doppler shifts in smaller vessels such as the posterior ciliary arteries (diameter of ~40 microns).

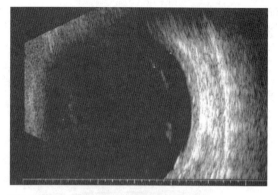

Fig. 2.11 US (B-scan) of PVD.
Note: posterior hyaloid face is only faintly reflective and appears incomplete on a static image.

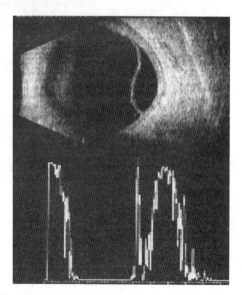

Fig. 2.12 US (B-scan + A-scan) of retinal detachment.
Note: retina appears as a highly reflective convex membrane which is complete but irregular.

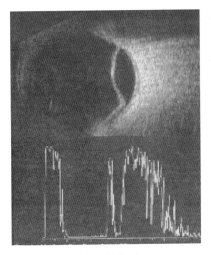

Fig. 2.13 US (B-scan + A-scan) of choroidal detachment.
Note: retina/choroid appears as a highly reflective regular dome-shaped membrane.

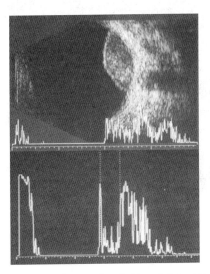

Fig. 2.14 US (B-scan, vector A-scan, and standard A-scan) of choroidal melanoma.
Note: dome-shaped membrane with low internal reflectivity on standard A-scan.

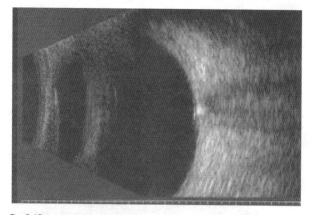

Fig. 2.15 US (B-scan) of buried drusen.
Note: highly reflective bodies overlying the optic nerve.

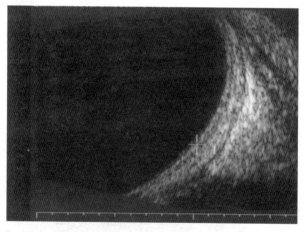

Fig. 2.16 US (B-scan) of posterior scleritis.
Note: well-defined thickened sclera and fluid in Tenon's space.

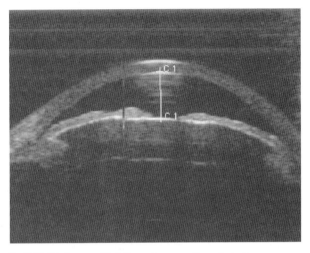

Fig. 2.17 High-frequency US of the anterior segment in a patient with phakomorphic glaucoma.

Note: anteriorly displaced iris with 2° narrowing of the angles.

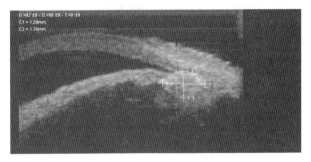

Fig. 2.18 High-frequency US of the anterior segment in a patient with ciliary body melanoma.

Electrodiagnostic tests (1)

EDTs are aimed at providing an objective evaluation of visual pathway function. They are useful for diagnostic and prognostic purposes and are increasingly important in correlating genotypes with specific phenotypes and in the context of new treatment modalities (e.g. gene therapy).

The basic tests used in the electrophysiology lab are the full-field electro-retinogram (ERG), the pattern ERG (PERG), the multifocal ERG (mFERG), the electro-oculogram (EOG), the VEP, and dark adaptation (DA). The results of each test are interpreted by the polarity and amplitude of the electrophysical deflections and their latency (implicit time). Other useful technologies are available, such as long duration stimulus ERG (on/off ERG), S-cone ERG, focal ERG, and multifocal VEP (mfVEP).

All tests should be performed to the International Society for Clinical Electrophysiology of Vision (ISCEV) standards, if possible, so that comparable tests can be recorded throughout the world, as the responses and normal values can still differ between centres due to variation in equipment and technique.

Full-field ERG

The ERG records the mass electrical activity from the retina when stimulated by a flash of light.

Indications

- Clinical presentation does not correlate with severity of visual symptoms.
- A specific diagnosis has to be confirmed or excluded [e.g. RP, Leber's congenital amaurosis (LCA), choroideraemia, gyrate atrophy, achromatopsia, congenital stationary night blindness (CSNB), cone dystrophies].
- Prognostic information is required for the management of the patient.
- Assessment of retinal function in specific cases such as investigating family members for known hereditary retinal dystrophies, carrier states of retinal dystrophies, evaluation of suspected functional visual loss, evaluation of retinal function in the context of opaque media, and evaluation of retinal function in uncooperative cases (e.g. paediatric cases and patients with learning difficulties).

Method

A full-field (ganzfeld) stimulation should be used and the retinal response recorded, when possible, using electrodes that contact the cornea or nearby bulbar conjunctiva (CL electrodes, conductive fibres and foils, conjunctival loop electrodes, and corneal wicks).

The rod-response ERG is recorded in dark-adapted eyes (after 30min in the dark) with a dim white flash which is below cone sensitivity and comprises only a b-wave. The maximal ERG is obtained in dark-adapted eyes using a bright white flash and is a mixed rod and cone response. Photopic responses are acquired with a background that suppresses rod activity; the photopic single-flash cone response is obtained in light-adapted eyes (after 10min in the light); the cone-derived flicker response is acquired using a 30Hz white light flicker stimulus (rods are unable to respond due to poor temporal resolution).

Results

A bright single-flash stimulus is followed by an initial negative 'a wave' and then a positive 'b wave', with superimposed oscillatory potentials (OPs); this usually takes <250ms. Amplitude (microvolts) and implicit time (ms) of these waves are the two major parameters that are used to interpret the ERG response.

- a-wave arises primarily from the photoreceptors.
- b-wave arises primarily from the bipolar and Müller cells.
- OPs arise primarily from amacrine cells.

By varying the parameters of the stimulus (intensity and frequency) and the adaptive state of the eye, different parts of the retina can be selectively stimulated, and the ISCEV recordings allow localization of abnormal function.

- *Example*: ERG can be useful in CRVO distinguishing between non-ischaemic and ischaemic CRVO. The b-wave is affected by large areas of ischaemia. This produces a reduced b-wave amplitude, reduced b:a wave ratio, and/or a prolonged b-wave implicit time.

Interpretation

All EDTs must be interpreted in the context of clinical presentation (history, clinical examination, and progression over time). It is rare the tests are pathognomonic for a specific pathological entity (see Table 2.7).

Table 2.7 Interpreting ERG results

Reduced a- and b-waves	Rod–cone dystrophies (including RP)
	Total retinal detachment
	Metallosis
	Drug toxicity (e.g. phenothiazines)
	Autoimmune retinopathy
	Cancer-associated retinopathy (CAR)
	Ophthalmic artery occlusion
Normal a-wave, reduced scotopic b-wave	CSNB
	X-linked retinoschisis (XLRS)
	CRAO or CRVO
	Myotonic dystrophy
	Oguchi's disease
	Quinine toxicity
	Melanoma Associated Retinopathy (MAR)
Abnormal phototopic and normal scotopic ERGs	Achromatopsia
	Cone dystrophy
Reduced OPs	In diabetic patients, can correlate with an increased risk of developing severe proliferative diabetic retinopathy (PDR)
	Drug toxicity (e.g. vigabatrin)

Electrodiagnostic tests (2)

PERG

Indication
- Objective assessment of macular function.

Method A reversing chequerboard evokes small potentials that arise from the inner retina.

Results A normal PERG, evoked according to ISCEV standards, comprises a prominent positive component at around 50ms (P50) and a larger negative component at ~95ms (N95).

Interpretation
P50 is photoreceptor-driven and is key to assessing macular cone function; N95 originates from the macular ganglion cells.

Amplitudes, peak times, and N95/P50 ratio (typically >1.1) are evaluated in interpreting the PERG.

mfERG

Unlike standard ERG, which sums the electrical potentials from the whole retina, the mfERG creates a topographical functional map of the stimulated retina.

Indication
- Can be used in almost any retinal disorder; especially useful where retinal dysfunction is localized or patchy (e.g. early hydroxychloroquine toxicity).

Method Multiple small areas of the retina are stimulated with appropriately scaled stimuli. Fourier transformation of the responses results in topographical localization of retinal function as it varies across the stimulated retina.

Results A two-dimensional map demonstrates the topographical variation in ERG responses across the retina.

Interpretation
The multifocal ERG can be transformed into a three-dimensional map of retinal function that resembles the hill of vision. A further transformation showing the differences between the recorded mfERG and a reference mfERG (from normal subjects) can be used to highlight areas of loss of function.

EOG

The EOG reflects activity of the RPE and photoreceptors of the entire retina; it measures the standing potential at the RPE–photoreceptor interface, which typically varies according to whether the eye is dark-adapted (low potential) or light-adapted (high potential).

Indications
- Diagnosis of certain macular dystrophies (e.g. Best's disease).
- Early detection/screening of individuals at risk (e.g. Best's disease)
- Aid diagnosis of certain inherited or acquired retinopathies/maculopathies [e.g. CSR, acute zonal occult outer retinopathy (AZOOR), drug toxicity].

Method Electrodes are placed at the medial and lateral canthi, and patients intermittently follow targets that move from right to left over a 30° horizontal plane. The cornea makes the nearest electrode more positive, compared to the other, and the difference between the two electrodes is measured. It is performed in dark- and light-adapted states.

Results Results are expressed, based on Arden index (light peak / dark trough × 100), and inform regarding RPE function.

Interpretation
Normally, the potential doubles from the dark-adapted to the light-adapted eye; >180% is considered to be normal, subnormal if 140–180%, abnormal if <140%.

VEP

The VEP is a gross electrical response recorded from the visual cortex in response to a changing visual stimulus such as multiple flash or pattern stimuli. It requires relatively normal retinal/macular function to be a reliable test of visual pathway function.

   The pattern reversal VEP (PR-VEP) gives the most clinical information; a flash VEP is useful in poorly cooperative patients.

Indications
- Optic nerve disease, particularly subclinical demyelination.
- Chiasmal and retrochiasmal dysfunction.
- Suspicion of non-organic visual loss.

Method
The PR-VEP measures activity over the visual cortex, following a reversing high-contrast black and white chequerboard. The nature of the stimulus and the size of the VF stimulated (central 15°) imply the PR-VEP predominantly reflects macular cone activity. The occipital cortex voltage changes over time are plotted as waveforms.

Results
A positive deflection occurs at about 100ms (P100). Negative deflections occur at ~75ms (N75) and 135ms (N135).

Interpretation
Decreased amplitude and increased peak-time of P100 typically occur in optic neuropathies/optic neuritis; however, they also occur in maculopathies; therefore, a delayed/reduced PR-VEP should not be considered pathognomonic of optic nerve disease and must be interpreted in conjunction with retinal function tests (PERG, ERG).

Electrodiagnostic tests (3)

Dark adaptometry (DA)

DA measures the absolute threshold of photoreceptor activity with time in the dark-adapted eye. It is used in conjunction with the EOG and ERG (see Fig. 2.19 and Fig. 2.20).

Goldmann–Weekers adaptometry

Indications
- Retinal disorders causing night blindness (e.g. vitamin A deficiency).
- Cone dysfunction.
- Evaluation of drugs affecting dark adaptation (vitamin A analogues such as isotretinoin).

Method
Photoreceptors are totally bleached by a bright background light, which is then extinguished. In the dark, subjects are then presented with a series of dim flashes of increasing intensity; the threshold at which the light is perceived is then plotted against time.

Results
A biphasic curve is typically plotted; the first curve represents cone threshold (reached at 5–10min); the second curve represents rod threshold, reached at ~30min (at which stage rhodopsin has fully regenerated and retinal sensitivity has reached its peak).

Interpretation
Defects in rhodopsin metabolism produce high thresholds, with abnormal DA curve.

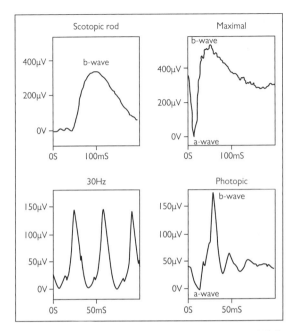

Fig. 2.19 Normal full field ERGs (courtesy of Dr Anthony Robson, Moorfields Eye Hospital.).

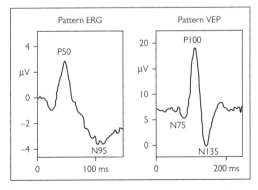

Fig. 2.20 Normal pattern ERG and pattern reversal VEP (courtesy of Dr Anthony Robson, Moorfields Eye Hospital).

Ophthalmic radiology: X-ray, dacryocystography (DCG), and dacryoscintigraphy (DSG)

X-ray orbits

Indications

Although plain X-rays have been largely superseded by computerized tomography (CT) and magnetic resonance imaging (MRI), plain films may be useful in excluding a radio-opaque FB (which may preclude an MRI). Other pathology (e.g. orbital fractures) may be identifiable on plain X-ray but generally require further characterization by CT or MRI.

Method

Commonly used views include occipitomental (Water's view), overtilted occipitomental, and lateral. If an intraocular FB (IOFB) is suspected, upgaze and downgaze views may show a change in position of a radio-opaque IOFB.

DCG

Requires the injection of radio-opaque contrast medium (oil-based) into the lacrimal drainage system. The technique is similar to syringing the tear ducts. A DCG causes a typical effective dose of X-ray irradiation equal to 6–12mo of natural atmospheric radiation.

Indications

- Aids diagnosis of epiphora.
- Plans surgical procedures.

Method

The puncta are intubated with a thin plastic cannula. A plain film X-ray (control film) is taken. With the patient supine, a radio-opaque contrast is then injected simultaneously into both lacrimal systems, and further series of X-ray films is taken.

Results

Contrast is seen in the fornices, canaliculi, common canaliculi, and nasolacrimal ducts if bilateral systems are patent. Can identify the level of obstruction and distinguish masses, stenosis, or fistulae.

Interpretation

A blockage or filling defect at any level will be seen if pathology is present. Reflux of contrast is nearly always pathological.

DSG

This lacrimal drainage scintigraphic technique is useful as a physiological test of tear flow through the lacrimal system.

Indications
- Aids diagnosis of 'functional' epiphora.
- Helps plan surgical procedures.

Method

The patient is sitting upright in front of a pinhole collimator and camera. A drop of a radioactive tracer isotope (usually technetium-99m) is placed in the inferior fornix of both eyes. The patient remains still and blinks normally. The distribution of the tracer is imaged every 10s for the first 2–3min, then at 5, 10, 15, and 20min.

Results

Time–activity curves for asymptomatic normals have a large variation. Abnormal tests are split into 'presac', 'preductal', or 'intraductal' delay. Failure for the tracer to reach the lacrimal sac by the end of the study is termed presac delay. Preductal delay is early filling of the lacrimal sac, but no sign of sac emptying at 5min. Intraductal delay is defined as tracer in the upper part of the lacrimal system, but no further drainage over 15min.[4]

Interpretation

DSG is useful for proximal obstruction, which may be masked in the DCG by overvigorous injection of dye into the lacrimal system.

4. Wearne MJ et al. Comparision of dacryocystography and lacrimal seintigraphy in the diagnosis of functional nasolacrimal duct obstruction *Br J Ophthalmol* 1999;**83**:1032–5.

Ophthalmic radiology: CT and CT angiography (CTA)

CT

CT is useful for detecting a wide range of orbital and intracranial pathology. A CT head causes a typical effective dose of X-ray irradiation equal to 10mo of natural background radiation. In comparison to MRI, CT is quick, reliable, reproducible, cheap, and appropriate in the setting of trauma.

Indications
- Orbital cellulitis.*
- Orbital lesions.*
- Orbital trauma.
- Intracranial lesions.*
- Detection of FB.
- Cerebrovascular accidents (CVA).
- Contraindication to MRI.*

Method

CT involves the rotation of a tightly collimated X-ray beam and detector around the patient. From the data gained in different projections, an image of a single plane ('slice') is reconstructed. A series of slices is recorded through the area of interest. Three-dimensional reconstructions can then be produced.

Interpretation

Visualization of the bony orbit and lesions with calcification makes this a good technique for the orbit and globe.

Caution

IV contrast[5]

The iodinated contrast media used for contrast-enhanced CT studies is potentially nephrotoxic. The following are risk factors:
- Combination of renal failure and diabetes (significant risk).
- Age >70y.
- Nephrotoxic medications.
- Congestive cardiac failure.

NB Estimated glomerular filtration rate (eGFR) is more reliable than serum creatinine in assessing renal function. eGFR <60mL/min is taken as impaired renal function.

---

* May need IV contrast.

Metformin

Metformin does NOT need to be stopped after iodinated IV contrast in patients with normal serum creatinine or eGFR. If impaired renal function prescan, the decision to stop metformin for 48h post-scan should be made WITH the referring clinician or diabetologist.

CTA

Indications

- Intracranial aneurysms.
- Vascular lesions.
- Neurosurgical planning.

Method

High-resolution thin-cut CT scan, combined with IV contrast media injection (see ➲ Caution, p. 92 for cautions of IV contrast use).

Results

Excellent vasculature anatomy in three dimensions combined with adjacent bony structure. Helps delineate borders of aneurysms and neck size to aid endovascular treatment planning. Useful in small aneurysms of the circle of Willis (see Table 2.8).

Table 2.8 Comparison of MR and CT imaging

	CT	MR
Bony detail	Excellent	Inferior to CT
Soft tissue contrast	Inferior to MR	Excellent
Ionizing radiation	Yes	None
Cost	£	£££
Time	+	+++
Contraindications during pregnancy	Not recommended	1st trimester of pregnancy not recommended
Contraindications		Metallic orbital FB, cochlear implants, neural stimulators, pacemakers, some aneurysm clips, recent surgical metallic implant (within 8wk) Claustrophobia

5. Royal College of Radiologists. *Standards for intravascular contrast agent administration to adult patients*, 2nd edition. (2010). London: The Royal College of Radiologists. Available at: ✆ http://www.rcr.ac.uk

Ophthalmic radiology: MRI and MR angiography (MRA)/MR venography (MRV)

MRI

Tissue exposed to a short electromagnetic pulse undergoes rearrangement of its hydrogen nuclei. When the pulse subsides, the nuclei return to their normal resting state, re-radiating some energy they have absorbed. Sensitive receivers pick up this electromagnetic echo. T1 and T2 times are two complex parameters that depend on proton density, tissue components, and their magnetic properties (see Fig. 2.21 and Fig. 2.22).

Indications

- Orbital masses or tumours.
- Optic nerve tumours such as glioma or meningioma.
- Intracranial extension of orbital tumours.
- Suspected compressive optic neuropathy.
- In retrobulbar neuritis, the presence of multiple white matter plaques is predictive of the development of clinical multiple sclerosis (MS).
- Suspected lesions of the chiasm such as pituitary tumours.
- Intracranial aneurysms.

Method

Conventional sequences are T1- and T2-weighted. Protocols are determined by the examining radiologist, based on the clinical situation. In addition, orbital imaging uses specialized fat suppression techniques, which is useful for optic nerve visualization, usually masked by the high signals from orbital fat.

Diffusion weighted, or diffusion tensor, MRI sequences (image Brownian motion within tissues) were initially found to be useful in acute strokes. More recently, the technique has been shown to be useful for intracranial abscesses and distinguishing an epidermoid from an arachnoid cyst.

IV paramagnetic gadolinium is used as 'contrast'. Gadolinium-enhanced scans are useful in the detection of blood–brain barrier abnormalities, inflammatory changes, and increased vascularity.

NB In tumour staging around the skull base and orbits, CT and MRI are often complementary.

Interpretation

Always review your own scans in conjunction with the radiology team. It is also important to consider the quality of the scan (e.g. adequate slices, appropriate use of contrast/processing), especially when unexpectedly 'normal'.

MRA

MRA is a non-invasive method of imaging the intra- and extracranial carotid and vertebrobasilar circulations. The principle of the computerized image construction is based on the haemodynamic properties of flowing blood, rather than on vessel anatomy.

Indications

Demonstrates abnormalities such as stenosis, occlusion, AVMs, and aneurysms.

Methods

MRA is usually a static evaluation; however, time-resolved MRA can be useful, as it highlights the separate arterial and venous supplies to an intracranial AVM.

Disadvantages

Cannot detect aneurysms <5mm in diameter; long acquisition time; suboptimal detection of intravascular calcifications.

MRV

MRV is similar to MRA, but the imaging is 'gated' to the speed of venous flow. It is useful in identifying cerebral sinus venous thromboses (see ➔ Cerebral venous sinus thrombosis (CVST), p. 683). It is therefore commonly performed for investigation of papilloedema.

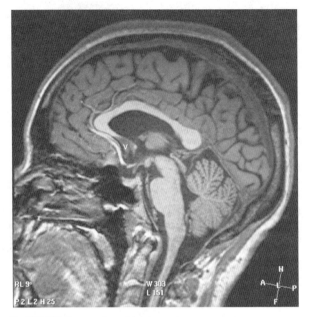

Fig. 2.21 MRI of a normal brain (sagittal section).

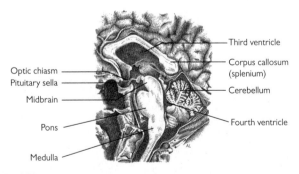

Fig. 2.22 Illustration corresponding to Fig, 2.21, with key structures identified.

Ocular trauma

Ocular trauma: assessment

See Box 3.1 for assessment approach.

Box 3.1 An approach to assessing ocular trauma

Incident	Date, time, place, witness history (if assault or paediatric case), mechanism of injury, associated head injury (loss of consciousness, nausea, vomiting, fits), other injuries
Symptoms	↓VA (sudden/gradual), floaters, flashes, field defects, diplopia, pain
POH	Previous/current eye disease
PMH	Any systemic disease, tetanus status
SH	Family support, alcohol/drug abuse
FH	Family history of eye disease
Dx	Drugs
Ax	Allergies
GCS	Conscious level
Visual function	VA, RAPD, colour vision, VF to confrontation ± formal perimetry
Orbits	Continuity of orbital rim, infraorbital sensation
Soft tissues	Periorbital bruising/oedema/surgical emphysema, lid lacerations
Globes	Proptosis/enophthalmos/hypoglobus, pulsatility
Mobility	Mechanical restriction or paretic muscle
Conjunctiva	Diffuse/defined subconjunctival haemorrhage, laceration, ischaemia
Cornea	Abrasion or full-thickness laceration (sealed/leaking), FB, rust ring, infiltrate, oedema, limbitis
AC	Depth, flare, cells (erythrocytes, leucocytes), pigment
Gonioscopy	(May need to be deferred) angle recession/dialysis, FB in angle
Iris	Anisocoria, traumatic mydriasis, iridodialysis, iridodonesis, transillumination defect, FB
Lens	Cataract, FB, phacodonesis, subluxation, Vossius ring (iris pigment imprinted on anterior capsule)
Tonometry	Applanation (may need to be deferred); if ↓IOP, consider penetrating injury, retinal detachment
Vitreous	Haemorrhage, pigment, posterior vitreous detachment
Fundus	Retinal oedema (commotio retinae), haemorrhage, tear, detachment, dialysis; choroidal rupture; exit wound; optic nerve avulsion
Indirect ophthalmoscopy	(Indentation may need to be deferred)

Documentation

Careful assessment and accurate documentation are critical. Legal proceedings often follow trauma cases. Clinical photographs can be very helpful.

Investigations

- If the eye cannot be examined due to soft tissue swelling or no fundal view is possible due to opaque media, consider B-scan US (use water bath) ± CT scan to identify gross intraocular/orbital pathology.
- CT orbits/face/head is also valuable in IOFBs, orbital/maxillofacial fractures, and associated cerebral injuries. Ask for 2mm slices to reduce the risk of missing a small IOFB. MRI should be avoided in cases where a ferromagnetic IOFB is suspected. Facial X-rays may assist in diagnosing radio-opaque IOFB (upgaze/downgaze views) and orbital fractures; it has largely been replaced by CT.
- If there is suspected globe rupture, manipulation must be kept to a minimum. This includes deferring gonioscopy, scleral indentation, and even tonometry.

Tetanus status and prophylaxis

Current UK immunization protocol

Tetanus vaccines

- *For children*: adsorbed tetanus vaccine is given as part of DTaP/IPV/Hib at 2mo, 3mo, and 4mo of age, followed by booster doses at three years four months (dTaP/IPV) and 14yrs (Td/IPV).
- *For non-immune adolescents/adults*: three doses of 0.5mL IM (Td/IPV), separated by 4wk, with a booster after 10y.

Definitions

- *Immune*: 1° immunization is complete (three doses) and within 10y of a booster dose, or if the patient has received a total of five doses.
- *Tetanus-prone wound*: wound is septic, devitalized, soil-contaminated, puncture wound, or significant delay before surgery (>6h).
- *Very high-risk wound*: unusual in ophthalmology but would include injuries such as major facial trauma with soil contamination.

Treatment

See Table 3.1 for treatment and Table 3.2 for prophylaxis.

Table 3.1 Treatment of open wounds

Patient	Wound	Action
Immune	Clean	Nil needed
	Tetanus-prone	Clean/debride wound, as required
		Give tetanus immunoglobulin only if very high risk. Consider antibiotic prophylaxis (e.g. co-amoxiclav)
Non-immune	Clean	Immediate dose of vaccine, followed by completion of standard schedule (by general practitioner (GP))
	Tetanus-prone	Clean/debride wound, as required
		Immediate dose of vaccine (as above) and tetanus immunoglobulin (at a different site), followed by completion of standard schedule (by GP). Consider antibiotic prophylaxis (e.g. co-amoxiclav)
Uncertain of vaccination status	Clean	As for non-immune patients with clean wounds. Request GP to check medical records, and complete standard schedule, if necessary
	Tetanus-prone	As for non-immune patients with tetanus-prone wounds. Request GP to check medical records, and complete standard schedule, if necessary

If tetanus vaccine indicated, it should be given immediately. Immunoglobulin should be given at a different site to vaccine.

Table 3.2 Summary of indications for tetanus prophylaxis

Risk		Treatment required		
Patient	Wound	Vaccine	Immunoglobulin	Completion of course by GP
Immune	Clean	No	No	No
	Tetanus-prone	No	Yes if very high risk	No
Non-immune	Clean	Yes	No	Yes
	Tetanus-prone	Yes	Yes	Yes
Uncertain of vaccination status	Clean	Yes	No	Yes if needed
	Tetanus-prone	Yes	Yes	Yes if needed

Chemical injury: assessment

For chemical injuries, treat first; ask questions later (see ➲ Chemical injury: treatment, p. 104).

Chemical injuries are among the most destructive of all traumatic insults suffered by the eye. They may occur in domestic, industrial, and military settings. Alkalis cause liquefactive necrosis and thus penetrate the eye to a greater extent than acids, which cause coagulative necrosis and so impede their own progress.

Prognostic factors

The severity of a chemical corneal injury is determined by the following:

- *pH*: alkaline agents generally cause more severe injuries than acids, although very acidic solutions may behave similarly; most domestic chemical agents are alkaline (or neutral), rather than acidic.
- *Duration of contact.*
- *Corneal involvement*: surface area, duration of contact.
- *Limbal involvement*: corneal re-epithelialization relies on migration of the limbal stem cells.
- *Conjunctival involvement*: blind-ended sacs that may retain chemical and cause continuing ocular damage.
- *Associated non-chemical injury*: blunt trauma, thermal injury.

Clinical features

- Conjunctival injection or ischaemia (beware the 'white' eye) ± chemosis, haemorrhage, epithelial defects, ulceration, necrosis, or complete loss of conjunctiva; perilimbal ischaemia/limbitis (blanched vessels with no visible blood flow); corneal epitheliopathy (punctate to complete loss; **NB** may stain poorly with fluorescein); corneal oedema; corneal stromal necrosis; AC activity and fibrin; traumatic mydriasis, ↑IOP (consider Tonopen, rather than Goldmann); rarely, scleral necrosis, vitritis, necrotic retinopathy.

Classification of severity

The Roper-Hall classification (see Table 3.3) assesses the state of the cornea and limbus, whereas the Dua classification (see Table 3.4) assesses the limbus and conjunctiva (with a view to predicting prognosis from the extent of stem cell loss).

Complications

- *Conjunctival burns*: cicatrization (scarring), symblepharon formation, loss of goblet cells, keratinization.
- *Significant limbal ischaemia*: conjunctivalization, vascularization, and opacification of the cornea.
- *Full-thickness burns*: scleritis, vitritis, retinitis, glaucomatous optic neuropathy or hypotony, iris, ciliary, and lenticular damage; may progress to phthisis bulbi; very poor prognosis.
- *Periorbital burns*: first-/second-/third-degree chemical burns of periorbital tissues.

Table 3.3 Classification of severity of ocular surface burns (Roper-Hall classification)*

Grade	Corneal appearance	Limbal ischaemia	Prognosis
I	Clear cornea	Nil	Good
II	Hazy cornea: iris details visible	<1/3	Good
III	Opaque cornea: iris details obscured	1/3 to 1/2	Guarded
IV	Opaque cornea: Iris details obscured	>1/2	Poor

* Roper-Hall MJ. Thermal and chemical burns. *Trans Ophthalmol Soc UK* 1965;**85**:631–53.

Table 3.4 Alternative classification of ocular surface burns, highlighting limbal involvement (Dua classification)*

Grade	Limbal involvement (clock hours)	Conjunctival involvement (%)	Prognosis
I	0	0	Very good
II	≤3	≤30	Good
III	>3–6	>30–50	Good
IV	>6–9	>50–75	Good to guarded
V	>9–12	>75–<100	Guarded to poor
VI	12 (total)	100 (total)	Very poor

This information can also be presented in component form, e.g. 4.5/40 indicates 4.5 clock hours of limbus and 40% conjunctiva involved. Conjunctiva refers to bulbar conjunctiva up to, and including, the fornices.

* Dua HS *et al.* A new classification of ocular surface burns. *Br J Ophthalmol* 2001;**85**:1379–83.

Chemical injury: treatment

Immediate
- Neutralization of pH by irrigation before full history and examination (see Table 3.5 for common substances).

Immediate irrigation
This is probably the most important determinant of outcome.
- Test pH, then instil topical anaesthetic (e.g. proxymetacaine); insert a speculum, and irrigate with water, normal saline, or Hartmann's solution through IV tubing, and deliver a minimum of 2L or until normal pH is restored. Delay to obtain irrigants other than water is not warranted.

Inspection
Evert the lids (double-evert the upper lid), and inspect the fornices. Remove retained particulate matter that may perpetuate alkalinity (e.g. lime, cement).

Indicator test
Test pH at end of irrigation and 5min after completion of irrigation.
- *If pH neutral/near neutral* (normal tears may be slightly alkaline; up to about 7.4), then you may begin examination and initiate further treatment. However, recheck pH after 20min.
- *If pH abnormal,* then repeat irrigation cycle (with another 2L) until pH normal.
- pH should be recorded on a daily basis until ocular surface is healed (to exclude release of chemical from inherent forniceal particles of chemical).

Acute: all injuries
- *Admit*: if severe or any other concerns.
- *Topical antibiotics*: prophylaxis (e.g. preservative-free chloramphenicol 0.5% 4×/d).
- *Topical cycloplegia*: for comfort/AC activity (e.g. preservative-free cyclopentolate 1% 3×/d or atropine 1% once daily).
- *Topical lubricants* (preservative free, e.g. carmellose 1%) 1–4-hourly day and night + liquid paraffin nocte).
- *Oral analgesia* (e.g. paracetamol ± codeine).

Topical medication should be preservative-free where possible.

Table 3.5 Strong acids and alkalis in common use

Substance	Chemical	pH
Common alkalis		
Oven cleaning fluid	Sodium hydroxide	14
Drain cleaning fluid	Sodium (or potassium) hydroxide	14
Plaster	Calcium hydroxide	14
Fertilizers (some)	Ammonium hydroxide	13
Common acids		
Battery fluid	Sulfuric acid	1
Lavatory cleaning fluid	Sulfuric acid	1
Bleach	Sodium hypochlorite	1
Pool cleaning fluid	Sodium (or calcium) hypochlorite	1

Acute: severe injuries

Admit and consider:
- Topical steroids (e.g. prednisolone 0.5–1% initially 4–8×/d for <10d).
- Topical ascorbic acid (e.g. sodium ascorbate 10% up to 2-hourly for <10d).
- Oral ascorbic acid (e.g. 1g 2×/d).
- Systemic tetracyclines, e.g. doxycycline 50–100mg 1×/d or oxytetracycline 500mg 4×/d for 3mo (tetracyclines contraindicated in children <12, in pregnant/breastfeeding women, and in hepatic and renal impairment).

Ascorbic acid is essential for collagen formation and is an effective scavenger of damaging free radicals; it should not be used in acid chemical burns. Doxycycline is a proteinase inhibitor and serves to not only prevent tissue necrosis and facilitate healing, but also has anti-inflammatory properties.

Less commonly used are topical sodium citrate 10% (reduces neutrophil chemotaxis and inhibits collagenases but is painful). Paracentesis and replacement of aqueous with a buffered phosphate solution can help to normalize the AC pH more quickly.[1]

Acute: injuries with ↑IOP

Acetazolamide 250mg 4×/d ± topical β-blocker (e.g. preservative-free timolol 0.5% 2×/d).

Long-term: complicated cases

Poor corneal healing

Medical treatment as for persistent epithelial defects (see ➲ Persistent epithelial defects, p. 242). Surgical treatment includes techniques to assist epithelial migration (amniotic membrane (AM) transplantation) and re-epithelialization of the cornea (limbal stem cell transplantation; see ➲ Limbal epithelial stem cell deficiency, p. 244).

Obliterated fornices and pseudopterygium formation

Consider:

• Pseudopterygium excision, together with conjunctival autograft (if adequate host conjunctiva) or AM facilitated by anti-proliferatives (intraoperative mitomycin C (MMC)), and

• Forniceal reconstructive surgery, including division of symblepharon and mucous membrane or amniotic membrane grafting (AMG).

Corneal opacification

Consider limbal epithelial stem cell transplantation followed by penetrating keratoplasty (PK) if adequate tear film. In bilateral cases, keratoprosthesis remains a surgical option in severely damaged eyes.

1. Paterson CA et al. Aqueous humor pH changes after experimental alkali burns. *Am J Ophthalmol* 1975;**79**:414–19.

Thermal injury/burns: assessment

It is vital to first assess the extent of the burns injury. If there is any suspicion from the history or examination that the mouth/airways may have been involved, immediate anaesthetic assistance is mandatory with a view to assessing and stabilizing the airway. Inhalational burns injuries can lead to airway oedema and fatal airways/respiratory compromise.

Assessment

Thermal injuries most commonly affect the lids, but cornea and conjunctiva may also be involved, They range from the mild and visually insignificant to the severe and blinding.

Assessment of burns to the lids is performed in the standard manner used for cutaneous burns elsewhere: superficial/partial thickness/full thickness. Assessment of burns to the globe requires careful slit-lamp examination in a manner similar to that used for chemical injuries (see ➔ Chemical injury: assessment, p. 102).

Assessment of the ocular thermal burns must be taken in context with whole body involvement, i.e. estimation of total body surface area (BSA) involvement. *Proportion of each body area is dependent on age*: face is 19% total BSA of child <1y of age, 13% of a 5–9y old, and only 7% of an adult.

Clinical features

Corneal and ocular surface

Direct contact thermal injury
- Keratopathy:
  - Spectrum ranges from mild punctate/confluent defects (e.g. most cigarette ash injuries) to severe limbitis and permanent opacification, stromal melting or perforation (e.g. from molten metal, which may form a complete cast between lid and globe).
  - Associated features include conjunctival injection, ischaemia (the eye may be white), chemosis, necrosis, and cataract (if severe).

2°exposure
- Exposure keratopathy may occur acutely if there is significant loss of lid tissue, or as a late complication of lid cicatrization.

Lids

- *Superficial (1st degree) burns:* commonly caused by sunburn or short-duration flash burns. Dry burns with oedema and no blistering; erythema and pain are common; heals in ≤1wk, accompanied by superficial peeling and no scar formation (although discoloration may occur).
- *Partial thickness (2nd degree) burns:* causes include longer-duration scalds and flame injury. Blisters and weeping of the skin, intense erythema, significant pain, and temperature sensitivity. Heals in 1–4wk, with little scarring, but pigmentary changes common.
- *Full-thickness (3rd degree) burns:* commonly caused by chemical, electrical, flame, and scald injuries. Skin appears dry, inflexible, and leathery, with little/no pain. Heals with significant cicatrization and scarring.

Thermal injury/burns: management

Management

Systemic

Liaise with a burns specialist to optimize systemic care and preferably for admission to a specialist burns unit. Some general principles are included here.

Resuscitation with IV fluids

Fluid resuscitation is critical within the first 24h. The amount of fluid resuscitation can be determined from the % BSA involved.

- Estimate % BSA by the 'rule of 9s':
  - Rule of 9s for adults: 9% for each arm, 18% for each leg, 9% for head, 18% for front torso, 18% for back torso.
  - Rule of 9s for children: 9% for each arm, 14% for each leg, 18% for head, 18% for front torso, 18% for back torso.
- Estimate fluid replacement by the Parkland Formula:
  - Fluid for first 24h (mL) = 4 × patient's weight in kg × % BSA.
  - Give 50% of this fluid in the first 8h, and the remaining 50% in the next 16h.

General skin care

- Air-fluidized bed if large BSA involved.
- Reverse barrier nursing.
- Leave intact blisters, and gently remove necrotic skin only.
- Simple emollients, e.g. 50:50 white soft paraffin:liquid paraffin applied to the burns.
- *Dressings*: non-adherent, e.g. Acticoat Silver® (change every 2–3d).
- Isotonic, sterile saline to irrigate mouth, nostrils, eyes, and anogenital areas frequently.

Management of corneal and ocular surface thermal injuries

Essentially as for chemical injuries (see ➔ Chemical injury: treatment, p. 104), but limited role for irrigation. In summary:

- *Topical antibiotics:* prophylaxis (e.g. preservative-free chloramphenicol 0.5% 4×/d).
- *Topical cycloplegia*: for comfort/AC activity (e.g. preservative-free cyclopentolate 1% 3×/d or atropine 1% 2×/d).
- *Topical lubricants* (preservative-free, e.g. carmellose 1–4-hourly + liquid paraffin nocte).
- *Oral analgesia* (e.g. paracetamol ± codeine).
- *Consider topical steroids*, especially in the presence of significant oedema (preservative-free, e.g. prednisolone 0.5–1% initially 4–8×/d for <10d).

Topical medication should be preservative-free where possible. In more severe cases, consider similar strategies to those used for chemical injuries, including systemic ascorbic acid, tetracyclines, and ocular surface protection, including the use of AM overlay (see ➔ Amniotic membrane transplantation, p. 283).

NB Symblepharon formation can occur, and early removal of pseudomembrane formation and surgical division of acute forniceal adhesions may be necessary.

Management of lid thermal injuries
- *Superficial burns*: cool compresses; lubrication; pain control.
- *Partial-thickness burns*: topical antibiotic ointment; copious lubrication ± occlusion dressing or moisture chamber; trim eyelashes if singed (lash particles cause irritation); consider lid suture or temporary tarsorrhaphy if risk of corneal exposure.
- *Full-thickness burns*: as for partial-thickness burns + debride dead tissue and eschar; protect the eye with lubrication, Jelonet® and Geliperm® dressings, and tarsorrhaphy. Refer to oculoplastic team for specialist assessment, including skin grafting.

Complications
- *Loss of lid tissue*: leads to corneal exposure.
- *Lid cicatrization*: leads to entropion/ectropion, trichiasis, and corneal exposure.
- *Epiphora*: from damage to the punctae/lacrimal ducts.
- *Conjunctival burns*: cicatricial changes, symblepharon, and severe dry eye (through damage to goblet cells, accessory lacrimal and meibomian glands (MGs)).
- *Significant limbal ischaemia*: conjunctivalization, vascularization, and opacification of the cornea.

Orbital fractures: assessment

Assessment

See Table 3.6 for assessment features.

Table 3.6 Specific features in assessment of potential orbital fractures

Hx	Mechanism of injury
	Diplopia, areas of numbness, pain, epistaxis, visual symptoms (associated ocular injury), dental malocclusion
O/E	Periorbital bruising/oedema/haemorrhage, surgical emphysema, globe position (proptosis, enophthalmos, dystopia), globe pulsation, pupillary responses and RAPD, resistance to retropulsion, ocular motility, subconjunctival haemorrhage, discontinuity of orbital rim
	Any associated ocular injury
	Any potential cervical or head injury (refer to trauma team); collapse may be due to oculocardiac reflex 2° to extraocular muscle (EOM) entrapment
Ix	CT (2mm axial and coronal slices): identify fractures (bony windows), prolapsed orbital fat/EOM, and haemorrhage
	Facial X-rays: droplet sign (soft tissue prolapse in orbital floor fracture); fluid level in maxillary sinus, visible fracture. However, CT is preferable
	Hess/Lees and fields of binocular vision tests show characteristic mechanical restrictive patterns and allow monitoring of recovery

Clinical features

Orbital floor (maxillary bone)

This is the commonest orbital fracture in those of Caucasian or Asian (Oriental or Indian) ethnic origin.[2] It usually follows a blow from an object >5cm (e.g. tennis ball/fist). The force may be transmitted by hydraulic compression of the globe/orbital structures ('blowout') or may be directly transmitted along the orbital rim.

- *Soft tissue*: periorbital bruising/oedema/haemorrhage, surgical emphysema.
- *Vertical diplopia due to mechanical restriction of upgaze*: this may be 2° to tissue entrapment following prolapse through the bony defect (persistent) or soft tissue swelling tenting the EOM insertion (transient).
- *Enophthalmos.*
- *Infraorbital anaesthesia*: due to nerve damage in infraorbital canal.
- Beware 'white eye blowout' fractures in children—a 'greenstick' fracture may result in minimal signs but significant EOM entrapment.

Medial wall (ethmoidal)

Medial wall fractures are rare as an isolated feature but may accompany orbital floor fractures. This is the most common form of orbital fracture in those of Afro-Caribbean origin.[2]

- Soft tissue signs as for orbital floor fractures, but surgical emphysema may be prominent.
- Horizontal diplopia due to mechanical restriction from medial rectus (MR) entrapment.

Orbital roof (frontal)

Orbital roof fractures are very rare as an isolated feature. They are most commonly seen in children following brow trauma.

- Soft tissue signs as for orbital floor fractures, but bruising may spread across midline.
- Superior subconjunctival haemorrhage, with no distinct posterior limit.
- Inferior/axial globe displacement.
- May have bruit/pulsation due to communication with cerebrospinal fluid (CSF); carry risk of meningitis.

Lateral wall (zygomatic arch)

The lateral wall is very robust and acts as a protective shield to the globe. Lateral wall fractures are usually only seen following major maxillofacial trauma.

The tense orbit

Orbital injuries resulting in soft tissue oedema and retrobulbar haemorrhage (occurring in 0.3–3.5% of facial traumas) within the non-expansile bony orbit. This may result in an acute rise in intraorbital pressure, compromising blood flow and resulting in ischaemia and optic nerve damage (orbital compartment syndrome). This which can lead to catastrophic, irreversible loss of vision if not managed appropriately.[3]

Clinical features

- Painful proptosis.
- Reduced vision.
- Resistance to retropulsion.
- Elevated IOP (>35mmHg).
- Sluggish pupil or RAPD.
- Restricted ocular movements.
- Ptosis.
- Retinal arterial pulsations.

Treatment

- *Immediate:* IV mannitol (0.5–2g), IV acetazolamide (500mg), and IV methylprednisolone (IVMP; 0.5–1g) (if no contraindications).
- *If no improvement or if/worsens:* canthotomy (incision of the lateral canthal tendon) and cantholysis (canthotomy combined with disinsertion of the lateral canthal tendon).
- *If no improvement or if/worsens:* orbital decompression or drainage.
- *If responds to IV mannitol and IV acetazolamide* (reduced features of tense orbit): half-hourly reassessment for 3h (most orbital haemorrhages are self-limiting). If deterioration during the reassessment period: proceed to canthotomy/cantholysis. If stable after reassessment period, then proceed with conservative management.

2. de Silva DJ et al. Orbital blowout fractures and race. Ophthalmology 2011;**118**:1677–80.

3. McClenaghan FC et al. Mechanisms and management of vision loss following orbital and facial trauma. Curr Opin Ophthalmol 2011;**22**:426–31.

Orbital fractures: treatment

All orbital fractures

- Advise patients to refrain from nose blowing, which may contribute to surgical emphysema, herniation of orbital contents, or spread of upper respiratory organisms into the orbit.
- Consider antibiotic prophylaxis; commonly, anaerobic cover is prescribed (e.g. co-amoxiclav), but limited evidence for any benefit.
- Refer to orbital or maxillofacial team for consideration of surgical repair.
- Arrange orthoptic follow-up with serial Hess charts to monitor recovery/post-operative course.
- Some studies have demonstrated that effective fracture repair can be performed up to 29d after trauma.[4]
- Persisting diplopia, even following orbital fracture repair, may require squint surgery.

Fractures of the orbital floor

See Table 3.7 for indications for surgical interventions and Box 3.2 for outline of repair.

Table 3.7 Indications for surgical intervention in orbital floor fractures

Immediate	Persistent oculocardiac reflex
	Young patient with 'white-eyed' trapdoor fracture (orbital floor buckling occurring in children)
	Significant facial asymmetry
Early (<2wk)	Persistent symptomatic diplopia
	Significant enophthalmos (>2mm and symptomatic)
	Hypoglobus
	Progressive infraorbital hypoaesthesia
Observation	Minimal diplopia (e.g. just in upgaze)
	Minimal restriction
	Minimal enophthalmos

Box 3.2 Outline of repair for orbital floor fractures

- Use a transconjunctival or 'swinging eyelid' approach to expose the inferior orbital rim.
- Incise the periosteum, 2mm outside the orbital rim, and dissect posteriorly, elevating the periorbita/periosteum off the orbital floor.
- Carefully release all herniated orbital contents, taking care to separate from the infraorbital nerve and vessels.
- Continue until the whole fracture has been exposed.
- Repair bony defect with an implant (e.g. polyethylene-coated titanium), with an overlap of ≥5mm, which should be fixed in position.
- Close periosteum with absorbable suture (e.g. 4-0 vicryl).
- Close subciliary/transconjunctival incision.

4. Dal Canto AJ et al. Comparison of orbital fracture repair performed within 14 days versus 15 to 29 days after trauma. *Ophthal Plast Reconstr Surg* 2008;24:437–43.

Lid lacerations

Lacerations involving the eyelid are common, occurring in the context of both blunt and sharp injuries. They carry morbidity in their own right and may be associated with significant injuries of globe or orbit.

Lid lacerations require careful exploration and precise closure, particularly at the lid margin (see Box 3.3 for assessment).

Assessment

Box 3.3 Specific features in assessment of lid lacerations

Hx	Mechanism of injury and likelihood of associated injuries (e.g. stab injuries), likely infective risk (e.g. bites)
O/E	Lid laceration (depth, length, tissue viability), lid position, orbicularis function, lagophthalmos, intercanthal distance
	Canalicular involvement, nasolacrimal drainage
	Beware: associated injury of globe or orbit
Ix	All stab injuries should have orbital X-ray and/or orbital and head CT (FBs, pneumocranium)

Treatment

- *Prophylaxis*: protect cornea with generous lubrication; administer tetanus vaccine/immunoglobulin, if indicated (see ➔ Tetanus status and prophylaxis, p. 100).
- *Surgery*: assess for surgical repair, according to depth, extent of tissue loss, involvement of lid margin, and involvement of canaliculus.
- Complicated lid lacerations (e.g. involving lid margin or canaliculi) should be repaired in theatre by an experienced surgeon (see Table 3.8).

Table 3.8 Outline of repair for lid lacerations

Simple superficial not involving margin	Close with interrupted 6-0 sutures parallel to lid margin; absorbable (e.g. Vicryl®) are often preferred (especially for children), but non-absorbable (e.g. silk) may be used
Partial thickness	Small defect restricted to anterior lamella; consider allowing repair by granulation
	Larger defect requires a reconstructive procedure
Full thickness with tissue loss	*Small defect (0–25% tissue loss):*
	Debride/freshen up wound edges; close with interrupted absorbable (e.g. 6-0 Vicryl®) sutures in one layer to tarsus and one layer to skin
	Large defect (25–60% tissue loss):
	Consider lateral canthotomy/cantholysis, Tenzel or McGregor myocutaneous flap
	Very large defect (>60% tissue loss):
	For lower lids, consider Hughes tarsoconjunctival flap and skin graft or transposition skin flap or Mustarde myocutaneous flap
	For upper eyelids, consider Cutler–Beard flap or Mustarde lid-switch (2-stage)
Involving margin	Debride/freshen up wound edges
	Place grey line suture (non-absorbable or absorbable, e.g. 6-0 Vicryl®); leave long
	Close tarsus with interrupted absorbable suture (e.g. 6-0 Vicryl®)
	Place additional marginal suture (lash line), if required; leave long
	Close overlying skin with interrupted absorbable suture (e.g. 6-0 Vicryl®); these sutures should also catch the long ends of the marginal sutures to prevent corneal abrasion
Canalicular laceration	Internally splint the opened duct with silicone tubing, e.g. Mini Monoka stent
	For upper and lower canalicular laceration, consider bicanalicular intubation
	For lower lids, consider reapposing medial edge of eyelid to posterior lacrimal crest
	Close laceration with 6-0 Vicryl®
	Leave silicone tubes *in situ* for 3mo
Post-operative	Topical antibiotic/lubrication (e.g. Oc chloramphenicol 3×/d to wound and fornix for 1wk)
	Remove skin sutures at 5–7d

Blunt trauma: assessment

Traumatic eye injuries account for about 4,500 admissions in the UK per year. They are commonly associated with more extensive injuries; ocular involvement occurs in about 10% of all non-fatal casualties. Most ocular trauma is blunt (80%), rather than penetrating (20%), with IOFBs occurring in 1%. (See Box 3.4 for assessment.)

In the UK, legislation (notably the compulsory wearing of seatbelts and health and safety at work) has effectively reduced some sources of eye injuries, such that now most are related to sport or other leisure activities.

Assessment

> **Box 3.4 Specific features in assessment of blunt injury**
>
> Hx Mechanism, associated injuries, tetanus status
>
> O/E *Globe:* look for anterior or posterior rupture
>
> *Cornea:* check fluorescein staining, clarity
>
> *AC:* check for cells/flare and depth (compare with other eye)
>
> *Iris/ciliary body:* note abnormalities of pupil, and examine iris root/ angle by gonioscopy (if stable)
>
> *Lens:* opacity, position, stability
>
> *Vitreous:* PVD, haemorrhage
>
> *Fundus:* note commotio retinae (usually temporal); check macular pathology (e.g. hole); examine equator/periphery for retinal tears/ dialysis; consider choroidal rupture (often masked by blood)
>
> *Optic nerve:* check function and disc appearance
>
> *IOP*
>
> *Beware:* 'occult' posterior rupture; check for associated orbital/ adnexal injuries
>
> Ix *Consider orbital/facial X-ray, B-scan US, CT orbits/brain (assess extent of damage, particularly where clinical assessment limited)*

Clinical features

Globe

- *Anterior rupture:* usually obvious with herniation of uveal tissue, lens and vitreous, and other signs of injury (e.g. severe subconjunctival haemorrhage, hyphaema, etc.).
- *Posterior rupture:* suspect if deep AC ± low IOP (compare with contralateral eye).

Anterior segment

- Corneal abrasion (epithelial defect; see ➥ Corneal foreign bodies and abrasions, p. 126), corneal oedema (transient endothelial decompensation, spontaneously resolves).
- *Hyphaema*: red blood cells in the AC (see ➥ Hyphaema, p. 128).
- *Iris*: miosis (usually transient), mydriasis (often permanent), and sphincter rupture (irregular pupil; permanent); iris root abnormalities include iridodialysis (dehiscence from ciliary body) and angle recession (late risk of glaucoma; see ➥ Other secondary open-angle glaucoma, p. 378).
- *Lens*: Vossius ring (imprint of iris pigment on anterior capsule), cataract (anterior or posterior subcapsular); subluxation/luxation of the lens.

Posterior segment

- *Vitreous*: PVD, vitreous haemorrhage.
- *Commotio retinae*: grey-white retinal opaqueness as a result of fragmentation of the photoreceptor outer segments and intracellular oedema (photoreceptors and pigment epithelium); with increasing severity intraretinal haemorrhages:
  - In most cases, commotio retinae completely resolves, but, in a minority, macular hole/pigmentary change ensues.
  - In extreme cases, such as where a projectile has grazed but not penetrated the globe, haemorrhagic necrosis of the choroid and retina may occur (chorioretinitis sclopetaria; *syn* chorioretinitis sclopteria).
- *Retinal dialysis*: full-thickness circumferential break at the ora serrata; commonly superonasal (when traumatic). It is not related to PVD, and thus progression to any retinal detachment is slow (several months); irregular retinal tear(s) may occur at the equator (see ➥ Retinal breaks, p. 482).
- *Macular holes*: acute or late (see ➥ Macular hole, p. 500).
- *Choroidal rupture*: rupture through choroid/Bruch's membrane/RPE but sclera intact; the rupture is usually concentric to the disc; it is usually obscured initially by overlying subretinal blood; later a white streak of sclera may be visible; CNV is a late complication.
- *Traumatic optic neuropathy*: acutely ↓optic nerve function (including RAPD) in presence of normal disc appearance; later disc pallor.
- *Optic nerve avulsion*: ↓/absent optic nerve function, depending on completeness of avulsion; defect in place of optic disc; confirm on B-scan US if dense vitreous haemorrhage prevents clinical view.

Blunt trauma: treatment

1° repair of globe rupture

- *Admit and prepare for general anaesthesia (GA)*: nil by mouth; determine last meal/drink; liaise with anaesthetist, ECG/bloods (if indicated).
- *Prophylaxis*: protect globe with clear plastic shield, systemic antibiotic (e.g. ciprofloxacin PO 750mg 2×/d) ± preservative-free topical antibiotic; administer tetanus vaccine/toxoid, if indicated (see ➔ Tetanus status and prophylaxis, p. 100).
- *Surgery*: assess and proceed with 1° repair (see Table 3.9).

2° repair

- *Iris*: most injuries involving the iris (other than herniation through a ruptured globe) do not require surgical intervention.
- *Lens*: significant lens injuries resulting in ↓VA (opacity, subluxation), ↑IOP (for lens-related glaucoma, see ➔ p. 376), or inflammation (breached capsule) warrant removal of the lens; some cases may require a vitreoretinal approach.
- *Vitreoretinal*: retinal tears or retinal dialysis require urgent referral for vitreoretinal assessment and repair; macular holes should also be referred but can generally be seen electively.

Other

- *Commotio retinae*: no treatment usually indicated, as most spontaneously recover; some have persistent/late ↓VA due to macular hole/ pigmentary change.
- *Choroidal rupture*: no treatment is indicated; however, if a CNV develops, this can be treated in the conventional manner.
- *Traumatic optic neuropathy*: liaise with a neuro-ophthalmologist; 'megadose' systemic corticosteroids are sometimes given, which, while of proven benefit in spinal injuries, are unproven in traumatic optic neuropathy.

Penetrating trauma/intraocular foreign bodies: assessment

Small (<2mm) FBs may leave a sealed wound and minimal clinical signs. Penetrating trauma should be excluded, following injury from sharp objects and projectiles with high mass and/or velocity.

An IOFB must be excluded in all cases of penetration. Multiple IOFBs are not uncommon, and some form of X-ray imaging should be carried out, even in cases where an IOFB has been identified under direct vision.[5] Double perforation (through and through injury) should be considered, even if IOFB is now within the globe. Posterior rupture following significant blunt trauma should always be considered (see Box 3.5 for assessment).

Complications of IOFB injury (infection, retinal detachment, and toxicity) may have a more severe impact on visual outcome than the initial physical injury.[6] Occasionally, iatrogenic penetrating injuries occur, e.g. in up to 1 in 1,000 peribulbar injections.

Assessment

> **Box 3.5 Specific features in assessment of penetrating injury and IOFBs**
>
> Hx   *Source* (e.g. hammer on steel, machinery, explosive), probable IOFB material, likely toxicity and infective risk, tetanus status
>
> O/E *Entry site:* identify location and integrity (leak) of wound
>
>   ↓IOP
>
>   *Trajectory:* look for iris hole (transillumination), focal cataract/lens tract, retinal haemorrhage
>
>   *Location:* including gonioscopy and dilated fundoscopy
>
>   *Beware:* occult IOFB in angle, ciliary body, pars plana
>
> Ix   X-ray examination: orbital X-ray (in upgaze and downgaze) or CT with 2mm slices in all cases, even if an IOFB is clearly visible
>
>   US, VEP (chronic retained IOFB → reduced b-wave)

Clinical features

Mechanical injury

- *Globe*: penetration, perforation, or double perforation ('through and through') of corneosclera and uvea.
- *Anterior segment*: angle recession (late risk of glaucoma; see ➲ Other secondary open-angle glaucoma, p. 378); hyphaema (see ➲ Hyphaema, p. 128); lens capsule injury, cataract formation, zonular dehiscence, subluxation.
- *Posterior segment*: vitreous liquefaction, vitreous haemorrhage, abnormal vitreoretinal traction, retinal haemorrhage, retinal tear, retinal detachment.

Introduction of infection
- Endophthalmitis, panophthalmitis.

Toxicity
- Siderosis, chalcosis (see Box 3.6).

Siderosis (ferrous FB)
- Dissociated iron has a predilection for deposition in epithelial tissue (lens, RPE), causing metabolic toxicity and cellular death.
- RPE toxicity results in ↓VA, constricted VF, and RAPD.
- Clinical features include injection, heterochromia (iris reddish brown), ↑IOP (2° glaucoma), anterior capsular cataract, reddish ferrous deposits at lens epithelium, coarse degenerative pigment dispersion, retinal detachment. VEP shows b-wave attenuation.

Chalcosis (copper FB)
- Pure copper IOFBs result in rapid fulminant endophthalmitis.
- Chalcosis results from FB of alloys of copper (brass, bronze) and mirror the ocular signs of Wilson's disease: Kayser–Fleischer ring, anterior 'sunflower' cataract, yellow retinal plaques.

Box 3.6 Toxicity and IOFB

Inert ← - → Toxic			
Platinum	Aluminium	Iron	Copper
Silver	Zinc		Organic material
Gold	Nickel		Soil
Lead	Mercury		
Glass			
Plastic			
Stone			
Carbon			

5. Woodcock M *et al.* Mass and shape factors in intraocular foreign body injuries. *Ophthalmology* 2006;**113**:2262–9.

6. Roper-Hall MJ. Review of 555 cases of intra-ocular foreign body with special reference to prognosis. *Br J Ophthalmol* 1954;**38**:65–98.

Penetrating trauma/intraocular foreign bodies: treatment

With penetrating injuries, the urgent priority is to repair the integrity of the globe.

If present, IOFBs are ideally removed at the time of 1° repair, but closure of the globe should not be delayed if vitreoretinal expertise is not readily available. Similarly, additional procedures (e.g. lensectomy, vitrectomy, retinal detachment repair) may be carried out at the time of 1° repair but are commonly deferred to a planned 2° rehabilitative procedure.[7,8]

General

- *Admit and prepare for GA*: nil by mouth; determine last meal/drink; liaise with anaesthetist; ECG/bloods (if indicated).
- *Prophylaxis*: protect globe with clear plastic shield, systemic antibiotic (e.g. ciprofloxacin PO 750mg bd) ± preservative-free topical antibiotic; administer tetanus vaccine/toxoid, if indicated (see ➜ Tetanus status and prophylaxis, p. 100).
- *Surgery*: assess and proceed with 1° repair, IOFB removal, and any additional procedures required (see Table 3.9 and Table 3.10).

1° repair

Table 3.9 An approach to 1° repair

All wounds	Debride contaminated non-viable tissue
	Carefully maintain the AC to avoid expulsion of ocular contents
Small self-sealing corneal wound	Shelved corneal laceration with formed AC may not require formal closure
	Observe until healed; consider BCL, and cover with adequate antibiotic cover
Corneal wound	May require AC deepening/stabilization with viscoelastic
	Return exposed viable iris tissue through perforation; abscise exposed tissue if non-viable
	Directly close corneal wound with perpendicular deep 10-0 nylon sutures, and rotate sutures to bury knots
	Remove viscoelastic
Involving limbus	Expose adjacent sclera to determine full posterior extent of wound
	Start closure at limbus, and proceed posteriorly
Scleral	Conjunctival peritomy; expose and explore sclera
	Return exposed viable uveal tissue through perforation
	Cut prolapsed vitreous flush to wound, taking care not to induce vitreous traction
	Direct scleral closure

IOFB removal

Table 3.10 IOFB removal

AC IOFB	Corneal approach; removal with fine forceps
Angle IOFB	Scleral trapdoor approach
Lenticular IOFB	If in clear lens matter, consider leaving *in situ* or remove with lens at cautious cataract surgery (potential capsular and zonular instability)
Ciliary body IOFB	Cannot be directly visualized, so consider using an electroacoustic locator and electromagnetic removal through scleral trapdoor approach
Posterior segment IOFB	IOFB removal should be undertaken as soon as optimal surgical expertise and operating room conditions are available
	Use an intraocular magnet or vitrectomy forceps
	Reserve direct trans-scleral delivery for those IOFB that are easily accessible

2° procedures

Planned 2° repair of posterior segment trauma has traditionally been performed 4–10d after initial injury, in part, to allow for the formation of a PVD.

2° repair may be performed earlier in the presence of an IOFB (not removed at the 1° repair), retinal detachment, or endophthalmitis. The timing of IOFB removal is a balance between the risk of infection and the ease of surgically inducing a PVD. However, in a recent large case series, delayed IOFB removal was not found to be associated with increased presence of a PVD. It is therefore suggested that IOFB removal should not be delayed for this reason. However, the risk of infection is significantly reduced by the use of systemic antibiotics and, so long as these have been given, surgery can be delayed until optimal surgical expertise and/or conditions are available.[7,8]

2° repair may include vitrectomy, membrane dissection (if proliferative vitreoretinopathy), encircling buckle (if breaks), lensectomy (if cataract; IOL commonly deferred), intravitreal antibiotics (if endophthalmitis), and tamponade (usually C3F8 or silicone oil).

Sympathetic ophthalmia

Sympathetic ophthalmia is a rare bilateral granulomatous panuveitis in which trauma to one eye may cause sight-threatening inflammation in the untraumatized 'sympathizing' eye. Its nature, clinical features, prophylaxis, and treatment are discussed elsewhere (see Sympathetic ophthalmia, ➔ p. 444).

7. Woodcock M *et al.* Mass and shape factors in intraocular foreign body injuries. *Ophthalmology* 2006;**113**:2262–9.

8. Colyer MH *et al.* Delayed intraocular foreign body removal without endophthalmitis during Operations Iraqi Freedom and Enduring Freedom. *Ophthalmology* 2007;**114**:1439–47.

Corneal foreign bodies and abrasions

Corneal FBs

Most corneal FBs are metallic and only rarely cause infection. Microbial keratitis more commonly follows stone, ceramic, and organic FBs. Remember to exclude additional intraocular or subtarsal FB.

Clinical features

- Photophobia, pain, injection, lacrimation, blurred vision; history of projectile striking eye; failure to wear protective eye-wear while working, welding, hammering.
- FB ± rust ring (forms within 48h) or infiltrate; ± anterior uveitis.

Treatment

- Corneal FBs should only be removed under slit-lamp visualization. The previously common practice of removing them under direct vision with a cotton bud is strongly discouraged.
- *Removal*: explain what you are about to do, and give them a target to stare at; instil topical anaesthetic (e.g. oxybuprocaine 0.4%); remove FB and rust ring under slit-lamp visualization (e.g. with 26G needle).
- Topical antibiotic (e.g. chloramphenicol oc 1% 4×/d for 5d); consider short-term cycloplegic (for comfort/AC activity) and non-steroidal anti-inflammatory preparations.
- Warn the patient that their eye will be uncomfortable once the anaesthetic has worn off.

Corneal abrasions

Corneal abrasions are superficial corneal wounds. Corneal abrasions are common and often innocuous but may cause severe pain and distress. Epithelial denuding exposes the stromal nocioreceptors, triggering pain, photophobia, lacrimation and increasing the risk of bacterial invasion.

Clinical features

- *Superficial/partial-thickness corneal laceration*: differentiate from deeper partial-/full-thickness lacerations by careful oblique illumination of the wound tract and by the Seidel's test (identifies leaking full-thickness wounds); note depth + dimensions.
- *Complications*: microbial keratitis (see ➔ Microbial keratitis: assessment, p. 222), recurrent erosions (especially if abrasion is large, ragged, involving the basement membrane (BM), and in a predisposed patient) (see ➔ Recurrent corneal erosion syndrome (RCES), p. 240).

Treatment

- Topical antibiotic (e.g. chloramphenicol oc 1% 4×/d for 3d); if there is associated infiltration, treat as a microbial keratitis. Debride any rough devitalized (grey) tissue that may hamper re-epithelialization from ingrowth of neighbouring epithelium.
- *Supportive*: consider short-term topical cycloplegic (for comfort/AC activity) and topical non-steroidal anti-inflammatory drugs (NSAIDs). Patching is not advisable for most abrasions, as it has been shown to delay closure for abrasions <10mm. However, it may help make larger abrasions more comfortable.

Hyphaema

Blood in the AC is most commonly seen in the context of blunt trauma. It ranges from a relatively mild microhyphaema (erythrocytes suspended in the aqueous) to a total '8-ball' hyphaema where the AC fill is complete (see Box 3.7 for assessment).

Box 3.7 Specific features in assessment of hyphaema

Hx   Mechanism of injury (potential for IOFB, globe rupture), ↓VA (stable, worsening may suggest rebleed), sickle cell status, risk factors, drug history (e.g. aspirin, NSAIDs, warfarin, etc.)

O/E Note depth/distribution of hyphaema, IOP, iris trauma/abnormality (defer gonioscopy where possible)
     Dilated fundoscopy: rule out any posterior segment injury

Ix   Sickle cell status
     Consider B-scan US and CT to rule out additional globe/orbital injuries (particularly if adequate clinical assessment not possible)

Causes
- *Trauma*: blunt or penetrating.
- *Surgery*: e.g. trabeculectomy, iris manipulation procedures.
- *Spontaneous*: iris/angle neovascularization, haematological disease, tumour (e.g. juvenile xanthogranuloma), IOL erosion of iris (uveitis-glaucoma-hyphaema (UGH) syndrome).

Clinical features
- *Erythrocytes in the AC*: in minor bleeds, most erythrocytes fail to settle and are only visible with the slit-lamp (microhyphaema); larger bleeds result in a macroscopically visible layer (hyphaema).
- *Complications*: rebleeds, corneal staining (especially if ↑IOP), red cell glaucoma.

Treatment
- Admit high-risk cases (see Box 3.8).
- Strict bed rest and globe protection (e.g. shield/glasses).
- Avoid aspirin/antiplatelet agents, NSAIDs, warfarin, if possible (liaise with prescribing physician).
- Topical steroid (e.g. dexamethasone 0.1% 4×/d), and consider cycloplegia (e.g. atropine 1% 2×/d, but controversial).

Monitoring/follow-up
- Daily review (inpatient or outpatient) for IOP check and to rule out rebleeds while hyphaema resolving; as improves, can be discharged and follow-up become less frequent.
- From 2wk after resolution, the patient can usually return to normal levels of activity and gonioscopy ± indented indirect ophthalmoscopy can be performed.
- Annual IOP checks (risk of angle recession glaucoma).

Red cell glaucoma

Hyphaema (usually traumatic) leads to blockage of the trabecular meshwork by red blood cells.

In 10% of cases, a rebleed may occur, usually at about 5d. Patients with sickle cell disease/trait do worse and are harder to treat (e.g. sickling may be worsened by the acidosis from carbonic anhydrase inhibitors).

Treatment

- *Of hyphaema*: as described under ➔ Treatment, p. 128.
- *Of ↑ IOP*: topical (e.g. β-blocker, α2-agonist, carbonic anhydrase inhibitor) or systemic (e.g. acetazolamide) agents, as required, but avoid topical and systemic carbonic anhydrase inhibitors in sickle cell disease/ trait.

If medical treatment fails, consider AC paracentesis ± AC washout. If all else fails, trabeculectomy is an effective treatment. Although a trabeculectomy's 'life expectancy' in these circumstances is short, it usually works long enough for the blood to clear.

Box 3.8 High-risk features in hyphaema

- Children and others with increased risk of non-compliance.
- Rebleed.
- Large hyphaema (>1/3).
- Sickle cell disease/trait..
- On antiplatelets (e.g. aspirin) or anticoagulants (e.g. warfarin).
- Significant associated injury.

Laser trauma

Even a relatively low-output laser can produce serious eye injury, simply because the eye focuses the beam and increases the retinal irradiance by a factor of over 100,000 times over that which is incident at the cornea. High-powered lasers have been in use by the military for many years. There are reports of unintentional injuries from the 1960s onwards and reports of adversarial use from 1980s. The consequence of these events was the 1995 Protocol to the Geneva Convention which specifically regulates laser use to decrease the chance of deliberate injury and bans the use of lasers designated to be blinding weapons.

The risk has not been eliminated; pilots were attacked with laser targeting designators in Bosnia in the late 1990s. With relatively cheap, readily available, and easily portable devices, insurgents, terrorists, and criminals are learning from military laser use, and rapidly increasing numbers of incidents are occurring.

Laser effects on vision

Glare/dazzle

Visible laser light can interfere with vision, even at low energies which do not produce eye damage. Exposure to continuous wave or rapidly pulsed, visible laser light can cause a significant distraction which can have serious consequences for people with vision critical tasks such as pilots or drivers.

Flash blindness and after-image

Visible laser light can also produce a lingering, yet temporary, visual loss associated with spatially localized after-effects, similar to that produced by flashbulbs. These after-effects can occur at exposure levels which do not cause eye damage.

- *Flash blindness*: the inability to detect or resolve a visual target, following exposure to a bright light.
- *After-image*: the perception of light, dark, or coloured spots after exposure to a bright light. These may persist for minutes, hours, or days. After-images are very dynamic and can change in colour ('flight of colour'), size, and intensity, depending upon the background being viewed. While they are often annoying and distracting, they are unlikely to cause a significant reduction in VA.

Visual loss from damage

Lasers can cause permanent visual loss. The degree of loss is dependent on the power and type of laser used (see Table 3.11).

Table 3.11 Laser damage according to wavelength

Wavelength range*	Pathological effect
180–315nm (UVB, UVC)	Photokeratitis
315–400nm (UVA)	Photochemical cataract
400–780nm (visible)	Retinal burn
780–1400nm (near-infrared)	Cataract, retinal burn
1.4–3.0 microns (infrared)	Aqueous flare, cataract, corneal burn
3.0 microns–1 mm	Corneal burn

* *Safety of laser products—part 1: equipment classification and requirements* (2nd edition). (2007). Geneva: International Electrotechnical Commission.

- *Anterior segment damage*: photokeratitis can significantly degrade vision due to increased light scatter from opacities. This may be transient with injuries much like those seen with arc eye or snow blindness or permanent if stomal scarring occurs. High-power injuries can lead to gross rupture. In addition, iritis can be seen in association with corneal injuries, causing photophobia, pain, and miosis.
- *Posterior segment damage*: in the case of retinal damage, functionally significant loss of vision usually occurs only if the burn directly affects the fovea. A laser's light energy may well affect both eyes, unless one is occluded or otherwise protected, because the laser beam's diameter, when shone from a significant distance, will be wider than the IPD. Low-power exposure to the fovea will have variable effects on VA, with either no effect or a mild reduction in vision to ~6/12. However, a direct high-power exposure to the foveola, leading to a significant thermal burn, will significantly reduce vision. If the retinal damage includes haemorrhage, the visual loss may be even more profound because of the initial masking effect of the haemorhage and then later toxic effects of the breakdown of haemoglobin on the surrounding photoreceptors.

Treatment
- *Corneal injuries*: the treatment for laser-induced corneal burns is the same as for thermal burns (see ➜ Thermal injury/burns: management, p. 110).
- *Retinal injuries*: at present, the treatment for laser injuries to the retina/choroid is not well defined. Ocular and oral corticosteroids have not proven effective for the treatment of retinal burns or haemorrhages. Significant vitreous or preretinal haemorrhages may benefit from vitreoretinal surgery.

Chapter 4

Lids

Anatomy and physiology (1)

The eyelids are vital to the maintenance of ocular surface integrity. Their functions include a mechanical barrier to a variety of insults, a sweeping mechanism to remove debris from the cornea (e.g. blink reflex), and a vital contribution to the production and drainage of the tear film. They also contribute to facial expression, and even minor aberrations or asymmetry may affect cosmesis.

General

- At their simplest, the lids comprise a layered structure of skin, orbicularis oculi, tarsal plates/septum, and conjunctiva (see Fig. 4.1).
- The orbital portion is more complex, with preaponeurotic fat and retractors lying deep to the septum.
- The interpalpebral fissure is usually 30mm wide and 10mm high (slightly higher in ♀).
- The resting position of the upper lid is 2mm below the superior limbus (higher in children); for the lower lid, the resting position is level with, or just above, the inferior limbus.

Skin and eyelashes

- The skin of eyelids is very thin and has loose connective tissue but no subcutaneous fat.
- It contains eccrine sweat glands and sebaceous glands.
- The lashes are arranged in 2–3 rows along the lid margins, with about 150 on the upper and 75 on the lower lid. They are replaced every 4–6mo but can grow back faster if cut. The lash follicles have apocrine sweat glands (of Moll) and modified sebaceous glands (of Zeis).

Orbicularis oculi

- This sheet of striated muscle is divided into orbital and palpebral portions; the latter is further divided into preseptal and pretarsal parts. Innervation is by temporal and zygomatic branches of VIIn for the orbicularis overlying the upper lid, and by the zygomatic branch alone for the lower lid.
- The *orbital* portion forms a ring of muscle arising from the medial canthal tendon and parts of the orbital rim.
- The *preseptal* part of each lid runs from the medial canthal tendon, arches over the anterior surface of the orbital septum, and inserts into the lateral horizontal raphe. Similarly, each *pretarsal* part arises from the medial canthal tendon, arches over the tarsal plates, and inserts into the lateral canthal tendon and horizontal raphe.
- Horner muscle is formed by deep pretarsal fibres running medially to insert on to the lacrimal crest.
- Functions of the orbicularis oculi include lid closure and the lacrimal pump mechanism.

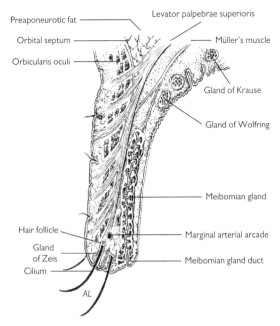

Preaponeurotic fat

Orbital septum

Orbicularis oculi

Levator palpebrae superioris

Müller's muscle

Gland of Krause

Gland of Wolfring

Meibomian gland

Hair follicle

Gland of Zeis

Cilium

Marginal arterial arcade

Meibomian gland duct

AL

Fig. 4.1 Anatomical section of the lid.

Anatomy and physiology (2)

Orbital septum and tarsal plates

The septum is a sheet of tissue that arises from the orbital rim where it is continuous with orbital fascia and periosteum.

Towards the palpebral margin, it is thickened, forming the tarsal plates that maintain the shape of the lid. These are 25mm long, 1mm thick, and of variable height: about 10mm high for the upper lid, 5mm for the lower lid. They also contain MGs (about 35 in the upper lid, 25 in the lower lid) which secrete the lipid component of the tear film.

Canthal tendons

- At each end, the tarsal plates are stabilized by a horizontal canthal tendon.
- The medial canthal tendon is well developed with an anterior limb arising from the anterior lacrimal crest, and a posterior limb from the posterior lacrimal crest.
- The lateral canthal tendon lies just posterior to the horizontal raphe and inserts into the zygomatic bone (Whitnall's tubercle) and merges posteriorly with the lateral check ligament (from the sheath of lateral rectus).

Fat pads

The preaponeurotic fat pads are extensions of orbital fat lying just posterior to the orbital septum.

Lid retractors

- The upper lid retractors comprise levator palpebrae superioris (LPS) and Müller's muscle. LPS originates from the orbital apex and runs forward over superior rectus (SR) to the orbital rim. At this point, it is stabilized by the superior transverse ligament of Whitnall (a fascial bridge running between the trochlea and the lacrimal gland fascia), permitting the distal LPS to run steeply downward and insert as an aponeurosis into the septum, tarsus, and orbicularis.
- Innervation is by IIIn; Müller's muscle is an accessory retractor muscle supplied by the sympathetic system.
- Overaction is demonstrated in sympathetic overdrive and TED; underaction is seen in Horner's syndrome.
- The lower lid retractors are more rudimentary but are similarly divided into voluntary and sympathetic groups.

Conjunctiva

See ➲ Anatomy and physiology, p. 178. The conjunctiva is a mucous membrane comprising non-keratinized epithelium, BM, and stroma. The epithelium of the palpebral conjunctiva is of stratified squamous form. It contains mucin-secreting goblet cells and crypts of Henle.

Nerves, arteries, veins, and lymphatics

Nerves

- *Sensation to the lower lid* is mainly by the infraorbital nerve (Vb), with infratrochlear branch of the nasociliary nerve (Va) innervating the medial canthal area.
- *Sensation to the upper lid* is by lacrimal, supraorbital, and supratrochlear nerve (all Va).
- Orbicularis oculi is innervated by VIIn, LPS by IIIn, and Müller's muscle by the sympathetic system.

Arteries

- Arterial supply is by three arcades that form anastomoses between the medial palpebral artery (from the terminal ophthalmic artery) and the lateral palpebral artery (from the lacrimal artery).
- *In the upper lid*, there is a marginal arcade 2mm above the margin and a peripheral arcade at the top of the tarsal plate.
- *In the lower lid*, the arcade lies 4mm below the margin.

Veins

Venous drainage is to superficial temporal vein laterally and to the ophthalmic and angular veins medially.

Lymphatics

Lymphatic drainage is to the parotid glands laterally, the submandibular glands inferiorly, and the anterior cervical chain inferomedially.

Eyelash disorders

Misdirected lashes

Misdirection of the eyelashes is a common source of ocular irritation.

Corneal changes range from mild punctate epitheliopathy to ulceration, $2°$ infection, scarring, and perforation.

Classification

Trichiasis may be classified as:

Misdirected eyelashes

Lashes arise from their normal position but are posteriorly directed, normally due to minor scarring of the lid margin or lash orifice.

Metaplastic lashes: congenital (distichiasis)

Lashes arise from an abnormal position (e.g. from, or slightly posterior to, the MGs). It is an uncommon congenital abnormality that may be sporadic or autosomal dominant (AD). Can rarely be associated with Meige's (lymphoedema-distichiasis) syndrome.

Metaplastic lashes: acquired

Lashes arise from an abnormal position $2°$ to chronic injury, e.g. meibomitis, cicatrizing conjunctivitis (see ➲ Cicatricial conjunctivitis (1), p. 193), or surgical trauma.

Pseudotrichiasis

Lashes arise from the normal position but are posteriorly directed due to marginal entropion.

Treatment options

Preventative

- Prevention is better than cure—management of MG disease, immunosuppression of cicatricial conjunctival disease, and meticulous surgical eyelid margin reapposition to prevent notches.

Lash removal

- Epilation.

Lash destruction

- Electrolysis, cryotherapy (double freeze–thaw technique; 25s freeze, 4min thaw, with or without grey line split), lash root trephination, photoablation, argon or diode laser are all useful techniques for small numbers of lashes. These techniques need to be used with caution and attention to the underlying condition, as they can cause inflammation, scarring, and loss of tarsal plate that can exacerbate the condition.

Surgery

In marginal entropion, surgical correction is required, with technique depending on degree of entropion and underlying cause:

- Jones retractor plication ± horizontal lid tightening.
- Anterior lamellar repositioning ± grey line split ± mucous membrane or hard palate graft.
- Anterior lamellar excision of lash roots.
- Tarsal fracture with 180° rotation ± mucous membrane graft.

Lash infestations

Infestation of the lashes by lice causes itching, blepharitis, and a follicular conjunctivitis. The lice and nits (eggs) are easily identified on slit-lamp examination.

Treatment options include mechanical removal or destruction (e.g. cryotherapy) for localized cases, and chemical for generalized cases. Chemical options (e.g. malathion or permethrin) require a 12h application to the whole body and repeated 7d later; aqueous malathion is effective in treating lash phthiarisis (unlicensed use), but ocular contact is contraindicated with all these agents.

Generalized infestation also requires laundry of all clothes and linen to >50° C.

Phthiriasis

Infestation by *Phthirus pubis* ('crab louse'). It is most commonly seen in adults in whom it is usually acquired as a sexually transmitted infection.

Pediculosis

Infestation by *Pediculus humanus corporis* or *capitis* ('head-louse'). If heavily infested, the lice may spread to involve lashes.

Madarosis

This is partial or complete loss of lashes. It may be a purely local phenomenon or associated with systemic disease (see Table 4.1).

Table 4.1 Causes of madarosis

Local	Chronic meibomian gland disease or anterior blepharitis
	Cicatrizing conjunctivitis
	Iatrogenic (cryotherapy/radiotherapy/surgery)
Systemic	Alopecia (patchy/totalis/universalis)
	Psoriasis
	Hypothyroidism
	Leprosy

Lash poliosis

This is whitening of the lashes. It may be associated with premature greying of the hair, a purely local phenomenon, or be associated with systemic pathology (see Table 4.2).

Table 4.2 Causes of poliosis

Local	Chronic lid margin disease
Systemic	Sympathetic ophthalmia
	Vogt–Koyanagi–Harada (VKH) syndrome
	Waardenburg syndrome
	Hypogonadism

Blepharitis and Meibomian gland dysfunction (MGD) (1)

The term blepharitis is frequently used as shorthand for chronic lid margin disease. Blepharitis refers to any inflammation of the lid and includes a wide range of diseases such as preseptal cellulitis, internal and external hordeola, herpes simplex virus (HSV)/varicella-zoster virus (VZV) infections, etc.

The descriptive terms anterior and posterior blepharitis are sometimes used to indicate the distribution of disease.

MGD is defined as a chronic, diffuse abnormality of the MGs, commonly characterized by terminal duct obstruction and/or qualitative and quantitative changes in the glandular secretion.[1]

MG function

MG-derived lipids contain cholesterol, wax esters, diesters, triacylglycerol, free cholesterol, free fatty acids, and phospholipids. These interact with tear film aqueous proteins in a complex of:

- Proteins (lipocalin, lysozyme, surfactant proteins) intercalated with an outer non-polar lipid layer mediate tear film physical properties, including surface tension.
- Long chain (O-acyl)-hydroxy fatty acids form intermediate surfactant polar lipid sublayer adjacent to the aqueous phase of the underlying muco-aqueous gradient.
- This lipoprotein construction confers tear film stability by minimizing evaporation and maintaining tear film integrity; it also forms an effective barrier, protecting the eye from bacterial agents and organic matter.

MGD

- *Causes*: intrinsic (Meibomian oil deficiency, disorders of lid aperture, low blink rate (Parkinson's disease), drug action) and extrinsic (ocular surface disease, eye drop preservatives, vitamin A deficiency).
- *Pathology*: reservoir of lid oil is reduced, with delayed spreading. Stagnation of the oils in the MGs → alteration of lipid structure, conferring pro-inflammatory properties → aggravated by lid margin hypercolonization of staphylococcal species that secrete esterases, lipases. Release fatty acids, mono/diglycerides, together with exotoxins, giving rise to characteristic tear film 'foam', chronic inflammation, lid margin hyperkeratinization, cicatrization, and irreversible blockage of MGs.
- *Clinical features*: staging of MGD is based upon the quality of MG secretions expressed from the glands, changes in lid morphology defined by the internal migration of the mucocutaneous junction, changes in the MG orifices, acini structure, and glandular dropout. (See Table 4.3.)
- The stage of disease is used to direct treatment protocols which include modulating diet, lid margin hygiene, warm glandular expression, topical emollient lubrication, tetracyclines, and topical anti-inflammatory therapy (see Table 4.3).

Table 4.3 Clinical stages of MGD with therapeutic options[*]

Stage of MGD	Clinical description	Treatment
1	No symptoms Minimally altered secretions No ocular surface staining	Inform patient about MGD Alter diet; reduce environmental stress Consider lid hygiene and warm expressions
2	Minimal to mild symptoms of discomfort, itching, and photophobia Minimal to mild altered secretions None or limited ocular surface staining and TFBUT <10s	Improve ambient humidity; increase dietary omega-3 intake Lid hygiene and warm expression (minimum of 4min twice daily) Lubricants, topical azithromycin, emollient lubricant, liposomal spray Consider tetracycline derivatives
3	Moderate symptoms with definite limitation of activity Moderately altered secretions with increased lid margin vascularity, telangiectasia, and orifice plugging Mild to moderate conjunctival and peripheral corneal staining and TFBUT ≈ 5s	All of stage 2 treatment Plus oral tetracycline derivatives Lubricant ointment Consider anti-inflammatory therapy for dry eye
4	Marked symptoms with definite limitation of activity Severely altered secretions with MG dropout and displacement Central corneal staining and conjunctival inflammation and TFBUT ≈ 0–5s	All of stage 3 treatment Plus anti-inflammatory therapy for dry eye
Plus disease	Exacerbated inflammatory ocular surface disease Mucosal keratinization Phlyctenular keratitis Trichiasis MG cysts Anterior blepharitis Demodex-related anterior blepharitis, with cylindrical dandruff	Pulsed soft steroid, as indicated Therapeutic CL/scleral CL Steroid therapy Epilation, cryotherapy Intralesional steroid or excision Topical antibiotic or antibiotic-steroid combination Tea tree oil scrubs

[*] Adapted from Geerling G et al. The International Workshop on Meibomian Gland Dysfunction: Report of the Subcommittee on Management and Treatment of Meibomian Gland Dysfunction. Invest Ophthalmol Vis Sci 2011;**52**:2050–649.

1. Nichols KK et al. The International Workshop on Meibomian Gland Dysfunction: executive summary. Invest Ophthalmol Vis Sci 2011;**52**:1922–9.

Blepharitis and Meibomian gland dysfunction (2)

Treatment of MGD[2]

- *Lid hygiene*: effective lid margin hygiene is paramount, requiring application of warm compresses for up to 30min twice daily to increase the fluidity of the stagnant oils within the glands which eases expression when lids are massaged by a firm stroking motion towards the lid margins. Expressed matter is cleansed lightly with a cotton-tipped applicator, moistened with boiled, cooled water with bicarbonate, tea tree oil, or commercially available lid wipes. In mild to moderate MGD, hygiene improves symptoms/clinical signs. In extensive glandular and duct atrophy associated with thickened and indurated lids, cicatrization, and negligible excreta, response may only be partial or even refractory.

NB Do not use baby shampoo, as this contains perfume and irritates the eyes.

- *Topical treatments*: antibiotics, lubrication (guar gum substitutes, e.g. Systane® preparations, are beneficial in evaporative dry eye), corticosteroids if severe inflammation. Non-preserved drops, ointments.
- *Liposomal sprays*: e.g. Actimist™, Clarymist (OTC preparations). Liposomes are sprayed on the closed eyelid margins. When the eyes open, the liposomes spread across the surface of the eye, creating a new oily film.
- *Oral tetracyclines*: doxycycline 100mg 1×/day (protease inhibitor, lipid soluble, penetrates into MG). Doses as low as 20mg 1×/day are effective.
- *Environmental factors*: increased humidity (cool mist humidifiers); wrap around glasses; avoid wind, hot air, smoke.
- *Diet*: there is increasing evidence a diet high in omega-3 fats can help improve ocular surface health, MG function, and dry eye disease (see Box 4.1).

Box 4.1 **Role of diet in MGD**

- Aim for omega-3:omega-6 ratio of 1:1. In the western diet, this is currently ~1:25. Improving the omega-3 index has wide implications (heart disease, joint problems, macular degeneration).
- The most important omega-3s are eicosapentaenoic acid (EPA) and docosahexaenoic acid (DHA) (source: wild fish). Alphalinolenic acid (ALA) (source: green leafy vegetables, flaxseed, soya beans, canola oil, and walnuts) is also an omega-3 and can be converted to EPA and DHA, but the conversion rate is very low in humans (about 1%).
- Omega-6 fatty acids include linolenic acid (LA), γ-linolenic acid (GLA), arachidonic acid (ARA) (source: vegetable oils, red meat-derived saturated fats, fast foods, evening primrose oil, and borage oil).
- Redress omega-3 vs omega-6 balance, and improve the omega-3 index. Increase oily fish intake (mackerel, salmon, sardines, herring, fresh tuna (not canned because the canning process removes the beneficial oils)), flaxseed oil, omega-3 supplements (better consumed as 're-esterified' omega-3 (soon available in the UK)). Increase omega-7 (sea buckthorn oil).

Meibomianitis

Meibomianitis describes a subset of MGD in which inflammation is a major feature. It is often associated with facial rosacea.

Clinical features
- Burning, worse in mornings.
- Inflamed MG openings, thickened secretions; glands may become obstructed ± chalazia (lipogranulomatous inflammation within MG) ± internal hordeolum (acute abscess formation within MG).

Treatment
- As for MGD (see Table 4.3), with tetracyclines, lid hygiene, and topical therapies, as needed.

Bacterial blepharitis

This results in a mainly anterior blepharitis. It is usually due to lid commensals, most commonly staphylococci, but may also arise from streptococci, *Propionibacterium acnes*, and *Moraxella*.

Clinical features
- Burning, gritty, crusted.
- Injected lid margins, scales at lash bases ± external hordeolum (abscess of lash follicle and associated glands) ± preseptal cellulitis.

Treatment
- *Lid hygiene*: regular lid margin cleaning (see ➲ Treatment of MGD, p. 142).
- *Ocular lubricants*: tear film instability is common.
- *Antibiotics*: topical antibiotics may be required for acute exacerbations; external hordeola and preseptal cellulitis also require oral antibiotics.
- *Topical steroids (weak)*: may be required in severe cases with corneal involvement.

Seborrhoeic blepharitis

This results in a mixed anterior/posterior blepharitis arising from excessive Meibomian secretions. It is commonly associated with seborrhoeic dermatitis of the scalp.

Clinical features
- Burning, gritty, crusted.
- Lashes stuck together by soft scales, oily lid margin, foamy tear film.

Treatment
As for MGD (see Table 4.3), with tetracyclines, lid hygiene, and topical therapies, as needed.

NB Unilateral blepharitis (and recurrent chalazia) should be treated with extreme suspicion, as lid tumours (e.g. sebaceous cell carcinoma) may present in this way.

2. Geerling G et al. The International Workshop on Meibomian Gland Dysfunction: Report of the Subcommittee on Management and Treatment of Meibomian Gland Dysfunction. *Invest Ophthalmol Vis Sci* 2011;**52**:2050–64.

Lid lumps: cysts and abscesses

Anterior lamella

External hordeolum (stye)

- This is an acute abscess within a lash follicle and its associated glands of Zeis and Moll.
- It results in a tender lump, with associated inflammation.
- Is usually staphylococcal in origin.
- *Treatment*: warm compresses; if associated with preseptal cellulitis, add in oral antibiotics (see ➲ Orbital and preseptal cellulitis, p. 596), e.g. flucloxacillin 250–500mg 4×/d for 1wk).

Cyst of Moll

These chronic cysts (or apocrine hidrocystomas) are markedly translucent and arise from blockage of the apocrine duct of the gland of Moll. There is likely to be recurrence with incision and drainage. More definitive treatments are deroofing with diathermy to the cyst base or total excision. Similar lesions may arise from blockage of the eccrine ducts of sweat glands of the eyelid skin.

Cyst of Zeis

These chronic cysts are poorly translucent and arise from blockage of the gland of Zeis. Similar sebaceous cysts may arise in the periorbital skin but rarely from the lids.

Xanthelasma

These common lesions result from the deposition of lipids within perivascular xanthoid cells and may be a sign of hyperlipidaemia. Clinically, they appear as yellowish subcutaneous deposits located on the medial aspect of the lids and periorbit.

Molluscum contagiosum

- These pearly, umbilicated nodules are common in children/young adults. They are caused by a double-stranded DNA (dsDNA) virus of the pox virus group; profuse lesions are seen with HIV infection and chemotherapy.
- Transmission is by close contact. If at the lid margin, they may cause a persistent follicular conjunctivitis (see ➲ Viral conjunctivitis, p. 186). A unilateral follicular conjunctivitis should lead the clinician to search the eyelid margins for such lesions.
- *Treatment*: if troublesome, the lesions may be removed by cryotherapy, cauterization, shave excision, or expression/curettage.

Posterior lamella

Internal hordeolum

- This is an acute abscess within an MG. It results in a tender lump, with associated inflammation. It is usually staphylococcal in origin.
- *Treatment*: acute—warm compresses; acute with preseptal cellulitis—add in oral antibiotics (see ➲ Orbital and preseptal cellulitis, p. 596); chronic (or large acute lesion)—also perform incision and curettage.

Chalazion
- This is the commonest of all lid lumps. They arise from chronic lipogranulomatous inflammation of blocked MGs. They are usually located on the upper lid and are commoner in patients with chronic marginal blepharitis, rosacea, or seborrhoeic dermatitis.
- *Treatment*: small chalazia are often ignored by the patient and resolve with time. Hot compresses can be effective in encouraging drainage. Persistent or symptomatic lesions may be treated surgically by incision and curettage. Any recurrence of the lesion should be regarded as suspicious and a biopsy sent for histology (see Box 4.2).

Box 4.2 Outline of incision and curettage of a chalazion
- *Consent*: discuss what the procedure involves, likelihood of further chalazia/recurrence, and risks, including bruising, bleeding, and infection.
- Identify location of chalazion (it will be less obvious after instillation of anaesthetic).
- Instil topical anaesthesia (e.g. oxybuprocaine) in the fornix of the affected eye.
- Prepare surgical area with 5% povidone iodine.
- Inject local anaesthetic (e.g. 1–2% lidocaine with adrenaline 1 in 200,000) SC to the affected lid.
- Evert lid with guarded lid clamp.
- Incise chalazion vertically with surgical blade (e.g. No. 11) from the conjunctival surface.
- Curette to remove the chalazion contents and to break down any loculations.
- Instil topical antibiotic (e.g. Oc chloramphenicol 1%).
- Remove clamp, and apply pressure to ensure haemostasis.
- Apply eye patch; this can be removed after 2–3h.
- Advise patient not to drive with eye patch.
- *Post-procedure*: topical antibiotic (e.g. Oc chloramphenicol 1% 4×/d for 1wk ± topical steroid); if atypical or recurrent chalazion, then curettings/biopsy should be sent for histology.

Lid lumps: benign and premalignant tumours

Benign tumours

Anterior lamella

Papillomas
- Skin papillomas are very common.
- They are derived from squamous cells.
- May be non-specific or related to human papillomavirus (HPV) (viral wart or verruca vulgaris).
- They are either broad-based (sessile) or narrow-based (pedunculated) protrusions with irregular surfaces formed from finger-like extensions.

Seborrhoeic keratosis (basal cell papilloma)
- Common, especially in the elderly.
- Derived from basal cells.
- Are broad-based protrusions, usually brown in colour, with a greasy irregular surface.

Keratoacanthoma
- Uncommon tumours that grow rapidly for 2–6wk and then may involute over 4–6mo. Most pathologists now consider keratoacanthoma to be one end of a spectrum of squamous cell carcinoma (SCC).
- They are non-pigmented protrusions with a keratin-filled central crater.
- Some cases cannot be distinguished clinically from an SCC with malignant potential. In these cases, complete excision is necessary, as an incomplete specimen may be indistinguishable from an SCC on histological examination.

Naevi
- Common cutaneous lesions that are classified according to depth.
- They arise from arrested epidermal melanocytes.
- *Junctional naevi* are flat, brown and are located at the epidermis/dermis junction. *Dermal naevi* are elevated, may not be visibly pigmented, and are located within the dermis. *Compound naevi* are slightly elevated and share features of junctional and dermal types.
- Overall, there is a low risk of transformation that is slightly higher for the more superficial naevi.

Vascular
- Congenital vascular anomalies, such as capillary haemangiomas (strawberry naevi) and port-wine stain, may involve the lids.
- Capillary haemangiomas usually involute by the age of 5. If lesions are potentially amblyogenic, the treatment options are oral propranolol, intralesional steroid, or excision. The commonest dose of oral propranolol is 2mg/kg/d. Treatment is continued until the end of the proliferative period (6–12mo) or until stabilization of astigmatism. Propranolol should be used in conjunction with paediatricians—the complications of hypoglycaemia and hypotension are more common in young infants.

Posterior lamella

Pyogenic granuloma

This is an abnormal response to injury such as trauma or, less commonly, inflammation. It is a red, highly vascular mass that appears to be a haemangioma with associated granulation tissue.

Premalignant tumours

Actinic keratosis

This common lesion of sun-exposed skin is relatively uncommon on the lids. Clinically, it is a flat, scaly lesion with hyperkeratosis and may have a keratin horn. Histologically, it shows parakeratosis and cellular atypia but no invasion. Rarely develops into SCC.

Lid lumps: malignant tumours (1)

Basal cell carcinoma (BCC)

- This is the *commonest lid malignancy* (90% of lid malignancies).
- Preferentially affects the lower lid, followed by medial canthus, upper lid, and then lateral canthus.
- *Risk factors include*: increasing age, white skin, sun exposure, some cutaneous syndromes (xeroderma pigmentosa, basal cell naevus syndrome), and albinism.
- Can be locally invasive and destructive but very rarely metastasizes (<0.1%).

Clinical features

- *Nodular type (rodent ulcer)*: firm nodule, rolled pearly edges, fine telangiectasia, surface ulceration.
- *Morpheiform (sclerosing) and infiltrative types*: often minimal surface changes or scar-like plaques overlying extensive infiltration, so may mimic chronic inflammation/scarring (e.g. chronic marginal blepharitis).
- *Superficial type*: reddish, scaly plaques. Can resemble Bowen's disease, nummular eczema, or fungal infection.
- *Other clinical subtypes*: micronodular, pigmented, differentiated BCCs such as cystic, keratotic (pilar), follicular.

Histological subtypes

- Nodular, superficial, and pigmented—more benign.
- Morphoeic, micronodular, infiltrative, basosquamous—more associated with aggressive invasion and destruction.
- *Typical histological features are*: nests of basaloid tumour cells with hyperchromatic nuclei and sparse cytoplasm, with peripheral palisading of nuclei, cleft artefacts, and variable inflammation and necrosis.
- Perivascular and perineural invasion are features of the most aggressive tumours.

Treatment

- Wide local excision may be achieved by Mohs' micrographical technique (especially for morpheiform type) or by excisional biopsy with histological (e.g. slow Mohs or paraffin or frozen section) control. A 2–4mm margin is recommended. Lesions incompletely excised at the deep margins are at greatest risk of recurrence. Recurrent tumours are more difficult to treat.
- When non-surgical treatments are used, diagnosis should be confirmed by incisional biopsy.
- Cryotherapy in double or triple freeze-thaw technique (−50 to −60° C for 30s ×3)—useful for low-risk BCCs, such as small nodular BCCs, or in patients with multiple lesions.
- Topical imiquimod 5% cream (an immune response modifier that stimulates apoptosis)—indicated for small superficial BCC. Applied 5 × weekly for 6–12wk; 82–90% response rate with estimated 2y recurrence of 20.6%

- Photodynamic therapy (PDT)—for superficial BCC, average clearance 85%.
- Vismodegib—approved in the USA, Jan 2012, for recurrent or metastatic BCC not amenable to surgery or irradiation. It is the first Hedgehog pathway inhibitor.

SCC

This is much less common (2–5% of lid malignancies) but has a much higher risk of metastasis, often by lymphatic spread. It preferentially affects the lower lid.

- *Risk factors include*: increasing age, white skin (Fitzpatrick skin types I and II), sun exposure, X-ray and chemical exposure, immunosuppression, and xeroderma pigmentosa.

Clinical features

- *Nodular type*: hyperkeratotic, with irregular margins; resemble BCC.
- *Plaque type*: erythematous, scaly, hyperkeratotic plaque.
- *Both types*: may ulcerate, show lymphatic and perineural spread, and metastasize.
- *Cutaneous horn*: may be hyperkeratotic actinic keratosis or well-differentiated SCC.
- *Bowen's disease*: squamous carcinoma *in situ* (without invasion through the epidermal BM).

Histology

- Epidermal cell proliferation, with dermis invasion by atypical keratinocytes and epithelial/keratinous pearls or squamous eddies.

Treatment

Wide local excision may be achieved by Mohs' micrographical technique or by excisional biopsy with histological (e.g. paraffin or frozen section) control. This is usually curative for early lesions. Orbital involvement may require exenteration. SCC *in situ* may be treated surgically or with cryotherapy, imiquimod cream, 5-fluorouracil (5-FU), mitomycin, or PDT.

Sebaceous gland carcinoma

This uncommon tumour (1–2% of lid malignancies) usually arises from the MGs or occasionally the glands of Zeis. It is aggressive and carries a significant mortality rate (10% overall mortality rate, but up to 67% 5y mortality if metastasizes). It is commoner in the upper lid. It may also develop in the caruncle.

- *Risk factors include*: increasing age and ♀ sex. May occur as part of the Muir–Torre (sebaceous neoplasia-visceral carcinoma) syndrome.

Clinical features
- *Nodular type*: firm nodule resembling chalazion (so biopsy 'recurrent chalazion').
- *Spreading type*: diffuse infiltration may involve the conjunctiva and resemble chronic blepharoconjunctivitis. Loss of lashes is common.

Treatment
Perform mapping biopsies of conjunctiva to assess extent of tumour, because of the risk of pagetoid spread, and confirm diagnosis with full-thickness lid biopsy (histology; cytoplasmic lipid vacuolization—warn histopathologist, and send fresh tissue to assist with fat staining). Wide local excision is essential but may be difficult to achieve due to pagetoid and multicentric spread.

Regional lymph node clearance and exenteration may be performed, depending on tumour extent.

Lid lumps: malignant tumours (2)

Malignant melanoma

- Melanoma only rarely affects the lids (<1% lid malignancies). However, it must be considered when assessing pigmented lesions, as it can be fatal.
- It has a non-invasive, horizontal growth phase, followed by an invasive, vertical growth phase.
- *Risk factors include:* increasing age, white skin, sun exposure and sunburn, and some cutaneous syndromes (dysplastic naevus syndrome, xeroderma pigmentosa).
- *ABCD rule:* Asymmetry, Border irregularities, Colour heterogeneity, Dynamics (evolution in colour, elevation, or size).

Clinical features

- *Lentigo maligna type:* initially flat pigmented lesion with well-defined margins (lentigo maligna) that starts to show elevation as it invades dermis (malignant transformation).
- *Superficial spreading type:* smaller pigmented lesion with irregular margins and mild elevation ± nodules, induration; more aggressive.
- *Nodular type:* nodule (may not be visibly pigmented) with rapid growth, ulceration, and bleeding.

Treatment

Wide local excision with 10mm margins (confirmed on histology) is recommended but not always possible. Recommended excision margins depend on tumour thickness. Some recommend regional lymph node dissection for tumours >1.5mm thick or with evidence of haematogenous or lymphatic spread.

Novel treatments for unresectable tumours include vemurafenib which has received Food and Drug Administration (FDA) approval for late-stage melanoma. It is a kinase inhibitor with specific activity against malignant melanoma with the V600E mutation in BRAF.

Prognosis

Poor prognosis correlates with histological depth of invasion (by Clark's levels) and thickness (by the Breslow system). Thus, 5y survival post-excision is 100% for tumours ≤0.75mm thick, but only 50% for those >1.5mm thick. Depending on tumour invasion and thickness, sentinel lymph node biopsy may need to be considered.

Kaposi's sarcoma

This is a rare tumour arising from human herpesvirus 8 (HHV8) in the general population but is relatively common in patients with acquired immune deficiency syndrome (AIDS). Clinically, it is a vascular purple-red nodule that may also affect the conjunctiva.

Treatment for symptomatic lesions is usually radiotherapy; it is not curative.

Merkel cell carcinoma

This is a very rare tumour that is more common in the elderly. It shows rapid growth and is highly malignant. Clinically, it is a non-tender purple nodule, usually on the upper lid.

Repair of eyelid defects

Technique will depend on the extent, depth, and location of tissue loss.

Periocular skin and anterior lamella only

- Healing by 2° intention/laisser-faire/granulation (particularly suited to the medial canthus).
- Direct closure, with or without undermining.
- *Other useful techniques for the medial canthus*: rhomboid flap, bilobed flap, glabellar flap, skin graft.
- Advancement flaps and skin grafts.

Full-thickness eyelid defects

These should be repaired without undue tension. Technique will not only depend on tissue loss and whether upper or lower lid is affected, but also on pre-existing tissue laxity. General guidelines are:

- Small—direct closure.
- Medium—lateral canthotomy/cantholysis, periosteal flap, Tenzel or MacGregor flaps.
- Large—Hughes tarsoconjunctival flap from upper to lower lid with full-thickness skin graft or free tarsal graft with skin-muscle flap. Hewes upper to lower lid tarsal transposition flap. The Cutler–Beard flap can be used for similar upper lid defects.
- Occasionally, larger flaps are required for vertically deep defects, e.g. Mustarde cheek rotation flap.

Skin graft considerations

Non-hair-bearing skin: skin from the same or opposite upper lid provides the best match, if available. A minimum of 21mm vertical residual skin should be left. If not available, good matches can be harvested from the pre- or post-auricular areas, supraclavicular, or inner arm. Post-operatively, pressure should be applied to assist graft attachment and prevent haematoma formation between graft and bed.

Ectropion

Ectropion is the abnormal eversion of the eyelid (usually the lower) away from the globe. This disruption frequently causes irritation and may threaten the integrity of the ocular surface. It is usually acquired as a result of involutional, cicatricial, mechanical, or paralytic processes, e.g. VIIn palsy, but may occasionally be congenital.

Involutional ectropion

This is the commonest form and results from age-related tissue laxity.

Clinical features (non-specific)

These are present in most ectropia:
- Variable irritation, epiphora, recurrent infections.
- Everted lid (varies from slightly everted punctum to eversion of the whole lid—tarsal/shelf ectropion), conjunctival irritation/inflammation, and keratinization.

Clinical features (specific)
- Test for lid laxity and speed of snap-back (pull away from globe; >10mm is abnormal), lateral canthal tendon laxity (pull lid medially; >2mm movement of canthal angle is abnormal; lateral canthus also has rounded appearance), medial canthal tendon laxity (pull lid laterally; >2mm movement of punctum is abnormal (although treatment is usually reserved for cases where the punctum can be distracted to the level of the centre of the pupil), inferior retractor weakness.

Treatment

Surgery is directed towards the specific defect. Most commonly, this requires lid shortening for horizontal laxity, but the procedure of choice will depend on the relative contribution of lid, tendons, canthal position, etc. (see Table 4.4).

Cicatricial ectropion

This is uncommon. It occurs when scarring vertically shortens the anterior lamella. Causes include trauma, burns, radiotherapy, and dermatitis (ocular medications) and epiphora.

Clinical features (specific)
- Scarring, no skin laxity, tension lines in skin when lid put into position; features of underlying disease.

Treatment
- *Medical*: the cicatrizing process should be controlled as best possible.
- *Surgical*: skin-gaining procedures (see Table 4.4); treatment for epiphora (see Chapter 5).

Mechanical ectropion

This is uncommon. It occurs when masses (e.g. tumours) displace the lid away from the globe.

Clinical features (specific)
- Visible/palpable mass, e.g. tumour, cyst, oedema.

Treatment

Removal of the cause may lead to complete resolution; if residual lid laxity, treat as for involutional (see Table 4.4). However, occasionally, an autogenous fascia lata sling may be required.

Table 4.4 Overview of common ectropion operations

Operation	Indication	Procedure
Horizontal lid shortening		
Lateral tarsal strip	Lateral/generalized laxity	Lid shortened laterally, tightened, and elevated at lateral canthus
Wedge excision	Lid laxity, no tendon laxity	Full-thickness pentagon excised
Kuhnt–Szymanowski	As above + excess skin	Wedge excision + lower lid blepharoplasty
Medial canthal resection	Significant medial laxity only	Lid shortened laterally and tightened at medial canthus
Transconjunctival retractor plication +LTS	Shelf ectropion poorly repositioned with lid shortening alone	Retractors identified and reattached to lower border of tarsus
Vertical lid shortening		
Diamond excision	Mild medial ectropion	Diamond of tarsoconjunctiva excised just inferior to punctum
Combined shortening procedures		
Lazy-T procedure	Medial ectropion with lid laxity	Diamond excision + wedge excision
Skin-gaining procedures		
Z-plasty	Focal scars	Z-incision with middle stroke excising scar gains vertical height
Skin flap/graft	Congenital/cicatricial skin loss	Transposition flap with pedicle or full-thickness autologous graft
SOOF or mid-face lift	Midface descent	Sub-periosteal or sub-orbicularis oculi fascia elevation and fixation to orbital rim
Horizontal fissure shortening		
Medial canthoplasty combined with lateral tarsal strip or lateral tarsorrhaphy	Cornea threatened by lagophthalmos	Fuses the lids at lateral and medial aspect

Paralytic ectropion

This is uncommon. It occurs when VIIn palsy causes orbicularis weakness.

Clinical features (specific)
- Weakness of orbicularis and other facial muscles; lagophthalmos, corneal exposure likely.

NB Corneal sensation may be compromised by underlying disease. These patients must be taught their only warning of exposure-related problems might be redness of the eye or reduced VA.

Treatment
- *Topical*: ocular lubricants; consider taping eye shut at night.
- *Surgical*: depends on severity and associated laxity; options include medial canthoplasty, lateral canthal sling, lateral tarsorrhaphy, upper lid lowering by botulinum toxin injection, anterior levator recession with mullerectomy, or placement of gold or titanium weight. Orbicularis or nerve transfer procedures are occasionally performed.

Congenital

This is rare but may be seen in Down's syndrome and blepharophimosis syndrome. It may occur in both the lower and upper lids and is due to a shortage of skin.

Entropion

Entropion is abnormal inversion of the eyelid (usually the lower) toward the globe. Abrasion of the cornea by the inwardly directed lashes can result in ulceration and 2° infection.

Usually acquired as a result of involutional or cicatricial processes but may occasionally be congenital.

Involutional entropion

This is the commonest form and results from inferior retractor dysfunction with tissue laxity and possibly override of preseptal orbicularis over pretarsal orbicularis.

Clinical features (non-specific)

These are present in most entropia:
- FB sensation, photophobia, blepharospasm, epiphora.
- Inverted lid (transient/permanent), pseudotrichiasis, keratopathy, pannus formation.

Clinical features (specific)

Test for inferior retractor weakness/dehiscence (reduced movement of lower lid in downgaze); test for lid laxity as for ectropion (see ➜ Clinical features (specific), p. 154).

Treatment

Surgery is directed towards the specific defect. Most commonly, this requires lid shortening for horizontal laxity and reattachment of the retractors (see Table 4.5). Botox can be considered while awaiting surgery.

Orbicularis (Wies) type procedures are no longer considered effective.

Cicatricial entropion

This is uncommon. It occurs when scarring vertically shortens the posterior lamella. It is caused by cicatrizing conjunctivitis, most commonly due to trachoma, ocular cicatricial pemphigoid and other bullous diseases, chemical injuries, radiotherapy, trauma, and severe blepharitis. (see Cicatricial conjunctivitis (1), ➜ p. 193).

Clinical features (specific)

- *Chronic*: loss of plica semilunaris, loss of forniceal depth, formation of symblepharon/ankyloblepharon, dry eye signs. In trachoma, subtarsal fibrosis is likely to be evident.
- *Acute*: papillary conjunctivitis, subconjunctival vesicles, injection, evolving picture.

Treatment

- *Medical*: the cicatrizing process should be optimally controlled, especially before surgical intervention (see Cicatricial conjunctivitis (1), ➜ p. 193).
- *Surgical*: retractor reattachment may suffice in mild cases; transverse tarsotomy (tarsal fracture) or mucosal graft if moderate/severe loss of posterior lamella (see Table 4.5). Recently, anterior lamellar excision has been proposed as a simple treatment that does not appear to aggravate the inflammatory process.

Table 4.5 Overview of common entropion operations

Operation	Indication	Procedure
Retractor reattachment		
Everting sutures ± horizontal shortening	Retractor dehiscence, with or without lid laxity	Everting sutures from fornix to below lash line ± lateral tarsal strip
Jones plication (modified)	Retractor dehiscence, with no horizontal lid laxity. Usually reserved for recurrence	Reattachment/tightening of the retractors via subciliary incision
Horizontal lid shortening		
Lateral tarsal strip	Lateral/generalized laxity	Lid shortened laterally and tightened at lateral canthus, elevated at lateral canthus
Wedge excision	Lid laxity, no tendon laxity	Full-thickness pentagon excised
Kuhnt–Szymanowski	As above + excess skin	Wedge excision + lower lid blepharoplasty
Medial canthal resection	Medial laxity only	Lid shortened laterally and tightened at medial canthus
Posterior lamellar reconstruction		
Transverse tarsotomy	Moderate loss of posterior lamella	Tarsal fracture and eversion of distal tarsus
Hard palate mucosal graft	Severe loss of posterior lamella	As above + limited separation of lamellae + graft to posterior lamella
Limitation of orbicularis override		
Quickert procedure	Lid laxity and retractor dehiscence	Everting sutures and full-thickness lid split + wedge excision to shorten lid
Upper lid entropion		
Anterior lamellar repositioning ± grey line split or anterior lamellar excision	Upper lid entropion	Anterior lamellar everted with lashes to prevent corneal abrasion

Congenital entropion

This is very rare and often resolves with time, without the need for intervention. Pretarsal orbicularis is hypertrophied, forming a marked ridge. The lashes do not usually damage the cornea, but recurrent infections are common.

Upper lid entropion

This is most commonly seen in cicatricial disease, notably trachoma. As with lower lid entropion, it may threaten corneal integrity.

Treatment depends on the underlying disease and severity of entropion.

Ptosis: acquired

Ptosis is an abnormal low position of the upper lid. Normal lid position, and therefore lid measurements, vary slightly, according to age, sex, and ethnicity. Table 4.6 shows average values:

Table 4.6 Normal lid measurements

Palpebral aperture	8–11mm (♀> ♂)
Upper margin reflex distance	4–5mm
Upper lid excursion (levator function)	13–16mm
Upper lid crease position	8–10mm from margin (♀> ♂)

An appearance of ptosis may be simulated by a number of conditions (pseudoptosis). True ptosis may be congenital (either isolated or syndromic) but is most commonly acquired as an involutional degeneration. It may also be the presenting feature of a number of serious conditions.

Involutional ptosis

This very common condition arises from disinsertion of the LPS. It increases with age and is more common after ophthalmic surgery (more so with use of excessive traction with a speculum), trauma, chronic CL use, and periocular corticosteroid injections.

Clinical features

Uni-/bilateral ptosis, high upper lid crease, compensatory brow lift, normal levator function, deep upper sulcus, low relative eyelid position in downgaze.

Treatment

- *Surgery*: anterior levator advancement (see Box 4.3), or posterior approach with white line advancement or conjunctival mullerectomy.

Neurogenic ptosis

- *IIIn palsy*: ptosis may arise as part of a IIIn palsy, a potential ophthalmic emergency (see ● Third nerve disorders, p. 700). It is classically a complete ptosis due to loss of levator function, usually associated with ocular motility abnormalities and sometimes with mydriasis. Aberrant regeneration is common in chronic compressive lesions. Surgery (frontalis suspension) is delayed for at least 6mo (spontaneous improvement is common) and until any motility disturbance has been successfully corrected.
- *Horner's syndrome*: causes a partial ptosis (see ● Anisocoria: sympathetic chain, p. 710). It may be associated with ipsilateral miosis, lower lid elevation, and, in some cases, anhydrosis. *Surgery* for persistent and significant ptosis is by anterior or posterior levator resection or posterior mullerectomy without tarsal resection.

Myasthenic ptosis

Myasthenia gravis (MG) may cause variable and fatiguable uni-/bilateral ptosis and/or ocular motility disturbance (see ➲ Myasthenia gravis, p. 722). It should be considered as a serious possibility in ptosis with normal skin crease height. Consider using the ice-pack test (see ➲ Investigations, p. 722) to look for an improvement in >2mm after 2min; the Tensilon test should only be performed by trained specialists (with appropriate resuscitation facilities).

Usually treated medically. Surgical repair should be avoided, except in refractory disease causing severe visual disability.

Myopathic ptosis

The chronic progressive external ophthalmoplegia group cause a bilateral, usually symmetric ptosis, associated with restricted ocular motility commonly without diplopia.

Surgical repair (usually frontalis suspension) requires caution, as lid closure is also abnormal and Bell's phenomenon may be reduced. It is therefore delayed until ptosis is visually significant. Over time, brow function may also be reduced, limiting the effectiveness of surgery.

Non-surgical management includes spectacle or scleral CL mounted ptosis props.

Mechanical ptosis

Masses, infiltrations, or oedema of the upper lid may cause ptosis. The ptosis often resolves with correction of the underlying disease.

Pseudoptosis

- *Brow ptosis*: a lowering of the eyebrow due to frontalis dysfunction.
- *Dermatochalasis*: a common condition where upper eyelid skin hangs in folds from the lid; it is commoner in the elderly.
- *Blepharochalasis*: abnormal lid elastic tissue permits recurrent episodes of lid oedema that lead to abnormal redundant skinfolds.

Other simulators of ptosis are listed in Table 4.7.

Table 4.7 Causes of pseudoptosis

Ipsilateral pathology	Excessive skin	Brow ptosis
		Dermatochalasis
	Inadequate globe size	Microphthalmos
		Phthisis bulbi
		Prosthesis
	Incorrect globe position	Enophthalmos
		Hypotropia
Contralateral pathology		Contralateral lid retraction
		Contralateral large globe
		Contralateral proptosis

Ptosis: congenital

Isolated congenital ptosis

This is a developmental myopathy of the levator. It is usually unilateral, with absent skin crease, reduced levator function, and the lid fails to drop normally in downgaze.

Treatment

Surgery: if levator function is reasonable, then anterior levator resection ± cutting of the LPS horns will suffice. For poor levator function, frontalis suspension should be performed. To optimize symmetry and to encourage brow elevation, this may be bilateral with excision of the uninvolved levator (see Box 4.3).

Blepharophimosis syndrome

This AD condition is characterized by horizontally shortened palpebral fissures, telecanthus, severe bilateral ptosis with poor levator function, and commonly epicanthus inversus and ectropia.

Treatment

Surgery is first directed towards correcting the telecanthus and epicanthus. Bilateral frontalis slings are performed later.

Marcus Gunn jaw-winking syndrome

This is a synkinesis in which innervation of the ipsilateral pterygoids causes elevation of the ptotic lid during chewing.

Treatment

Surgery requires levator resection (mild) or bilateral levator excision with frontalis suspension (severe).

Box 4.3 Outline of anterior levator advancement

- Mark level of desired post-operative lid crease and postion of desired peak.
- Administer SC local anaesthetic.
- Make skin incision at level of predetermined skin crease.
- Dissect to expose superior tarsus.
- Divide orbicularis and septum, and retract the preaponeurotic fat pads up to expose LPS.
- Free LPS both from any remaining overlying or underlying attachments to the tarsus and from the underlying Müller muscle.
- Advance the aponeurosis, and suture to tarsus (partial thickness—evert lid to check, e.g. 6-0 Vicryl®).
- In the awake patient, the resultant position should be observed and adjusted accordingly.
- Reform the lid crease by suturing the skin to the advanced edge of the levator (e.g. 6-0 Vicryl®).
- Close skin incision (e.g. 6-0 or 7-0 Vicryl®—remove at 1wk).

Miscellaneous lid disorders

Congenital

Epiblepharon

This is a common horizontal fold of skin running just below the lower lid. It may cause the lid to invert, with pseudotrichiasis. It is rarely significant and usually resolves.

Epicanthic folds

These are common folds of skin that may arise in one of four patterns around the medial canthus:
- *Epicanthus palpebraris*: medial vertical fold between upper and lower lids; present in 20% normal children, usually resolves.
- *Epicanthus tarsalis*: primarily upper lid fold, typical of oriental races.
- *Epicanthus inversus*: primarily lower lid fold seen in blepharophimosis and Down's syndrome.
- *Epicanthus superciliaris*: fold arising above the brow, rare.

Telecanthus

This is wide separation of the medial canthi, despite normally positioned orbits (i.e. normal IPD), in contrast to hypertelorism where the whole orbits are widely separated. It may be isolated or syndromic (e.g. blepharophimosis).

Cryptophthalmos

This is a failure of lid development so that the surface ectoderm remains continuous over the surface of an often poorly developed eye. Even with cosmetic improvement, visual prognosis is often poor. It is sometimes autosomal dominantly inherited.

Ankyloblepharon

These are abnormal areas of upper and lower lid fusion and are of variable severity. They may be isolated or syndromic.

Coloboma

These are focal lid defects arising from failure of lid development or interference of amniotic bands. They are usually located medially in the upper lid and laterally in the lower lid.

Acquired

Floppy eyelid syndrome

In this underdiagnosed condition, an excessively lax upper lid can spontaneously evert during sleep, resulting in exposure and chronic papillary conjunctivitis.

It is more common in the obese and may be associated with sleep apnoea (with risk of pulmonary hypertension and other cardiovascular complications). Sleep studies are therefore recommended.

Severe lid and corneal disease, such as recurrent corneal erosion/scarring, may be cured by a combination of sleeping habit advice, appropriate management of sleep apnoea, lubrication, and lid-shortening procedures.

Lid retraction

See Table 4.8 for causes.

Table 4.8 Causes of lid retraction

Congenital		Isolated
		Down's syndrome
		Duane syndrome
Acquired	Systemic	TED
		Uraemia
	Neurological	VIIn palsy
		IIIn misdirection
		Marcus Gunn syndrome
		Parinaud syndrome
		Hydrocephalus
		Sympathetic drive (including medication)
	Mechanical	Cicatricial
		Surgical
		Globe (buphthalmos/myopia/proptosis)

Lacrimal

Anatomy and physiology

The lacrimal system comprises a secretory component (tear production by the lacrimal gland) and an excretory component (tear drainage by the nasolacrimal system) (see Fig. 5.1).

Anatomy

Lacrimal gland

This almond-shaped bilobar gland is located in the shallow lacrimal fossa of the superolateral orbit. It is held in place by fascial septae and divided into palpebral (smaller superficial part) and orbital (larger deeper part) lobes by the LPS aponeurosis. Around 12 ducts run from the orbital lobe through the aponeurosis and palpebral lobe to open into the superolateral fornix. The gland is of serous type but also contains mucopolysaccharide granules.

It is innervated by the parasympathetic system: superior salivary nucleus (pons) → greater petrosal n. → synapse at pterygopalatine ganglion → zygomatic n. (Vb) → lacrimal n. (Va) → lacrimal gland.

Nasolacrimal system

Tear drainage starts with the upper and lower lacrimal puncta (0.3mm diameter) which are located around 6mm lateral to the medial canthus. These are angled backward and are located within the slightly elevated lacrimal papillae.

The superior and inferior canaliculi comprise a vertical part (the ampulla: 2mm long, up to 3mm wide) and a horizontal part (8mm long, up to 2mm wide). The terminal canaliculi usually fuse to form the common canaliculus, on average 2mm, before entering the lacrimal sac. The sac is around 12mm in length and lies within the lacrimal fossa. The lacrimal fossa lies posterior to the medial canthal tendon and lateral to the ethmoid sinus (although this is variable). From the nasal aspect, the lacrimal sac lies anterolateral to the head of the middle turbinate and extends superiorly above the axilla. It is located behind the maxillary line.

The nasolacrimal duct is around 18mm long and runs parallel to the nasojugal fold (i.e. inferolaterally). The first 12mm lies in the bony nasolacrimal canal and the last 6mm within the mucous membrane of the lateral wall of the nose. It opens into the inferior meatus via the ostium lacrimale just beneath the inferior turbinate.

There are a number of valves along the system, of which the most important are the valves of Rosenmuller (entry into the lacrimal sac) and Hasner (exit from the nasolacrimal duct).

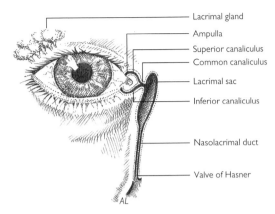

Lacrimal gland
Ampulla
Superior canaliculus
Common canaliculus
Lacrimal sac
Inferior canaliculus
Nasolacrimal duct
Valve of Hasner

AL

Fig. 5.1 Anatomy of the nasolacrimal system.

Physiology

Production (secretion) of tears may be basic or reflex.

Basal secretion

- *Lid*: MGs (around 60) → outer lipid layer which reduces evaporation.
- *Conjunctiva*: glands of Krause (around 28) and glands of Wolfring (around 3) → middle aqueous layer which has washing and antimicrobial functions.
- *Goblet cells* → inner mucin layer which helps stabilize the tear film.
- *Lacrimal gland*: may also contribute to basal secretion.

Reflex secretion

- *Lacrimal gland*: innervated by the parasympathetic system.

Excretion

Tears flow along the marginal tear strips and are drained into the distensible ampullae. This is probably both passive (70% is drained via the inferior canaliculus vs 30% via the superior) and active (i.e. suction). From the ampullae, an active lacrimal pump then drives the tears, first into the sac and then down the nasolacrimal duct into the nose. Contraction of the pretarsal orbicularis oculi (superficial and deep heads) compresses the loaded ampullae, while contraction of the preseptal orbicularis (deep head which inserts onto lacrimal fascia) forcibly expands the sac, creating a wave of suction towards the sac. With relaxation of orbicularis, the ampullae reopen and the sac collapses, expelling the tears down the nasolacrimal duct.

The watery eye: assessment

This is a common complaint, particularly in the elderly population. It ranges from the transient and trivial (e.g. associated with a local irritant) to the permanent and disabling. Objective quantification is difficult, but the main issue is how much of a problem it is for the patient (see Box 5.1 and Table 5.1).

Box 5.1 An approach to assessing the watery eye

Symptoms	Episodic/permanent, frequency of wiping eyes, exacerbating factors (in/outside, cold/warm), site where tears spill over (laterally/medially)
POH	Previous surgery/trauma; concurrent eye disease; herpes simplex blepharoconjunctivitis
PMH	Previous ear, nose, and throat (ENT) problems (e.g. sinusitis, surgery/nasal fracture, granulomatous disease)
Dx	Pro-secretory drugs (e.g. pilocarpine)
Ax	Allergies or relevant drug contraindications
VA	Best corrected/pinhole
Facies	Scars (previous trauma/surgery), asymmetry, prominent nasal bridge, mid-face hypoplasia, or age-related sag
Lacrimal sac	Swelling, any punctal regurgitation on palpation
Lids	MG disease, lash malposition, lid position (ectropion/entropion/low lateral canthus), laxity (lid/canthal tendons)
Puncta	Position, scarring, concretions, patency
Conjunctiva	Irritation (e.g. chronic conjunctivitis)
Cornea	Inflammation, chronic corneal disease
Tear film	Meniscus high/low, TBUT, dry eye (Schirmer's test)
Fluorescein dye disappearance test (FDT)—tear film height, symmetry, dilution	
Dye recovery	Jones I (physiological—without syringing), Jones II (non-physiological—after syringing), retrieve dye with cotton bud under inferior turbinate or ideally visualize with nasendoscope
Cannulation	Patency of puncta
Syringing	Do gently with lateral distraction of lid to avoid false passage; do not advance through an obstruction. Careful assessment will indicate site of obstruction—assess flow, regurgitation through upper or lower punctum, and presence of fluorescein or mucous in the fluid

Perform nasendoscopy where possible. CT DCG if previous trauma/destructive disease/suspected tumour. Lacrimal scintigraphy is more useful than DCG, as it simulates physiologic tear drainage conditions.

Table 5.1 Causes of the watery eye (common causes in bold)

Increased production	Basal	Autonomic disturbance
		Pro-secretory drugs
	Reflex	**Chronic lid disease (e.g. blepharitis)**
		Local irritant (e.g. FB, trichiasis)
		Systemic disease (e.g. TED)
		Chronic conjunctival disease (e.g. OcMMP)
		Chronic corneal disease (e.g. keratoconjunctivitis sicca (KCS))
Lacrimal pump failure	Lid tone	**Lid laxity**
		Orbicularis weakness (e.g. VIIn palsy)
	Lid position	**Ectropion**
Decreased drainage	Punctal obstruction	Congenital: punctal atresia, accessory punctum
		Idiopathic stenosis (elderly)
		2° to punctal eversion
		HSV infection
		Post-irradiation
		Trachoma
		Cicatricial conjunctivitis
	Canalicular obstruction	**Idiopathic fibrosis**
		HSV infection, *Actinomyces*
		Chronic dacrocystitis
		Cicatricial conjunctivitis
		5-FU administration (systemic)
	Lacrimal sac obstruction	Granuloma, sarcoid, syphilis, fungi
		Papillomas
		Epithelial papillary (squamous and transitional cell) carcinomas
		Lymphoma
		Invasive pharyngeal or sinus carcinoma
	Nasolacrimal duct obstruction	Congenital: **delayed canalization**
		Idiopathic stenosis
		Trauma (nasal/orbital fracture)
		Nasal pathology (chronic inflammation polyps)
		Post-irradiation
		Granulomatosis with Polyangiitis (GPA)
		Tumours (e.g. nasopharyngeal carcinoma)

The watery eye: treatment

Increased production

This is usually due to reflex tearing in response to a chronic irritant or disease. Treatment is directed towards controlling the disease process, e.g. ocular lubricants for KCS. It is important to explain this to the patient, since it will seem counterintuitive to be treating a watery eye with drops. For MG disease, prescribe hot compresses, massage, lid cleaning ± lubricants/topical steroid/antibiotic/oral doxycycline. See ⟴ Blepharitis and Meibomian gland dysfuntion (MGD) (1), p. 140.

Lacrimal pump failure

This is usually a function of lid laxity and ectropion causing punctal eversion. This often leads to 2° punctal stenosis. Treatment is directed towards restoring the position of lid and punctum, often with a lid shortening procedure (see Table 5.2 and ⟴ Ectropion, p. 154).

Decreased drainage

Obstruction may arise at the level of the punctum, the canaliculi, the sac, or the nasolacrimal duct. The extent of surgery required will depend on the level of blockage, but most cases arising distal to the puncta require a dacryocystorhinostomy (DCR) (see Table 5.2).

Table 5.2 Overview of operations to improve nasolacrimal drainage

Operation	Indication	Procedure
Punctal position		
Ziegler cautery	Very mild medial ectropion	Cauterize tissue 5mm inferior to punctum: causes scarring/inversion
Diamond excision	Mild medial ectropion	Diamond of tarsoconjunctiva excised just inferior to punctum + inverting suture
Lazy-T procedure	Medial ectropion with lid laxity	Diamond excision + wedge excision
LTS	Ectropion with generalized laxity	Lid shortened laterally and tightened + elevated at lateral canthus
Lateral canthopexy	Mild laxity with intact LCT	Lid tightened laterally + elevated
Punctal obstruction		
1-, 2-, or 3-snip procedure	Isolated punctal stenosis	Vertical and small medial cut in the punctal ampulla enlarges opening
Canalicular obstruction		
Silastic tube insertion	Partial obstruction	Canaliculi intubated with silastic tube secured at nasal end; left for 6mo. May require opening by trephination
DCR with Jones tube	Complete obstruction	DCR + carunculectomy with a Jones (pyrex) tube from sac to medial canthus
Nasolacrimal duct obstruction		
DCR	Most nasolacrimal duct obstructions	The lacrimal sac is opened directly to nasal mucosa by a rhinostomy + membranectomy if there is a membrane over the common canalicular opening

Dacryocystorhinostomy

A DCR aims to create an epithelium-lined tract from the lacrimal sac to the nasal mucosa. The conventional external route is the gold standard, with a success rate of 90–95%. Endonasal DCR has the advantage of no external scar, and, with modern mechanically assisted techniques with good-sized osteotomy, success rates rival those of external DCR. Endonasal DCR can also offer a simple solution in patients requiring redo surgery. Laser-assisted endonasal DCR is an obsolete technique with low success rates, probably due to the smaller ostium created and scarring due to heat dissipated by the laser.

Indication

Acquired nasolacrimal duct obstruction (± dacryocystitis), congenital nasolacrimal obstruction in which a probe cannot be passed. In distal or common canalicular obstruction, a canalicular DCR (C-DCR) is performed, with membrane/scar excision or trephination, if necessary.

Preoperative preparation

With external and endonasal DCR, bleeding can be reduced with preoperative nasal decongestant spray, e.g. xylometazoline, nasal packing with cocaine 5–10%, Moffat's solution (**NB** cardiac effects), or simply cocaine or lidocaine with adrenaline nasal spray.

Local anaesthetic with adrenaline infiltration is advised with both.

Intraoperative prophylactic antibiotics, such as co-amoxiclav or cefalexin, are commonly used.

Method

See Box 5.2 and Box 5.3.

Post-operative care

If the nose has been packed at the end of the operation, this can usually be removed on the first day after surgery. Prescribe prophylactic oral antibiotics if intraoperative IV antibiotics were not given. Advise no hot food or drinks for 12h, to sleep propped up for first night, no nose blowing for 2wk.

Complications

Haemorrhage with epistaxis may occur early (within 24h) or late (4–7d) when clot retraction occurs. Treat with nasal packing (± thrombin-soaked packs). If haemostasis still not achieved, the vessel may need embolization. Haemorrhage can also occur 2° to infection.

Other complications include failure (closure of the ostium), scar formation, infection, very rarely, orbital haemorrhage, and even more rarely meningitis.

Box 5.2 Outline of external DCR

1. Cutaneous incision on flat aspect of nose and inferior to medial canthal tendon (around 10mm long).
2. Blunt dissect down to periosteum; reflect periosteum from anterior lacrimal crest, and divide the superficial limb of the medial canthal tendon.
3. Reflect the lacrimal sac laterally.
4. Use Traquair's periosteal elevator to open suture between nasal and lacrimal bones.
5. Use Kerrison punches to create a good-sized opening (rhinostomy) through the bone of the sac fossa to the nasal cavity taking care to avoid nasal mucosa.
6. Use curved artery forceps or bone nibbler to do anterior ethmoidectomy.
7. Vertically fully divide the lacrimal sac and exposed nasal mucosa anterior to the root of the middle turbinate to form posterior and larger anterior flaps.
8. Anastamose mucosa of the sac and the nose by suturing the posterior, then the anterior, flaps together. Anterior flaps may be suspended from orbicularis.
9. Prior to suturing the anterior flaps silastic tubes can be inserted to keep the ostium open.
10. Close skin incision.

Box 5.3 Outline of endonasal DCR

1. Use 30° nasal endoscope.
2. Inject lignocaine with adrenaline 1:80,000 into nasal mucosa overlying the lacrimal sac.
3. Open nasal mucosa, starting above the insertion of the middle turbinate, curving forwards, anterior to the maxillary line, vertically down towards the insertion of the inferior turbinate, then backwards—creating a posteriorly hinged nasal mucosa flap.
4. Elevate nasal mucosa from underlying bone with a Freer periosteal elevator or similar, exposing the frontal process of maxilla and the thin lacrimal bone. Reflect mucosa over middle turbinate to protect it during osteotomy.
5. Osteotomy is performed inferiorly, using Kerrison punch or similar; superiorly, the anterior aspect and fundus of the sac are exposed, using a 15° diamond burr drill.
6. Insert Bowman's probe to tent up lacrimal sac, ensuring adequate bony removal.
7. Incise medial wall of sac vertically. Trim nasal mucosal flap, if too large.
8. Insert silastic tubes, tying over triamcinolone-soaked Spongistan or Gelfoam may reduce scarring in initial healing period.

Lacrimal system infections

Canaliculitis

This uncommon chronic condition usually arises from the Gram-positive bacteria *Actinomyces israelii* (streptothrix) but may be due to *Nocardia*, fungi (*Candida, Aspergillus*), and viruses (HSV, VZV).

Clinical features

- Unilateral epiphora, recurrent 'nasal' conjunctivitis, canalicular inflammation, 'pouting' of the punctum, expression of discharge, or concretions from the canaliculi. In *Actinomyces* infection these concretions are bright yellow ('sulfur granules'). The lacrimal sac is not swollen, and both sac and nasolacrimal duct are patent.

Investigation and treatment

Perform an extended 1-snip procedure, fully opening up the affected canaliculus, and remove concretions with curette (send for microbiological analysis) and consider irrigation (e.g. with benzylpencillin 100,000U/mL or iodine 1%—ensure drainage out through nose, not nasopharynx) and topical antibiotics.

Acute dacryocystitis

This condition is relatively common in patients with complete or partial nasolacrimal duct obstruction. It is usually due to staphylococci or streptococci. Acute dacryocystitis is easily identified and requires urgent treatment to prevent a spreading cellulitis.

Clinical features

- Pain around sac, worsening epiphora.
- Tender, erythematous lump, just inferior to medial canthus, may express pus from puncta on palpation + preseptal cellulitis.

Investigation and treatment

- Send discharge to microbiology.
- *Antibiotics*: systemic (e.g. co-amoxiclav 625mg 3×/d for 1wk) and topical (e.g. chloramphenicol 1% Oc 4×/d for 1wk).
- Consider warm compress, gentle massage (encourages expression), and incision and drainage if pointing (but may not heal until DCR performed). Spontaneous or surgical drainage through the skin risks the formation of a fistula.
- *Surgery*: most cases have associated nasolacrimal duct obstruction requiring DCR; this can be done endonasally at the time of acute infection or delayed until after the inflammation has settled.

Chronic dacryocystitis

In chronic dacryocystitis, there may be recurrent ipsilateral conjunctivitis, epiphora, and a mucocele. It may be identified by demonstration of nasolacrimal duct obstruction and expression of the contents of the mucocele or regurgitation of mucous on syringing. Surgical treatment is with DCR. In elderly frail patients not fit enough for DCR, particularly when symptoms of epiphora are mild, dacryocystectomy may be performed instead.

Chapter 6

Conjunctiva

Anatomy and physiology

The conjunctiva is a mucous membrane that is essential for a healthy eye. At the histological level, it comprises epithelium, BM, and stroma. At the macroscopic clinical level, it is divided into palpebral, forniceal, and bulbar parts.

Microscopic

Epithelium

This is a 2–5-layered, non-keratinized epithelium that may be stratified squamous (palpebral and limbal) or stratified columnar (bulbar conjunctiva).

The microvilli on the apical surface harbour glycoproteins that form a hydrophilic glycocalyx layer that helps stabilize the tear film. The epithelial layer also contains goblet cells (constituting about 10% of epithelial cells).

Epithelial BM

The BM consists mainly of type IV collagen, anchoring fibrils, and hemidesmosomes linking to the conjunctival epithelial cells.

Stroma

This consists of a superficial lymphoid layer and a deeper fibrous layer. The superficial layer is attached to the epithelium via the BM and contains lymphoid tissue. The deeper fibrous layer is attached to the episclera/Tenon's layer and comprises collagenous elastic tissue interspersed with neurovascular tissue.

Macroscopic

Palpebral

This is firmly adherent to the posterior lamella of the lid; contains the crypts of Henle and goblet cells (both secrete mucin).

Forniceal

This is loose and relatively mobile. It contains accessory lacrimal glands of Krause and Wolfring (secrete aqueous component of tears) and goblet cells.

Bulbar

This is loosely attached to Tenon's layer but firmly attached at the limbus. It contains glands of Manz (secrete mucin) and goblet cells.

The tear film

Although conventionally described as a defined trilaminar structure, it is becoming apparent that the tear film is rather more complex. The layers blend together, forming a muco-aqueous gradient on the surface of the eye (see Fig. 6.1).

Phospholipid	Meibomian glands
	Glands of Zeis
Aqueous	Lacrimal gland
	Glands of Krause
	Glands of Wolfring
Mucin	Goblet cells
	Glands of Manz
	Crypts of Henle
Epithelium	

Fig. 6.1 Tear film components and their origins.

Mucin layer

The mucin layer (secreted primarily by the goblet cells) abuts the surface epithelium and provides a smooth hydrophilic surface that stabilizes the aqueous against the otherwise hydrophobic epithelium.

Aqueous layer

The aqueous component (secreted by the lacrimal gland and the accessory glands) consists primarily of water, but also proteins such as epidermal growth factor, lactoferrin, lysozyme, immunoglobulins, and cytokines.

Phospholipid layer

The aqueous layer is supported by a phospholipid layer (secreted primarily by the MGs) that resists evaporative loss of aqueous and stabilizes the tear film by increasing surface tension.

Conjunctival signs

See Table 6.1 for pathophysiology of signs.

Table 6.1 Conjunctival signs and their pathophysiology

Sign	Pathology	Causes
Hyperaemia	Dilated blood vessels, non-specific sign of inflammation	• *Generalized*—e.g. conjunctivitis, dry eye, drop hypersensitivity, CL wear, scleritis • *Localized*—e.g. episcleritis, scleritis, marginal keratitis, superior limbic keratitis, corneal abrasion, FB • *Circumcorneal*—e.g. anterior uveitis, keratitis
Discharge	Inflammatory exudate	• *Purulent*—bacterial conjunctivitis • *Mucopurulent*—bacterial or chlamydial conjunctivitis • *Mucoid*—vernal conjunctivitis, atopic keratoconjunctivitis, dry eye syndrome • *Watery*—viral or allergic conjunctivitis
Papillae	Vascular response: projections of a core of vessels, surrounded by oedematous stroma and hyperplastic epithelium; also chronic inflammatory cells	• Bacterial conjunctivitis • Allergic conjunctivitis (perennial/seasonal) • Atopic keratoconjunctivitis • Vernal keratoconjunctivitis (VKC) • Blepharitis • Floppy eyelid syndrome • Superior limbic keratoconjunctivitis • CL
Giant papillae	Papillae which, due to chronic inflammation, have lost the normal fibrous septae that divide them	• VKC • Atopic keratoconjunctivitis • CL-related giant papillary conjunctivitis • Exposed suture • Prosthesis • Floppy eyelid syndrome
Follicles	Lymphoid hyperplasia, with each follicle comprising an active germinal centre	• Viral conjunctivitis • Chlamydial conjunctivitis • Drop hypersensitivity • Parinaud oculoglandular syndrome
Lymph-adenopathy	Temporal 2/3 drains to the preauricular nodes, nasal 1/3 to the submandibular nodes	• Viral conjunctivitis • Chlamydial conjunctivitis • Gonococcal conjunctivitis • Parinaud oculoglandular syndrome

(Continued)

Table 6.1 (*Cont.*)

Sign	Pathology	Causes
Pseudo-membrane	Exudate of fibrin and cellular debris; loosely attached to the underlying epithelium; easily removed without bleeding	• Infective conjunctivitis: • Adenovirus • *Streptococcus pyogenes* • *Corynebacterium diphtheriae* • *Neisseria gonorrhoeae* • SJS (acute) • Graft-versus-host disease (GVHD) • Vernal conjunctivitis • Ligneous conjunctivitis • Thermal burn
Membrane	Exudate of fibrin and cellular debris; firmly attached to the underlying epithelium; attempted removal strips off the epithelium, causing bleeding	• Infective conjunctivitis: • Adenovirus • *Streptococcus pneumoniae* • *Staphylococcus aureus* • *Corynebacterium diphtheriae* • SJS (acute) • Ligneous conjunctivitis
Cicatrization	Scarring	• Drug-induced (topical medication) • Chemical injury (acid/alkali) • OcMMP • SJS/TEN • Other immunobullous disease (e.g. linear IgA disease, epidermolysis bullosa) • Trachoma • Atopic keratoconjunctivitis • Sjögren's syndrome • Trauma/surgery • GVHD
Haemorrhagic conjunctivitis	Subconjunctival haemorrhages	• Infective conjunctivitis: • Adenovirus • Enterovirus 70 • Coxsackie virus A24 • *Streptococcus pneumoniae* • *Haemophilus aegyptius* • Neonatal chlamydial conjunctivitis

Bacterial conjunctivitis (1)

Acute bacterial conjunctivitis

This is one of the commonest ocular problems seen in the community and is usually successfully treated by GPs.

The commonest conjunctival bacterial pathogens are *Staphylococcus epidermidis*, *Staphylococcus aureus*, *Streptococcus pneumoniae*, *Haemophilus influenzae*, and *Moraxella lacunata*. There is some variation, according to climate (*Haemophillus aegyptius* in warm climates, *Haemophilus influenzae* and *Streptococcus* in cool climates) and age (classically *Haemophilus influenzae* in children). Atypical bacteria may be seen in immunocompromised patients.

Bacteria have to overcome the protective mechanisms of the eye: lids (physical barrier, blink reflex), tears (flushing effect, lysozyme, β-lysin, lactoferrin, IgG, IgA), and conjunctiva (physical barrier, conjunctiva-associated lymphoid tissue) (see Table 6.2).

Clinical features
- Acute, red, gritty, sticky eye; usually bilateral but may be sequential.
- Purulent discharge, crusted lids, diffusely injected conjunctiva with papillae; may have mild chemosis.

Investigation
Reserve microbiological investigation for cases that are severe, recurrent, resistant to treatment, atypical, or occur in the vulnerable (e.g. immunosuppressed, neonate). For these, take conjunctival swabs for culture/sensitivities.

Treatment
- *Topical antibiotics* (e.g. chloramphenicol 1% Oc 4×/d, sodium fusidate 1% 2×/d or trimethoprim/polymyxin B Oc 4×/d for 1wk). Patients may find drops easier than ointment. For guttae, more frequent administration is required (*British National Formulary (BNF)* recommends ≥q 2h), reducing frequency as the infection is controlled and continuing for 48h after healing.
- *Advise patient*: follow-up if condition worsens or persists after treatment; measures to reduce spread such as frequent hand washing, minimal touching of eyes, not sharing towels/flannels, not shaking hands, etc. **NB** Wash hands and clean equipment before the next patient.

Chronic or recurrent bacterial conjunctivitis

Chronic or recurrent bacterial conjunctivitis usually reflects a neighbouring reservoir of infection. Such sites include the lids (staphylococcal blepharitis), lacrimal sac (chronic dacryocystitis), or the upper fornices of the elderly. Giant fornix syndrome[1] occurs when there is sequestration of bacteria (including *Staphylococcus aureus*) in a proteinaceous coagulum in a deep upper fornix. It is more common in the elderly and typically results in a chronic relapsing, copiously purulent conjunctivitis.

---

1. Rose GE. The giant fornix syndrome. *Ophthalmology* 2004;**111**:1539–45.

Table 6.2 Different types of insults

Insult	Main symptom	Onset	Uni-/bilateral	VA	Hx	Discharge	Chemosis	Tarsal conjunctiva	Preauricular lymphadenopathy
Bacterial	Red Sticky Gritty	Acute/ hyperacute	Uni- or bilateral		Known contact	Purulent	Mild	Papillae	Occasional
Viral	Red Watery Gritty	Acute	Uni- or bilateral	Should be normal/near normal when discharge blinked away. Reduced acuity and photophobia suggest additional involvement such as keratitis.	Known contact	Watery	Moderate	Follicles	Common
Chlamydial	Red Persistent discharge	Subacute	Unilateral		Sexual hx	Mucopurulent	Mild	Follicles	Common
Allergic	Red Itchy Swelling	Acute/ subacute/ recurrent	Bilateral		Atopy; exposure to antigen	Watery	Severe	Papillae	No
Toxic (drops)	Discomfort + redness worse with drop instillation	Acute	Uni- or biawlateral		Medication	Minimal	Mild	Follicles	No

Bacterial conjunctivitis (2)

Gonococcus (adult)

Now rare, this important Gram-negative diplococcus is found in adults (sexual transmission) and neonates (born to infected mothers). The incubation period is 3–5d in adults and 1–3d in neonates. Gonococcus (*Neisseria gonorrhoeae*) may penetrate cornea in the absence of an epithelial defect.

Clinical features
- Hyperacute onset (<24h) with severe purulent discharge, marked lid swelling and chemosis, papillae, preauricular lymphadenopathy, pseudomembrane ± keratitis.
- *Keratitis*: marginal ulceration may progress rapidly, resulting in a ring ulcer, perforation, and endophthalmitis.
- *Systemic*: history of (unprotected) sexual activity, urethritis, proctitis, vaginitis; although often asymptomatic in women, it is a significant cause of infertility.

Investigation
- Conjunctival scrapings/swabs for immediate Gram stain, culture, and sensitivities.
- After appropriate explanation to the patient, refer to a genitourinary (GU) clinic for assessment, treatment, and contact tracing.

Treatment
- Local microbiological/infectious disease advice is vital.
- Topical antibiotic (e.g. ofloxacin 0.3% 2-hourly), saline irrigation of discharge 4×/d.
- *With keratitis*: consider admission, ceftriaxone 1g IV 2×/d for 3d, topical antibiotic (e.g. ofloxacin 0.3% hourly), saline irrigation; treat chlamydial co-infection.
- Systemic treatment, usually by GU physician, may include ceftriaxone 1g IM stat and co-treatment for possible chlamydial co-infection (e.g. azithromycin 1g single dose).

Gonococcus (neonate)

See ⟴ Ophthalmia neonatorum, p. 788.

Viral conjunctivitis

Adenovirus

Over 40 serotypes of this dsDNA virus have been identified. The incubation period is ~1wk, and virus shedding continues for a further 2wk, during which it is highly contagious. The spectrum of presentation may be generalized into two distinct syndromes:

- *Pharyngoconjunctival fever*: serotypes 3, 7, and many others; aerosol transmission; common in children/young adults; systemic upset (typically upper respiratory tract infection) is common; keratitis is only present in up to 30% and is usually mild.
- *Epidemic keratoconjunctivitis*: serotypes 8, 19, 37; transmission by contact (fingers, instruments); keratitis may occur in up to 80% and can be severe; systemic features are rare. Epidemics may be nosocomial (e.g. arising from eye clinics/casualty) or generalized.

Clinical features

- Acute onset (7–10d), watering, burning, itching ± photophobia/blurred vision (if keratitis).
- Watery discharge, lid oedema, moderate chemosis, follicles (inferior > superior), tender preauricular lymphadenopathy ± subconjunctival petechial haemorrhage ± pseudomembrane ± symblepharon, keratitis.
- *Keratitis*: first diffuse epithelial keratitis (days 1–7; fluorescein staining), then focal epithelial keratitis (days 7–30; fluorescein staining), and finally subepithelial opacities (day 11 onwards, may last years; non-staining).

Investigation

- Conjunctival swabs (viral transport medium) for viral antigen determination or polymerase chain reaction (PCR).

Treatment

- Supportive (cool compresses and artificial tears) ± topical antibiotics (supposedly to prevent 2° bacterial infection). Where subepithelial opacities significantly affect vision, some authors advocate low-dose topical steroids. However, the opacities recur on cessation of steroids, encouraging long-term steroid dependency.
- *Advise patient*: follow-up if condition worsens or persists after treatment; measures to reduce spread such as frequent hand washing, minimal touching of eyes, not sharing towels/flannels, not shaking hands, etc.
- Wash hands and clean equipment before the next patient.

Molluscum contagiosum

This dsDNA virus of the pox virus group is common in children/young adults; profuse lesions are seen with HIV infection or severe immunosuppression. Transmission is by close contact. The lesions may be missed if buried in the lash margin. Shedding of viral particles from the lesion may cause a persistent follicular conjunctivitis.

Clinical features
- Chronic history, pearly, umbilicated nodule at lid margin, mucoid discharge, follicles.

Treatment
- Remove the lid lesion (e.g. cryotherapy, cauterization, shave excision, expression).

Herpes simplex (type 1)

Blepharokeratoconjunctivitis usually occurs as a 1° infection of this dsDNA virus.

Clinical features
- Burning, FB sensation; unilateral follicular conjunctivitis, preauricular lymphadenopathy ± lid vesicles ± keratitis (e.g. dendritic ulcer) (see ➋ Herpes simplex keratitis (1), p. 232).

Treatment
Topical (e.g. aciclovir 3% Oc 5×/d for 3wk; *BNF* recommends treatment until 3d after complete healing). If keratitis, then treat accordingly (see ➋ Fungal keratitis: treatment, p. 230).

Other viruses

Other viruses causing follicular conjunctivitis include other members of the herpes group, enterovirus 70, coxsackie A24. influenza A, and the Newcastle disease virus.

Chlamydial conjunctivitis

Chlamydiae are Gram-negative bacteria that exist in two forms:
- A spore-like infectious particle (elementary body), and
- The obligate intracellular reproductive stage (reticular body) that replicates within the host cell (seen as an inclusion body).

Adult inclusion conjunctivitis

This disease of *Chlamydia trachomatis* serotypes D–K is almost always sexually transmitted, although occasional eye-to-eye infection is reported. It is commonest in young adults (♂> ♀). It may be associated with keratitis.

Clinical features
- Subacute onset (2–3wk), usually unilateral (but may be bilateral), mucopurulent discharge, lid oedema ± ptosis, follicles (papillae initially), non-tender lymphadenopathy, superior pannus (late sign); signs are usually most severe on the superior tarsus and the bulbar conjunctiva, with relatively mild disease elsewhere.
- *Keratitis*: punctate epithelial erosions, subepithelial opacities, marginal infiltrates.
- *Systemic* (common but often asymptomatic): cervicitis (♀), urethritis (♂).

Investigation
- *Conjunctival swabs*: firmly swab superior tarsus to remove sufficient cells for immunofluorescent staining; cell culture, PCR, and enzyme-linked immunosorbent assay (ELISA) may also be used.
- After appropriate explanation to the patient, refer to a GU clinic for assessment, treatment, and contact tracing.

Treatment
- *First line*: chloramphenicol Oc 1% 4×/d (bacteriostatic for *Chlamydia*). Systemic (oral) treatment is usually best administered by the GU clinic (after appropriate investigation). Options include oral azithromycin 1g stat or doxycycline 100mg 2×/d for 1wk; if pregnant, erythromycin (e.g. 500mg 2×/d for 2wk) is usually given.

Neonatal chlamydial conjunctivitis

See ➜ Ophthalmia neonatorum, p. 788.

Trachoma

Trachoma accounts for 10–15% of global blindness and is the leading preventable cause. It is caused by *Chlamydia trachomatis* serotypes A, B, Ba, and C in conditions of crowding and poor hygiene, in which the common fly acts as the vector. In endemic areas, it may start in infancy; in non-endemic areas (such as the UK), patients usually present with the complications of chronic scarring (see Table 6.3 for classification).

The World Health Organization (WHO) is aiming to eliminate trachoma as a blinding disease by 2020. Party to this is the SAFE strategy—Surgery for in-turned eyelashes, Antibiotics for active disease, Face washing (or promotion of facial cleanliness), and Environmental improvement to reduce transmission.

Clinical features
- Distinctive follicular reaction (more marked in the upper, rather than lower, lid), conjunctival scarring (with ensuing Arlt lines on the superior tarsus, trichiasis, entropion, dry eyes), limbal follicles (which may scar to form Herbert pits).
- *Keratitis:* superficial, subepithelial, ulceration, 2° microbial keratitis, pannus formation.

Investigation (if acute)
- *Swabs:* usually for immunofluorescent staining, but cell culture, PCR, and ELISA may be used.

Treatment
- Azithromycin 1g PO stat.
- Ocular lubricants, surgical correction of lid/lashes position.

Table 6.3 WHO classification

TF	Trachomatous inflammation: follicular	>5 follicles on upper tarsus
TI	Trachomatous inflammation: intense	Tarsal inflammation sufficient to obscure >50% of the tarsal vessels
TS	Trachomatous scarring	Conjunctival scarring
TT	Trachomatous trichiasis	Trichiasis
CO	Corneal opacity	Corneal opacity involving at least part of the pupillary margin

Allergic conjunctivitis (1)

Seasonal and perennial allergic rhinoconjunctivitis

These extremely common ocular disorders arise due to type I hypersensitivity reactions to airborne allergens. These may be seasonal (grass, tree, weed pollens (UK), ragweed (USA)) or perennial (animal dander, house dust mite).

Clinical features
- Itching, watery discharge; history of atopy.
- Chemosis, lid oedema, papillae, mild diffuse injection.

Investigation
- Consider conjunctival swabs (microbiology), skin prick testing, serum IgE, radioallergosorbent test (RAST).

Treatment
- Identify and eliminate allergen where possible (e.g. change bedding; reduce pet contact; introduce air conditioning).
- If *mild*: artificial tears (dilutes allergen).
- If *moderate*: mast cell stabilizer (e.g. sodium cromoglicate 2% g 4 x /d, lodoxamide 0.1% 4×/d) or topical antihistamine (azelastine 0.05% 2–4×/d for 6wk maximum, levocabastine 0.05% 2–4×/d); and oral antihistamine (e.g. chlorphenamine 4mg 3–6×/d or cetirizine 10mg 1×/d).
- If *severe*: add in short course of mild topical steroid (e.g. fluorometholone 0.1% 4×/d for 1wk); consider referral to clinical immunologist in severe cases for consideration of desensitization therapy.

VKC

This is an uncommon, but serious, condition of children and young adults (onset age 5–15y; duration 5–10y). Before puberty, it is commoner in ♂ but subsequently shows no gender bias.

Although its incidence is decreasing among the white population, it is increasing in Asians. Paler-skinned Caucasians more commonly exhibit the tarsal/palpebral form, whereas the limbal form is commoner in darker races; however, a mixed picture is often seen. It is commoner in warm climates and is usually seasonal (spring/summer).

Over 80% have an atopic history. There is both type I hypersensitivity and a cell-mediated role with a predominantly Th2 cell type. It has been proposed that the Th2 cytokines inhibit matrix metalloproteinases (MMPs), resulting in build-up of conjunctival collagens.

Clinical features
- Itching, thick mucous discharge; typically young ♂, presenting in spring with history of atopy.
- *Tarsal signs*: flat-topped giant ('cobblestone') papillae on superior tarsus.
- *Limbal signs*: limbal papillae, white Trantas dots (eosinophil aggregates).
- *Keratitis*: superior punctate epithelial erosions, vernal ulcer with adherent mucus plaque (may result in subepithelial scar), pseudogerontoxon.

Treatment
- *Topical*: mast cell stabilizer (e.g. sodium cromoglicate 2% g 4×/d) ± topical steroid ± ciclosporin (either 2% g or 0.2% Oc 3–4×/d); consider mucolytic (e.g. acetylcysteine 5% 4×/d).
- **NB** Acute exacerbations may require intensive treatment with topical steroids (e.g. dexamethasone 0.1% PF hourly), but then titrate down to the minimum potency/frequency required to control exacerbations, e.g. fluorometholone 0.1% 1–2×/d). Topical ciclosporin may be used as an adjunct with a 'steroid-sparing' role. It is available in two preparations: 2% ciclosporin drops and 0.2% ciclosporin ointment. The latter is only licensed for veterinary use ('target species dog') but has been widely used in humans (off label).
- *Systemic*: if severe, consider systemic immunosuppression, in conjunction with dermatologist/clinical immunologist; if using immunosuppressants, consider antiviral (e.g. aciclovir 200mg 5×/d or 400mg 2×/d), as these patients are vulnerable to herpes simplex keratitis.
- *Surgical*: debridement or superficial lamellar keratectomy to remove plaques/shield ulcers.

Allergic conjunctivitis (2)

Atopic keratoconjunctivitis

This is a rare, but serious, condition of adults (onset 25–30y). Patients are usually atopic, commonly with eczema of the lids and staphylococcal lid disease. Control of lid disease is an important aspect of treatment. This is a mixed types I and IV hypersensitivity response, but with a higher Th1 cell type component than in vernal disease.

Clinical features
- Itching, redness; photophobia ± blurred vision (if keratitis); history of atopy.
- Lid eczema (often severe), staphylococcal lid disease (anterior blepharitis), small tightly packed papillae, otherwise featureless tarsal conjunctiva (due to inflammation); chemosis + limbal hyperaemia (acute exacerbations); may develop slowly progressive conjunctival scarring (chronic) with forniceal shortening.
- *Keratitis*: inferior punctate epithelial erosions, shield ulcers, pannus, corneal vascularization, herpes simplex, or microbial keratitis.
- *Associations*: keratoconus, cataract (anterior subcapsular type).

Treatment
- *Topical*: as for VKC, including preservative-free ocular lubricants + mast cell stabilizer (usually less effective than in VKC) ± topical steroid (e.g. initially dexamethasone 0.1% PF hourly) ± ciclosporin (2% g or 0.2% Oc 3–4 x /d).
- *Systemic:* consider oral antihistamines (may help with itching) and for severe exacerbations corticosteroids/immunosuppressants—calcineurin inhibitors are particularly effective; if using immunosuppressants, consider antiviral (e.g. aciclovir 200mg 5×/d or 400mg 2×/d), as patients are vulnerable to herpetic (HSV) disease.
- *Surgical*: consider debridement or superficial lamellar keratectomy to remove plaques.
- *For lid disease*: consider topical (e.g. chloramphenicol 1% Oc 4×/d) and oral (e.g. doxycycline 50–100mg 1×/d 3mo—note contraindications. Doses as low as 20mg 1x/d 3mo may also be effective) antibiotics.
- *For 2° infective keratitis*: topical antivirals and antibiotics.
- *Skin disease*: liaise with dermatologist; consider topical tacrolimus to facial skin, periocular regions to the lid margins.

Cicatricial conjunctivitis (1)

Cicatrizing conjunctivitis (conjunctival inflammation associated with scarring) is a rare, usually bilateral, sight-threatening group of disorders for which early diagnosis and appropriate treatment are essential. Loss of goblet cells, ocular surface failure (from chronic limbitis, limbal epithelial stem cell (LESC) failure → blinding keratopathy), and progressive conjunctival scarring = hallmark of the disease. Onset may be insidious, delaying diagnosis (see Table 6.4). *Get expert help early*—it is very easy to underestimate these conditions.

Table 6.4 Classification of progressive conjunctival scarring

Aetiology	Cause	Pattern
Physical	• Heat	• SSP
	• Ionizing radiation	• SSP
Chemical	• Alkali	• SSP
	• Acid	• SSP
Infection	• Trachoma	• SSP
	• Membranous conjunctivitis (e.g. *Streptococcus* and adenovirus)	• SSP
	• *Corynebacterium diphtheriae*	• SSP
	• Chronic mucocutaneous candidiasis	
Oculocutaneous disorders	• Mucous membrane pemphigoid (MMP)	• Prog
	• Bullous pemphigoid (BP)	• SSP
	• Linear IgA disease	• SSP or Prog
	• Dermatitis herpetiformis	• SSP
	• Pemphigus	• Prog
	• Systemic lupus erythematosus (SLE)	• SSP
	• Epidermolysis bullosa aquista (EBA)	• Prog
	• Ectodermal dysplasia	• SSP or Prog
	• SJS	• SSP or Prog
	• TEN	• SSP or Prog
	• Lichen planus	• Prog
	• Chronic atopic keratoconjunctivitis	• SSP
Other associated systemic disorders	• Rosacea	• SSP
	• Sjögren's syndrome	• SSP
	• Inflammatory bowel disease (IBD)	• SSP
	• GVHD	• SSP
	• Immune complex diseases	• SSP
	• Paraneoplastic syndrome	• SSP or Prog
	• Sarcoid	• SSP
	• Porphyria	• SSP
Drug-induced	• Drug-induced cicatrizing conjunctivitis (antiglaucoma medication)	• SSP or Prog
Neoplasia	• Ocular surface squamous neoplasia (squamous cell or sebaceous cell carcinoma)	• Prog • SSP
	• Lymphoma	

SSP, static or slowly progressive; Prog, progressive.

Cicatricial conjunctivitis (2)

Ocular Mucous Membrane Pemphigoid (OcMMP)

MMP is a chronic inflammatory subepithelial blistering disease of the mucous membranes. It usually occurs >60y of age but may occur in adolescents, in whom the disease is more severe;[2] it is slightly more common in ♀.

There is an association with other autoimmune disease (e.g. rheumatoid arthritis (RA) and pernicious anaemia).

MMP is thought to be a type II hypersensitivity reaction, with linear deposition of immunoglobulin and complement at the BM zone of mucosal surfaces. Although the target antigens are known (the antibodies are specific to components of the BM and hemidesmesomes), the triggering agents for the disease are not clear. Oral mucosa and conjunctiva are most commonly affected, although skin and other mucous membranes may be involved. Involvement of the trachea or oesophagus is potentially life-threatening.

According to International Consensus,[3] the diagnosis of MMP requires direct immunopathological confirmation as well as typical clinical features, but, for OcMMP, diagnosis is primarily clinical, with immunopathology providing supporting evidence only.

Clinical features
- Irritation.
- Acute and chronic papillary conjunctivitis, subconjunctival bulla →
  ulceration, progressive cicatrization (loss of plica semilunaris and
  fornices, formation of symblepharon/ankyloblepharon, trichiasis,
  cicatricial entropion), dry eye, 2° microbial keratitis, corneal
  neovascularization, ulcerative keratitis, perforation, LESC failure,
  keratinization.

NB Exclude infection as a cause of inflammation before attributing inflammation to the disease process; risk factors include poor ocular surface, lid trauma, and immunosuppression.

Treatment
- Early diagnosis and treatment improves outcome.[4] Refer early for
  specialist help.
- *Adnexa*: ensure lids and lashes are not a cause of inflammation. Early
  conjunctiva-sparing lid surgery is vital.
- *Maximize tear film stability*: punctal occlusion, tear substitutes; treat
  MGD and blepharitis.
- *Exclude infection*.

Once all 2° causes of inflammation (dry eye, lash/lid trauma, infection) are treated), any residual inflammation is disease-related:

- *Immunomodulation*:
  - *General*: topical corticosteroids—use with caution; may mask disease. Doxycycline 50–100mg 1×/d for 3mo, reduce to 50mg 1×/d thereafter (MMP inhibitor; note contraindications).
  - *Disease-modifying agents*: 'step-up strategies' from dapsone if mild inflammation or 'step-down strategies' from cyclophosphamide if patient has severe inflammation. Hierarchy—mild: dapsone; moderate: mycophenolate, methotrexate, or azathioprine; severe: high-dose IVMP ± cyclophosphamide (PO or IV); combination treatments, according to drug action, may be required. All need monitoring; systemic immunosuppression is generally required for >1y.[4] For persistent/resistant cases IV immunoglobulin, anti-CD20 or anti-tumour necrosis factor (anti-TNF) therapies.

NB Clinically quiescent eyes may have occult inflammation, resulting in disease progression. Monitor scarring with photography and measurements (e.g. fornix depth measurer).

- *Treat complications*: entropion, trichiasis, fornix obliteration (may require oral mucosal grafting to reconstruct fornix), persistent epithelial defects (exclude infection first), limbal stem cell failure, corneal exposure (botulinum toxin is of limited use, due to mechanical restriction, but can be effective in a few), corneal perforations. End-stage disease may require osteo-odonto-keratoprosthesis.

2. Rauz S *et al.* Evaluation of mucous membrane pemphigoid with ocular involvement in young patients. *Ophthalmology* 2005;**112**:1268–74.

3. Chan LS *et al.* The first international consensus of mucous membrane pemphigoid—definition, diagnostic criteria, pathogenic factors, medical treatment, and prognostic indicators. *Arch Dermatol* 2002;**138**:370–9.

4. Radford CF *et al.* The incidence of cicatrising conjunctival disorders in the United Kingdom. *Eye (Lond)* 2012;**26**:1199–208.

Cicatricial conjunctivitis (3)

Other causes of cicatrizing conjunctivitis

Erythema multiforme, SJS, and TEN (Lyell disease)

These are acute vasculitides of the mucous membranes and skin, associated with drug hypersensitivity (sulfonamides, anticonvulsants, allopurinol) or infections (e.g. mycoplasma, HSV). Triggers cause T-cell activation and immunological cascades, delivering various disease phenotypes where TEN is systemically the most severe, characterized histologically by keratinocyte apoptosis and clinically by >30% body involvement. Mortality rates are 30–40%. In those who survive, ocular disease may be persistent, whilst the systemic disease subsides. **NB** Systemic disease severity predictors do not predict acute or chronic ocular disease.

Clinical features

- Acute fever/malaise and skin rash (e.g. target lesions or bullae) ± haemorrhagic inflammation of mucous membranes (SJS and TEN).
- Sloughing of epidermal surfaces (seen in TEN) is called Nikolsky's sign.
- Papillary or pseudomembranous conjunctivitis cicatrization (as for OcMMP).[5,6]
- Ocular disease progression, including ocular surface failure, can occur years after the acute illness.[5]

Treatment

- Acute phase
  - Expert multidisciplinary care is required; should be treated in regional burns unit where possible.
  - *Topical*: tear substitutes, corticosteroids, and antibiotics (PF).
  - *Systemic immunosuppression*: controversy surrounds the use of corticosteroids (systemic), as they have a role for ocular disease but may have a negative effect on general disease and prognosis. There is a possible role for IV immunoglobulin and IV ciclosporin.
  - Consider surgical division of adhesions and careful removal of membranes *(controversial: may become locked in conjunctival fibrosis if forgotten)*, gas-permeable scleral CL, or conformers (vault lids away from bulbar conjunctiva), AMG to protect ocular surfaces and lids (John's procedure), or at the bedside use amnion mounted on a scleral skirt (ProKera®) or an amnion-wrapped conformer; all combined with or without subtarsal triamcinolone 20mg each tarsus.
- Chronic phase
  - Sequelae include persistent chronic inflammation, scleritis, ocular surface failure, and cicatrizing conjunctival changes with OcMMP phenotype.
  - Management of chronic sequelae are as outlined for OcMMP or scleritis.

Injury

Thermal, radiation, chemical (especially alkali), and surgical injuries (e.g. glaucoma surgery) may all cause cicatrization.

Anterior blepharitis (staphylococcal)

Limited cicatrization and keratinization of the lid margin with reduced tear film quality may cause chronic irritation.

Infective conjunctivitis

Cicatrization is most common with *Chlamydia trachomatis* but may also occur after membranous and pseudomembranous conjunctivitis.

Drugs

This may vary from mild irritation to drug-induced cicatrizing conjunctivitis, clinically indistinguishable from OcMMP. Drugs implicated may be systemic (practolol (discontinued), penicillamine) and topical (propine (discontinued), pilocarpine, timolol, idoxuridine, gentamicin (particularly 1.5%), guanethidine).

Inherited

This includes ectodermal dysplasia (associated abnormalities of hair and teeth) and epidermolysis bullosa (inherited hemidesmosome disease).

Systemic

Consider rosacea, Sjögren's syndrome, and GVHD.

GVHD

GVHD occurs in some allogeneic bone marrow transplant patients where the donor's leucocytes attack the immunosuppressed recipient. GVHD most commonly affects the ocular surface, although rarely posterior segment features (e.g. posterior scleritis, choroidal thickening) during the acute stage.

- In the acute response, there is TEN-like response, which may include a pseudomembranous conjunctivitis. It may be graded: stage I, hyperaemia; stage II, hyperaemia with serosanguineous chemosis; stage III, pseudomembranous conjunctivitis; and stage IV, pseudomembranous conjunctivitis with corneal epithelial sloughing.[7]
- In chronic GVHD, there are scleroderma-like changes of the skin and Sjögren's-like changes of the glands to cause dry eye and cicatricial changes of the conjunctiva.

Neoplastic

Unilateral cicatrizing conjunctivitis may be due to sebaceous cell carcinoma, conjunctival intraepithelial neoplasia, or SCC.

5. Da Rojas MV *et al.* The natural history of Stevens–Johnson syndrome: patterns of chronic ocular disease and the role of systemic immunosuppressive therapy. *Ophthalmology* 2007;**91**:1048–53.

6. Sotozona C *et al.* New grading system for the evaluation of chronic ocular manifestations in patients with Stevens–Johnson syndrome. *Ophthalmology* 2007;**114**:1294–302.

7. Jabs DA *et al.* The eye in bone marrow transplantation. III. Conjunctival graft-vs-host disease. *Arch Ophthalmol* 1989;**107**:1343–8.

Dry eyes: clinical features

Although patients report 'dry eyes' extremely commonly, most often they are describing mild tear film instability associated with blepharitis or MGD. While some symptomatic relief will be obtained from ocular lubricants, in these cases, the blepharitis itself should be the focus of treatment. However, true dry eyes (*syn* KCS) may be severe, very painful, and threaten vision (see Table 6.5 for grading).

Causes

The major causes of dry eyes (see Table 6.6) may be classified according to the Dry Eye Workshop (known as the DEWS report).[8,9]

Clinical features

Symptoms are 2° to a combination of decreased lubrication (rapid tear film break-up, increased mechanical shear stresses between the lids and globe, reduced expression of mucins), alteration of tear film composition (hyperosmolarity, presence of inflammatory mediators), together with hypersensitivity of the nociceptive sensory nerves subserving the ocular surface.

- Burning (may be very painful) ± blurred vision (corneal involvement).
- Mucus strands; small/absent concave tear meniscus; punctate epitheliopathy; filaments; mucus plaques; TBUT <10s; Lissamine green <o> pattern; Schirmer test <5mm over 5min (without topical anaesthetic).

Scoring severity

Table 6.5 Grading of severity in dry eye disease (DEWS)*

Level Feature	1	2	3	4
Discomfort (severity/ frequency)	Mild and/ or episodic; response to environment	Moderate episodic or chronic; stress or no stress	Severe frequent or constant without stress	Severe and/or disabling and constant
Visual symptoms	None or episodic mild fatigue	Annoying and/or activity-limiting episodic	Annoying, chronic and/ or constant, limiting activity	Constant and/ or possibly disabling
Conjunctival injection	None to mild	None to mild	+/−	+/++
Conjunctival staining	None to mild	Variable	Moderate to marked	Marked
Corneal staining	None to mild	Variable	Marked central	Severe punctate erosions
Corneal/tear signs	None to mild	Mild debris, ↓ meniscus	Filamentary keratitis, mucus clumping, ↑ tear debris	As for (3) + ulceration
Lids/MG disease	MG disease variably present	MG disease variably present	Frequent	Trichiasis, keratinization, symblepharon
TFBUT	Variable	≤10s	≤5s	Immediate
Schirmer score	Variable	≤10mm/5min	≤5mm/5min	≤2mm/5min

For level 4, symptoms and signs are required.

* 2007 Report of the Dry Eye WorkShop. *Ocul Surf* 2007;5:65–204. Available at: ℘ http://www.tearfilm.org/dewsreport

8. 2007 Report of the Dry Eye WorkShop. *Ocul Surf* 2007;5:65–204. Available at: ℘ http://www.tearfilm.org/dewsreport

9. Behrens A *et al.* Dysfunctional tear syndrome. A Delphi approach to treatment recommendations. *Cornea* 2006;**25**:900–7.

Table 6.6 Causes of dry eyes

Aqueous-deficient		
Sjögren's syndrome	1° Sjögren's syndrome	KCS with xerostomia (dry mouth)
	2° Sjögren's syndrome	KCS with xerostomia associated with connective tissue disease such as RA, SLE, systemic sclerosis, GVHD
Lacrimal gland deficiencies	1°	Age-related dry eye
		Congenital alacrima
		Familial dysautonomia
	2°	Lacrimal gland infiltration
		• Sarcoidosis
		• Lymphoma
		• AIDS
		• GVHD
		Lacrimal gland ablation
		Lacrimal gland denervation
Lacrimal gland duct obstruction		Trachoma
		OcMMP
		Erythema multiforme
		Chemical and thermal burns
Reflex hyposecretion		Reflex sensory block
		CL wear
		Diabetes
		Neurotrophic keratitis
		Reflex motor block
		VIIn damage
		Multiple neuromatosis
Systemic drugs		
Evaporative		
Intrinsic (direct effect on evaporation)		Meibomian oil deficiency
		Lid aperture problems
		Low blink rate
		Drugs
Extrinsic (indirect effect via changes to ocular surface)		Vitamin A deficiency
		Topical drugs/preservatives
		CL wear
		Ocular surface disease (e.g. allergies)

Dry eyes: treatment (1)

Treatment

General

Treat ocular disease according to its severity[10,11] (see Table 6.7), and ensure that any underlying systemic disease is optimally controlled.

Table 6.7 Treatment according to severity level*

Level 1	Level 2	Level 3	Level 4
	If level 1 treatment inadequate, add:	If level 2 treatment inadequate, add:	If level 3 treatment inadequate, add:
Education and environmental/dietary modifications	Topical anti-inflammatories	Autologous serum	Systemic anti-inflammatory drugs
Elimination of offending systemic medications	Tetracyclines (for meibomianitis or rosacea)	CL	Surgery (lid surgery, tarsorrhaphy; salivary gland transposition, mucous membrane/AM)
Artificial tear substitutes, gels/ointments	Punctal plugs	Permanent punctal occlusion	
Lid hygiene	Secretagogues		

* Behrens A et al. Dysfunctional tear syndrome. A Delphi approch to treatment recommendations. *Cornea* 2006;25:900–7.

Tear substitutes
- *Consider viscosity*: low viscosity drops require frequent administration (sometimes more than hourly) but have minimal effect on vision; more viscous gels will transiently blur the vision but are longer lasting and may be effective when used only 4–6×/d; highly viscous paraffin-based ointments significantly blur vision and may only be suitable for night use (see Table 6.8 for common tear substitutes; for a more extensive list see ➔ Topical tear replacement, p. 988).
- *Consider preservative-free preparations*: to reduce the risk of epithelial toxicity, if frequent (>6×/d) administration required.
- *Consider physiological tear substitutes*:
  - Hyaluronic acid is a natural component of tears. Sodium hyaluronate preparations are available for topical application (e.g. Vismed®, Clinitas™, Hylo-forte™). It improves the symptoms of dry eye and is cytoprotective, promotes BM hemidesmosome formation, and has improved surface retention in inflamed eyes due to specific ligand binding to exaggerated CD44 (a cell surface adhesion molecule) expression on the ocular surface during inflammation (see Box 7.6).

- Carmellose (carboxymethylcellulose) is a widely used agent that appears to provide cytoprotection (in addition to lubrication).
- *Autologous serum*: in severe cases, autologous serum may be used (in the UK, this is only available on a named patient basis after Clinical Commissioning Group (CCG) funding approval, from the National Health Service Blood and Transplant (NHSBT)—Tissue Services).

Table 6.8 Commonly used artificial tears and lubricants (selected)

Viscosity	Frequency	Preserved examples	PF examples
Low Hypromellose/ polyvinyl alcohol	q 4h–q 1/2h	Hypromellose Hypotears® Sno Tears®	Liquifilm® (PF) Refresh®
Medium Carbomer/ cellulose/guar gum	1–6×/d	Viscotears® GelTears® Systane®	Celluvisc® (0.5%/1%) Viscotears PF® Systane Ultra SDU®
High Paraffins	1–4×/d		Lacri-Lube® Vit-A-Pos® Simple eye ointment

10. 2007 Report of the Dry Eye WorkShop. *Ocul Surf* 2007;5:65–204. Available at: ℛ http://www.tearfilm.org/dewsreport

11. Behrens A *et al*. Dysfunctional tear syndrome. A Delphi approch to treatment recommendations. *Cornea* 2006;25:900–7.

Dry eyes: treatment (2)

Lid treatments

- *Treat any blepharitis*: lid hygiene ± oral antibiotic (e.g. doxycycline 50–100mg 1×/d 3mo; doxycycline also has significant anti-inflammatory role and is a proteinase inhibitor; note contraindications) (see ➔ Treatment of MGD, p. 142).

Anti-inflammatories

- *Treat any active inflammation*: consider topical corticosteroids; if responsive, these patients may benefit from topical ciclosporin (e.g. Restasis®, a 0.05% preparation of ciclosporin licensed for dry eyes, currently only available on a named patient basis from international pharmacies). As discussed under ➔ Lid treatments, p. 204, doxycycline has an anti-inflammatory role.

Secretagogues

- *Increase secretion*: pilocarpine hydrochloride 2.5mg 1–4×/d (increase slowly from 5mg/d to try to reduce anticholinergic side effects).
- Pilocarpine is licensed for dry mouth and dry eyes in Sjögren's syndrome but is only effective if some residual lacrimal gland function.

Interventional/surgical

- *Punctal occlusion*: plugs can be intracanalicular or punctal, and either temporary (collagen-based) or permanent (silicone-based); permanent occlusion can also be achieved by cauterization of the puncta.
- *Therapeutic CL*: consider silicone hydrogel or, less commonly, scleral CL (scleral CL require expert fitting) to retain a protective tear lake over the cornea.
- *Surgery*: occasionally salivary gland transposition (the parotid or submandibular glands—**beware** severe reflex gustatory epiphora).

Other therapeutic options

- *Mucolytic* (if filaments, mucus plaques): acetylcysteine 5% 4×/d (warn that it stings).
- *Environmental*: lower room temperature, moist chamber goggles, room humidifier (limited success).
- *Dietary*: intake of fish high in omega-3 fatty acids or re-esterified triglycerides is associated with ↓dry eye symptoms in women.
- *Pain relief*: for symptomatology disproportionate to the clinical signs related to hyperalgesia[12]—tramadol, carbamazepine, amitriptyline, gabapentin, and pregabalin (but potential to compound sicca symptoms).

---

12. Rosenthal P *et al.* Corneal pain without stain: is it real? *Ocul Surf* 2009;7:28–40.

Miscellaneous conjunctivitis and conjunctival degenerations

Toxic conjunctivitis

Topical medication (e.g. aminoglycosides, antivirals, glaucoma treatments, preservatives, and CL solutions) may result in an inferior papillary reaction. With chronic usage, topical medication (e.g. glaucoma treatments, antibiotics, and antivirals) may cause a follicular reaction and conjunctival cicatrization. Inferior punctate epitheliopathy may be seen.

- *Treatment*: discontinue precipitating agent, and consider preservative-free ocular lubricant (e.g. Celluvisc®).

Parinaud oculoglandular syndrome

This is a rare unilateral conjunctivitis with granulomatous nodules (+ follicles) on the palpebral conjunctiva, ipsilateral lymphadenopathy (preauricular/submandibular), and systemic upset (malaise, fever). Most commonly due to cat-scratch disease (*Bartonella henselae*), but also consider tularaemia, mycobacteria (e.g. TB), sarcoid, syphilis, lymphoproliferative disorders, infectious mononucleosis, fungi, etc.

Investigations will be dictated by history but consider conjunctival biopsy, conjunctival swabs, FBC, venereal disease research laboratory (VDRL), CXR, Mantoux testing, serology (cat-scratch and tularaemia).

Ligneous conjunctivitis

This is a rare idiopathic chronic conjunctivitis of children (especially girls), characterized by recurrent pseudomembranes or membranes of the 'wood-like' tarsal conjunctiva and often of other mucous membranes (e.g. oropharynx, trachea, etc.). Histologically, these comprise fibrin, albumin, IgG, T- and B-cells. Treat with topical ciclosporin. It is available in two preparations: 2% ciclosporin drops and 0.2% ciclosporin ointment. The latter is only licensed for veterinary use ('target species dog') but has been widely used in humans (off label).

Pinguecula

Extremely common, this yellow-white patch of interpalpebral bulbar conjunctiva is located just nasal or temporal to the limbus. It represents elastotic degeneration of collagen.

Reassurance, and occasionally ocular lubrication, is usually all that is required.

Pterygium

This triangular fibrovascular band is commonest in ♂ exposed to dry climates and high UV light. It usually arises from the nasal limbus, grows slowly across the cornea, and ceases before causing any significant visual impact. Histologically, it is akin to pinguecula, with elastotic degeneration of collagen but with additional destruction of Bowman's layer. It is adherent to underlying tissue for the whole length, compared to pseudopterygium, which is a fold of conjunctiva, only attached at the base and apex, usually resulting from corneal ulceration with adherence of local conjunctiva.

Clinical features

- Cosmetic issues, astigmatism, may encroach on visual axis, FB sensation.
- Triangular pink-white fibrovascular band:
    - *Signs of activity:* rapid growth, engorged vessels, inflammation, grey leading edge in the cornea, punctate epitheliopathy.
    - *Signs of stability:* iron line (Stocker line) just anterior to the margin.

Treatment

- Reserve for progressive, vision-threatening lesions, as recurrence is common and may be aggressive.
- Excise, with conjunctival autograft. AMG or MMC may be used when removing recurrent or large pterygia/pseudopterygia; if the visual axis is involved, lamellar keratoplasty may also be required.

Concretions

Common in the elderly and those with chronic blepharitis, these yellow-white deposits may erode through the palpebral conjunctiva, causing an FB sensation. If troublesome, they can be removed with a needle (at the slit-lamp under topical anaesthetic).

Retention cyst

Very common, this thin-walled, fluid-filled conjunctival cyst occasionally causes symptoms if it disturbs the corneal tear film. It can be punctured with a needle (at the slit-lamp under topical anaesthetic) but may recur, in which case consider excision.

Pigmented conjunctival lesions

Benign

Congenital

Conjunctival epithelial melanosis

Common, racial, bilateral, flat, patchy, freely moving brown pigmentation, which may be diffuse (usually denser around the limbus and anterior ciliary nerves) or focal, e.g. round an intrascleral nerve (Axenfield loop).

Conjunctival freckle

Common, tiny, flat, freely moving pigmented area.

Melanocytoma

Rare, black pigmentation, fixed, slowly growing.

Acquired

Deposits, e.g. mascara in the inferior fornix, coal dust tattoos, adreno-chrome on forniceal/palpebral conjunctiva (from chronic adrenaline administration).

Premalignant

1° acquired melanosis (PAM)

Uncommon; very rare in African-Caribbeans. Histological differentiation is vital, as PAM without atypia is a benign melanocytic proliferation, whereas PAM with atypia has a 50% risk of transformation to melanoma by 5y.

Clinical features
- Unilateral, single/multifocal, flat, freely moving area of irregular brown pigmentation. Pigmentation and size of lesion may increase, decrease, or remain constant over time.
- Nodules within PAM suggest malignant transformation to melanoma.

Treatment
- *For PAM with atypia*: excision + cryotherapy/radiotherapy/ antimetabolite.

Conjunctival naevus

Uncommon; very low risk of transformation.

Clinical features

Single, defined, freely moving brown pigmentation ± cysts; most commonly at the limbus, followed by the caruncle/plica; may increase in pigmentation/size at puberty. Extension into the cornea may indicate malignant transformation.

Congenital ocular melanocytosis

Uncommon. Oculodermal melanocytosis (naevus of Ota) is the most common variant, followed by the limited dermal and ocular forms. Oculodermal melanocytosis is more common in ♀ and orientals.

Clinical features

Subconjunctival, flat, grey lesions; associated unilateral hyperpigmentation of the face (most commonly in a Va/b distribution; ipsilateral iris hyperchromia, iris mamillations, glaucoma (10%) associated with trabecular hyperpigmentation); melanoma (ocular, dermal, or central nervous system (CNS)).

Malignant

Melanoma

Consider this first when confronted with abnormal conjunctival pigmentation. Although rare, it may be fatal. Commoner in middle age. It most commonly arises from atypical PAM but may arise from a naevus or *de novo.*

Clinical features

- Solitary grey/black/non-pigmented, vascularized nodule fixed to episclera; most commonly at the limbus.
- May metastasize to draining lymph nodes, lung, liver, brain.

Prognosis

5y mortality is 13%. Poor prognostic factors include: multifocal lesion; caruncle, fornix, or palpebral location; thickness >1mm; recurrence; lymphatic or orbital spread.

Treatment

- Wide local excision + double freeze-thaw cryotherapy to excised margins. Consider adjunctive radiotherapy/antimetabolite, if incomplete excision/diffuse.
- Exenteration may be necessary, if unresectable.

Key points

- Congenital pigmented lesions that are stable, regular, flat, and asymptomatic (i.e. not bleeding, discharging, inflamed, or affecting vision) are likely to be benign.
- Acquired pigmented lesions that are growing, irregular, elevated, or symptomatic (e.g. bleeding, itchy, painful, inflamed) are more likely to be malignant.
- *Specialist advice should be sought for all potentially malignant/ premalignant lesions.*

Non-pigmented conjunctival lesions (1)

Benign

Papilloma
- *Pedunculated form*: common from teenage onwards, associated with HPV 6, 11, 16, and 18; most commonly arise from palebral/forniceal/caruncular conjunctiva and are often bilateral and multiple.
  - *Treatment*: they often resolve spontaneously, but surgery, cryotherapy, oral cimetidine, topical MMC, or intralesional interferon may be used for large/persistent lesions. Send tissue for HPV PCR.
- *Sessile form*: common in middle age; most commonly arise from bulbar/limbal conjunctiva and are usually unilateral and solitary.
  - *Treatment*: excision. Send tissue for HPV PCR.

Transmission may be vertical, through sexual contact or autoinfection from distant papillomas. There is an important association with human immune deficiency virus (HIV) infection. The potential for malignant transformation is controversial.[13]

Epibulbar choristoma
- *Dermoids*: uncommon choristoma of childhood; associated with Goldenhar syndrome. A soft yellow limbal mass that is usually unilateral; it may encircle the limbus.
  - *Treatment*: can be excised with lamellar graft if limbal, but forniceal require CT scan to rule out intraorbital/intracranial extension.
- *Lipodermoid*: uncommon choristoma of adults. This is a soft white mass at the lateral canthus.
- *Ectopic lashes*: rare choristomas seen as subconjunctival cilia.

Pyogenic granuloma
Typically a rapidly growing red vascular mass after previous trauma/surgery.

13. Karcioglu ZA *et al.* Human papilloma virus in neoplastic and non-neoplastic conditions of the external eye. *Br J Ophthalmol* 1997;**81**:595–8.

Non-pigmented conjunctival lesions (2)

Premalignant

Conjunctival intraepithelial neoplasia (carcinoma in situ, dysplasia)

Rare; commoner over age 50y. It is usually conjunctival in origin but may arise from the cornea. It may transform to SCC (with breaching of the BM).

- *Clinical features*: it appears as a fleshy, freely moving mass, with tufted vessels located at the limbus.
- *Treatment*: excision + MMC ± cryotherapy to affected limbus. Followed by three cycles (1wk on/1wk off) MMC/5-FU eye drops. Ensure lower punctum plugged during cytotoxic treatment.

Malignant

Conjunctival SCC

- The commonest malignant conjunctival tumour worldwide but rare in temperate climates.
- Commoner over 50y of age.
- UV light and HPV are risk factors, and it may be associated with HIV in younger patients.
- It may arise from intraepithelial hyperplasia or *de novo*;[14] although usually conjunctival, it may also arise from corneal epithelium.

Clinical features

Persistent unilateral keratoconjunctivitis; ranges from atypical 'dysplastic' epithelium to limbal gelatinous mass, which may infiltrate cornea, sclera, and penetrate the globe; rarely metastasizes.

Treatment

Excision (2–3mm clear margins) + MMC, double freeze-thaw cryotherapy to margins, followed by three cycles (1wk on/1wk off) MMC/5-FU eye drops. Ensure lower punctum plugged during cytotoxic treatment. Enucleation/exenteration (only required for very advanced).

Conjunctival Kaposi's sarcoma

Typically a bright red mass, usually in the inferior fornix, which may mimic a persistent subconjunctival haemorrhage.

May be caused by HHV8 (commonly in the presence of HIV)—biopsy. Send tissue for HHV8 PCR.

- *Treatment*: focal radiotherapy, if large/aggressive.

Conjunctival lymphoma

Typically, a salmon-pink subconjunctival infiltrate, often bilateral. They are usually located in the fornices.

Histology is essential, as it may be benign or malignant.

Most commonly, it represents extranodal B-cell non-Hodgkin's lymphoma, although it may also arise in the orbit (anterior spread) or in mucosa-associated lymphoid tissue (MALToma).

Imaging and haematological/oncological referral are required in confirmed cases.

- *Treatment*: excision ± cryotherapy or subconjunctival interferon α-2b may be employed[15] ± local radiotherapy. Send tissue for Epstein–Barr virus (EBV) PCR and histology.

Muco-epidermoid carcinoma

This is a very rare, aggressive tumour that may mimic a pterygium. It arises from conjunctival mucus-secreting cells and squamous cells.

Infiltration from lid tumours

Sebaceous cell carcinoma of the lid may spread to involve the conjunctiva, so presenting as a unilateral cicatrizing conjunctivitis.

Key point

- *Specialist advice should be sought for all potentially malignant/premalignant lesions.*

14. Tulvatana W et al. Risk factors for conjunctival squamous cell neoplasia: a matched case-control study. Br J Ophthalmol 2003;**87**:396–8.

15. Ross JJ et al. Systemic remission of non-Hodgkin's lymphoma after intralesional interferon α-2b to bilateral conjunctival lymphomas. Am J Ophthalmol 2004;**138**:672–3.

Chapter 7

Cornea

Anatomy and physiology

The cornea acts as a clear refractive surface and a protective barrier to infection and trauma. Its anterior surface is elliptical (11.7mm horizontally, 10.6mm vertically), whereas its posterior surface is circular (11.7mm). It is thinnest centrally (around 535 microns)[1] and thickest in the periphery (660 microns). The tear film is discussed elsewhere (see ➲ Anatomy and physiology, p. 178).

Anatomy

The cornea consists of five layers. From anterior to posterior, these are:

Epithelium

The corneal epithelium is divided into two areas: the limbus (containing the LESC) and the central cornea (containing the terminally differentiated epithelial cells).

Epithelium of the central cornea

This is a non-keratinized stratified squamous epithelium (5–7 cell layers thick), which accounts for around 10% of the thickness of the adult cornea. It is of ectodermal origin. Cells are firmly adherent to the underlying BM and corneal stroma by highly specific molecular building blocks known as hemidesmosomes. More superficially, the cells flatten to become wing cells, and apical cells are characterized by microvilli coated by a negatively charged glycoprotein facilitating tear film stability.

Limbal Epithelial Stem Cells (LESC)

The corneoscleral limbus is the anatomical location of the corneal epithelial stem cell niche (higher density superiorly and inferiorly). Stem cell progenitors amplify, proliferate, and differentiate into corneal epithelium. Damage to this area results in conjunctivalization of the corneal surface.

BM zone

The BM zone consists of the epithelial BM and Bowman's layer. Bowman's layer is a strong, but thin, avascular superficial stromal layer of collagen fibrils. Hemidesmosomes link the corneal epithelium to the BM. It is also of ectodermal origin. It is unable to regenerate and, if injured, heals by scarring.

Stroma

The stroma accounts for around 90% of corneal thickness. Despite active deturgence, its main component is water (75%). Of its dry weight, 70% is collagen (types I, IV, V, VI), and the remainder is proteoglycan ground substance (chondroitin sulfate and keratan sulfate). Keratocytes are a resident population of dormant fibroblasts that are activated during innate immune responses and are involved in remodelling, following injury. It is of mesodermal origin. Collagen fibres are arranged to confer transparency. The avascular cornea derives nutrition from the tear film and aqueous humour.

Descemet's membrane

Descemet's membrane consists of a fetal anterior banded zone (present at birth) and a posterior non-banded zone (produced later by the endothelium). There is a pre-descemet's layer (Dua's layer). It is of mesodermal origin. It is not capable of regeneration.

Endothelium

This is a monolayer of hexagonal cells characterized histologically by an epithelial phenotype, forming a continuous mosaic, best seen with specular microscopy. It is of mesodermal origin, with the apical border in direct contact with the aqueous humour and the basolateral border with the Descemet's membrane. It is unable to regenerate. Cell loss with age is compensated by enlargement (polymegathism) and migration of neighbouring cells. The endothelial sodium-transporting capacity is critical for corneal deturgescence.

Physiology

Corneal transparency

Corneal transparency is dependent on:

- *Active deturgence*: the *endothelium* is relatively permeable. A passive flow of water and nutrients from the aqueous is drawn across into the stroma ('stromal swelling pressure'). To prevent overload (oedema) and maintain its transparency, the endothelium pumps Na^+ back out into the aqueous by active $Na^+K^+ATPase$, together with a passive movement of water. Water may also pass through hormonally mediated aquaporins, e.g. AQP1. The *epithelium* is relatively impermeable due to the presence of apical tight junctions.
- *Regular orientation and spacing of stromal collagen fibres*: this reduces diffractive scatter of light. After injury, loss of architecture may result in opacity and scarring and increased light scatter.

Refraction

The cornea accounts for 70% of the eye's total dioptric power. The radii of curvature of the anterior surface is 7.7mm; the posterior surface is 6.8mm. The cornea is a robust, elastic surface. Its shape is maintained by structural rigidity and IOP.

Nutrition and nerve supply

The cornea is avascular and relies upon diffusion from the limbus and aqueous for nutrition. Langerhans cells (antigen-presenting cells) are present in the epithelium but are usually restricted to the outer third. The first division of the trigeminal nerve forms stromal and subepithelial plexi responsible for corneal sensation.

1. Doughty MJ *et al.* Human corneal thickness and its impact on intraocular pressure measures: a review and meta-analysis approach. *Surv Ophthalmol* 2000;**44**:367–408.

Corneal signs

See Tables 7.1–7.4 for signs and their pathophysiology.

Table 7.1 Epithelial signs and their pathophysiology

Sign	Pathology	Causes
Punctate epithelial erosions	*Multiple fine areas of epithelial loss; stain well with F, poorly with LG*	*Superior*—e.g. VKC, superior limbic keratitis, floppy eyelid syndrome, poor CL fit
		Interpalpebral—e.g. KCS, UV exposure, corneal anaesthesia
		Inferior—e.g. MGD, exposure keratopathy, ectropion, poor blink, poor Bell's phenomenon, rosacea, preservative toxicity
Corneal filaments	*Mucus strands adherent to cornea, with mobile free tails; stain poorly with F, well with LG*	KCS, recurrent erosion syndrome, corneal anaesthesia, exposure keratopathy, herpes zoster ophthalmicus (HZO)
Punctate epithelial keratitis	*Tiny white spots of epithelial and inflammatory cells; stain poorly with F, well with LG*	Viral keratitis (adenovirus, HSV, molluscum contagiosum)
		Thygeson's superficial punctate keratopathy
Epithelial oedema	*Loss of lustre + translucency; microvesicles and bullae*	↑IOP, post-operative, CL overwear, aphakic/pseudophakic bullous keratopathy, Fuchs' endothelial dystrophy, trauma, acute hydrops, herpetic keratitis, congenital corneal clouding

F, fluorescein; LG, lissamine green.

Table 7.2 Iron lines (best visualized with cobalt blue light on the slit-lamp)

Line	Location	Causes
Ferry	*At trabeculectomy margin, so usually superior*	Trabeculectomy
Stocker	*At pterygium margin, so usually lateral*	Pterygium
Hudson–Stahli	*Usually horizontal inferior 1/3 of cornea*	Idiopathic (common in elderly)
Fleischer	*Ring around base of cone, so usually inferocentral*	Keratoconus

Table 7.3 Stromal signs and their pathophysiology

Sign	Pathology	Causes
Pannus	Subepithelial fibrovascular ingrowth	Trachoma, tight CL, phlycten, herpetic keratitis, rosacea keratitis, chemical keratopathy, marginal keratitis, VKC, atopic keratoconjunctivitis, superior limbal keratoconjunctivitis
Stromal infiltrate	Focal opacification due to leucocyte aggregations (sterile) or microbial colonization	Sterile—marginal keratitis, CL-related Infective—bacteria, fungi, viruses, protozoa
Stromal oedema	Thickened, grey opaque stroma	Post-operative, keratoconus, Fuchs' endothelial dystrophy, herpetic disciform keratitis
Cornea farinata	Deep stromal faint flour-like opacities	Idiopathic (innocuous)
Crocodile shagreen	Reticular polygonal network of stromal opacity	Idiopathic (innocuous)

Table 7.4 Endothelial signs and their pathophysiology

Sign	Pathology	Causes
Descemet's folds	Folds in intact DM	Post-operative, ↓IOP, disciform keratitis, congenital syphilis
Descemet's breaks	Breaks through DM 🔗⁺ associated oedema of overlying stroma	Birth trauma, keratoconus/keratoglobus (hydrops), infantile glaucoma (Haab's striae)
Guttata	Wart-like protuberances at endothelium	Peripheral: Hassall–Henle bodies (physiological in the elderly) Central: Fuchs' endothelial dystrophy
Pigment on endothelium	Dusting of pigment from iris on endothelium	Pigment dispersion syndrome (PDS) (Krukenberg spindle), post-operative, trauma
Keratic precipitates (KPs)	Aggregates of inflammatory cells on endothelium	Keratitis (e.g. disciform, microbial, marginal) Anterior uveitis (e.g. idiopathic, HLA-B27, Fuchs' heterochromic cyclitis, sarcoidosis, etc.)

DM, Descemet's membrane.

Corneal diagrams

Accurate documentation of corneal disease is important for assessing disease progression and response to treatment. Pictorial representation is generally the easiest. Note height, width, and depth of any lesions and any areas of corneal thickening or thinning. Using standardized shading schemes can be useful but, since a number of different schemes have been described,[2] include additional identifying labels to prevent any misunderstanding (see Fig. 7.1.)

2. Bron AJ. A simple scheme for documenting corneal disease. *Br J Ophthalmol* 1973;**57**:629–34.

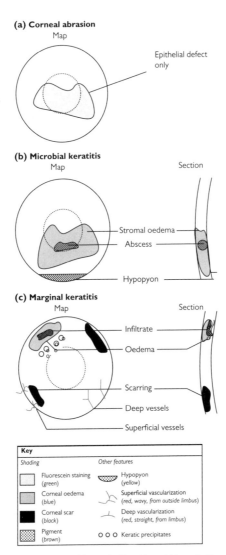

Fig. 7.1 (a) Corneal abrasion, (b) microbial keratitis, and (c) marginal keratitis.

Microbial keratitis: assessment

This is a common sight-threatening, mostly treatable, ophthalmic emergency. Common pitfalls include delay in diagnosis, inappropriate sample collection, injudicious or inadequate therapy, drug toxicity, and delayed follow-up, all of which may result in suboptimal visual outcome (see Table 7.5 for risk factors).

Risk factors

Table 7.5 Risk factors for microbial keratitis

Ocular	Trauma	Corneal abrasion
	CL	Extended wear > soft > daily disposable > rigid gas permeable (RGP); poor hygiene
	Iatrogenic	Corneal surgery (e.g. LASIK)
		Removal of suture
		Loose suture
		Long-term topical steroids/antibiotics
	Ocular surface disease	Dry eyes
		Bullous keratopathy
		Immune-mediated ocular surface disease
		Progressive conjunctival scarring disorders
		Chronic blepharokeratoconjunctivitis
		Chronic keratitis (e.g. HSV)
		Neurotrophic keratitis (e.g. HSV, VZV, tumours of the cerebellopontine angle)
	Lid disease	Entropion
		Lagophthalmos
		Trichiasis
	Nasolacrimal disease	Chronic dacryocystitis
Systemic	Immunosuppression	Drugs
		Immunodeficiency syndromes
		Diabetes
		RA
	Nutritional	Vitamin A deficiency

Clinical features

- Pain, FB sensation, redness, photophobia, tearing, discharge (may be purulent), ↓VA.
- Circumlimbal/diffuse injection, single or multiple foci of white opacity within stroma ± oedema, usually associated epithelial defect and anterior uveitis.
- *Complications*: limbal and scleral extension, corneal perforation, endophthalmitis (rare unless perforation or in the context of organisms, such as gonococcus or fungi, that can penetrate intact epithelia), panophthalmitis.

NB May present insidiously as infectious crystalline keratopathy (see ➲ Deposition keratopathies, p. 272).

Investigations

- Perform early and adequate corneal scrapes (see Box 7.1 and Table 7.6).
- If patient wears CL, send lenses, solutions, and cases for culture, but warn patient that they will be destroyed.
- Liaise with microbiologists, especially with regards to length of incubation required, antibiotic sensitivities required, and if unusual clinical features.
- If herpetic disease is considered to be an underlying risk factor, take a swab for molecular diagnostics (PCR).

Box 7.1 How to perform a corneal scrape

- Instil preservative-free topical anaesthesia (and perform scrape prior to use of fluorescein).
- Use a Kimura spatula, No. 15 blade or 25G needle.
- Scrape both the base and leading edge of the ulcer (from uninvolved to involved cornea).
- Place material onto glass slide for microscopy and staining (Gram stain, Ziehl–Neelsen, methenamine silver, etc.).
- Plate onto blood agar (aerobes), chocolate agar (*Neisseria, Haemophilus*), Sabouraud agar (fungi), and consider non-nutrient *E. coli*-enriched agar (if *Acanthamoeba* suspected); when plating small samples, rows of 'C streaks' are more effective than the traditional technique; use separate needles for each agar dish.
- Consider also culture in thioglycollate (anaerobes) and enrichment (bacteria) broths.

Table 7.6 Microbiological processing of corneal scrapes

Routine stains	Gram stain	B	F	A		
Additional stains	Giemsa stain	B	F	A		
	Gomori/methenamine silver		F	A		
	PAS					
	Calcofluor white		F	A		
	Ziehl–Neelsen		F	A	M	N
Routine media	Blood agar	B				
	Chocolate agar	B				
	Sabouraud dextrose agar		F			
	Thioglycollate broth	B(an)				
Additional media	Lowenstein–Jensen					
	Non-nutrient *E.coli*-enriched agar			A	M	N

B, bacteria; B(an), anaerobic bacteria; F, fungi; A, *Acanthamoeba*; M, mycobacteria; N, *Nocardia*.

Microbial keratitis: treatment

The treatment of microbial keratitis can be divided into a sterilization phase, followed by a healing phase. During the sterilization phase, appropriate topical antibiotics are administered intensively for 48–72h. During the healing phase, topical corticosteroids may be added, and the topical antibiotics are reduced (see Table 7.7 for common bacterial causes).

Initial treatment

- Stop CL wear.
- Admit patient if severe infection, poor compliance, or other concern (see Box 7.2).
- *Intensive topical antibiotics*: initially use an hourly empirical broad-spectrum regimen with either one or two topical antibiotics. If underlying ocular surface disease or immunocompromised, then treatment should be combined therapy (e.g. cefuroxime + ofloxacin) and non-preserved (see Box 7.3).

Consider oral antibiotics: if limbal lesion or corneal perforation, then add systemic ciprofloxacin (e.g. PO 750mg 2×/d).

- Cycloplegia (e.g. cyclopentolate 1% 2×/d) for photophobia and ciliary spasm and oral analgesia, if severe pain.

NB If stromal necrosis or threatened/actual perforation, consider oral tetracyclines and oral vitamin C (inhibit MMPs and pro-inflammatory cytokines and ↓ toxic-free radicals). If dry eye, consider additional lubrication and punctal occlusion. Correct lid deformities and trichiasis.

Box 7.2 Indications for admission

- *Severe infection*: >1.5mm diameter infiltrate, central corneal ulcer, hypopyon, purulent exudate, or complicated disease.
- *Poor compliance likely*: either with administering drops or returning for daily review.
- *Other concern*: only eye, failing to improve, etc.

Box 7.3 Combined therapy vs monotherapy in empirical treatment of microbial keratitis

- *Combined therapy*: commonly 'fortified' preparations of a cephalosporin (cefuroxime 5%) with a fluoroquinolone (e.g. ofloxacin). Penicillin 0.3% may be substituted for the cephalosporin if streptococcal infection suspected. Use aminoglycoside with caution (e.g. gentamicin 1.5%—beware toxicity and necrosis), particularly in patients with pre-existing ocular surface disease.
- *Monotherapy*: with fluoroquinolones (e.g. ofloxacin, levofloxacin) may be adequate for most cases of microbial keratitis but is insufficient for resistant species of *Staphylococcus aureus* and *Pseudomonas aeruginosa*.

NB Always use non-preserved therapy, wherever possible, in patients with existing ocular surface disease.

Table 7.7 Common bacterial causes of keratitis

		Frequency	Penetration of intact epithelium	Virulence
Gram +ve	Staphylococcus aureus	Common	–	+
	Staphylococcus epidermidis	Common	–	+/–
	Streptococcus pneumoniae	Common	–	++
Gram –ve	Pseudomonas aeruginosa	↑in CL wearers	–	+++
	Neisseria gonorrhoea	↑in neonates	+	+++
	Haemophilus	↑in children	+	+

Ongoing treatment

- Monitor response/progression at daily review (inpatient and outpatient) by degree of inflammation, size of epithelial defect (measured on slit-lamp), size of infiltrate and hypoyon, extent of corneal oedema, and degree of anterior uveitis. Taper frequency, and switch to non-fortified preparations with clinical improvement; add lubricants to promote healing; introduce topical steroids (e.g. dexamethasone 0.1%, prednisolone 0.5%) to treat residual inflammation.
- If initial scrape results in no growth and current regimen proves clinically ineffective, consider withholding treatment for 12h before rescraping or performing a formal corneal biopsy. The original slides can be restained with a view to identifying less common organisms (e.g. mycobacteria, fungi, etc.).
- *Consider topical steroids*: use carefully following re-epithelialization, and in the presence of sterile culture, to reduce stromal scarring and improve visual outcome. Initiation requires frequent (often inpatient) follow-up.

Treatment of complications

Persistent epithelial defect

If epithelial defect persists for >2wk, then consider switching to non preserved preparations of topical medication (if not already pres-free), reducing frequency of topical medication, adding ocular lubrication, and assisting lid closure (medical or surgical tarsorrhaphy).

Resistant or progressive keratitis

Seek specialist advice. In threatened scleral extension, consider oral ciprofloxacin which has high bioavailability at the limbus. In threatened corneal perforation, consider oral ciprofloxacin, therapeutic CL (cyanoacrylate glue), or emergency PK. Emergency PK is usually only performed after a minimum of 2d intensive treatment.

Endophthalmitis

Perform diagnostic vitrectomy, and administer intravitreal antibiotics (see ➲ Post-operative endophthalmitis, p. 336).

Microbial keratitis: *Acanthamoeba*

Isolated from soil, dust, sea, fresh and chlorinated water, *Acanthamoeba* are ubiquitous free-living protozoa. Capable of encystment in unfavourable conditions, the organisms can survive extremes of temperature, desiccation, and pH. *Acanthamoeba* keratitis remains rare (0.14 per 1,000 000 UK population in 1996), but incidence is rising with increased CL use. Largely resistant to normal first-line broad-spectrum antibiotics, late suspicion/ diagnosis can lead to devastating and irrevocable corneal scarring.

Risk factors

- **CL wear**: especially with extended wear CL, poor CL hygiene (e.g. rinsing in tap water), or after swimming with CL *in situ* (ponds, hot tubs, swimming pools).
- **Corneal trauma**: notably in a rural or agricultural setting.

Clinical features

- *Variable*: ranges from asymptomatic, FB sensation, ↓VA, or tearing to a severe pain (disproportionate to often relatively mild clinical findings); may occasionally be bilateral.
- Epithelial ridges, pseudo- and true dendrites; stromal infiltrates (may progress circumferentially to form a ring); perineural infiltrates; ↓corneal sensation.

NB Beware of missing this diagnosis—it is commonly misdiagnosed as herpes simplex keratitis.

- **Complications**: limbal and scleral extension, corneal perforation, intractable scleritis.

Investigation

- If *in vivo* confocal microscopy available, direct visualization of cysts are diagnostic.
- Perform early and adequate corneal scrapes (see Box 7.1). The epithelium is often fairly loose, and some practitioners deliberately debride all the affected epithelium. Send additional samples for DNA detection (PCR), culture, and histology, fixed in 10% formalin.
- If patient wears CL, send lenses, solutions, and cases for culture, but warn patient that they will be destroyed.
  - *Stains*: Gram (stains organisms), Giemsa (stains the organism and cysts), Calcofluor white (stains cysts visualized under UV light); also send a sample to histology (in formalin).
  - *Culture*: non-nutrient agar with *E. coli* overlay, at 25 and 37°C, may require up to 14d.

If strong clinical suspicion, but negative investigations, consider corneal biopsy for culture, together with light and electron microscopy of acanthamoebal cysts.

Treatment

Initial treatment

- Admit.
- Stop CL wear.
- Intensive topical anti-amoebic agents, commonly a biguanide (polyhexamethylene biguanide (PHMB) 0.02% or chlorhexidine 0.02%) and an aromatic diamidine (e.g. propamidine isethionate 0.1% or hexamidine 0.1%), administered hourly. Aminoglycosides or imidazoles (e.g. oral itraconazole or fluconazole may give additional benefit).
- Oral analgesia and cycloplegia.

Ongoing treatment

- Taper treatment, according to clinical improvement. Relapse is common and may signify incomplete sterilization of active *Acanthamoeba* trophozoites or reactivation of resistant intrastromal cysts. Treatment is prolonged (20–40wk).
- Consider cautious use of topical steroids (while continuing anti-amoebic agents) to reduce corneal scarring; see Table 7.8.

Treatment of complications

- *If scleritis*: consider immunosuppression with systemic steroids and a steroid-sparing agent such as ciclosporin.
- *If severe corneal scarring*: consider PK once treatment is completed and cornea is sterile.
- *If extensive necrosis*: consider emergency PK. Note high risk of persistent or recurrent disease in grafted tissue.
- *If severe, intractable pain*: patients may occasionally require enucleation for severe pain.

Prevention

- *Education*: a known avoidable and predisposing practice is easily identified in >90% of cases of *Acanthamoeba* keratitis.

Table 7.8 Anti-amoebic agents

Class	Mechanism	Examples
Aminoglycosides	Inhibit protein synthesis	Neomycin; paromomycin
Aromatic diamidines	Inhibit DNA synthesis	Propamidine isethionate; hexamidine
Biguanide	Inhibit function of membrane	PHMB; chlorhexidine
Imidazoles	Destabilize cell wall	Clotrimazole; fluconazole; ketoconazoles

Fungal keratitis: assessment

Fungal infection of the cornea is rare. It is usually seen only in the context of trauma (including contact with organic material) or where there is underlying susceptibility such as tissue devitalization or immunosuppression (including topical corticosteroid use). *Candida*, *Fusarium*, and *Aspergillus* spp. are the most common infectious agents.

Risk factors

Risk factors include trauma (including LASIK), immunosuppression (e.g. topical corticosteroids, alcoholism, diabetes, systemic immunosuppression), ocular surface disease (e.g. dry eye, neurotrophic cornea), hot humid climate, and contamination with organic matter (e.g. agricultural work, gardening, etc.).

Yeast vs filamentary fungal infections

The presentation of fungal keratitis and its treatment are dependent on the type of fungus responsible.

- *Yeast infection*: usually *Candida* species. Frequently associated with immunosuppression (topical or systemic) and those who have a compromised ocular surface, e.g. autoimmune cicatrizing conjunctivitis, neurotrophic corneas, and severe dry eye.
- *Filamentary fungal infection*: usually *Fusarium* and *Aspergillus* species.

Clinical features

- *General*: variable presentation, with onset ranging from insidious to rapid; symptoms range from none to pain, photophobia, tearing, and ↓VA.
- *Yeast infection*: insidious or rapid; often localized with 'button' appearance, expanding stromal infiltrate, and a relatively small epithelial ulceration.
- *Filamentary fungal infection*: usually insidious. Early: may be asymptomatic, intact epithelium, minimal corneal stromal infiltrate, and mild AC inflammation. Later: satellite lesions, feathery branching infiltrate, and immune ring. In severe infection: ulceration, involvement of deeper corneal layers and Descemet's membrane, white plaque on the endothelium, and severe AC inflammation (e.g. hypopyon).
- *Complications*: limbal and scleral extension, corneal perforation, endophthalmitis (see ➲ Post-operative endophthalmitis, p. 336), 2° bacterial infections, infectious crystalline keratopathy.

NB In late infection, these distinctive patterns may be lost, and the clinical appearance may resemble an advanced bacterial keratitis.

Investigation
- Perform early and adequate corneal scrapes (see Box 7.1).
- *Stains*: Gram (stains fungal walls), Giemsa (stains walls and cytoplasm); Grocott's methenamine silver (GMS) stain, periodic acid–Schiff (PAS) stain, and Calcofluor white may also be used.
- *Culture*: Sabouraud dextrose agar (for most fungi) and blood agar (for *Fusarium*); may require up to 14d; *in vitro* sensitivities are poorly predictive of *in vivo* sensitivity and so is little used clinically.

If strong clinical suspicion, but negative investigations, consider confocal microscopy or corneal biopsy for histopathology, and PCR for fungal DNA.

Fungal keratitis: treatment

Effective eradication of fungi is frequently difficult because of the deeply invasive nature of the infectious process. Identification of the organism (see ➲ Fungal keratitis: assessment, p. 228) must be a priority so as to ensure the optimal choice of therapy.

Treatment

Initial treatment

- Admit.
- Intensive topical broad-spectrum antifungal agents such as non-preserved clotrimazole 1%, natamycin 5% (preserved only), voriconazole 1% hourly day and night for the first 72h; voriconazole is the preferred agent for suspected/proven candidal infection, natamycin for filamentary fungal infection. For severe or unresponsive disease, add a second agent (e.g. preservative-free amphotericin 0.15% hourly day and night for first 24h, then reducing to day only).
- Avoid corticosteroids (reduce/stop them if already on them); may cautiously be used during healing phase (see ➲ Ongoing treatment, p. 231).
- Oral analgesia and cycloplegia (e.g. preservative-free cyclopentolate 1% 3×/d).

Systemic treatment

Consider the addition of systemic antifungal treatment (e.g. oral fluconazole or itraconazole) (see Box 7.4) which should be considered for:

- Severe disease (e.g. deep stromal lesions, threatened perforation, endophthalmitis), and in
- All immunocompromised patients.

Box 7.4 Systemic treatment in fungal keratitis

- *First line*: consider oral fluconazole (50–100mg 1×/d for 7–14d) which is effective against *Candida* and *Aspergillus*.
- *In resistant cases or where Aspergillus has been identified*: consider voriconazole (PO 400mg 2×/d for two doses, then 200mg 2×/d, but can ↑ to 300mg 2×/d; IV 6mg/kg 2×/d for two doses, then 4mg/kg 2×/d).
- An alternative for invasive yeast infections is IV flucytosine (50mg/kg 4×/d; adjust as per plasma level monitoring).

- Topical treatment should be continued.
- Liaise with a microbiologist for advice re drug selection, dosing, and monitoring.

NB Systemic antifungals are associated with significant side effects, including renal dysfunction (voriconazole), hepatotoxicity (fluconazole, voriconazole), blood disorders (flucytosine, voriconazole). Monitoring should include FBC, U+E, and LFT prior to starting treatment and at least weekly during treatment. In addition, dosing may need to be reduced in the presence of renal dysfunction, and plasma level monitoring is required for flucytosine (see Table 7.9).

Ongoing treatment
- Taper treatment, according to clinical improvement. Relapse is common and may signify incomplete sterilization or reactivation. Treatment is prolonged (12wk). In the healing phase, topical corticosteroids (e.g. preservative-free dexamethasone 0.1% 1×/d) are sometimes used; this should be at the direction of a corneal specialist and carefully monitored.
- Consider PK for progressive disease (to remove fungus/prevent perforation) or in the quiet, but visually compromised, eye.

Table 7.9 Antifungal agents

Class	Mechanism	Examples
Polyene	Destabilize cell wall	Natamycin, amphotericin
Imidazole	Destabilize cell wall	Clotrimazole, econazole, ketoconazole, miconazole
Triazole	Destabilize cell wall	Itraconazole, voriconazole, fluconazole
Pyrimidine	Cytotoxic	Flucytosine

Herpes simplex keratitis (1)

HSV is a dsDNA virus with two serotypes. HSV1 shows airborne transmission and classically causes infection of the eyes, face, and trunk; HSV2 infection is sexually transmitted and usually causes genital herpes with rare ophthalmic involvement.

1° infection is usually with a blepharoconjunctivitis, occasionally with corneal involvement. Following this, the virus ascends the sensory nerve axon to reside in latency in the trigeminal ganglion. Viral reactivation, replication, and retrograde migration to the cornea results in recurrent keratitis, which may be epithelial, stromal, endothelial (discoid), or neurotrophic. Potential intraocular involvement includes anterior uveitis and retinitis. Additionally, the resultant neurotrophic cornea is vulnerable to bacterial and fungal keratitis.

Blepharoconjunctivitis

HSV1 infection is common (90% of the population are seropositive). 1° infection occurs in childhood with generalized viral malaise and is usually ophthalmically silent. The most common ocular manifestation is a self-limiting blepharoconjunctivitis, characterized by periorbital vesicular rash, follicular conjunctivitis, and preauricular lymphadenopathy. HSV keratitis in 1° infection is rare; however, prophylactic topical (Oc) aciclovir 3% 5×/d or oral aciclovir prophylaxis may be considered. The skin is treated with topical aciclovir 5% cream 3×/d.

Epithelial keratitis

Clinical features

- FB sensation, pain, blurred vision, lacrimation.
- Superficial punctate keratitis → stellate erosion → dendritic ulcer (branching morphology with terminal bulbs, cf. pseudodendrites) → geographic ulcer (large amoeboid ulcer with dendritic advancing edges; more common if immunosuppressed/topical steroids). Ulcer base stains with fluorescein (de-epithelialized); ulcer margins stain with Rose Bengal (devitalized viral-infected epithelial cells); ↓ corneal sensation.
- *Systemic*: may have associated orofacial or genital ulceration.

Investigation

- This is usually a clinical diagnosis, but, where diagnostic uncertainty, investigate both for viral and other microbial causes (see ➔ Microbial keratitis: assessment, p. 222).
- Conjunctival and corneal swabs for molecular diagnosis (PCR and ELISA).
- *Corneal scrapings*: Giemsa stain (multinuclear giant cells).

Treatment
- *Topical antiviral*: aciclovir 3% Oc initially 5×/d for 10–14 days and continued for at least 3d after complete healing; if resistant, consider trifluorothymidine 1% initially 9×/d, but beware epithelial toxicity.
- Consider cycloplegia (e.g. cyclopentolate 1% 2×/d) for comfort/AC inflammation.
- If patient is on topical steroids for coexistent ocular disease, reduce steroid dose (potency and frequency) where possible. Where HSV keratitis is occurring in a corneal graft, reduction of topical steroids may increase the risk of graft rejection.
- If recurrent attacks, consider oral antivirals (e.g. aciclovir 400mg PO 2×/d, with an aim of providing a prolonged remission period) as prophylaxis.

Stromal keratitis
Stromal keratitis may occur with or without epithelial ulceration.

Clinical features
- Multiple or diffuse opacities → corneal vascularization, lipid exudation, and scarring; or may → thinning; AC activity.
- *Complications*: ↑ IOP; rarely perforation.

Treatment
- *Topical steroid*: defer (where possible) until epithelium intact; aim for minimum effective dose (e.g. prednisolone 0.1–1% 1–4×/d, titrating down in frequency and strength).
- *Antiviral*: systemic aciclovir (initially 400mg 5×/d, then reduce; prophylactic dose is 400mg 2×/d). There is clear evidence that systemic aciclovir is beneficial and useful in prevention of recurrence. Consider in all patients with atopic keratoconjunctivitis, ocular surface disease, or frequent recurrences. Use of topical aciclovir (3% Oc 5×/d) is controversial but may be of benefit if stromal keratitis is associated with epithelial breakdown. Valaciclovir or famciclovir may be considered in cases intolerant to aciclovir.
- Cycloplegia (e.g. cyclopentolate 1% 2×/d) for comfort/AC activity.
- Monitor IOP and treat, as necessary.
- *Surgery*: may be indicated acutely for perforation (tectonic graft) or in the long term for scarring (deep anterior lamellar keratoplasty preferred to PK where possible).

NB If facilities available, quantify and delineate corneal neovascularization, using fluorescein and ICG angiography, to monitor treatment.

Herpes simplex keratitis (2)

Disciform keratitis (endotheliitis)

Disciform keratitis probably results from viral antigen hypersensitivity, rather than reactivation.

Clinical features
- Painless, ↓VA, haloes.
- Central/paracentral disc of corneal oedema, Descemet's folds, mild AC activity, fine KPs; Wessely ring (stromal halo of precipitated viral antigen/host antibody).
- *Complications*: ↑IOP, chronic anterior uveitis.

Investigation
- If presentation is atypical and there is no previous history of herpetic keratitis, AC paracentesis and PCR of aqueous are of diagnostic benefit. Beware false negatives, as long-term aciclovir will reduce HSV DNA copy number.

Treatment
- *Topical steroid*: defer (where possible) until epithelium intact; aim for minimum effective dose (e.g. dexamethasone 0.1% or prednisolone 0.5% 1–4×/d, titrating down in frequency and strength); some patients may require low dose (e.g. prednisolone 0.1% alt—1×/d) for months or even maintenance. Use preservative-free treatment if coexistent ocular surface disease.
- *Antiviral*: aciclovir, systemic (initially 400mg 5x /d, then reduce; prophylactic dose is 400mg 2x/d); continue as prophylaxis (can ↓ frequency) until on low-frequency/low-strength topical steroid.
- Cycloplegia (e.g. cyclopentolate 1% 2×/d) for comfort/AC activity.
- Monitor IOP and treat, as necessary (see **➲** Treatment, p. 372).

Herpes zoster ophthalmicus

VZV is a dsDNA virus of the herpes group. 1° infection of VZV results in chickenpox (varicella). Reactivation of virus dormant in the sensory ganglion results in shingles (herpes zoster) of the innervated dermatome. Involvement of the ophthalmic branch of the trigeminal nerve occurs in 15% of shingles cases and results in HZO.

Transmission is by direct contact or droplet spread. Those never previously infected with VZV may contract chickenpox from contact with shingles. VZV infection may be more severe in the immunosuppressed, the elderly, pregnant women, and neonates. Maternal infection may also cause fetal malformations (3% risk in first trimester).

Systemic and cutaneous disease

Clinical features

Viral prodrome, preherpetic neuralgia (mild intermittent tingling to severe constant electric pain), rash (papules → vesicles → pustules → scabs) predominantly within the one dermatome (Va); Hutchinson's sign (cutaneous involvement of the tip of the nose, indicating nasociliary nerve involvement and likelihood of ocular complications); may be disseminated in the immunocompromised. Additionally, the resultant neurotrophic cornea is vulnerable to bacterial and fungal keratitis.

Treatment

- *Systemic antiviral*: start as soon as rash appears, either aciclovir PO 800mg 5×/d for 5d, valaciclovir PO 1g 3×/d for 7d, or famciclovir PO 750mg 1×/d for 7d; if immunosuppressed, then aciclovir IV 10mg/kg 3×/d.
- Post-herpetic neuralgia may cause depression (even suicide); treatments include amitriptyline, gabapentin, and topical capsaicin cream.

Keratitis

Clinical features

- *Epithelial*: superficial punctate keratitis + pseudodendrites, often with anterior stromal infiltrates; acute (onset 2–3d after rash; resolve in few week); common.
- *Stromal*: nummular keratitis with anterior stromal granular deposits is uncommon and occurs early (10d); necrotizing interstitial keratitis with stromal infiltrates, thinning, and even perforation (cf. HSV) is rare and occurs late (3mo–years).
- *Disciform*: endotheliitis with disc of corneal oedema, Descemet's folds, mild AC activity, fine KPs (cf. HSV); late onset (3mo–years); chronic; uncommon.
- *Neurotrophic*: corneal nerve damage causes persistent epithelial defect, thinning, and even perforation; late onset; chronic; uncommon.
- *Mucus plaques*: linear grey elevations, loosely adherent to underlying diseased epithelium/stroma; late onset (3mo–years); chronic.

Treatment
- Ensure adequate systemic antiviral treatment.

Additionally:
- *Epithelial*: topical lubricants, usually preservative-free (e.g. Celluvisc® 0.5–1% 8×/d).
- *Stromal and disciform*: topical steroid treatment (e.g. prednisolone 0.1–1% 1–4×/d, titrating down in frequency and strength); some patients may require low dose (e.g. prednisolone 0.1% alt—1×/d) for months or even maintenance; threatened perforation may require gluing, BCL, or tectonic grafting.
- *Neurotrophic*: preservative-free topical lubricants (e.g. Celluvisc® 0.5–1% 8×/d + Lacri-Lube® nocte), and consider tarsorrhaphy (surgical or medical with botulinum toxin-induced ptosis), AMG, or conjunctival flap.
- *Mucus plaques*: require mucolytics (e.g. acetylcysteine 5–10% non-preserved 3×/d) or surgical debridement.
- *Anterior uveitis*: topical steroid treatment (e.g. dexamethasone 0.1%) and cycloplegia (e.g. cyclopentolate 1% 2×/d) for comfort/AC activity.
- *Monitor IOP*: assess whether due to inflammation or steroids, and treat accordingly.
- *Corneal scarring*: axial scarring may require PK.

Other complications associated with HZO

- *Ocular*: conjunctivitis, 2° microbial keratitis, glaucoma, anterior uveitis, necrotizing retinitis (acute retinal necrosis (ARN), progressive outer retinal necrosis (PORN)), episcleritis, scleritis, optic neuritis, cranial nerve palsies.
- *Systemic*: strokes (cerebral vasculitis), neuralgia.

Thygeson's superficial punctate keratopathy

A rare condition, most commonly arising in young adulthood, which may last anywhere from 1mo to 24y. The aetiology is idiopathic, but a viral cause is suspected. It is bilateral but often asymmetric.[3,4]

Clinical features
- Bilateral recurrent FB sensation, photophobia, and tearing.
- Coarse, stellate grey-white epithelial opacities in a white, quiet eye; the opacities appear slightly elevated but are classically non-staining with fluorescein or lissamine green. There may be a slight epithelial haze.

Treatment
- Topical corticosteroids (e.g. fluorometholone 0.1%) which can be rapidly tapered; sometimes a mild maintenance dose (even 1×/wk) is required to prevent further episodes.
- *Consider therapeutic CL*: for vision and comfort.

3. Thygeson P. Superficial punctate keratitis. *J Am Med Assoc* 1950;**144**:1544–9.

4. Nagra PK *et al*. Thygeson's superficial punctate keratitis: ten years' experience. *Ophthalmology* 2004;**111**:34–7.

Recurrent corneal erosion syndrome (RCES)

As clinical features may have resolved by the time the patient sees an ophthalmologist, a provisional diagnosis of RCES may be made on history alone. RCES is indicative of failure of epithelial to BM readhesion and is defined as recurrent episodes of spontaneous breakdown of the corneal epithelium.

Risk factors

- Sharp trauma.
- *Corneal dystrophies*: anterior (especially epithelial BM dystrophy and Reis–Bucklers dystrophy) or stromal dystrophies.
- Post-keratoplasty.
- Diabetes, dry eye, ocular rosacea.

Clinical features

- Recurrent episodes of severe pain and photophobia, usually starting on opening eyes after sleep; aggravated by blinking; resolves within hours; history of corneal trauma (often forgotten).
- Variable degree of epithelial irregularities (including loose epithelium without staining) or frank epithelial defects; may also have signs of underlying disease, e.g. microcysts, maps, dots, fingerprints, or stromal changes. When severe, may last for several days, with pain accompanied by lid oedema, ciliary injection, extreme photophobia, and reduced vision.

NB May predispose to infection.

Pathology

Abnormalities of epithelial adhesion, defects in hemidesmosomes, BM which may exhibit thinning and reduplication. Excessive MMPs result in enzymatic degradation of adhesion complexes.

Treatment

Conservative

- *Topical*: lubricants (e.g. carmellose 0.5–1% hourly during the day, Oc Lacri-Lube® nocte ± cycloplegia (e.g. cyclopentolate 1% 2×/d), NSAID (e.g. ketorolac 3×/d) for comfort.
- *Therapeutic CL*: extended wear silicone hydrogel or high water content hydrogel.
- Tetracyclines (e.g. doxycyline 50–100mg 1×/d for 3mo or oxytetracycline 250mg 2×/d for 3mo) may be beneficial, since they inhibit MMP activity and promote epithelial stability (contraindicated in children under 12 (alternatively erythromycin 250mg 2×/d 8–12y, 125mg 2×/d 2–8y), in pregnant/breastfeeding women, or in hepatic or renal impairment).

Surgical
- *Mechanical debridement*: consider mechanical debridement if heaped up, devitalized epithelium. Anaesthetize cornea; gently break away non-adherent grey epithelium with moistened cotton bud or sponge; use post-procedure therapeutic CL with topical non-preserved chloramphenicol eye drops (0.5% 4×/d for 1wk to prevent 2° infection).
- *Alcohol delamination of the epithelium*: this promotes 'smoothing' of the stromal bed to improve epithelial adhesion. Technique involves 4–5 drops of 18% alcohol applied within a circular corneal well placed on top of the cornea for 30–40s. This is then drained from the well (e.g. by a surgical sponge), followed by epithelial debridement of entire corneal epithelium with a cotton-tipped applicator.
- *Excimer laser phototherapeutic keratectomy*: consider this procedure for refractory or severe cases of RCES. Where therapeutic laser is not available, anterior stromal micropuncture may be considered for RCES outside the visual axis. Anterior stromal micropuncture is performed at the slit-lamp (if cooperative patient) or in theatre with topical anaesthesia, and using a bent 25G needle to cover the defective area with closely packed micropunctures through epithelium and Bowman's layer.

Persistent epithelial defects

An epithelial defect is defined as persistent when it has failed to heal within a 2wk period. Persistent corneal epithelial defects arise when there is a failure of the mechanisms promoting corneal epithelialization, resulting in disassembly of hemidesmosomes. This is accompanied by degradation of Bowman's layer and stroma as a consequence of the disruption of the normally protective corneal microenvironment during a disease process.

Risk factors

Neurotrophic corneas, limbal stem cell deficiency such as chemical injury or hereditary conditions (aniridia); and immune-mediated ocular surface disorders, including atopic keratoconjunctivitis, OcMMP, SJS, and peripheral ulcerative sclerokeratitis.

Treatment

The treatment strategy must consider both the healing phase and then the maintenance phase (i.e. prevention of future epithelial defects). Treatment may include some of the following:

- *Topical treatment*:
  - Oc chloramphenicol 1% with double pad.
  - Lubricants (e.g. carmellose 0.5–1% hourly during the day, Oc paraffin eye ointment nocte ± sodium hyaluronate preparations 4×/d).
  - If there is contributing ocular surface inflammation (e.g. OcMMP, granulomatosis with polyangiitis (GPA, previously Wegener's)), then consider topical steroids (± systemic steroids/immunosuppression).
  - For severe cases, consider autologous serum drops.
- Systemic doxycycline 100mg 1×/d, ascorbic acid 1g 2×/d.
- *CL*: extended wear silicone hydrogel, high water content hydrogel, or gas-permeable scleral CL.
- *Lid procedures*: botulinum toxin-induced tarsorrhaphy or surgical tarsorrhaphy; punctal plugs; punctal occlusion.
- *Grafting procedures*: AM transplant, LESC transplantation, Gunderson flap, buccal mucous membrane graft (see Box 7.5 and Box 7.6).

Box 7.5 The role of AM transplantation in persistent epithelial defects

See also ➲ Amniotic membrane transplantation, p. 283.

- The use of AMG is usually reserved for cases where 1° conservative measures (ocular lubricants, therapeutic CL, and autologous serum (if available)) have failed and/or when there has been loss of Bowman's layer, when AM is used as a BM substrate, enabling corneal epithelial cell migration and closure of the epithelial defect.
- Beneficial effects of AMG appear to be independent of surgical technique employed (patch, bandage, or overlay).

Box 7.6 Developments in ocular lubricants

Most commercially available artificial tears do little more than lubricate and fail to recapitulate other properties of natural tears such as nutrition, promoting ocular surface renewal, and immunological defence. However, there is evidence that newer agents, such as those containing carboxy-methylcellulose or sodium hyaluronate preparations, do appear to have advantages beyond simple lubrication.

- *Carboxymethylcellulose (syn carmellose)*: these preparations have improved ocular surface retention and appear to be cytoprotective.
- *Sodium hyaluronate (hyaluronic acid)*: there is evidence that these preparations may be cytoprotective, promote BM hemidesmosome formation, and have improved surface retention in inflamed eyes due to specific ligand binding to exaggerated CD44 (a transmembrane cell surface adhesion molecule) expression on the ocular surface during inflammation.[*,†] Hyaluronic acid itself is a ubiquitous naturally occurring extracellular matrix glycosaminoglycan, which plays an important role in wound healing, inflammation, and lubrication.

[*] Haider AS et al. In vitro model of 'wound healing' analyzed by laser scanning cytometry: accelerated healing of epithelial cell monolayers in the presence of hyaluronate. *Cytometry A* 2003;**53**:1–8.

[†] Gomes JA et al. Sodium hyaluronate (hyaluronic acid) promotes migration of human corneal epithelial cells *in vitro*. *Br J Ophthalmol* 2004;**88**:821–5.

Limbal epithelial stem cell deficiency

The corneal limbus is thought to contain small numbers of LESC, resident within a specialized stem cell niche. The stem cells generate a continuous supply of daughter cells which, outside the stem cell niche, follow the normal paths of differentiation to replenish the ocular surface. This is vital to the maintenance of a healthy ocular surface, not only in terms of recovery from trauma, but also in the face of daily wear and tear. Deficiency of LESC leads to poor epithelialization, inflammation, vascularization, and scarring.

The presence of stem cells residing in a limbal niche explains a number of interesting clinical observations, notably the centripetal migration of healing epithelium, the circumferential migration of limbal epithelium, and that the columns of migration correspond to palisades of Vogt. Although there is no specific marker for LESC, identification may be assisted by the absence of markers typical of corneal epithelium (such as cytokeratins K3 or K12) and the presence of progenitor markers such as ABCG2 (an ATP-binding cassette transporter protein) and P63 (a transcription factor) (see Table 7.10 for causes).

Causes

Table 7.10 Causes of LESC deficiency

- Aniridia.
- Chemical injury.
- Thermal injury.
- UV/ionizing irradiation.
- CL wear.
- Preservative toxicity.
- Ocular surface malignancy.
- Neurotrophic cornea.
- Peripheral ulcerative keratitis.
- Inflammation:
  - OcMMP.
  - Atopic keratoconjunctivitis.
  - SJS/TEN.

Clinical features

- Conjunctivalization (invasion of conjunctival epithelium onto the corneal surface); 'corneal' epithelium which is opaque, irregular, thickened, and unstable after even minor trauma; persistent epithelial defects + corneal vascularization, inflammation, calcification.
- *Complications*: 2° corneal infection, perforation, and intraocular infection may render the eye permanently blind.

Investigations

Diagnosis can be confirmed on immunohistological studies (e.g. from impression cytology), demonstrating the presence of mucin-containing goblet cells on the cornea and the absence of normal differentiation markers of corneal epithelium (such as cytokeratins 3 and 12).

Treatment

See Table 7.11 for an approach to treatment.

Table 7.11 An approach to the treatment of LESC deficiency

Deficiency	Additional features	Treatment options
Partial	Conjunctivalized metaplastic epithelium on cornea	*If visual axis not involved:* Sequential sector conjunctival epitheliectomy
		If visual axis involved: Sequential sector conjunctival epitheliectomy + AMG
	With fibrovascular pannus	Sector limbal transplant + AMG
Total	Unilateral	Conjunctival limbal autograft (CLAU) from contralateral better eye
		Cultivated limbal corneal epithelial cells from contralateral better eye using carrier, e.g. AMG
	Bilateral	Living-related keratolimbal allograft (KLAL)
		Cadaveric KLAL
		Cultivated limbal corneal epithelial cells from cadaveric limbus using carrier, e.g. AMG

Allografts

Potential allograft donors are screened for hepatitis serology (HBsAg, antibodies to hepatitis C virus (HCV), HCV nucleic acid testing), HIV I/II, human T-cell lymphoma virus, and syphilis. Patients receiving allografts will require systemic immunosuppression (e.g. mycophenolate ± ciclosporin/rapamycin).

Cultivated limbal corneal epithelial cells

Cultivation of limbal corneal epithelial cells for transplantation into humans is an exciting development which requires meticulous care and is stringently regulated. In the UK, for example, the following requirements have to be met: Class 100 clean room facilities, compliance with the Human Tissue Act 2004 and the European Union Tissues and Cells Directive, compliance with Good Manufacturing Practice, and approval of the Medicines and Healthcare products Regulatory Agency (MHRA).

Corneal degenerative disease (1)

Arcus

A common bilateral degeneration, 2° to progressive deposition of lipid in the peripheral stroma. It is usually age-related but may be associated with hyperlipidaemia.

Causes

Most bilateral cases have no systemic association, but hyperlipidaemia (notably type II) should be ruled out in those presenting at a young age (arcus juvenilis). Unilateral arcus is rare and may signify ipsilateral carotid compromise or previous ocular hypotony.

Clinical features

Progressive peripheral opacity starts (and remains thickest) at 3 and 9 o'clock but spreads circumferentially to form a complete ring of around 1mm thickness; typically, the central margin is blurred, but the peripheral margin is sharp, leaving a zone of clear perilimbal cornea (which may show thinning).

Cornea farinata

A bilateral symmetrical degeneration of deep stromal, faint flour-like opacities which are prominent centrally but remain visually insignificant.

Crocodile shagreen

A faint reticular, polygonal network of stromal opacities, resembling crocodile skin. Anterior stromal shagreen is more common than posterior, but both forms are innocuous and asymptomatic.

Vogt's limbal girdle

A common bilateral degeneration. There is chalky white peripheral corneal deposition at 3 and 9 o'clock. It may be separated from the limbus by a clear perilimbal zone (type I), or it may extend to the limbus (type II). Both types are innocuous and asymptomatic.

1° lipid keratopathy

A rare idiopathic corneal deposition of cholesterol, fat, and phospholipids, appearing as yellow-white stromal deposits, with no associated vascularization. It is usually innocuous and non-progressive and requires no treatment.

2° lipid keratopathy

Causes

This may accompany corneal vascularization, following ocular injury or inflammation. Common causes include previous herpetic (simplex or zoster disciform) keratitis, trauma, and interstitial keratitis.

Clinical features

Corneal vascularization with associated yellow-white stromal deposition.

Investigations

If facilities available, quantify and delineate corneal neovascularization, using fluorescein and ICG angiography, to enable targeted vessel treatment and for monitoring of treatment.

Treatment

Treat underlying cause of ocular inflammation. Long-term mild corticosteroid (e.g. fluorometholone) is occasionally useful. Consider feeder vessel occlusion or PK.

- *Occlusion of the feeder vessel*: may be by argon laser photocoagulation or direct needle point cautery under the operating microscope. Anterior segment fluorescein angiography may help identify the feeder vessel.
- *PK*: it is performed if the disease is severe, persistent, and once the eye is quiet. However, prognosis is guarded due to the poor condition of host tissue and preoperative vascularization.
- There is some evidence that topical or subconjunctival anti-vascular endothelial growth factor (anti-VEGF) therapy may be of benefit.

Corneal degenerative disease (2)

Band keratopathy

A common progressive subepithelial deposition of calcium phosphate salts which may be due to ocular or systemic causes (see Table 7.12 for cause).

Causes

Table 7.12 Causes of band keratopathy

Ocular	Anterior segment inflammation	Chronic anterior uveitis
		Chronic keratitis
		Chronic corneal oedema
		Silicone oil in AC
	Phthisis bulbi	
Systemic		1° (familial)
		Senile
		Ichthyosis
		Hypercalcaemia
		Hyperphosphataemia
		Hyperuricaemia
		Chronic renal failure

Clinical features
- Often asymptomatic; FB sensation, pain, ↓VA.
- White opacities starting at 3 and 9 o'clock, progressing centrally to coalesce to form a band.

Treatment
- Identify and treat underlying cause, as appropriate.
- Consider therapeutic CL for comfort (often as a temporary measure).
- Remove calcium salts by: *chemical chelation* (disodium ethylenediamine tetra-acetic acid), followed by mechanical debridement (e.g. gentle scraping with No. 15 blade), followed by insertion of therapeutic CL; or *excimer therapeutic laser keratectomy*.

Salzmann nodular degeneration

An uncommon slowly progressive degeneration, usually seen as a complication of chronic keratitis. It arises from replacement of Bowman's layer by eosinophilic material.

Causes

Chronic keratitis, including trachoma, phlyctenular keratitis, vernal keratitis, interstitial keratitis; post-corneal surgery; idiopathic.

Clinical features

- Glare, ↓VA, pain (if loss of overlying epithelium).
- Well-defined grey-white elevated nodules ± iron lines (indicate chronicity). There may be associated epithelial breakthrough and discomfort.

Treatment

Identify and treat underlying keratitis. Consider lubrication, therapeutic CL, or excimer laser keratectomy.

Corneal dystrophies: anterior

Epithelial basement membrane dystrophy (*syn* map-dot-fingerprint dystrophy, Cogan's microcystic dystrophy)

The most common corneal dystrophy, with a prevalence of around 2.5%. Although there are pedigrees demonstrating AD inheritance, most clinical presentations appear to be non-familial. There is a slight ♀ predilection. It usually presents in early adulthood.

Pathophysiology

The basic defect appears to lie in epithelium–BM interaction. In the absence of normal hemidesmosomes and anchoring fibrils, there is continued secretion and intraepithelial extension of BM (maps), breakdown of desmosomes, degeneration of sequestered epithelial cells (dots or microcysts), and deposition of fibrillar material (fingerprints).

Clinical features

- Bilateral, asymmetrical; may be asymptomatic, but recurrent erosions in 10–33% (pain, lacrimation, photophobia).
- Epithelial maps (faint opacities), dots/microcysts, fingerprints (curvilinear ridges).

Treatment

- As for RCES (see ➲ Treatment, p. 240).

Reis–Bucklers dystrophy

A relatively common AD progressive dystrophy. It usually presents with recurrent erosions in early childhood. With age, these become less painful (due to ↓ corneal sensation), but central opacity may lead to ↓ VA.

Pathophysiology

This is caused by a mutation in the keratoepithilin gene *BIGH3* (also known as *TGFBI*; Chr 5q). There is progressive degeneration of Bowman's layer, with subepithelial collagen deposition (stains blue with Masson trichome). Thiel–Behnke (honeycomb dystrophy) is a similar, but milder, condition arising from a different mutation in *BIGH3*.

Clinical features

- Bilateral recurrent erosions (pain, lacrimation, photophobia); later ↓ VA.
- Multiple subepithelial grey reticular opacities, usually starting centrally.

Treatment

- As for RCES (see ➲ Treatment, p. 240).
- Consider excimer laser superficial keratectomy, or lamellar/PK if ↓ VA.

Meesman's dystrophy

A rare AD dystrophy. It usually presents in adulthood.

Pathophysiology

This is caused by mutations in the genes for cytokeratins CK3 (Chr 12) and CK12 (Chr 17) which normally form the cytoskeleton of the epithelial cell.

Clinical features

- Initially asymptomatic; mild ocular irritation, photophobia, and mild ↓VA in adulthood.
- Discrete clear epithelial vesicles; initially central but spread peripherally (sparing the limbus).

Treatment

- Treatment is not usually required; however, rarely lamellar keratoplasty may be considered in significant photophobia or visual impairment.

Corneal dystrophies: stromal (1)

Lattice dystrophy types I, II, III

Rare AD dystrophies, involving the progressive deposition of amyloid in the corneal stroma and sometimes elsewhere in the body. Type I is the commonest form and is isolated to the eye. Type II forms part of familial systemic amyloidosis (Meretoja's syndrome). Type III is rare, isolated to the eye, and is seen in those of Japanese origin.

Pathophysiology

Type I lattice dystrophy is caused by a mutation in the keratoepithilin gene *BIGH3* (also known as *TGFBI*; Chr 5q). Type II results from a mutation in the gene for the plasma protein gelsolin (Chr 9q). In all types, amyloid is deposited in the stroma, but, in types I and II, it may also disrupt the BM and epithelium. Amyloid stains with Congo red and demonstrates apple green birefringence and dichroism at polarizing microscopy.

Clinical features

- ↓VA, recurrent erosions (pain, lacrimation, photophobia).
- Bilateral (often asymmetric) criss-cross refractile lines; later, these may be obscured by a progressive central corneal haze (types I and II).
  In type III, the lines are thicker and more prominent. The peripheral cornea is usually spared.

Systemic features

- *In type II lattice dystrophy with familial amyloidosis (Meretoja's syndrome)*: mask-like facies, skin laxity, cranial nerve palsies (commonly VIIn, with additional risk of corneal exposure), peripheral neuropathy, renal failure, and cardiac failure.

Treatment

- As for RCES (see ➜ Treatment, p. 240).
- Consider PK or excimer laser keratectomy if ↓ VA. Recurrence after either procedure is common. If type II disease suspected, refer to physician for assessment of systemic involvement.

Granular dystrophy

A rare AD dystrophy, involving deposition of hyaline material in the corneal stroma. It presents in adulthood.

Pathophysiology

Granular dystrophy is caused by a mutation in the keratoepithilin gene *BIGH3* (Chr 5q). Hyaline material (probably phospholipids) deposited in the stroma stains red with Masson trichrome.

Clinical features

- ↓VA; occasionally recurrent erosions.
- Bilateral (often asymmetric) white, crumb-like opacities in otherwise clear stroma; initially central but progressively coalesce.

Treatment
- As for RCES (see ➲ Treatment, p. 240).
- If ↓ VA, consider PK or lamellar keratoplasty if relatively superficial disease. Recurrence is common.

Avellino dystrophy

A very rare AD dystrophy with some features of both granular and lattice dystrophies. It is usually seen in those originating out of Avellino, Italy.

Pathophysiology
Avellino dystrophy is caused by a mutation in the keratoepithilin gene *BIGH3* (Chr 5q). The stromal deposit stains both for hyaline (Masson trichrome) and amyloid (Congo red; birefringence and dichroism at polarizing microscopy).

Clinical features
- ↓VA; recurrent erosions (pain, lacrimation, photophobia).
- Bilateral (often asymmetric) granular-type opacities in anterior stroma and lattice-type lines in deeper stroma; may have a central subepithelial haze later.

Treatment
- As for RCES (see ➲ Treatment, p. 240).
- Consider PK if ↓ VA. Recurrence is common.

Corneal dystrophies: stromal (2)

Macular dystrophy

A rare autosomal recessive (AR) dystrophy, involving deposition of a glycosaminoglycan in the stroma. Abnormal stromal collagen packing causes loss of corneal translucency, usually from early adulthood.

Pathophysiology

This is effectively an ocular-specific mucopolysaccharidosis, arising from mutations in the gene for carbohydrate sulfotransferase (*CHST6*; Chr 16q). Abnormal glycosaminoglycans, similar to keratan sulfate, accumulate. These stain with alcian blue or colloidal iron. Macular dystrophy may be subclassified as type I (no keratan sulfate) and type II (low keratan sulfate).

Clinical features

- Gradual painless ↓VA; often incidental finding.
- Bilateral (often asymmetric) focal, ill-defined grey-white stromal opacities, superimposed on diffuse clouding; it may involve the whole cornea being superficial centrally, but potentially involving full stromal thickness peripherally. Cornea may be thinned.

Treatment

- If ↓VA, consider PK, or lamellar keratoplasty if relatively superficial disease. Recurrence is rare.

Schnyder's crystalline dystrophy

This is a rare progressive dystrophy presenting in childhood, with an AD inheritance pattern arising from mutations in the *UBIAD1* gene (Chr 1p). Stromal crystals contain cholesterol and neutral fat (stains red with Oil red O). It may be associated with systemic hypercholesterolaemia.

Clinical features

- ↓VA, glare.
- Central anterior stromal yellow-white (often scintillating) crystals ± corneal haze, and arcus.

Treatment

- Consider excimer laser keratectomy or PK if ↓ VA. Recurrence may occur. Check fasting lipids.

Congenital stromal corneal dystrophy

This is a very rare AD dystrophy, arising from a mutation in the decorin gene (*DCN*; Chr 12q); it was previously known as congenital hereditary stromal dystrophy (CHSD). It presents at birth with bilateral corneal clouding, due to 'snowflake' whitish opacities, without oedema throughout the entire cornea. It is static or slowly progressive. It appears to arise due to abnormalities of stromal collagen, but with normal anterior and posterior corneal layers. Corneal thickness is normal. Treatment requires PK.

Other dystrophies of the corneal stroma

- *Central cloudy dystrophy*: AD, similar changes to posterior crocodile shagreen, visually insignificant.
- *Fleck dystrophy*: AD, white flecks throughout stroma, visually insignificant.
- *Posterior amorphous corneal dystrophy*: AD, grey sheets in deep stroma, non-progressive, rarely visually significant.

Corneal dystrophies: posterior

Fuchs' endothelial dystrophy

A common corneal dystrophy that may be AD or sporadic. It is more commonly seen in ♀ (♀:♂ 4:1) and with increasing age. Presentation is usually gradual, with ↓VA from middle age, but may be acute after endothelial injury (e.g. intraocular surgery). There appears to be an increased incidence of 1° open-angle glaucoma (POAG).

Pathogenesis

1° endothelial dysfunction associated with $Na^+K^+ATPase$ pump failure allows the accumulation of fluid. Early-onset Fuchs' endothelial dystrophy has been associated with collagen VIII α2 gene (*COL8A2*; Chr 1p); more common late-onset forms arise from a number of genes, including *SLC4A11* (Chr 20p) and the homeobox gene *ZEB1* (Chr 10p). Microscopically, there is irregular thickening of Descemet's membrane, protuberances (guttata) and flattening, irregularity in size, and loss of endothelial cells.

Clinical features

- Gradual ↓VA (often worse in morning); may arise after intraocular surgery.
- *Stage 1*: corneal guttata (appear centrally, cf. the peripheral Hassall–Henle bodies which are normal with age); may extend to give 'beaten metal' appearance; pigment on endothelium.
- *Stage 2*: stromal oedema → Descemet's folds and epithelial bullae.
- *Stage 3*: recurrent corneal erosions → subepithelial vascular pannus and stromal haze.

Investigations

- *Specular microscopy*: ↓cell count, ↑average cell diameter, ↓hexagons, ↑variation in cell size.
- *Pachymetry*: ↑CCT.

Treatment

Relieve corneal oedema and improve comfort

- Topical hypertonic agents: 5% NaCl.
- Treat ocular hypertension (OHT).
- Warm air blown on the eyes (e.g. hair dryer).
- BCL for bullous change.

Visual rehabilitation

- Persistent corneal oedema—patient may require endothelial replacement surgery, e.g. Descemet's stripping automated endothelial keratoplasty, Descemet's membrane endothelial keratoplasty (DMEK); or, if there is corneal scarring, patients may require PK.

Prevention

Corneal decompensation may be inadvertently accelerated by the ophthalmologist:

- *Cataract surgery*: consider: (1) protecting the endothelium with additional heavy viscoelastic (soft-shell technique) and (as always) minimizing phako-time and (2) referring more severe cases to a corneal specialist for elective cataract surgery, followed by endothelial replacement surgery. Occasionally, simultaneous cataract and endothelial surgery may be performed. Rarely, if there is corneal scarring, a keratoplasty/cataract extraction/IOL (triple procedure). NB Careful counselling re risk of decompensation is essential prior to cataract surgery and is preferred.
- *OHT/glaucoma*: topical β-blocker preferred; topical carbonic anhydrase inhibitors may theoretically induce endothelial failure.

Congenital hereditary endothelial dystrophy (CHED)

CHED is an important cause of bilateral corneal oedema in otherwise healthy term neonates. The AR form (CHED2) is more common and more severe than the AD form (CHED1). The gene for CHED1 has been linked to the same region (Chr 20p) as the commonest form of posterior polymorphous corneal dystrophy (*PPCD1*); the gene for CHED2 has now been identified as *SLC4A11*, a sodium borate cotransporter essential for cell growth and proliferation in mammalian cells.

Clinical features

AR type

- Bilateral marked corneal oedema from birth; stroma up to 3× normal thickness; severe ↓VA, amblyopia and nystagmus; not usually painful.

AD type

- Bilateral mild corneal oedema from infancy, with tearing and photophobia; milder ↓VA and no nystagmus; gradually progressive.

Treatment

- *PK*: visual outcome is often limited by amblyopia.

Posterior polymorphous corneal dystrophy (PPCD)

PPCD is usually AD but has a very variable expression. There are three forms: PPCD1 (*VSX1*; Chr 20p), PPCD2 (*COL8A2*; Chr 1p), and PPCD3 (*ZEB1*; Chr 10p). It is often asymptomatic and may in fact be much commoner than currently appreciated. It shares features with iridocorneal endothelial (ICE) syndrome and the anterior segment dysgeneses.

Clinical features

- Clusters or lines of vesicles, irregular broad bands or diffuse haze of the posterior cornea ± iridocorneal adhesion, corectopia, glaucoma (closed or open angle).

Treatment

- Treatment is not usually necessary. Consider penetrating keratoplasty if significant ↓VA.

Keratoconus

A common corneal ectasia characterized by progressive *conical* distortion of the cornea, with irregular astigmatism, axial stromal thinning, apical protrusion, and increasing myopia. Prevalence estimates vary widely (0.05–5%), according to the population studied, the techniques used, and the definition adopted.

The aetiology is unclear but may be a combination of repeated trauma (e.g. eye rubbing) and abnormalities of corneal stroma (e.g. in connective tissue disorders). Previously, only 10% cases were thought to be familial. However, analysis by videokeratography suggests a high prevalence among asymptomatic family members, consistent with AD inheritance with variable penetrance.

Keratoconus usually presents in early adulthood; an earlier presentation is associated with a worse prognosis (see Table 7.13 for associations).

Risk factors

Table 7.13 Associations of keratoconus

Ocular		Leber's congenital amaurosis (LCA)
		VKC
		Floppy eyelid syndrome
		Retinitis Pigmentosa (RP)
		Retinopathy of prematurity (ROP)
Systemic	Atopy	Eczema
		Asthma
		Hay fever
	Connective tissue	Ehlers–Danlos syndrome
		Marfan's syndrome
		Osteogenesis imperfecta
	Other	Down's syndrome
		Crouzon's syndrome
		Apert's syndrome

Clinical features

- Usually bilateral (but asymmetric) progressive irregular astigmatism with ↓VA; progression continues into early adulthood but usually stabilizes by mid 30s.
- Corneal steepening/thinning (cone), Vogt's striae (vertical lines in the stroma which may disappear on pressure), Fleischer ring (iron deposition at base of cone), conical distortion of lower lid on downward gaze (Munson's sign), abnormal focusing of a slit-lamp beam orientated obliquely across the cone from the temporal side (Rizutti's sign), scissoring reflex on retinoscopy, oil droplet reflex on ophthalmoscopy.
- *Complications*: acute hydrops (Descemet's membrane rupture → acute corneal oedema, may result in scarring); corneal scar.

Investigations
- *Videokeratography/corneal topography*: this has largely replaced manual keratometry. It is used for diagnosis and monitoring of disease. It may also classify keratoconic changes according to:
  - *Severity*: mild (<48D), moderate (48–54D), and severe (>54D).
  - *Morphology*: cone, nipple, oval, bow tie, and globus.

Treatment
- *Counselling*: progressive nature of disease, frequent change in refractive error, potential impact on lifestyle (notably driving) and career. Since disease usually stabilizes by mid 30s, a patient with good VA at age 35 is unlikely to need a keratoplasty.
- *Mild astigmatism*: spectacle or CL correction.
- *Moderate astigmatism*: RGP lens (8.7–14.5mm), scleral lens (RGP). In CL- intolerant patients, insertion of intracorneal ring segments (ICRS) can flatten the cornea to improve vision and CL tolerance and collagen cross-linking.
- *Severe astigmatism*: deep anterior lamellar keratoplasty (if normal Descemet's membrane) or PK. 90% of patients with 1° keratoconus achieve clear transplants, but post-operative astigmatism ± anisometropia often necessitate additional CL use. Coexistent atopy worsens prognosis.
- *Hydrops*: topical steroids, lubrication, and cycloplegia. If break or scroll in Descemet's can be visualized, intracameral air injection or long-lasting gas can be tried to tamponade Descemet's break; watch IOP.
- *Progression*: until recently, there was no specific treatment for preventing keratoconus progression. However, there is now significant evidence to show that corneal collagen cross-linking is effective in halting keratoconus progression (see ➔ Corneal collagen cross-linking, p. 282). A new approach to keratoconus management is cross-linking to stabilize the cornea, followed by insertion of ICRS (see ➔ Intracorneal ring segments, p. 868), phakic IOLs (see ➔ Phakic IOLs, p. 870), or even limited topography-guided photorefractive keratectomy (PRK) (see ➔ PRK, p. 858).

Other corneal ectasias

Keratoglobus

A very rare bilateral ectasia, characterized by global corneal thinning and significant risk of rupture at minor trauma. It may be acquired (probably as an end-stage keratoconus) or congenital (AR, associated with Ehlers–Danlos type VI and brittle cornea syndrome). Treatment includes protection from trauma, scleral CL, and sometimes lamellar epikeratoplasty.

Pellucid marginal degeneration

A rare bilateral progressive corneal ectasia of the peripheral cornea. It results in crescentic thinning inferiorly and marked against the rule astigmatism. It presents in the 3rd to 5th decade with non-inflammatory, painless visual distortion. Hydrops is rare. Treatment is by hard CL; it is usually uncorrectable with spectacles; surgical intervention is usually disappointing. Surgical techniques include eccentric PK, wedge resection, and lamellar keratoplasty.

Posterior keratoconus

A rare non-progressive congenital abnormality of the cornea in which there is abnormal steepening of the posterior cornea in the presence of normal anterior corneal surface. It is usually an isolated unilateral finding but may be associated with ocular (e.g. anterior lenticonus, anterior polar cataract) or systemic abnormalities. Treatment is not usually necessary but requires PK if significant ↓VA.

Peripheral ulcerative keratitis (PUK)

PUK is an aggressive sight-threatening form of keratitis which is sometimes associated with underlying systemic disease. The aetiology is uncertain, although the rheumatoid model suggests that immune complex deposition at the limbus causes an obliterative vasculitis, with subsequent corneal inflammation and stromal melt (see Box 7.7 for causes).

Causes

Box 7.7 Causes of PUK
- Organ-specific autoimmune PUK (idiopathic).
- RA.
- Granulomatosis with polyangiitis (GPA; formerly Wegener's granulomatosis).
- SLE.
- Relapsing polychondritis.
- Polyarteritis nodosa (PAN).
- Microscopic polyangiitis.
- Churg–Strauss syndrome.

Clinical features
- Variable pain and redness (may be none); ↓VA.
- Uni-/bilateral peripheral corneal ulceration with epithelial defect and stromal thinning; associated inflammation at the limbus (elevated, injected) and either sectoral or diffuse scleritis.

NB Do not underestimate associated dry eye (may be severe and → filamentary keratitis).

- *Systemic features (if associated disease)*: include degenerative joints (RA), saddle nose (GPA), skin changes (psoriasis, scleroderma, SLE), degenerative pinna cartilage (relapsing polychondritis) (see Table 7.14 for corneal complications of RA).

Table 7.14 Corneal complications of RA

Marginal furrow	Peripheral thinning without inflammation or loss of epithelium; 'CL cornea'; does not perforate
PUK	Peripheral inflammation, epithelial loss, infiltrate, and stromal loss; may perforate
Acute stromal keratitis	Acute-onset inflammation with stromal infiltrates, but epithelium often preserved
Sclerosing keratitis	Gradual juxtalimbal opacification of corneal stroma bordering an area of scleritis
Keratolysis	Stromal thinning ('corneal melt') ± associated inflammation

Investigations
- As directed by systemic review. Consider BP; FBC, ESR, U+E, LFT, Glu, CRP, vasculitis screen (including RF, ANA, ANCA, dsDNA), cryoglobulins, hepatitis C serology; urinalysis; CXR.

Treatment
- Emergency referral to corneal specialist, and involve patient's physician/ rheumatologist.
- *Ensure adequate tear film*: topical lubricants (e.g. carmellose or hyaluronate); if grossly reduced, consider punctal plugs/cautery ± autologous serum.
- *Systemic immunosuppression (liaise with physician/rheumatologist)*: may include corticosteroids (pulsed methylprednisolone or high-dose oral prednisolone), methotrexate, ciclosporin, mycophenolate, azathioprine, or cyclophosphamide. Severe disease may require pulsed IV cyclophosphamide with methylprednisolone (6–9 pulses), followed by a steroid-sparing agent.
- Doxycycline and oral vitamin C promote a healing stromal environment (inhibit proteases and free radicals, respectively).
- *Topical immunosuppression*: steroids (but use with caution in RA or if significant thinning, since keratolysis may be accelerated).
- Ocular lubricants, topical antibiotics to prevent 2° infection (e.g. chloramphenicol preservative-free 0.5% 4×/d), and cycloplegic (for pain and AC activity).
- Globe protection (e.g. glasses by day, shield at night, botulinum toxin ptosis, or tarsorrhaphy).
- Consider therapeutic CL + cyanoacrylate glue for pending/actual perforation. Surgical options include conjunctival recession, AMG, tectonic freehand lamellar keratoplasty, and occasionally conjunctival flaps.

Mooren's ulcer

This is a rare form of PUK which appears to be autoimmune. It is rarely associated with hepatitis C. It exists in two forms; the limited form is typically seen in middle-aged/elderly Caucasians, presents with unilateral disease, and is fairly responsive to treatment; the more aggressive form is typically seen in young Africans with bilateral disease and may relentlessly progress despite treatment.

Clinical features
- Pain, photophobia, ↓VA.
- Uni-/bilateral progressive peripheral ulceration; leading edge undermines epithelium; grey infiltrate at advancing margin; ulcer advances centrally and circumferentially; underlying stromal melt. **NB** No perilimbal clear zone and no associated scleritis (but conjunctival and episcleral inflammation).
- *Complications*: perforation; uveitis; cataract; at end-stage, the cornea is thinned and conjunctivalized.

Investigations
- Systemic work-up to rule out hepatitis C or any of the diseases associated with PUK (as described under ➲ Peripheral ulcerative keratitis (PUK) p. 262).

Treatment
- Topical steroids (e.g. dexamethasone 0.1% PF hourly).
- *Systemic immunosuppression*: corticosteroids, cyclophosphamide, or ciclosporin A (liaise with physician/rheumatologist); interferon if coexistent hepatitis C (as directed by a hepatologist).
- Also topical antibiotics, cycloplegia, globe protection, BCL ± glue, and surgical options, as for PUK with systemic disease.

Other peripheral corneal diseases

Marginal keratitis

A common inflammatory reaction due to hypersensitivity to staphylococcal exotoxin. Often seen in patients with atopy, rosacea, or chronic blepharitis.

Clinical features

- Pain, FB sensation, redness (may be sectoral or adjacent to lid margins), photophobia, tearing, ↓VA.
- Sterile, white, subepithelial peripheral corneal infiltrate; most commonly at 2, 4, 8, and 10 o'clock but may spread circumferentially to coalesce; a perilimbal clear zone of cornea is preserved; epithelial ulceration (stain with fluorescein) and vascularization may occur.

Treatment

- Topical steroid/antibiotic (e.g. betamethasone 0.1% 4×/d for 1wk, then 2×/d for 1wk, with chloramphenicol 0.5% 4×/d for 2wk) is commonly used to hasten resolution.
- Treat associated blepharitis or rosacea (see ➲ Treatment of MGD, p. 142).

Rosacea-associated keratitis

Acne rosacea is a chronic progressive disorder, characterized by cutaneous telangiectasia and sebaceous hyperplasia. Affecting the face and eyes, rosacea presents in middle age, shows a ♀ bias, and is more common in the fair-skinned.

Clinical features

- Telangiectasias at lids, meibomianitis, keratitis (ranges from inferior punctate epithelial erosions to marginal infiltrates to significant corneal thinning/perforation); facial flushing is characteristically worse when consuming alcohol or spicy food.

Treatment

- *Oral antibiotics*: either a tetracycline (e.g. doxycycline 100mg 1×/d for 3mo or oxytetracycline 500mg 2×/d for 12wk; tetracyclines are contraindicated in children under 12, pregnant/breastfeeding women, or in hepatic or renal impairment) or a macrolide (e.g. erythromycin 500mg 2×/d).
- *Treat associated blepharitis*: lid hygiene, ocular lubricants, topical antibiotics (for acute exacerbations).
- *If moderately severe*: consider topical steroids±antibiotics (e.g. dexamethasone 0.1%±chloramphenicol 0.5%). Use with caution if significant stromal thinning, since keratolysis may be accelerated.
- *If very severe* (threatened corneal perforation): systemic immunosuppression is usually necessary (e.g. azathioprine or mycophenolate).

Phlyctenulosis

These solitary limbal lesions are rare in the West but are relatively common in Africa. Children are more commonly affected than adults. Phlycten appear to be a hypersensitivity response, most commonly to staphylococcal or mycobacterial proteins and rarely to adenovirus, fungi, Neisseria, lymphogranuloma venereum, and leishmaniasis. They may be located at the conjunctiva or the cornea. Conjunctival phlycten are inflamed nodules, which may stain with fluorescein. They often resolve spontaneously. Corneal phlycten are grey nodules with associated superficial vascularization which may gradually move from limbus to central cornea. *Treatment*: topical steroid (e.g. betamethasone 0.1% 4×/d).

Dellen

This is non-ulcerative corneal thinning, seen adjacent to raised limbal lesions, due to local drying and tear film instability. It is usually asymptomatic. Scarring and vascularization are rare. *Treatment*: lubrication and removal of precipitant (e.g. cessation of CL wear; removal of limbal mass).

Terrien's marginal degeneration

This is a rare cause of bilateral asymmetrical peripheral thinning, most commonly seen in young to middle-aged ♂ (♂:♀ 3:1). It is non-inflammatory and is therefore sometimes considered as an ectasia or degeneration.

Clinical features
- Initially asymptomatic; painless ↓VA (against-the-rule astigmatism).
- Initially, there is yellow lipid deposition, with fine vascularization at the superior marginal cornea; thinning occurs on the limbal side of the lipid line, with a fairly steep leading edge; intact overlying epithelium; a perilimbal clear zone of cornea is preserved.
- *Complications*: opacification may spread circumferentially and rarely centrally. Rarely, there may be associated inflammation (usually in younger men).

Treatment
- Spectacles/CL for astigmatism.
- If severe thinning/risk of perforation, consider surgical options, including crescentic or eccentric lamellar/PK.

Neurotrophic keratopathy

The ophthalmic branch of the trigeminal nerve is responsible for corneal sensation. Reduction of corneal sensation leads to:
- Loss of the normal feedback responsible for maintaining a healthy epithelium.
- Predisposition to inadvertent trauma and opportunistic infection.
- Impairment of epithelial repair.
- Delayed clinical presentation (as may be asymptomatic).

See Table 7.15 for causes.

Causes

Table 7.15 Causes of corneal hypoesthesia/anaesthesia

Congenital		Familial dysautonomia (Riley–Day syndrome)
		Anhydrotic ectodermal dysplasia
Acquired	Ocular	Herpes simplex keratitis
		HZO
		Corneal scarring
		Corneal surgery (e.g. keratoplasty, refractive surgery)
		CL wear
		Drugs (topical anaesthetics)
	Extraocular	Traumatic/surgical section of Vn
		Irradiation of Vn
		Compressive/infiltrative of Vn (e.g. acoustic neuroma)
	Systemic	Drugs (e.g. systemic β-blockers)
		Diabetes
		Age

Clinical features

- Painless red eye, ↓VA.
- ↓corneal sensation; interpalpebral punctate epithelial erosions→larger defects with heaped grey edges, persistent epithelial defects; epithelial oedema; LESC failure; opportunistic microbial keratitis; perforation.

Investigation

If cause of corneal anaesthesia not yet established, patient will need full assessment (e.g. neurological referral, CT/MRI head scan, etc.).

Treatment

- *Ensure adequate lubrication with non-preserved preparations*: consider ↑frequency or ↑viscosity.
- Doxycycline 100mg 1×/d, vitamin C (ascorbate) 1g 2×/d.
- Treat any 2° microbial keratitis (see Microbial keratitis: treatment, p. 224).
- If significant ulcerative thinning, consider admission, protective measures such as globe protection (e.g. glasses by day, shield at night), therapeutic CL, or tectonic grafting with AM and measures to promote corneal healing such as tarsorrhaphy (surgical or botulinum toxin-induced), and topical application of autologous serum (with caution).
- Some evidence that nerve growth factor is of benefit.

Prevention

- *Assess corneal protective mechanisms*: check corneal sensation, tear film, lid closure (VIIn), Bell's phenomenon; correct where possible.
- Warn patient of risk of corneal disease and that a red eye or↓VA requires urgent ophthalmic assessment.

Exposure keratopathy

In exposure keratopathy, there is failure of the lids' normal wetting mechanism, with consequent drying and damage to the corneal epithelium. This most commonly arises due to incomplete closure of the eyelids at night (nocturnal lagophthalmos) (see Table 7.16 for causes).

Causes

Table 7.16 Causes of exposure keratopathy

VIIn palsy	Idiopathic (Bell's palsy)
	Stroke
	Tumour (e.g. acoustic neuroma, meningioma, choleastoma, parotid, nasopharyngeal)
	Demyelination
	Sarcoidosis
	Trauma (temporal bone fracture)
	Surgical section
	Otitis
	Ramsay–Hunt syndrome (herpes zoster)
	Guillain–Barré syndrome
	Lyme disease
Lid abnormality	Nocturnal lagophthalmos (commonest cause)
	Ectropion
	Traumatic defect in lid margin
	Surgical (e.g. overcorrection of ptosis)
	Floppy eyelid syndrome
Orbital disease	Proptosis
	TED

Clinical features

- Irritable red eye(s); may be worse in the mornings.
- Poor Bell's phenomenon, poor blink excursion or reduced blink rate, periocular muscle weakness, punctate epithelial erosions (usually inferior if underlying lagophthalmos; central if due to proptosis); → larger defects; opportunistic microbial keratitis; perforation.

Investigation

- If cause of exposure keratopathy not yet established, patient will need further investigation, as directed by full ophthalmic and systemic assessment.

Treatment

- *Ensure adequate lubrication*: consider ↑ frequency or ↑ viscosity; preservative-free preparations preferred if >6×/d.
- *Ensure adequate lid closure*: temporary measures if early resolution anticipated (tape lids shut at night), intermediate (temporary lateral/central tarsorrhaphy; botulinum toxin-induced ptosis) vs permanent surgical procedures (e.g. lid weights or permanent tarsorrhaphy for lagophthalmos; orbital decompression if proptosis).
- Treat 2° microbial keratitis (see ➜ Herpes simplex keratitis, p. 232).
- If significant ulcerative thinning, consider admission, globe protection with tarsorrhaphy, gluing, BCL, or lamellar grafting.

Prevention

- *Assess corneal protective mechanisms*: check corneal sensation, tear film, lid closure (VIIn), Bell's phenomenon; correct where possible.
- Warn patient of risk of corneal disease and that pain, photophobia, or ↓VA require urgent ophthalmic assessment.

Deposition keratopathies

Wilson's disease (syn hepatolenticular degeneration)

This rare AR condition arises due to deficiency in a copper-binding protein, leading to low levels of caeruloplasmin and copper deposition throughout the tissues, including the cornea.

Clinical features
- Kayser–Fleischer ring (brownish peripheral ring at level of Descemet's membrane); starts superiorly and usually continuous with limbus; sunflower cataract (anterior and posterior subcapsular opacities).
- *Systemic*: liver failure, choreoathetosis (basal ganglia deposition), and psychiatric problems.

Vortex keratopathy (syn cornea verticillata)

A number of drugs may result in deposits at the corneal epithelium. Similar appearances occur in Fabry's disease.

Causes
- *Drugs*: amiodarone, chloroquine, suramin, indometacin, tamoxifen, chlorpromazine, atovaquone.
- *Systemic disease*: Fabry's disease.

Clinical features
- Asymptomatic; not an indication for withdrawing treatment.
- Swirling grey lines radiating from infracentral cornea.

Crystalline keratopathies

- *Infectious crystalline keratopathy*: presents as feathery stromal opacities in the absence of significant inflammation. These are biofilms (i.e. slime) arising from the presence of *Streptococcus viridans* or rarely *Staphylococcus epidermidis*, *Pseudomonas aeruginosa*, or *Candida* spp. Most commonly seen in graft tissue after PK, they also occur in the presence of ocular surface disease (e.g. OcMMP, SJS).
- *Non-infectious crystalline keratopathy*: includes deposition of gold (chrysiasis due to systemic treatment in RA), immunoglobulin (multiple myeloma, Waldenström's macroglobulinaemia, lymphoma), urate (gout), cysteine (cystinosis), lipids (lipid keratopathy, Schnyder's crystalline dystrophy).

Mucopolysaccharidosis keratopathy

The mucopolysaccharidoses are a group of inherited enzyme deficiencies (usually AR), in which there is an accumulation and deposition of glycosaminoglycans. This may be widespread, causing skeletal abnormalities, organomegaly, and mental retardation (e.g. Hurler's syndrome, MPS I), or limited (e.g. corneal deposition in macular dystrophy) (see ➲ Macular dystrophy, p. 254) (see Table 7.17).

Table 7.17 Mucopolysaccharidoses associated with corneal clouding

Systemic	MPS I	Hurler, Scheie, Hurler–Scheie
	MPS IV	Morquio
	MPS VI	Maroteaux–Lamy
	MPS VII	Sly
Limited		Macular dystrophy

Keratoplasty: penetrating keratoplasty

Corneal grafting has been performed for over 100y and is the commonest of all transplantation procedures. It may be performed as an elective procedure to improve vision or as an emergency procedure for corneal perforation. It may involve full-thickness replacement of a button of corneal tissue (PK), partial-thickness replacement (lamellar keratoplasty), or of just the posterior layers (endothelial keratoplasty). Although not necessary for low-risk procedures, systemic immunosuppression should be considered for high-risk grafts.

Penetrating keratoplasty (PK)

Indications

- *Visual*: keratoconus, pseudophakic/aphakic bullous keratopathy, Fuchs' endothelial dystrophy, other corneal dystrophies, scarring 2° to trauma, chemical injury, or keratitis.
- *Tectonic*: corneal thinning, threatened perforation, or actual perforation.

Cautions

- *Poor prognostic factors*: corneal vascularization, reduced corneal sensation, active inflammation, peripheral corneal thinning, herpetic disease, ocular surface disease, uncontrolled glaucoma.

Method

- *Consent*: explain what the operation does, the need for frequent post-operative visits, long-term follow-up, and the importance of immediate attendance if there are problems. Explain the nature of organ donation, that the donors are screened, but that there is still a small risk of transmission of infectious agents. Explain the delay in visual rehabilitation and possible complications, including failure, graft rejection, infection, haemorrhage, worsened vision, and need for correction of astigmatism (CL ± refractive surgery).
- *Preoperative*: miotic (e.g. pilocarpine 1%).
- *Prep*: with 5% povidone iodine and drape.
- *Check donor material*: healthy-looking corneoscleral ring in clear media, good endothelial cell count.
- *Determine button sizes*: depends on corneal morphology and pathology, but commonly 7.5mm for the host and 0.25–0.5mm larger for the donor.
- *Mark cornea*: measure height and width of cornea with calipers, and mark centre with ink; consider marking periphery with radial keratotomy marker to assist with suture placement.
- Perform paracentesis, and fill AC with viscoelastic.
- *Excise donor button*: cut from endothelial side, using a trephine (types include handheld, gravity, and vacuum-driven).
- *Excise host button*: cutting with the trephine (numerous designs) may be full-thickness or stopped at the first release of aqueous to perform a slower decompression with blade or corneal scissors.

- *Place cardinal sutures*: 4×10-0 nylon sutures to secure the donor button in position.
- *Complete suturing*: either additional interrupted sutures (often 16 in total) or a continuous running suture. Aim for 90% suture depth. Ensure suture tension even, and attempt to minimize astigmatism.
- Refill AC with balanced salt solution (BSS).

Post-operative

- Topical steroid and antibiotic; if low risk of rejection, then a combined preparation may be sufficient; if higher risk, consider non-preserved dexamethasone 0.1% q2h and chloramphenicol 0.5% 4×/d; also consider oral acetazolamide in the immediate post-operative period (especially if coexistent glaucoma) and oral aciclovir (if HSV disease).

Follow-up

- As clinically indicated, but commonly at 1d, 1wk, 1mo, and then 2–3-monthly.
- Regular refraction/autorefraction and corneal topography permit adjustment/removal of sutures to minimize astigmatism. A continuous running suture should not usually be removed for at least a year.
- Use antibiotic/steroid cover to reduce risk of infection/rejection, and check for wound leaks.
- Patients require one drop of topical steroid for a minimum of 2y (following which rejection rates fall) and possibly lifelong thereafter.

Keratoplasty: lamellar and endothelial keratoplasty

Deep anterior lamellar keratoplasty (DALK)

Indications

- *Visual*: suitable for diseases in which host endothelium/Descemet's membrane is healthy, e.g. most keratoconus, stromal dystrophies, scarring; although longer surgical time than PK, there is a reduced risk of rejection.

Method

- *Outline*: a deep stromal pocket is formed from a superior scleral (or corneal) incision and filled with viscoelastic, so permitting a trephine to excise a deep, but partial, thickness button. Visualization of depth may be assisted by filling the AC with air.

Superficial lamellar keratoplasty

Indications

- *Tectonic*: reinforce thinned cornea in threatened perforation or post-pterygium excision.
- *Visual* (uncommon): anterior stromal scarring.

Method

- *Outline*: a trephine is used to cut to the desired depth before using a blade or microkeratome to separate the button at the base.

Endothelial keratoplasty

Indications

- Endothelial pathology such as Fuchs' endothelial dystrophy and pseudophakic bullous keratopathy.
- *Advantages*: include shorter surgical time, corneal structural integrity, stable refraction, and faster visual recovery.
- *Additional complications*: include pupillary block, donor endothelial damage, and donor graft detachment needing repositioning with air injection.

Method

- *Outline*: the Descemet's membrane and endothelium are stripped off the recipient cornea; the donor endothelial graft is prepared using an automated keratome. The donor is inserted through a small incision, using an injectable introducer or glide, and opposed to the recipient stroma by air tamponade.

Triple procedure

Indications

- *Visual*: visually significant cataract with disease that requires PK; most commonly, Fuchs' endothelial dystrophy.

Method

- *Outline*: PK is performed with cataract extraction (usually by extracapsular 'open sky', rather than phakoemulsification) and IOL implantation.

Keratoplasty: complications

See Table 7.18 for summary.

Early post-operative complications

- *Wound leak*: Seidel positive leak, shallow AC, soft eye.
  - Consider lubricants, BCL, patching, or resuturing.
- *↑IOP*: causes include retained viscoelastic, malignant glaucoma, choroidal effusion, choroidal haemorrhage.
  - Identify and treat cause.
- *Persistent epithelial defect* (i.e. defect >2wk duration) (see ➲ Persistent epithelial defects, p. 242): causes include ocular surface disease, such as dry eye, blepharitis, rosacea, exposure, or systemic disease such as diabetes or RA.
  - Identify and treat cause; ensure generous lubrication and that all drops are preservative-free; consider taping lid shut/tarsorrhaphy.
- *Endophthalmitis*: rare, but sight-threatening ophthalmic emergency.
  - Recognize and treat urgently (see ➲ Post-operative endophthalmitis, p. 336).
- *1° graft failure*: endothelial failure causes persistent graft oedema from day 1 in a quiet eye.
  - Observe for 2–4wk; consider regraft, if oedema persists.
- *Early graft rejection* (see ➲ Graft rejection, p. 279).
- *Urrets–Zavalia syndrome*: a fixed, dilated pupil may occur after either PK or DALK; it is presumed to be due to iris ischaemia.

Late post-operative complications

- *Astigmatism*: monitor with corneal topography; adjust running suture or remove interrupted sutures (at steepest axes), but ensure that wound is secure; can be improved with hard CL ± arcuate keratotomies.
- *Microbial keratitis*: risk increased due to epithelial disturbance, sutures, and chronic steroid use.
  - Recognize and treat urgently (see ➲ Microbial keratitis: assessment, p. 222).
- *Suture-related problems*:
  - Remove loose/broken sutures, and check for wound leaks; use antibiotic/steroid cover to reduce risk of infection/rejection; if wound leak, then may require resuturing; a continuous running suture should not usually be removed for at least a year.
- *Disease recurrence in graft*: this is common with viral keratitis (e.g. HSV) and some corneal dystrophies (e.g. macular dystrophy).
  - Identify and treat, if possible (e.g. aciclovir for HSV); may require further graft.
- *Late graft rejection* (see ➲ Graft rejection, p. 279).

Graft rejection

This is the commonest cause of graft failure. This is usually due to endothelial rejection which occurs in about 20% of grafts. Rejection is dependent on the presence of appropriate antigen-presenting cells and CD4+ T-cells. Due to redundancy within the immune system, multiple indepdent mechanisms may result in rejection, e.g. rejection is not restricted to a pure Th1 or Th2 response. Vigilant post-operative review and management are required. If the patient remains rejection-free for the first 24mo post-surgery, the risk of rejection decreases. However, a history of rejection increases the risk of further rejection episodes.

Have a low threshold for admission—prompt and adequate treatment may save the graft. Anterior uveitis occurring in a patient with a corneal graft should be considered as graft rejection until proven otherwise. Although, for most cases, topical steroid drops are sufficient, in severe rejection episodes or high-risk grafts, consider oral prednisolone ± pulsed IVMP.

Epithelial rejection

Graft epithelium is replaced by host epithelium, resulting in an epithelial demarcation line.

- ↑topical steroids to at least double current regimen (e.g. dexamethasone pres-free 0.1%, up to hourly).

Stromal/subepithelial rejection

This is indicated by subepithelial infiltrates.

- ↑topical steroids to at least double current regimen (e.g. dexamethasone pres-free 0.1%, up to hourly).

Endothelial rejection

This is indicated by corneal oedema, KPs, Khodadoust line (inflammatory cell/graft endothelium demarcation line), AC activity.

- Intensive topical steroids (e.g. dexamethasone pres-free 0.1% hourly day and night/steroid ointment at night); consider subconjunctival or systemic corticosteroids if fails to improve; cycloplegia (e.g. cyclopentolate 1% 3×/d).

Strategies for prolongation of graft survival

- Survival rates for corneal transplants at 5y are less than those of renal transplantation; survival rates for high-risk corneal transplantation are worse than those of liver transplantation. However, there is little evidence to support strategies for prolongation of corneal transplant survival in high-risk grafts.
- Induction with mycophenolate and adding sirolimus post-operatively to the maintenance regime. Supplementary, as required, subconjunctival treatment with antiangiogenic substances, i.e. bevacizumab—an anti-VEGF—for the management of acute vascular rejection episodes in the post-operative period.

Table 7.18 Summary of complications in keratoplasty

Early	Wound leak
	↑IOP
	Flat AC
	Iris prolapse
	Persistent epithelial defect
	Endophthalmitis
	1° graft failure
	Early graft rejection
	Urrets–Zavalia syndrome
Late	Astigmatism
	Graft rejection
	Microbial keratitis
	Suture-related problems (loose, abscess, endophthalmitis)
	Disease recurrence in graft
	Glaucoma

Corneal collagen cross-linking

Collagen fibres cross-link naturally during maturation and ageing. In the human cornea, the process can be modified by the use of topical riboflavin, followed by exposure to UVA light. It provides novel therapeutic options for stabilizing the progression of keratoconus, 2° ectatic responses (LASIK, microbial keratitis), fine-tuning results of previous refractive surgery (intrastromal rings, photorefractive keratectomy), or reducing spacial separation of collagen fibrils in the oedematous stroma (corneal decompensation).

Method

Outline

The original method described by Wollensak, Spoerl, Seiler, and co-workers is effective, safe, and proven both in laboratory and clinical trials. Under topical anaesthesia (g proxymetacaine 0.5%), the central 9mm corneal epithelium is removed, and the surface is treated with 0.1% iso-osmolar riboflavin (vitamin B2) solution every 1–5min for 30min. The central de-epithelialized cornea is then exposed to calibrated UVA (365nm wavelength, $3mW/cm^2$, at a distance of 5mm from the cornea for 30min, i.e. a total of $5.4J/cm^2$). Pachymetry should be performed, as the minimum safe corneal thickness for treatment is 400 microns. The procedure is completed with instillation of a topical broad-spectrum antibiotic and a therapeutic CL.

Long-term outcome

Delay in progression of disease has been shown in many observational studies. High-quality randomized controlled trials (RCTs) are under way and point to the sustained efficacy of treatment.

Complications (epithelial defects, infective keratitis, melts) and failure rates are generally low (<5%) and are more likely with age>35 and very steep pre-treatment Ks (>58D). This suggests higher efficacy and lower failure in younger patients with progression, rather than established advanced keratoconus.

Amniotic membrane transplantation

The AM is part of the mammalian placenta, which has found numerous applications in ocular surface rehabilitation. It is widely available and, unlike most allografts (i.e. grafts from another individual), does not result in immunological rejection.

Histology

The placenta comprises a fetal component (the amniochorion) and a maternal component (the decidua). The AM is an epithelial monolayer that secretes a thick BM which is adjacent to an avascular stroma. This stroma comprises three collagenous layers: a compact layer, a fibroblast layer (also contains resident macrophages and serves to secrete components of the compact layer), and an intermediate spongy layer (abundant in hydrated proteoglycans and glycoproteins). In preparing the AM for surgical use, it is separated from the chorion along the natural cleavage plane of the intermediate spongy layer.

Function

The biological properties of amnion in ocular surface rehabilitation are thought to be primarily related to the amnion matrix and BM substrate. AM has anti-inflammatory, anti-angiogenic, and anti-scarring properties that promote inflammatory cell apoptosis, suppression of myofibroblast differentiation, inhibition of proteases and transforming growth factor (TGF)-β signalling pathways. Other studies have indicated that AM may also possess bactericidal properties. There is large biological inter- and intra-amniotic membrane variation, and synthetic alternatives are being sought.

Applications (See Table 7.19)

Table 7.19 Applications of AM transplantation

Common	Persistent corneal defects
	Reconstruction of conjunctival defects
	Chemical and thermal burns
	Limbal stem cell deficiency
	Bullous keratopathy
	Glaucoma surgery
Uncommon	Band keratopathy
	Post-refractive surgery haze
	Corneal hydrops
	Encasement of orbital prostheses
	EOM surgery

Donor eye retrieval and eye banks

Corneal transplantation (see ➲ Keratoplasty: penetrating keratoplasty, p. 274) depends on the availability of screened deceased donor corneoscleral tissue, preserved in optimal condition by a dedicated eye bank. In the UK, the majority of corneas are stored by the Corneal Transplantation Service Eye Banks in Bristol and Manchester.

Retrieval

Eye retrieval should be carried out by somebody who is competent in enucleation or has been trained in eye retrieval (usually ophthalmic nurses, technicians, or doctors). Often there is a local transplant coordinator who will have already discussed consent and established the suitability of the donor. However, the person performing retrieval has a responsibility to check that both of these have been satisfactorily performed.

Consent

Consent should be obtained from the most relevant life partner or closest family member. Consent should include confirmation: (1) that they agree to donation and that the deceased had no known objection to donation, (2) that they agree that the tissue may be used for research (if not suitable for transplantation), (3) that a blood test can be taken (if no premortem blood test available) to check for infective risk, and (4) that further information about the deceased can be obtained from their medical records or relevant medical professionals.

Screening

Screening comprises gaining information on the likely suitability of the tissue for transplantation purposes, primarily with regard to avoiding transmission of infective agents or malignancy. Information may be gained from medical records, senior medical/nursing staff caring for the deceased, family of the deceased, 1° health care practitioner, and post-mortem. Serological tests for infective agents are also performed.

Enucleation

The procedure is carried out using aseptic technique and appropriate disinfection (e.g. povidone iodine 10%). A peritomy is performed to allow isolation and severing of the EOM (squint hook/strabismus scissors). A pair of enucleation scissors (closed) are then slid round the eye to sever the optic nerve and allow the globe to be removed. After packing the sockets with cotton wool, the lids can be closed over plastic eye caps to restore the normal appearance of the lids.

Processing

Processing procedures must pay regard to the potential infective risk of the donor material and follow codes of Good Laboratory Practice and Good Manufacturing Practice. Donor eyes are cleaned (e.g. povidone iodine 10%) and the corneoscleral disc excised under sterile conditions (e.g. class II biological safety cabinet).

Storage

Corneoscleral discs

Options include:

- *Suspension in organ culture medium at 34°C*: can be stored for 30d.
  Advantages: long storage time; infective risk can be screened for by
  routine sampling of culture medium at 7d.
- *Hypothermic storage at 4°C*: can be stored for 7–10d.
  Advantages: relatively simple. *Disadvantages*: shorter storage time;
  infective risk less easily identified.

Sclera

- Storage in 70% ethanol; can be stored for up to 1y.

Whole eyes

For short-term storage (e.g. between removal and arrival at the eye bank):

- *Moist chamber storage*: whole eye placed on a stand, with cornea
  uppermost, in a closed pot. Humidity is provided by moistened cotton
  wool. The pot is kept at 4°C (fridge or on ice during transit).

Issuing corneas

3d before the scheduled date of transplantation, the corneal endothelium
is examined. If endothelial cell count is ≥2,200 cells/mm², the cornea is
considered suitable for transplantation. It is placed back into medium and
returned to 34°C. 2d before transplantation, the medium may be sam-
pled again to assess for infection. On the day before transplantation, the
corneas are sent in medium at ambient temperature to the operating hospital (see Table 7.20 for contraindications to the use of ocular tissue in
transplantation).

Table 7.20 Summary of contraindications to the use of ocular tissue in transplantation as outlined in Annex 1 of the Royal College of Ophthalmologists *Standards for the retrieval of human ocular tissue used in transplantation*, 2008

Infection	*Known infection*: HIV, viral hepatitis (A, B, or C), viral encephalitis or encephalitis of unknown origin, viral meningitis, rabies, congenital rubella, TB, Reyes syndrome, progressive multifocal leukoencephalopathy, septicaemia, active malaria
	Seropositivity: HIV (1 or 2), HBsAg, HCV, syphilis
	Behaviour leading to risk of contracting HIV, hepatitis B or C
Previous surgery	Receipt of an organ transplant (including dura, corneal, scleral, or limbal graft) or human pituitary-derived hormones
	Brain/spinal surgery pre-August 1992
CNS disorders and disorders of unknown aetiology	Motor neurone disease, chronic fatigue syndrome (ME), CNS diseases of unknown aetiology (e.g. most dementias, MS, Parkinson's disease)
	Death from unknown cause
Malignant/premalignant disease	Leukaemia, lymphoma, myeloma, sideroblastic anaemia, polycythaemia
Ocular	Ocular inflammation, including known ocular involvement by systemic disease, e.g. sarcoidosis, RA
	Any ocular disorders that would preclude successful graft outcome (including previous refractive surgery)
	Malignant tumours

Sclera

Anatomy and physiology

The sclera is the tough outer coat of the globe covered by a loose connective tissue layer the episclera. The sclera develops from a condensation of mesenchymal tissue situated at the anterior rim of the optic cup. This forms first at the limbus at around wk 7 and proceeds posteriorly to surround the optic nerve and form a rudimentary lamina cribrosa at wk 12 (see Table 8.1 for perforations).

Sclera

Anatomy

The sclera is almost a complete sphere of 22mm diameter. Anteriorly, it is continuous with the cornea, and posteriorly with the optic nerve. It is thickest around the optic nerve (1.0mm), and thinnest just posterior to the recti insertions (0.3mm).

The sclera consists of collagen (mainly types I, III, and V, but also IV, VI, VIII), elastin, proteoglycans, and glycoproteins. The stroma consists of a roughly criss-cross arrangement of collagen bundles of varying sizes (10–15 micron thick, 100–150 micron long). This renders it opaque but strong. The inner layer (lamina fusca) blends with the uveal tract, separated by the potential suprachoroidal space. The sclera itself is effectively avascular but is pierced by a number of vessels. It is innervated by the long and short ciliary nerves.

Physiology

The sclera provides a tough protective coat that is rigid enough to prevent loss of shape (with its refractive implications) but can tolerate some fluctuation in IOP. Scleral opacity is due to the irregularity of collagen and its relative hydration. The limited metabolic demands are supported by episcleral and choroidal vasculature. Inflammation of the sclera leads to engorgement of mainly the deep vascular plexus. This is relatively unaffected by the administration of topical vasoconstrictors (e.g. phenylephrine).

Episclera

Anatomy

This layer of connective tissue comprises an inner layer apposed to the sclera, intermediate loose connective tissue, and an outer layer that fuses with the muscle sheaths and the conjunctiva juxtalimbally. It is heavily vascularized with a superficial and deep anterior plexus (which underlies and anastamoses with the conjunctival plexus) and a posterior episcleral plexus supplied by the short posterior ciliary vessels.

Physiology

The episclera gives nutrition to the sclera and provides a low friction surface, assisting the free movement of the globe within the orbit. Inflammation of the episclera leads to engorgement of the conjunctival and superficial vascular plexus. These blanch with administration of topical vasoconstrictors (e.g. phenylephrine), leading to visible whitening.

Table 8.1 Scleral perforations

Location	Transmits
Anterior	Anterior ciliary arteries
Middle	Vortex veins
Posterior	Long + short ciliary nerves Long + short posterior ciliary arteries
Lamina cribrosa	Optic nerve

Episcleritis

This common condition is a benign, recurrent inflammation of the episclera. It is commonest in young women. It is usually self-limiting and may require little or no treatment, the main reason its incidence is underestimated. It is not usually associated with any systemic disease, although around 10% may have a connective tissue disease.

Simple episcleritis

Clinical features

- Sudden onset of mild discomfort, tearing ± photophobia; may be recurrent.
- Sectoral (occasionally diffuse) redness which blanches with topical vasoconstrictor (e.g. phenylephrine 10%); globe non-tender; spontaneous resolution 1–2wk.

Investigation

Investigations are not usually required, unless there is a history suggestive of systemic disease.

Treatment

- *Supportive*: reassurance ± cold compresses.
- *Topical lubricants*.
- *Other topical medication*: the role of topical NSAIDs and corticosteroids is controversial. Topical NSAIDs (such as diclofenac, flurbiprofen, ketorolac, nepafenac, and bromfenac) have become popular, but evidence of benefit is lacking; they are licensed for perioperative indications, not for episcleritis. Topical corticosteroids appear effective for short-term control, but, given the benign nature of the condition, it is not clear that the benefits outweigh the risks. They may be useful in those cases showing a more prolonged course.
- *Systemic*: if severe/recurrent, consider oral NSAID (see Box 8.1).

Nodular episcleritis

Clinical features

- Sudden onset of FB sensation, discomfort, tearing ± photophobia; may be recurrent. Recurrences tend to develop in the same location.
- Red nodule arising from the episclera; can be moved separately from the sclera (cf. nodular scleritis) and conjunctiva (cf. conjunctival phlycten); blanches with topical vasoconstrictor (e.g. phenylephrine 10%); does not stain with fluorescein; globe non-tender (cf. scleritis); spontaneous resolution 5–6wk.

Investigation

Investigations are not usually required, unless there is a history suggestive of systemic disease.

Treatment

- As for simple episcleritis, but greater role for ocular lubricants.

Box 8.1 Systemic NSAIDs

Background

- NSAIDs are cyclo-oxygenase (COX) inhibitors. Most are non-selective, blocking both COX-1 (constitutively expressed throughout the body, with a number of important physiological roles, e.g. protecting the stomach mucosa) and COX-2 (induced during inflammation; constitutively expressed in kidney and brain).
- Selective COX-2 drugs are less gastrotoxic than the non-selective drugs but equally nephrotoxic; additionally, one of the first major COX-2 inhibitors (rofecoxib) was associated with elevated risk of myocardial infarction (MI) and stroke.

Prescribing principles

- There is significant variation in how an individual responds to different NSAIDs, both in efficacy and side effects: so be prepared to change drug, if ineffective.
- Although the analgesic effect should occur after the first dose, the anti-inflammatory effect may take up to 3wk.
- NSAIDs should be used with caution in the elderly, patients with cardiac failure, and in patients with previous gastrointestinal (GI) bleeding. In patients at high risk of developing NSAID-related GI complications (e.g. age >65y, previous peptic ulcer, significant comorbidity), consider prophylactic treatment with a proton pump inhibitor. Contraindication if previously documented NSAID hypersensitivity (e.g. worsening of asthma).

Examples

- Diclofenac sodium (25–50mg 3×/d), naproxen (250–500mg 2×/d), and flurbiprofen (50–100mg 3×/d) balance good efficacy with relatively low gastrotoxicity; ibuprofen has lower gastrotoxicity but is less effective.[*]

[*] See *BNF* for further information and updates.

Anterior scleritis

This uncommon condition is a potentially blinding inflammation of the sclera. It is associated with systemic disease in around 50%, of which most cases are of a connective tissue disease. It is commonest in middle-aged women. Scleritis is bilateral in 50% of cases, but both eyes may not be affected at the same time (see Table 8.2 for classification).

Classification

Table 8.2 Classification of scleritis and approximate frequency

Anterior	Non-necrotizing	Diffuse	50%
		Nodular	25%
	Necrotizing	With inflammation	10%
		Without inflammation	5%
Posterior			10%

A number of activity grading systems for anterior scleritis have been proposed, but, as yet, there is no consensus system of determining disease activity/severity. One recent proposal is based on scoring activity from 0 (no inflammation) to 4 (necrotizing scleritis), based on appearance 15min after instillation of 10% phenylephrine; the key feature is that this is done by comparison to a set of reference photographs, the introduction of which were found to substantially improve interobserver agreement ($\kappa = 0.29$ to $\kappa = 0.60$).[1] (See Box 8.2 for key points.)

Box 8.2 Anterior scleritis: key points
- Pain (constant/deep/boring) can be so severe that it wakes the patient at night; pain on eye movement; radiation to jaw, neck, and head.
- The globe may be very tender to touch.
- Examine the eye under room light or in daylight prior to using the slit-lamp.
- A bluish hue implies scleral thinning from previous active scleritis.
- Topical phenylephrine 2.5–10% causes blanching of the more superficial episcleral vessels but does not change the engorgement of deeper sclera vessels and can help differentiate between scleritis and episcleritis.
- Scleral thinning may result in high degrees of astigmatism.
- When seen in conjunction with peripheral corneal infiltrates, consider a diagnosis of GPA (formerly known as Wegener's granulomatosis).

Risk factors

- *Associated disease*: RA; vasculitis, including GPA (formerly Wegener's granulomatosis),[2] relapsing polychondritis, SLE, PAN, Cogan's syndrome (see Table 8.3); sarcoidosis, IBD, psoriatic arthritis, ankylosing spondylitis, rosacea, atopy, gout.
- *Infection*, e.g. syphilis, TB, VZV.
- *Local*: trauma, surgery (including surgery-induced necrotizing scleritis (SINS)).

Diffuse non-necrotizing anterior scleritis

Clinical features

- Subacute onset (over 1wk) of moderate/severe pain, redness, tearing, photophobia.
- Diffuse injection of deep vascular episcleral plexus which does not blanch with vasoconstrictors (e.g. phenylephrine 10%), oedema; globe tender; usually non-progressive but may last for several months, if untreated.

Investigations

- FBC, ESR, RF, anti-CCP, ANA, ANCA, CRP, U+E, LFT, ACE, uric acid, syphilis serology, CXR, urinalysis. Consider further tests as per clinical indication, e.g. Mantoux/interferon γ release assay (IGRA) for suspected TB.
- Anterior segment fluorescein angiography (ASFA) is performed in some centres; rapid arteriovenous (AV) transit time, rapid intense leakage from capillaries and venules. ICG angiography is another alternative, allowing for better visualization of the vascular bed throughout the test due to larger size of the molecule and no leakage. Helpful in identifying early areas of ischaemia, indicating conversion to a more severe form.

Treatment

- *Oral*: NSAID (e.g. diclofenac sodium, naproxen, flurbiprofen) (see Box 8.1).
- If not controlled on NSAID, consider systemic immunosuppression. 'Rescue' with corticosteroids (e.g. prednisolone 1mg/kg/d, tapering down, or three pulses of IV methylprednisolone (IVMP) 1g od, followed by oral corticosteroid. IVMP is typically given in 100mL normal saline over 1h; beware cardiac failure. Taper down corticosteroid, aiming for 'maintenance' dose, e.g. prednisolone ≤7.5mg od; if this is not possible without recurrence of disease, then introduce a 'second-line' immunosuppressant (see ➡ Treatment, p. 294).
- Topical corticosteroids will not control disease but may have symptomatic benefit.

Nodular non-necrotizing anterior scleritis

Clinical features

- Subacute onset (over 1wk) moderate/severe pain, FB sensation, redness, tearing ± photophobia.
- Red nodule arising from the sclera; cannot be moved separately from underlying tissue (cf. nodular episcleritis); does not blanch with topical vasoconstrictor (e.g. phenylephrine 10%); globe tender.

Investigations
- As for diffuse anterior scleritis.

Treatment
- As for diffuse anterior scleritis, but add topical lubricants.

Necrotizing anterior scleritis with inflammation

Clinical features
- Subacute onset (3–4d), severe pain, redness, tearing ± photophobia.
- White avascular areas surrounded by injected oedematous sclera; scleral necrosis → translucency, revealing blue-black uveal tissue; anterior uveitis suggests very advanced disease.

NB Scleral thinning and degree of scleral injection may be best appreciated under natural/room light.
- *Complications*: PUK, acute stromal keratitis, sclerosing keratitis, uveitis, cataract, astigmatism, glaucoma, globe perforation.

NB Necrotizing scleritis must be taken seriously, both in its own right but also because it indicates a high risk of an underlying systemic disease and high mortality in 5y, if untreated.

Investigations
- FBC, ESR, RF, anti-CCP, ANA, ANCA, CRP, U+E, LFT, ACE, uric acid, syphilis serology, CXR, urinalysis. Consider further tests as per clinical indication, e.g. Mantoux/IGRA for suspected TB.
- ASFA is performed in some centres; AV shunts with perfusion of veins before capillaries and islands of no blood flow. Same comment for ICG made previously.

Treatment
- *Systemic immunosuppression*: it is essential that these patients receive rapid adequate immunosuppression.
- *Rescue therapy*: corticosteroids (e.g. prednisolone 1mg/kg/d, tapering down, or three pulses of IVMP 1g od, followed by oral corticosteroid. IVMP is typically given in 100mL normal saline over 1h; beware cardiac failure.
- *Maintenance therapy*: requires the addition of immunosuppressants such as methotrexate, mycophenolate mofetil, ciclosporin, azathioprine, or cyclophosphamide; in severe disease, cyclophosphamide may be combined with IVMP as part of rescue therapy.[3] Cyclophosphamide is of particular value in severe disease and in the context of GPA (formerly Wegener's granulomatosis) and PAN; biologics, such as infliximab, adalimumab, rituximab, may also be considered.

These drugs require careful monitoring and should only be used by someone trained in their use; they are commonly coordinated with a physician/rheumatologist.
- If risk of perforation, protect globe (e.g. glasses by day, shield at night) and consider scleral patch graft.

Necrotizing anterior scleritis without inflammation (scleromalacia perforans)

Scleromalacia perforans is usually seen in severe chronic seropositive RA. Angiography shows that vascular occlusion is a key part of the pathogenesis.

Clinical features

- Asymptomatic.
- Gradual reduction of vision as a consequence of progressive astigmatism.
- Small yellow areas of necrotic sclera coalesce to reveal large areas of underlying uvea in a quiet eye.
- *Complications*: although this does not usually result in perforation, it may do so after minor trauma.

Investigations

- As for necrotizing anterior scleritis with inflammation (see ➲ Investigations, p. 294).

Treatment

Systemic immunosuppression

Immunosuppression may ameliorate this form of scleritis in its early stages, but, once established, the destructive process may continue despite adequate immunosuppression due to the underlying irreversible ischaemia. Immunosuppression is, however, usually required for the associated underlying systemic disease, Rescue and maintenance therapy may be given as for necrotizing anterior scleritis with inflammation (see ➲ Treatment, p. 294).

Other

- *Topical*: generous lubrication.
- If risk of perforation, protect globe (e.g. glasses by day, shield at night) and consider scleral patch graft, although this is very rarely required.

Relapsing polychondritis

Rare condition of recurrent inflammation of cartilage affecting the ear, nose, and, most seriously, trachea, larynx, and large cardiac vessels (risk of respiratory obstruction). The ophthalmic features include anterior uveitis, episcleritis, scleritis, and rarely corneal involvement (KCS or PUK). Scleritis is usually resistant to therapy and difficult to control.

1. Sen HN et al. A standardized grading system for uveitis. *Ophthalmology* 2011;**118**:768–71.

2. Falk RJ et al. Granulomatosis with polyangiitis (Wegener's): an alternative name for Wegener's granulomatosis. *Arthritis Rheum* 2011;**63**:863–4.

3. Khan IJ et al. Ten-year experience of pulsed intravenous cyclophosphamide and methylprednisolone protocol (PICM protocol) in severe ocular inflammatory disease. *Br J Ophthalmol* 2013;**97**:1118–22.

Posterior scleritis

Posterior scleritis is uncommon but is probably underdiagnosed. It is a potentially sight-threatening condition. It may be overlooked on account of more obvious anterior scleral inflammation or because there is isolated posterior disease, and thus the eye appears white and quiet (often despite severe symptoms). It is associated with systemic disease (usually RA or vasculitis (see Table 8.3)) in up to one-third of cases.

Any posterior scleritis may lead to visual loss and needs to be treated seriously.

Clinical features
- Mild to severe deep pain (may be referred to brow or jaw), ↓VA, diplopia, photopsia, hypermetropic shift; it may, however, sometimes be painless.
- White eye (unless anterior involvement), lid oedema, proptosis, lid retraction, restricted motility; shallow AC, choroidal folds, annular choroidal detachment, exudative retinal detachments (ERD), macular oedema, disc oedema.

Investigation
- *B-scan US*: scleral thickening (see Figs 2.3–2.10) with fluid in Tenon's space (T-sign). Scleral thickening will also be seen on CT and MRI.

Treatment
- *Oral*: NSAIDs (see Box 8.1). Increasing recognition of the risk of visual loss from posterior scleritis has led many practitioners to go directly to using corticosteroids, reserving NSAIDs for those cases where corticosteroids are contraindicated.
- If not controlled on NSAIDs and/or concern over the risk of posterior scleritis-induced visual loss, consider systemic immunosuppression. 'Rescue' with corticosteroids (e.g. prednisolone 1mg/kg/d, tapering down, or three pulses IVMP 1g od, followed by oral corticosteroid. IVMP is typically given in 100mL normal saline over 1h; beware cardiac failure. Taper down corticosteroid, aiming for 'maintenance' dose, e.g. prednisolone ≤7.5mg od; if this is not possible without recurrence of disease, then introduce a 'second-line' immunosuppressant (see ➔ Treatment, p. 294).
- The response to therapy may be monitored by measuring the posterior scleral thickness on serial B-scan US.

Table 8.3 Classification of vasculitides according to the Chapel Hill consensus[*]

1° vasculitides	Large artery	GCA
		Takayasu arteritis
	Medium artery	PAN
		Kawasaki disease
	Small artery and vein	Wegener's granulomatosis
		Microscopic polyangiitis
		Churg–Strauss syndrome
		Henoch–Schönlein purpura
		Leukocytoclastic vasculitis
		Essential cryoglobulinaemic vasculitis
	Other	Behçet's disease
		Cogan's syndrome
2° vasculitides		Connective tissue disease
		Hepatitis B/C
		HIV

[*] Jennette JC et al. Nomenclature of systemic vasculitides. Proposal of an international consensus conference. *Arthritis Rheum* 1994;**37**:187–92.

NB Recently, Watts et al. have suggested a possible fourth category, no predominant vessel size, to describe Behçet's syndrome, 1° CNS vasculitis, and Cogan's syndrome.[4]

4. Watts RA et al. Systemic vasculitis—is it time to reclassify? *Rheumatology (Oxf)* 2011;**50**:643–5.

Lens

Anatomy and physiology

The lens is a transparent, avascular biconvex structure, consisting of an outer acellular capsule, lens epithelium, cortex, and nucleus. It provides one-third of the refractive power of the eye (the remaining two-thirds by the cornea). In the unaccommodated state, the adult lens is 4–5mm thick, with a 10mm anterior radius of curvature, a –6mm posterior radius of curvature, a refractive index of 1.386 (1.406 centrally), and an overall dioptric power of 18D.

Anatomy

Capsule

Unusually thick BM, rich in type IV collagen; the anterior capsule arises from the epithelium, and the posterior capsule from the elongating fibre cells; the capsule is thicker at the equator than centrally, and thicker anteriorly (8–14 microns, increasing with age) than posteriorly (2–3 microns).

Epithelium and lens fibres

The lens epithelium lies just deep to the anterior capsule; centrally, the epithelium is cuboidal and non-mitotic; peripherally, the epithelium is columnar and mitotic, producing almost 2 million transparent lens fibres over an adult's life. As the cells elongate (up to 10mm long), transparency is attained by loss of organelles, a tight regular arrangement, and a 90% crystallin composition.

Nucleus and cortex

The nucleus (comprising embryonic and fetal parts) consists of the fibres laid down before birth—no cells are lost from the lens. The cortex contains the more recently formed fibres, whilst the nucleus contains the older non-dividing cells. Lens sutures are formed by interdigitation of the ends of the fibres. The most visible example are the two Y-shaped sutures of the fetal nucleus—anterior Y, posterior λ.

Zonules

These comprise sheets of suspensory fibres composed of fibrillin (Chr 15q) that arise at the ciliary body and attach to the lens pre-equatorially, equatorially, and post-equatorially.

Physiology

The lens has a low water (65%) and high protein (35%) content. It has a resting pH of 6.9, a relatively low temperature, and is relatively hypoxic. Most energy production and active transport occur at the epithelium, but peripheral lens fibres demonstrate significant protein synthesis (mainly of crystallins), and even central lens fibres show limited carbohydrate metabolism. Although oxidative phosphorylation occurs at the epithelium, most energy production is anaerobic (via glycolysis, pentose-phosphate pathway, and the α-glycerophosphate shuttle). Most glucose is thus converted to glucose-6-phosphate and, to a lesser degree, sorbitol.

The high refractive index of the lens results from the crystallin content of its fibres. These proteins, of which α-crystallin is the commonest, are extremely stable and provide good short-range order (predominantly β-sheet 2° structure).

Clarity of the lens is attained by minimizing lens fibre scatter with: (1) narrow lens fibre membranes; (2) small interfibre spaces; (3) tightly packed regular contents (crystallin); (4) absence of blood vessels; and (5) loss of organelles.

Detoxification of free radicals is achieved by glutathione, supported by ascorbic acid (cf. hydrogen peroxide catalase elsewhere in the body). In the process, glutathione is oxidized to glutathione disulfide (GSSG), which would potentially form disulfide bonds with lens proteins, were it not returned to its reduced state by glutathione reductase.

Cataract: introduction

Cataracts account for about 40% of global blindness, representing about 16 million people. While cataract is ubiquitous, occurring in almost every ageing population, the inequity of eye care means that 99% of these blinding cases are seen in developing countries.

Risk factors

The prevalence of cataract increases markedly with age. In the UK, a visually significant cataract (VA <6/12) was present in 16% of those aged 65–69y, in 42% of those aged 75–79y, and in 71% of those aged >85y.[1]

Other risk factors include: age, sunlight, smoking, alcohol, dehydration, radiation, corticosteroid use, diabetes mellitus.

Pathogenesis

How these factors cause cataracts is unclear, although a common pathway appears to be protein denaturation, e.g. by oxidation.

Metabolic disturbance (hyperglycaemia in diabetes mellitus or hyperuraemia in dehydration or renal failure), toxins (e.g. smoking, alcohol), loss of antioxidant enzymes, membrane disruption, reduced metabolism, failure of active transport, and loss of ionic/osmotic balance may all contribute to this process.

Clinical presentations

Common

- *Change in vision*: reducing acuity, contrast sensitivity, or colour appreciation, glare, monocular diplopia, polyplopia, or ghosting.
- *Change in refraction*: typically myopic shift in nuclear sclerosis or increased or changing astigmatism.
- *Change in fundal view*: optometrists and ophthalmologists may have difficulty 'looking in', long before the patient feels they have difficulties 'looking out'. This may be a problem when trying to monitor/treat posterior segment disease such as diabetic retinopathy.

Uncommon

Phacomorphic glaucoma

The large cataractous lens may cause anterior bowing of the iris with 2° angle closure. Presentation is as acute or chronic angle closure with high IOP, shallow AC, and fixed semi-dilated pupil. Distinguish it from 1° angle-closure glaucoma (PACG) by the presence of an ipsilateral swollen cataractous lens and contralateral open angle with deep AC.

Phacolytic glaucoma

The hypermature cataract loses soluble lens proteins through the intact anterior capsule, causing trabecular obstruction and subsequent 2° open-angle glaucoma. Note raised IOP, lens protein in a deep AC (may form a pseudohypopyon), open angles, and hypermature cataract.

Phacoanaphylactic uveitis

This is an inflammatory response to lens protein, usually following traumatic capsular rupture or post-operative retention of lens material (when it must be distinguished from endophthalmitis). The IOP may be high, normal, or low.

1. Reidy A *et al.* Prevalence of serious eye disease and visual impairment in a north London population: population based, cross sectional study. *BMJ* 1998;**316**:1643–6.

Cataract: types

Cataracts may be classified, according to age of onset, morphology, grade of opacification, and maturity.

Age of onset

Cataracts may be congenital (see ➲ Congenital cataract: assessment, p. 792), juvenile/presenile (see Table 18.29), or age-related (senile).

Morphology

Cataract morphology (see Table 9.1) may be divided into fibre-based (pattern relates to anatomical structure of the lens) or non-fibre-based (a more random distribution). Fibre-based cataracts may be divided into sutural (pattern relates to lens sutures) and non-sutural types (see Table 9.2).

Table 9.1 Classification of cataract morphology

Fibre-based	Sutural	Congenital sutural
		Concussion
		Storage disorder
		Deposition
	Non-sutural	Lamellar
		Nuclear
		Cortical
Non-fibre-based	Subcapsular	Lamellar
		Coronary
		Blue dot
		Christmas tree

Grade

Grading systems have been designed that aim to quantify the degree of opacification. These vary from simple assessment by direct ophthalmoscopy to more sophisticated methods such as the Lens Opacities Classification System II where slit-lamp examination is compared with a standard set of photographs (separate set for nuclear, cortical, and posterior subcapsular).

Maturity of cataract

- *Immature*: opacification is incomplete.
- *Mature*: opacification is total.
- *Hypermature*: lysis of cortex results in shrinkage, seen clinically as wrinkling of the capsule.
- *Morgagnian*: liquefaction of cortex allows the harder nucleus to drop inferiorly (but still within the capsule).

Table 9.2 Cataract types

Type		Properties	Cause
Sutural	Y	Congenital	Non-progressive
		Concussion	Often flower-shaped (lens fibre separation and fluid entry); anterior and posterior
		Storage disorder	Usually start posteriorly; Fabry's disease, mannosidosis
		Deposition	Usually start anteriorly; Copper, gold, silver, iron, chlorpromazine
Nuclear		Congenital	Non-progressive; limited to embryonic nucleus (cataracta centralis pulverulenta) or more extensive
		Age-related	Increased white scatter (light scattering) and brunescence (brown chromophores)
Lamellar		Congenital/infantile	Localized to a particular lamella (layer) ± extensions (riders) Inherited, rubella, diabetes, galactosaemia, hypocalcaemia
Coronary		Sporadic	Round opacities in the deep cortex forming a 'crown' Occasionally inherited
Cortical		Age-related	Spoke-like opacities in the superficial cortex, spreading along fibres at an unpredictable rate
Subcapsular		Age-related	Granular material just beneath capsule, posterior (more common and visually significant) or anterior Diabetes, corticosteroids, uveitis, radiation
Polar		Congenital	*Anterior*: with abnormalities of capsule ± anterior segment (persistent pupillary membrane, anterior lenticonus, Peter's anomaly) *Posterior*: with abnormalities of capsule ± posterior segment (persistent hyperplastic 1° vitreous, Mittendorf dots, posterior lenticonus)
Diffuse		Congenital	Focal blue dot opacities are common and visually insignificant Also present in Lowe syndrome carriers
		Age-related	Christmas tree cataracts are highly reflective crystalline opacities

Cataract surgery: assessment

There is no proven medical treatment of cataract. Surgical removal of cataracts is effective and safe. It is predominantly performed in elderly patients, with 90% of patients ≥60y old.[2] Overall, 92% patients attain best-corrected visual acuity (BCVA) ≥6/12 within 3mo of surgery, and >80% are within 1D of predicted refraction.

Sight-threatening complications are rare. However, this is, in part, due to careful preoperative preparation and post-operative assessment (see Table 9.3 for initial assessment).

Referral

Referral may be by the 1° care physician or, increasingly, directly from the optometrist.

Appropriate referral
- The cataract is likely to be responsible for the patient's visual complaint.
- The cataract is compromising the patient's lifestyle.
- The risks and benefits have been discussed with the patient and appropriate written information provided.
- The patient wants to have the operation.

All this information and a copy of a recent sight test should be included in the referral.

Outpatient appointment

Appropriate listing for cataract surgery
- There is visually significant cataract responsible for the patient's complaint and compromising their lifestyle.
- Although VA is the main indicator for surgery, other measures of visual functioning, including glare, contrast sensitivity, and functional disability, are increasingly being considered.
- There is no coexisting ocular disease precluding surgery; any disease that may affect surgery (e.g. pseudoexfoliation (PXF)) or outcome (e.g. AMD) has been discussed with the patient and an appropriately guarded prognosis given.
- The patient wants to proceed and understands the risks.
- Informed consent is taken, and a surgical plan is formulated (see ➋ Cataract surgery: consent and planning, p. 308).

The younger patient
In the younger patient, also consider why they might have developed presenile cataracts (trauma, steroids, etc.) (see Table 18.29).

Preoperative assessment

For patient convenience, this should be on the same day as the initial assessment. Aspects may be performed by suitably trained nursing staff, according to local protocol.

History
- *General health*: PMH, drugs, allergies.
- *SH*: support, telephone, transport, ability to manage topical medication.
- *Education*: surgery, post-operative care, information leaflet.

Investigation
- Biometry/IOL power calculations.
- Focimetry (unless recent copy of refraction).

Treatment
- Prescription of preoperative treatments, e.g. for blepharitis.
- Prescription of mydriatic drops, e.g. cyclopentolate 1% + phenylephrine 2.5% + diclofenac 0.1% to potentiate mydriasis.
- Prescription of post-operative treatment: steroid/antibiotic drops (e.g. Tobradex® 4×/d for 4wk); IOP-lowering agents (e.g. timolol 0.5% or acetazolamide 250mg stat dose post-operation).

Table 9.3 Initial assessment for cataract surgery

Visual symptoms	Blur at distance/near, glare, distortion, colour perception, 'second sight' (myopic shift)
POH	Previous acuity; history of amblyopia, strabismus, previous surgery (*especially* refractive surgery), trauma; concurrent eye disease; refraction from optometrist
PMH	Diabetes, hypertension, COPD; ability to lie flat and still for 30min; anaesthetic history (if GA considered)
SH	Occupation, driving, hobbies, daily tasks
Dx	Warfarin, antiplatelet agents, α1-adrenoreceptor blockers, e.g. tamsulosin; topical medication
VA	Distance/near, unaided/best corrected/pinhole
Pupils	Check for RAPD, adequate dilatation
Cataract	Morphology, density, maturity
Other factors	Globe (deep-set, small/large), lids (blepharitis, entropion, ectropion), nasolacrimal (mucocele), cornea (scarring, guttata), AC depth, IOP, iris (PXF), iridodonesis, posterior synechiae (PS), inducible mydriasis), lens (PXF, phacodonesis, lens–vitreous interface) optic disc (e.g. glaucoma, neuropathy), macula (e.g. AMD), fundus

2. HES online. *Main procedures and interventions: 2000–2008*. Available at: ℛ http://www.hesonline.nhs.uk

Cataract surgery: consent and planning

Nature of the operation

Explain what a cataract is, 'The clear lens in your eye has become cloudy', and what the operation does, 'It replaces the cataract with a new plastic lens'.

General risk

For all patients, warn of sight-threatening risks, notably endophthalmitis (0.1%), retinal detachment/tear (0.1%), and choroidal haemorrhage (0.1%). Also advise of the possibility of requiring a second operation ± GA (dropped nucleus/IOL (0.5%)). The commonest intraoperative complication is posterior capsule rupture with vitreous loss (4%), which may have a significant effect on outcome. The commonest post-operative complication is posterior capsule opacification (PCO) (10% in 2y).

Anaesthetic options include topical, local (peribulbar or subtenons) or GA (see ➲ Ocular anaesthesia (1), p. 928).

The risk of a GA will depend on the general health of the patient and, if necessary, should be discussed with the anaesthetist ± physician before the day of surgery. Risks of local anaesthesia include globe rupture (0.006–0.1%) and life-threatening events such as brainstem anaesthesia or the oculocardiac reflex (0.03%).

Specific risk

Assess and warn of any additional risk such as technical difficulties (see Table 9.4), guarded visual prognosis, and any increased risk of sight-threatening complications. Consider whether subspecialist review is indicated, e.g. for posterior polar cataracts or in the presence of endothelial dystrophies.

Common technical issues

Table 9.4 Common technical issues*

Feature	Risk	Strategy
Positional		
Cervical spondylosis	Head-up posture	Tilt feet up
Deep-set eye	Poor access	Temporal approach
View		
Oily tear film	Aberrant reflexes	External methylcellulose
Poor red reflex	Difficult capsulorhexis	Vision blue
Access		
Short axial length	Crowded AC	High viscosity viscoelastic
Poor dilation	Inadequate access	Iris hooks/stretch techniques
Zonular integrity		
Age >90y	Zonular dehiscence	Minimize lens movement
PXF	Zonular dehiscence	Minimize lens movement
Preoperative phacodonesis	Zonular dehiscence	Vitreoretinal approach
White cataract	Zonular dehiscence	Consider M-SICS/ECCE/chopping
Posterior capsule (PC) integrity		
Shallow AC depth	Iris/PC trauma	High viscosity viscoelastic
Posterior polar	PC rupture	Vitreoretinal approach

* See also *Cataract Surgery Guidelines 2010* of the Royal College of Ophthalmologists for further discussion of these and similar strategies for tackling common challenges in cataract surgery. Available at: ℜ http://www.rcophth.ac.uk

Guarded visual prognosis
Note history of amblyopia or evidence of pre-existing corneal opacity, vitreous opacities, macular or optic nerve disease.

Increased risk of sight-threatening complications
- *Endophthalmitis*: note lid disease (blepharitis, trichiasis, entropion, ectropion), conjunctivitis, nasolacrimal disease (obstruction, mucocele, etc.), diabetes; pre-treat where possible, e.g. lid hygiene/antibiotics for blepharitis/conjunctivitis, surgery for lid malposition/nasolacrimal obstruction.
- *Retinal detachment*: note high myopia, lattice degeneration
- *Choroidal haemorrhage*: possibly uncontrolled hypertension, age, arteriosclerosis.
- *Corneal decompensation*: note endothelial dystrophy (e.g. Fuchs').

Desired outcome
Consider the refractive needs of the patient.

When aiming for emmetropia (most patients), explain that, while they may need no/weak glasses for distance, they will need reading glasses. Patients with significant ametropia or astigmatism are more complex.

High ametropia
- *Complications*: anisometropia may lead to aniseikonia.
- *Preoperatively*: with bilateral cataracts, discuss options: (1) aim for emmetropia, and do the second eye within 6wk, or (2) aim to leave ametropic (but up to 2D nearer emmetropia than the other eye), with less immediate need for a second operation. If unilateral cataract, particularly where the second eye has good acuity and accommodative function, consider aiming for emmetropia and using a contact lens on the second eye until surgery is indicated.

Astigmatism
Pre-existing astigmatism can usually be reduced by choosing to operate 'on-meridian'. For higher degrees of astigmatism, additional refractive incisions can be placed at the time of cataract surgery (see ➔ Cataract surgery: perioperative, p. 312).

Cataract surgery: perioperative

Preoperative check (on the day of surgery)

Patient preparation
- Ensure mydriasis, e.g. cyclopentolate 1% + phenylephrine 2.5% + diclofenac 0.1%.
- Check consent form complete.
- Check any new ophthalmic problems, especially evidence of active infection.
- Mark side of operation.
- Operating surgeon to confirm IOL type/power and axis/operating position.

NB Inserting the incorrect IOL has become a Never Event in the NHS (Department of Health (UK), *Never Events List 2012–13*).

IOL selection
- Check that the biometry does indeed belong to your patient.
- Check for *intraocular* consistency in axial length and K values (i.e. that they are similar and the SD is low).
- Check for *interocular* consistency in axial length and K values. Most individuals have similar axial lengths and corneal curvatures in either eye; 92% of axial lengths are within the range 21.0–25.5mm; 99% of K readings are within the range 40–48D.
- Royal College of Ophthalmologists 2010 guidelines suggest repeating measurements if: (1) axial length is <21.20mm or >26.60mm, (2) mean corneal power is <41D or >47D, (3) delta K is >2.5D, (4) difference in axial length between fellow eyes of >0.7mm, (5) difference in mean corneal power of >0.9D.
- Check appropriate formula used (see Table 9.5).
- Select appropriate lens power (usually, but not always, aiming for emmetropia); if previous refractive surgery, enter corrected K values into SRK/T, Haigis, Haigis-L, Hoffer Q, and Holladay 2, and select the highest IOL power suggested.

Table 9.5 Royal College of Ophthalmologists recommendations 2004*

<22mm	Hoffer Q or SRK/T
22–24.5mm	SRK/T, Holladay, Haigis
>24.6	SRK/T

* The 2010 recommendations comment that all these formulae perform well in the normal axial length range, but the Haigis and Hoffer Q may be preferred for short axial lengths (<22mm). Most importantly, the IOL constants (A constant) should be optimized for the method of axial length measurement (whether optical or acoustic; and specific instrument). An international resource for this is provided by the User Group for Laser Interference Biometry (ULIB) at: ℬ http://www.augenklinik.uni-wuerzburg.de/ulib/index.htm

Astigmatic targeting

Some surgeons always operate 'from the top', but there are refractive advantages to a temporal clear corneal incision or scleral tunnel (relative astigmatic neutrality), or by operating 'on-meridian' (astigmatic targeting). If operating 'on-meridian', a clear corneal incision is placed on the steep corneal meridian. This should be based on keratometry, as the refractive astigmatism may include a lenticular component that will be dealt with by lens removal. The astigmatic effect of the incision increases with depth and length of wound. It can be enhanced by an opposite refractive incision (on-meridian surgery) or by single or paired incisions at another meridian (off-meridian surgery) (see Box 9.1 for IOL selection after refractive surgery).

Box 9.1 IOL selection after refractive surgery

Keratometric measurements performed after laser refractive surgery are unreliable in traditional biometric formulae and will result in substantial post-operative refractive errors (hyperopic surprise in patient who have undergone myopic correction and vice versa). Many methods developed to estimate the correct central corneal power include:

Historical methods

Uses pre-refractive data to calculate IOL power, such as the methods of Hoffer, and Feiz and Mannis.

CL method

- Measure refraction, with and without a 40D hard CL.
- Corrected K = 40 + (refraction with CL − refraction without CL).
- These corrected Ks are entered into SRK/T, Haigis, Hoffer Q, and Holladay 2 formulae, and the highest IOL power selected.

Topographical method

Topographer used to measure apical axial curvature (after Maloney).

Online calculators

Recently, web-based calculators have been developed e.g. American Society of Cataract and Refractive Surgery (ASCRS) IOL calculator (available at: http://www.iol.ascrs.org). The advantage of this calculator is that it is easy to use and incorporates multiple calculation methods. The predicted IOL represents an average of all the results that has increased accuracy over a single method.

NB It is vital to have a thorough discussion with any post-refractive laser patient undergoing cataract surgery regarding the difficulty in accurate IOL prediction. These patients should be warned of the higher risk of post-operative refractive surprise which may require further treatment. This should be documented in the notes and appropriate consent obtained.

Phacoemulsification (1)

Preparation

Povidone iodine (5% aqueous solution) cleansing of the skin and instillation into the conjunctival sac reduce bacterial load and risk of endophthalmitis. Careful draping maximizes surgical view, keeps lashes out of the surgical field, and prevents pooling of fluid.

Incision

Wound construction is critical. The wound needs to be large enough to allow easy access of instruments, but small enough to permit a stable AC and reduce risk of iris prolapse (e.g. 2.8mm). At the end of the operation, it must seal to become watertight.

Options for conventional phacoemulsification wounds include clear corneal incisions (which may be tri-, bi-, or uniplanar) and scleral tunnels. Scleral tunnels are fairly astigmatically neutral, whereas corneal incisions tend to cause flattening. This can be made use of by operating 'on-meridian' to reduce any pre-existing corneal astigmatism. With the advent of bimanual microincision cataract surgery (see Box 9.3), wounds may be as small as 1.4mm.

Subsequent instrumentation should respect the shape of the wound to reduce the risk of stripping off Descemet's membrane.

Ophthalmic viscosurgical devices (OVDs) (viscoelastics)

OVDs are solutions of long-chain polymers with a range of viscosity and cohesive properties (see Table 9.6). Higher-viscosity cohesive OVDs are used for stabilizing the AC and opening the bag prior to IOL insertion. Lower-viscosity dispersive OVDs are used to isolate part of the surgical field, e.g. protecting a vulnerable cornea in the 'soft-shell' technique[3] (see Box 9.2) or keeping the iris or vitreous out of the way. Viscoadaptives are more advanced OVDs that can behave like a higher-viscosity cohesive OVD or like a dispersive, according to AC fluid dynamics.

Table 9.6 OVDs

Group	Subgroup	Content	Example	Molecular weight
Viscoadaptive		Hyaluronic acid	Healon 5	4,000–8,000kDa
Higher viscosity	Superviscous	Hyaluronic acid	Healon GV	4,000–8,000kDa
	Viscous	Hyaluronic acid	Healon Provisc	1,000–2,000kDa
Lower viscosity	Medium viscosity	Hyaluronic acid	Viscoat	100–500kDa
	Very low viscosity	HPMC	Ocucoat	80–90kDa

Combination OVDs:

1. Cohesive and dispersive OVD combination—superior retention, space maintenance, and easy removal, e.g. DisCoVisc®

2. Viscoelastic with anaesthetic—for topical anaesthesia, e.g. Visthesia®.

Box 9.2 Options for the soft-shell technique

Traditional soft-shell technique[*]
- High-viscosity cohesive OVD to maintain AC.
- Low-viscosity dispersive OVD to coat cornea.

Viscoadaptive soft-shell technique
Viscoadaptive OVD to achieve both maintenance of AC and protection of cornea. It is either used in combination with BSS (known as the 'ultimate soft-shell technique') or with a viscodispersive OVD.

[*] Arshinoff SA. Dispersive-cohesive viscoelastic soft shell technique. *J Cataract Refract Surg* 1999;25:167–73.

3. Arshinoff SA. Dispersive-cohesive viscoelastic soft shell technique. *J Cataract Refract Surg* 1999;25:167–73.

Phacoemulsification (2)

Continuous curvilinear capsulorhexis

The aim is to achieve a 5–6mm continuous central anterior capsulectomy via cystotome and/or forceps under viscoelastic. This is large enough to assist lens removal (and reduce risk of post-operative capsular phimosis) and small enough to stabilize the lens (and reduce risk of post-operative capsular opacification).

In the presence of poor red reflex or significant cortical opacities, visibility may be assisted by the use of trypan blue (often injected under air and irrigated after <60s). Decompress intumescent cataracts by puncturing the AC and aspirating lens matter.

A capsulorhexis that is running out to the periphery may be rescuable by deepening the AC/pushing the iris back with more or higher viscosity viscolelastic, e.g. Healon 5. If unable to bring the capsulorhexis back in, consider: tearing in the opposite direction from the start position; capsulorhexis scissors or a can-opener capsulotomy. Review whether to continue with cautious phacoemulsification or convert to extracapsular cataract extraction (ECCE).

A small capsulorhexis can be extended after insertion of the posterior chamber IOL (PCIOL) by making a nick (e.g. with a cystotome) and then tearing with forceps as usual.

Hydrodissection

Injection of BSS under the anterior capsular rim separates the nucleus from the cortex and is seen as a wave passing posteriorly. If successful, it permits rotation of the nucleus. If overly aggressive, it may cause posterior capsule rupture, as may the use of a fine-bore cannula (smaller than 27G).

Managing the small pupil

Inadequate dilatation of pupil makes surgery technically more difficult and increases the risk of complications.

Causes

Common causes include diabetes, PXF, uveitis, the intraoperative floppy iris syndrome, and long-term pilocarpine usage.

Intraoperative strategies

- Pupil stretch.
- Iris hooks.
- Intracameral mydriatics, e.g. intracameral lidocaine + phenylephrine ± cyclopentolate.
- Pupil expansion device.
  - Benefits—round pupil, no sphincter damage, no need for additional paracentesis, and saves time, e.g. Malyugin ring.

Phacoemulsification (3)

Phacoemulsification

Rotate the probe to enter wound with minimal trauma.

Technique
- *Divide and conquer*: the groove should be about 1.5 phaco tips wide and as deep as safely possible (this is usually about 3mm deep centrally). An improving red reflex may assist in judging depth. Use a second instrument to rotate nucleus 90° to form the next groove, and continue until a cruciate configuration is formed. Insert both instruments deep into each groove, gently pulling apart to crack the nucleus into four segments. Use a higher vacuum setting to bring each segment centrally to be emulsified.
- *Phaco chop*: allows significant reduction in phaco power needed, compared to divide and conquer. Use high vacuum and sufficient phaco power to bury the phaco tip into the nucleus, just proximal to the centre and aiming steeply posterior. In *horizontal chop*, the second instrument is inserted under the anterior capsule and chopped through the stabilized nucleus against the phaco probe. This is repeated to generate wedges that can then be emulsified. Alternatively, in *vertical chop*, following the impaling of the nucleus, a sharp-tipped instrument is buried in the nucleus adjacent to the phaco probe. The phaco tip is lifted and the chopper depressed, allowing cleavage of the nucleus by separation of the probe and chopper.
- *Stop and chop*: central groove is made as for divide and conquer, but, after separation of the lens into two hemisegments, the latter are chopped with second instrument.
- *Chip and flip*: sculpt to form a bowl, and then flip it anteriorly to complete emulsification safely.

Pumps and fluidics

The traditional distinction between a vacuum pump (e.g. Venturi system) and a peristaltic pump has become blurred by hybrids such as the scroll pump.
- *Vacuum systems*: use a Venturi or a diaphragm pump to generate a low pressure relative to the AC. Flow is dependent on this pressure difference and thus cannot be altered independently of vacuum.
- *Peristaltic systems*: the pressure gradient is generated by milking fluid along compressible tubing by a series of rollers. Flow and vacuum can be set separately. A low-flow setting results in a more gradual, gentler response, so aiding cautious manipulation. This may be helpful in training. Higher flow results in a faster (but more aggressive) response from the phaco probe. Adjusting the vacuum level limits the maximum vacuum that will be generated once the tip is occluded.

Phaco power modulation

Phaco power can be delivered as continuous or intermittent. Intermittent modes are all directed at using phaco power more efficiently, so reducing the effective phaco time (EPT) (EPT = phaco time × % phaco power used). These modes include pulse (usually linear control of energy with fixed/varying pulse rate), burst mode (fixed phaco power with variable duration/interval), and assorted modifications such as sonolase, 'no burn', and 'cool' phaco.

Dual linear

This permits simultaneous foot control of both phaco power (pitch, i.e. up/down) and aspiration (yaw, i.e. left/right). This is particularly useful for the phaco chop technique.

Irrigation and aspiration

This is usually automated (straight/curved/45°/90° tips) and can be combined or split (bimanual). Manual irrigation and aspiration are an alternative (Simcoe). Cortex is engaged peripherally and dragged centrally where the vacuum can be increased under direct view.

IOL

Depending on the type of IOL and the original incision size, it may be necessary to enlarge the wound sufficiently to allow the introduction of the lens before introducing it via an injector or lens forceps. Pre-fill the bag with viscoelastic before implanting the lens, placing the lead haptic directly into the bag before dropping/dialling in the second haptic. The choice of lens will be affected by capsular integrity (and therefore type of operation) (see ➲ Intraocular lenses (1), p. 324).

Wound closure

Well-constructed wounds sized for foldable lenses are usually self-sealing but may be assisted by stromal hydration. If in any doubt, suture the wound closed.

Perioperative antibiotics

At the end of the procedure, antibiotics (± corticosteroids) are routinely given. Traditionally, this has been topical, subconjunctival, or subtenons; intracameral cefuroxime has been increasingly popular, since the ESCRS study reported a 5-fold reduction in the rate of endophthalmitis.[4]

Common regimens include: subconjunctival—cefuroxime or gentamicin ± dexamethasone; intracameral—cefuroxime (1mg).

Box 9.3 Bimanual microincision cataract surgery

In essence, bimanual microincision cataract surgery uses separate handpieces for irrigation and phacoemulsification/aspiration. The technique requires two limbal incisions of 1.2 × 1.4mm made with a trapezoidal blade.

Advantages include

- Smaller incision (e.g. 1.45mm) due to narrower handpieces, leading to fewer wound complications.
- More stable AC.
- Improved fluid dynamics: the irrigation does not propel the pieces of nucleus away from the tip of the phaco probe.
- Improved accessibility (e.g. easier removal of soft lens matter (SLM), as the probes can be interchanged between the two wounds).
- Reduced 'phaco time/power'.

---

4. Barry P et al. ESCRS study of prophylaxis of postoperative endophthalmitis after cataract surgery.

Femtosecond laser (FSL) cataract surgery

FSL technology has been recently introduced for use in cataract surgery. Stages of FSL-assisted cataract surgery include:
- Preoperative planning.
- Docking the eye.
- Intraoperative anterior segment imaging.
- Treatment stage.

FSL technology

Currently the main platforms available are
- Victus (Technolas/Bausch & Lomb).
- Lens Sx (Alcon).
- Catalys (Optmedica).
- LensAR (LensAR).

Detailed anterior segment imaging is key to effective and safe treatment and is achieved by Fourier domain OCT (LenSx, Catalys & Victus systems) or Scheimpflug related technology (LensAR system).

Applications of FSL

FSL is used for the following applications in cataract surgery:
- *Clear corneal incisions*. increased stability and reproducibility using FSL, compared to manual techniques.
- *Limbal relaxing incisions*: those created with FSL are more accurate, reliable, and have little or no risk of perforation, compared to manual.
- *Capsulorhexis*: ideally, anterior capsulotomy should be perfectly circular and just overlap the IOL optic by 0.5mm for 360°. Size and circularity of anterior capsulotomy are vital to positioning and performance of IOL—especially with toric, multifocal, and accommodating lenses. FSL capsulotomies are more accurate and reproducible in terms of size, circularity, and centration, compared to manual capsulorhexis (even in experienced hands).
- *Lens fragmentation*: FSL used to liquefy/fragment nucleus/soften hard lenses. Results in decreased intraocular instrumentation and movement and allows significant reduction in phaco time and power.

Results of FSL

Although published outcomes of FSL-assisted cataract surgery are still limited, emerging data suggest good visual outcomes, low complication rates, and no significant safety concerns. VA outcomes are not statistically significantly better than manual techniques so far. There is a statistically significant improvement in FSL capsulotomy outcomes, compared to manual techniques, which would specifically benefit toric and multifocal lens insertion. Some limitations, including poor patient compliance, patient characteristics (e.g. deep-set eyes, small palpebral apertures), small pupils, PS, and very dense cataracts which would still need conventional phaco methods. However, main limitation to widespread use of FSL-assisted cataract surgery currently is financial. Further evidence needed to support theoretical advantages over manual techniques before widespread adoption of technology.

Extracapsular, manual small incision, and intracapsular cataract extraction

See Table 9.7 for types of cataract extraction.

ECCE

This is removal of the lens while retaining the posterior capsule and integrity of the anterior vitreous face. The operation requires a superior 10mm biplanar corneal (or limbal) incision, injection of viscoelastic to form the AC, anterior capsulotomy (usually can-opener technique), hydrodissection, nucleus expression (gentle digital pressure or irrigating vectis), aspiration of cortex, and lens implantation (usually rigid polymethylmethacrylate (PMMA) lens into the bag).

Manual small incision cataract surgery (MSICS)

MSICS is an adaptation of ECCE, in which the nucleus is expressed through a self-sealing scleral tunnel wound (rather than a corneal wound). MSICS has become the operation of choice in most parts of the world where phacoemulsification is not generally available for cost reasons. A number of trials of MSICS vs phacoemulsifcation have been performed, with a meta-analysis showing phacoemulsification to be slightly superior to MSICS in terms of uncorrected VA (with less surgically induced astigmatism); there were no significant differences in visual rehabilitation, endothelial cell loss, or complication rates between the two techniques.[5]

Intracapsular cataract extraction

This is removal of the whole lens, including capsule, and was widely practised during the 1960s and 1970s. The operation requires a 150° corneal (or limbal) incision, a peripheral iridectomy, zonular digestion (α-chymotrypsin), forceps or cryoprobe removal of the lens, and insertion of an anterior chamber IOL (ACIOL) (angle or iris-supported), a sutured lens, or aphakic correction (spectacles or CL).

Table 9.7 Types of cataract extraction

Technique	Advantages	Disadvantages
Intracapsular	No PCO Can deal with zonular dialysis	Higher rates of CMO and retinal detachment Higher rate of rubeosis in diabetic eyes ACIOL, sutured lens, or aphakia Sutures required
Extracapsular	PCIOL Lower rate of CMO and retinal detachment	PCO Sutures required
Phacoemulsification	More stable AC/IOP PCIOL Lower rate of CMO, retinal detachment, and expulsive haemorrhage Sutureless wound Reduced astigmatism Faster visual rehabilitation Reduced post-operative inflammation Topical anaesthesia possible	PCO Expensive equipment Risk of dropped lens fragments
Manual small incision	Most of the same advantages as phacoemulsification No expensive equipment Sutureless wound Less astigmatism than ECCE	PCO More astigmatism than phacoemulsification

J Cataract Refract Surg 2006;**32**:407–10.

Intraocular lenses (1)

Choice of lens

Phacoemulsification with intact posterior capsule and anterior capsulorhexis permits use of a foldable PCIOL (smaller wound, usually sutureless), which can be placed in the bag (preferable optically and physiologically).

In the presence of a small tear in the anterior or posterior capsule, it may still be possible to implant the lens in the bag. If there is a significant PC tear, but intact anterior capsule, consider sulcus placement. If anterior and posterior capsular damage, consider ACIOL (angle supported or iris claw type). For ECCE, the larger incision is sufficient for implantation of a rigid PMMA lens into the bag or sulcus.

PCIOL

IOLs may be classified according to their material (silicone or acrylic), interaction with water (hydrophilic or hydrophobic), and design (one-piece or three-piece; spherical or toric; rounded or square-edged). Lens behaviour therefore arises from a number of contributing factors. For example, hydrophilic acrylic lenses appear to be the most biocompatible, with little attachment of inflammatory cells. However, the hydrophobic acrylic IOLs appear to have the lowest PCO rates, but this may be due to their square-edged design, rather than the material (see Table 9.8 for types and Table 9.9 for materials).

Material

Table 9.8 Types of PCIOL

Material	Advantages	Disadvantages
Rigid		
PMMA	Follow-up >50y	Large incision needed
	Stable	Higher rate of PCO
Foldable		
Silicone	Follow-up >15y	Rapid unfolding
	Folds easily	Poor handling when wet
		Adherence to silicone oil
Hydrophobic acrylic	Higher refractive index allows thinner lenses	Glistenings in optic (some lenses)
	Slow unfolding	
	Low PCO rate (some designs)	
Hydrophilic acrylic	Slow unfolding	Calcium deposition on/ in optic (some lenses)
	Low inflammatory cell attachment	
	Resistant to YAG laser damage	

Table 9.9 PCIOL materials

Lens type	Material	Refractive index (n)
Rigid		
PMMA	Polymethyl methacrylate	1.49
Flexible		
Silicone	Silicone polymers	1.41–1.46
Hydrophobic acrylic	Acrylate + methacrylate	1.54
Hydrophilic acrylic	Poly-hydroxyethyl-methylacrylate + hydrophilic acrylic monomer	1.47

Design

Square-edged vs rounded

IOL optics with square posterior edges appear to reduce PCO by reducing migration of lens epithelial cells, although dysphotopsia (crescentic glare in certain ambient light conditions) from edge reflections can be bothersome with 'very' square-edged lenses.

Toric vs spherical

Toric IOLs can correct for preoperative astigmatism but may cause problems, if not perfectly positioned.

Short wavelength filtration

Some recent IOLs filter out short wavelength blue light, as this may be linked to accelerated age-related macular changes in pseudophakic patients. They are also reported to increase contrast and reduce glare.

Aspheric

Aspheric design reduces spherical aberration, thus creating a crisp image. Negative spherical aberration in IOL can negate natural positive aberration and improve depth of focus. Patient customization is possible.

Preloaded

Advantages include minimization of external contamination, insertion through a small incision, saves time.

Thin vs standard

Thin IOLs are designed for use with the smaller incisions of microincision cataract surgery. They are reported as also causing less aberration, glare, and haloes than standard lenses.

Pseudo-accommodative and accommodative lenses

Pseudo-accommodative lenses are multifocals that may be diffractive or refractive in nature. *Accommodative IOLs* alter their focal length by anteroposterior movement within the capsular bag (see ➲ Accommodative/pseudo-accommodative IOL, p. 326).

Intraocular lenses (2)

Accommodative/pseudo-accommodative IOL

Pseudo-accommodative (multifocal)

Multifocal IOLs produce multiple focal points (usually two), resulting in a focused and defocused image on the retina for different object distances. This allows for clear unaided distance and near vision which is not possible with monofocal IOLs.

Types

- *Refractive type*: concentric zones of different optical power; may be near dominant or far dominant, e.g. AMO Rezoom.
- *Diffractive type*: annular grooves cut in surface of IOL cause diffraction and multiple foci, e.g. Acrysof Restor.

Disadvantages

Loss of contrast sensitivity, glare, night vision problems, visual adaptation, and good outcome rely on very accurate spherical targeting (just +0.125 side of emmetropia) and <0.50DC or residual astigmatism for the lenses to work. As these post-operative refractive errors increase, so the lens efficacy reduces; yet the side effects remain. Therefore, careful consideration should be exercised when using these lenses, and patients should be sufficiently counselled regarding limitations and potential side effects.

New models of multifocal IOL

- *Non-rotational symmetric multifocal IOL*: examples include Lentis MPlus. This has a sector shaped near vision segment, characterized by seamless transition between near and far vision zones. Advantages: excellent near, intermediate, and far vision; pupil independent, minimal haloes and glare; high contrast sensitivity.
- *New generation trifocal multifocal IOL*: examples include FineVision IOL(Physiol), AT LISA Trifocal (Zeiss). These IOLs allow for good *intermediate* vision as well as far and near vision. The optics have been modified to minimize glare and haloes. Toric versions of these multifocal IOLs will soon be available, allowing use in patients with significant astigmatism.

Accommodative

Accommodative IOLs alter their focal length by anteroposterior movement within the capsular bag due to their thin, flexible hinge at the haptic-optic junction that permits forward movement of the optic with haptic compression. Examples include 1 CU IOL, Crystalens.

Disadvantages

In general, longer-term results (1–2y) have so far been disappointing due to high levels of capsular fibrosis restricting optic movement. Glasses independence is therefore less than with modern multifocal IOLs.

New models of accommodative IOL

The Synchrony IOL is an unusual 'dual-optic' accommodative IOL with a high-plus power anterior optic connected via spring haptics to a minus-power posterior optic. Changes in ciliary body tone and capsular tension result in movement of the front optic.

Cataract surgery: post-operative

For most patients, this has largely been replaced by a telephone assessment by a trained nurse. The first-day review is now generally reserved for higher-risk patients (complicated surgery, coexistent ocular disease).

Examination
- *Cornea*: wounds sealed (Seidel test negative), clarity.
- *AC*: formed, activity.
- *Pupil*: round.
- *PCIOL*: centred and in the bag.
- *Consider*: IOP check.

Give clear instructions re post-operative drops, use of a clear shield, what to expect (1–2d discomfort, watering), what to worry about (increasing pain/redness, worsening vision), and where to get help (including telephone number).

Final review (usually 2–4wk later)

Examination
- *VA*: unaided/pinhole.
- *Cornea*: wounds sealed (Seidel test negative), clarity.
- *AC*: depth and activity.
- *Pupil*: round.
- *PCIOL*: centred and in the bag.
- *IOP*.
- *Fundus*: no CMO, flat retina.

If good result, then either list for second eye or discharge to optometrist for refraction, as appropriate.

If disappointing VA (unaided), perform refraction/autorefraction to look for 'refractive surprise' (see ➔ Refractive surprise, p. 340) and dilated fundoscopy to check for subtle CMO (especially if VA (pinhole) < VA (unaided)), and, if in doubt, consider OCT.

Cataract surgery and concurrent eye disease

Diabetes
- *Preoperative*: if severe preproliferative diabetic retinopathy (PPDR)/ PDR, then treat (PRP) prior to surgery where possible. Treat clinically significant macular oedema (focal/grid laser) 12wk before surgery.
- *Post-operative*: consider topical NSAID (e.g. ketorolac 0.3% 3×/d for 6wk). An extended course of topical steroids may be required. See at 1d, 1wk, and then 6wk.
- *Complications*: fibrinous anterior uveitis, PCO, progression of retinopathy, and macular oedema. Risk of complications increases with degree of retinopathy.

Glaucoma
- *Preoperative*: stabilize IOP control.
- *Post-operative*: consider extended use of post-operative acetazolamide to minimize post-operative pressure spike (and risk of 'wipe out' to a vulnerable optic nerve). Although there have been concerns re CMO, the continuation of prostaglandin analogues post-operatively is probably safe. In the short eye, beware aqueous misdirection syndrome. See at 1d, 1wk, and then 6wk.
- *Complications*: post-operative pressure spike, progression of field loss.
- A potential advantage with uncomplicated surgery is a small lowering of IOP.

Uveitis
- *Preoperative*: control inflammation and IOP as far as possible. In well-controlled anterior uveitis, consider intensive topical steroids for 2wk prior to surgery (e.g. dexamethasone 0.1% 2-hourly). In patients with chronic uveitis, consider 500mg IVMP 1h prior to surgery, or prednisolone 40mg 1x/d for 1wk prior to surgery.
- *Intraoperative*: ensure adequate pupillary access (synechiolysis, iris hooks, iris stretching), but avoid unnecessary iris manipulation. Ensure meticulous cortical clearance. Perform a well-centred 5–6mm capsulorhexis (vs post-operative phimosis, iris-capsule synechiae). Foldable lenses (e.g. acrylic or silicone) may be used. Give subconjunctival steroid (e.g. betamethasone 4mg).
- *Post-operative*: frequent potent topical steroid (e.g. dexamethasone 0.1% 2-hourly), and taper slowly; if oral steroids were started/increased preoperatively, these should be tapered slowly to zero/maintenance dose. Consider mydriatic (e.g. cyclopentolate 1% nocte). In persistent fibrinous uveitis, consider intracameral recombinant tissue plasminogen activator. See at 1d, 1wk, and then 6wk.
- *Complications*: exacerbation of inflammation, fibrinous anterior uveitis, synechiae, raised IOP, macular oedema, PCO.

Post-vitrectomy

- *Preoperative*: silicone oil slows sound transmission (estimated at 987m/s), and this must be incorporated when calculating axial length from an A-scan. Additionally, the axial length may not be stable within a year of encirclement procedures and may be unpredictable post-macular surgery.
- *Intraoperative*: use clear corneal incision (rather than scleral tunnel). Poor mydriasis may require iris hooks/stretching. Fluctuation of AC depth and the risk to the flaccid PC may be minimized by well-constructed wounds, lower bottle height, reduced vacuum, and lifting the iris with second instrument. Minimize nucleus manipulation to protect damaged zonules. Use acrylic or PMMA lenses (*not* silicone), placing in the bag or sulcus.
- *Post-operative*: give retinal detachment warning; dilate at follow-up review.
- *Complications*: PCO, retinal (re)detachment, vitreous haemorrhage.

Prostatism, α-blockers, and the intraoperative floppy iris syndrome

Intraoperative floppy iris syndrome occurs in patients using $\alpha 1$-adrenergic blocking agents, e.g. tamsulosin, alfuzosin used in the treatment of benign prostatic hypertrophy. It is characterized by iris prolapse and progressive narrowing of the pupil during surgery, thus increasing the risk of complications.

- *Preoperative*: identify relevant drugs.
- *Intraoperative*: strategies include use of iris hooks and intracameral phenylephrine (see Table 25.2). It can also be useful to keep the side port incision as small as possible, and consider moving both incisions anteriorly into the cornea to help with flow dynamics and reduce prolapse. This is also useful in the hypermetropic eye.
- *Complications*: iris trauma, iris prolapse, poor visualization, unstable AC.

Cataract surgery: complications

Intraoperative

Posterior capsule rupture without vitreous loss (about 2%)

The main aims, when confronted with a PC tear (± vitreous loss), are to maintain as much capsule as possible and to clear any vitreous. If PC tear is small and well defined, the PCIOL may still be placed in the bag, either at the time of surgery or as a 2° procedure. However, with larger, poorly defined PC tears, it is safer to place the lens in the sulcus, provided sufficient anterior capsule remains to stabilize it.

NB Assuming equal A-constants, a sulcus-fixated lens should be 0.5D lower power than that calculated for fixing in the bag.

Posterior capsule rupture with vitreous loss (1%)

Clear the wound and AC of vitreous with manual (sponge/scissors) and/or automated vitrectomy while maintaining as much posterior capsule as possible. If sufficient anterior capsule remains, place the lens in the sulcus, else consider an ACIOL (+ PI). The crucial role of the cataract surgeon under these circumstances is to:

- Maintain all the capsule possible (this may facilitate PCIOL insertion 4wk later), and
- Clear vitreous from the AC and wounds; intracameral triamcinolone can be very useful, as it will highlight any remaining vitreous.

Anterior capsule problems

The capsulorhexis has a tendency to 'run out' in a number of situations: shallow AC, positive posterior pressure, young patients, intumescent cataracts. Stabilize the AC with a more viscous viscoelastic, e.g. Healon 5. Decompress intumescent cataracts by puncturing the AC and aspirating lens matter. If unable to bring the capsulorhexis back in, options include returning to the start and attempting a second tear in the opposite direction, the use of capsulorhexis scissors, and switching to a can-opener technique. Depending on the security of the resulting capsulorhexis either continue with cautious phacoemulsification or convert to MSICS or ECCE.

Zonular dehiscence

Consider stabilizing with iris hooks (secure the capsule in the area of dialysis) or a capsular tension ring (stabilizes the bag and redistributes forces away from individual zonules). If associated with vitreous loss, an anterior vitrectomy will be required.

Loss of nuclear fragment posteriorly (0.3%)

Nuclear material is inflammatory. Very small fragments can be observed but may require prolonged topical steroids. Larger fragments require removal via a pars plana vitrectomy, ideally within 1–2wk. Refer immediately to a vitreoretinal surgeon. Start on their preferred regimen to control inflammation, reduce risk of infection, and prevent ↑IOP (partly to preserve corneal clarity). One example is dexamethasone 0.1% 2-hourly, chloramphenicol 0.5% 4×/d, acetazolamide SR 250mg bd.

Choroidal haemorrhage (0.1%)

- Suspect this if there is sudden increase in IOP, with AC shallowing, iris prolapse, loss of vitreous, and loss/darkening of the red reflex. This is often associated with patient complaining of severe pain.
- Immediately suture all wounds closed; give IV pressure-lowering treatment (e.g. acetazolamide or mannitol), and start on intensive topical steroids.
- Prognosis is poor, with only 45% achieving VA ≥6/60 in that eye.

Post-operative: early

Corneal oedema (10%)

- Control IOP and inflammation with topical treatment ± acetazolamide.

Elevated IOP (2–8%)

- Control with topical treatment ± acetazolamide.
- In extreme cases, consider releasing fluid from the paracentesis wound under aseptic conditions.

Increased anterior inflammation (2–6%)

- If greater than expected, increase topical steroids, maintaining normal antibiotic cover (e.g. chloramphenicol 0.5% 4×/d), but always have a low threshold of suspicion for toxic anterior segment syndrome (TASS) or endophthalmitis.

Wound leak (1%)

- Return to theatre, and suture wound closed if persistent or severe (AC shallow with iris prolapse or iridocorneal touch).

Iris prolapse (0.7%)

- Return to theatre; assess vitality of extruded iris (may need abscising); reform AC, and suture wound closed.

Endophthalmitis (0.1%) (See ➡ Post-operative endophthalmitis, p. 336)

Post-operative: late

PCO (10% by 2y)

- Consider YAG posterior capsulotomy if opacification is causing reduced vision, monocular diplopia, or is preventing assessment/treatment of fundal pathology.
- In uveitic patients, defer until opacification causing VA ≤6/12 or preventing fundal view and 6mo post-surgery and 2mo since last exacerbation.
- Do not perform a posterior capsulotomy if there is any question of lens replacement being required.

Cystoid macular oedema (1–12%) (See ➡ Post-operative cystoid macular oedema, p. 339)

Retained epinuclear fragment

Often in AC, causing late-onset corneal oedema; anterior segment OCT may aid diagnosis; prompt removal necessary.

Retinal detachment (0.7%)

Risk is increased in myopes, with lattice degeneration and particularly if there has been vitreous loss. Refer immediately to vitreoretinal surgeon.

Corneal decompensation

Risk is increased if pre-existing endothelial dystrophy, diabetes, intraoperative endothelial trauma/phacoburn, long phaco time/power or long irrigation time, or ACIOL. Control IOP and inflammation. Consider hypertonic drops (e.g. sodium chloride 5%), BCL (for comfort in bullous keratopathy), or penetrating/endothelial keratoplasty.

Chronic endophthalmitis (See ➲ Post-operative endophthalmitis, p. 336)

Diagnosis

Perform an AC tap, vitreous biopsy, and consider removal of posterior capsule. Send sample for smears (Gram, Giemsa, and methenamine-silver stain) and culture (blood, chocolate, Sabouraud, thioglycolate broth, and solid anaerobic medium; the last is especially important for *P. acnes*). PCR may also be helpful.

Treat

For *P. acnes* or low-grade *S. epidermidis*, consider vitrectomy, intravitreal vancomycin, and, if necessary, IOL removal. For suspected fungal infection, consider vitrectomy, intravitreal amphotericin (5–10 micrograms), and subsequent topical ± systemic antifungals, according to sensitivity.

Summary of Royal College of Ophthalmologists *Focus on Endophthalmitis 1996* and *2004* and *Cataract Surgery guidelines 2010*

Prophylaxis

- Skin and conjunctival sac preparation with 5% aqueous povidone iodine at least 5min before surgery. It is safe and effective in significantly reducing ocular surface flora. Additional benefit may be gained by post-operative instillation into the sac.
- Preoperative povidone iodine remains the only agent to be proven to provide a protective effect against post-operative endophthalmitis.
- Identifying and treating risk factors, such as blepharitis, conjunctivitis, or mucocele, are probably more useful than universal antibiotic prophylaxis. The use of antibiotics in irrigating solutions is controversial.
- The use of perioperative antibiotics is controversial. Antibiotics to prevent endophthalmitis are given either intraoperatively at the end of the procedure by the intracameral or subconjunctival route or topically at the end of the procedure.
- The national rate of endophthalmitis reported in the BOSU study (2004) was 0.14% and that in the Bolton study (2007) was 0.055%. The current advice is to continue with the local arrangements for preventative treatment of endophthalmitis if audited figures reveal a rate similar to the Bolton study. If figures are higher, the use of intracameral cefuroxime should be considered.

Treatment

- *VA > PL*: single-port vitreous biopsy via the pars plana should be performed using a vitreous cutting-suction device. The specimens are directly smeared, for Gram stain, etc., and plated for culture. Directly inject amikacin and vancomycin (or gentamicin and cefuroxime).
- *VA ≤ PL*: three-port pars plan vitrectomy and intravitreal antibiotics. High-dose systemic prednisolone may be given, e.g. 60–80mg daily, rapidly reducing to zero over a week to 10d. Steroids are contraindicated if there is a fungal infection.
- If the clinical course warrants it, the biopsy and intravitreal antibiotic injection may be repeated after 48–72h.

Toxic anterior segment syndrome

TASS is an acute post-operative, non-infectious, inflammatory reaction due to inadvertent entry of toxic substances in the AC. It can induce permanent corneal endothelial damage or trabecular meshwork damage.

Clinical features

- Rapid onset, 12–24h post-surgery (which often has been uneventful) of corneal oedema, moderate/severe AC inflammation ± fibrin/hypopyon, ↑IOP.
- Sometimes difficult to differentiate from infectious endophthalmitis. Distinguishing features of TASS (vs endophthalmitis) are: earlier onset, mild or no pain, limbus-to-limbus corneal oedema (classic finding), sudden increase in IOP; vitritis is rare, highly sensitive to topical steroids.

Treatment

- Intensive topical steroids; close monitoring of IOP.
- If diagnosis of TASS uncertain, then treat as infectious endophthalmitis.

Post-operative cystoid macular oedema

Irvine–Gass syndrome

Suspect if:

Worsening vision (may decrease with pinhole), perifoveal retinal thickening ± cystoid spaces. Increased risk in patients with diabetes, complicated surgery, post-operative uveitis, or previous CMO (in the other eye post-routine surgery). The classical presentation is excellent vision immediately post-operation and for a few days, then declining.

Diagnosis

Clinical appearance (but may be subclinical) and/or OCT/FFA findings:

- *Clinical appearance*: loss of foveal contour, retinal thickening, cystoid spaces; central yellow spot, small intraretinal haemorrhages, and telangiectasia (occasional).
- *OCT*: in addition to detecting cystoid spaces, can measure degree of retinal thickening and specific pathology, e.g. vitreomacular traction.
- *FFA*: typically dye leakage from both the parafovea into the cystoid spaces—petalloid pattern—and from the optic disc.

Prophylaxis

Consider adding topical NSAID (e.g. ketorolac 0.3% 3×/d 6wk) to usual post-operative steroid regimen for high-risk groups (diabetes, uveitis, previous CMO, complicated surgery with vitreous loss).

Treatment

A step-wise approach is recommended. Review the diagnosis (e.g. OCT, FFA) if atypical or slow to respond. One approach is as follows:

1. Topical: steroid (e.g. dexamethasone 0.1% 4×/d) + NSAID (e.g. ketorolac 0.3% 3×/d).

Review in 4–6wk; if persisting, then:

2. Periocular steroid (e.g. sub-Tenon's triamcinolone), and continue topical treatment.

Review in 4–6wk; if persisting, then:

3. Consider: repeating periocular or giving intravitreal steroid; vitrectomy; systemic steroids (e.g. prednisolone 40mg 1×/d, titrating over 3wk; or IVMP 500mg single dose); oral acetazolamide (500mg/d; limited evidence).

Refractive surprise

Failure to achieve the estimated/target refraction is disappointing for the patient and the surgeon. A careful systematic approach will help identify the source of the problem.

In patients where the refractive outcome is harder to predict (high ametropia, previous corneal refractive surgery), review patients early (1wk) with refraction to permit the option of an early IOL exchange if a large discrepancy noticed. It should be noted that retention of OVD (e.g. healon) in the capsular 'bag' in the early post-operative period may distort the true post-operative refraction (see Box 9.4 for assessment).

> Box 9.4 **An approach to the assessment of the patient with refractive surprise**
>
> *Verify the problem*
> * What is the post-operative refraction?
>   * Have it checked by a clinician experienced at refraction.
>
> *Case note review*
> * Was the correct IOL selected intraoperatively?
> * Was the preoperative biometry/lens selection valid?
>   * Check biometry used does indeed belong to your patient.
>   * Look for *intraocular* consistency in axial length and K values (i.e. that they are similar and the standard deviation is low).
>   * Look for *interocular* consistency in axial length and K values.
>   * Check appropriate formula used.
>   * Had they had previous refractive surgery?
>
> *Clinical examination*
> * Has there been a change in the corneal curvature (K readings) since the operation?
>   * Wounds: poorly constructed wounds or use of limbal relaxing incisions (LRIs); LRIs will rarely change the spherical equivalent when treating ≤3DC but have a hypermetropic effect when treating higher levels of astigmatism.
>   * Corneal oedema.
>   * Other corneal pathology (previously unrecognized), e.g. keratoconus, previous refractive surgery; CL use.
> * Is the IOL correctly positioned?
>   * Check IOL centred and completely in the bag.
>   * Is there retention of healon within the bag?
>   * Is early capsule healing/phimosis affecting IOL position?
>
> *Investigations*
> * Repeat biometry ± B-scan to confirm axial length (on pseudophakic mode).
> * Repeat keratometry ± corneal topography.

Treatment

Small errors

A stable refraction is essential before considering any treatment. Depending on the cause of the refractive surprise, the following options may be considered:

- *Observation*: post-operative change in corneal curvature may improve as oedema settles and wounds heal.
- *No treatment*: a small myopic refractive surprise in a non-dominant eye may be useful for reading.
- *Trial of spectacles.*
- *Intervention for specific problem*: surgical repositioning of poorly placed IOL, YAG laser for capsular phimosis.

Large errors

For large errors, the following may be considered:

- *CL.*
- *IOL exchange*: preferred option if recognized early but becomes increasingly difficult surgically, if delayed.
- 2° *piggyback IOL*: eliminates guesswork of IOL power, as power now based on post-operative refraction.
- *Laser refractive surgery for residual errors*: the most predictable surgical method.

NB It is important to recognize refractive surprise and accept—particularly with hypermetropic surprise—that the patient is unhappy for that reason. Do not be tempted to try to improve their vision by performing a YAG posterior capsulotomy, thereby reducing the surgeon's options and the patient's chance of a satisfactory outcome.

In general, unless the refractive surprise is very large, refractive surgery and piggyback IOLs are preferable to IOL exchange, as they carry a lower surgical risk and offer greater predictability.

Abnormalities of lens size, shape, and position

Abnormalities of size, shape, and position may affect both the refractive power of the lens and increase optical aberration. In addition, most of these abnormalities are associated with lens opacity. Commonest among this group are disorders of lens position, i.e. ectopia lentis (see Table 9.10).

Ectopia lentis

This may be complete (dislocation or luxation) or partial (displacement or subluxation). Do not neglect possible acquired causes of ectopia lentis.

Complications
- Refractive (edge effect, lenticular astigmatism, lenticular myopia, aphakic hypermetropia, diplopia).
- Anterior dislocation → glaucoma, corneal decompensation, uveitis.

Treatment
- *Refractive*: CLs, spectacles.
- *Dislocation*: into the posterior segment (followed by aphakic correction) either by: (1) YAG zonulolysis or (2) mydriatics + lie the patient on their back if lens already dislocated anteriorly.
- *Lensectomy* (followed by aphakic correction).

Causes
Congenital
- *Familial ectopa lentis (AD)*: uni-/bilateral superotemporal lens subluxation; no systemic abnormality.
- *Ectopia lentis et pupillae (AR)*: superotemporal dissociation with pupil displacement in the opposite direction; no systemic abnormality.
- *Marfan's syndrome (AD, Chr 15, fibrillin)*: bilateral superotemporal lens subluxation with some preservation of accommodation, lattice degeneration, retinal detachment, anomalous angles, glaucoma, keratoconus, blue sclera, axial myopia; musculoskeletal (arachnodactyly, disproportionately long-limbed, joint laxity, pectus excavatum, kyphoscoliosis, high-arched palate, herniae); cardiovascular (aortic dilatation, aortic regurgitation, aortic dissection, mitral valve prolapse).
- *Weill–Marchesani syndrome (AR)*: bilateral anteroinferior lens subluxation, microspherophakia, retinal detachment, anomalous angles; musculoskeletal (short stature, brachydactyly); neurological (reduced IQ).

- *Homocystinuria (AR, cystathionine synthetase abnormality → homocysteine and methionine accumulation)*: bilateral inferonasal lens subluxation, myopia, glaucoma; skeletal ('knock-kneed', marfanoid habitus, osteoporosis); haematological (thromboses, especially associated with general anaesthesia); facies (fine, fair hair); neurological (low IQ).
- *Hyperlysinaemia (AR, lysineα-ketoglutarate reductase)*: lens subluxation, microspherophakia; musculoskeletal (joint laxity, hypotonia); neurological (epilepsy, low IQ).
- *Sulfite oxidase deficiency (AR)*: lens subluxation; neurological (hypertonia, low IQ); life expectancy <5y.

Acquired
- These include trauma, high myopia, (hyper)mature cataract, PXF, buphthalmos, and ciliary body tumour.

Table 9.10 Abnormalities of lens size, shape, and position

Abnormality	Condition	Associations
Size	Microphakia (small lens)	Lowe syndrome (X)
	Microspherophakia (small spherical lens)	Familial microspherophakia (AD)
		Peters anomaly
		Marfan's syndrome (AD)
		Weill–Marchesani syndrome (AR)
		Hyperlysinaemia (AR)
		Alport syndrome (X-linked dominant, XD)
		Congenital rubella
Shape	Coloboma (inferior notch)	Iris/choroid colobomata
		Giant retinal tears
	Anterior lenticonus (bulge in anterior lens)	Alport syndrome
	Posterior lenticonus (bulge in posterior lens)	*Unilateral*: usually sporadic
		Bilateral: familial (AD/AR/X-linked, X)
		Lowe syndrome (X)
	Lentiglobus (extreme lenticonus)	Posterior polar cataract
Position	Ectopia lentis (congenital)	Familial ectopia lentis (AD)
		Marfan's syndrome (AD)
		Weill–Marchesani syndrome (AR)
		Homocystinuria (AR)
		Familial microspherophakia (AD)
		Hyperlysinaemia (AR)
		Sulfite oxidase deficiency (AR)
		Stickler syndrome (AD)
		Sturge–Weber syndrome (sporadic)
		Crouzon syndrome (sporadic)
		Ehlers–Danlos syndrome (AD/AR)
		Aniridia
	Ectopia lentis (acquired)	Trauma
		High myopia
		Buphthalmos
		Ciliary body tumour
		Hypermature cataract
		PXF

Glaucoma

Relevant pages
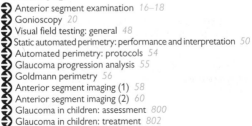

Anatomy and physiology

Glaucoma is a progressive optic neuropathy with characteristic changes in the optic nerve head and corresponding loss of VF. It represents a final common pathway for a number of conditions, for most of which raised IOP is the most important risk factor. In Western countries, glaucoma is present in 1% of those over 40 and 3% in those over 70y old. It is the second leading cause of blindness worldwide.

Anatomy

- *AC angle*: extends from Schwalbe's line (the termination of Descemet's membrane on the peripheral cornea) posteriorly to the trabecular meshwork, scleral spur, and, in some cases, ciliary body where an acute angle is formed with the peripheral iris.
- *Trabecular meshwork*: this is a reticulated band of fibrocellular sheets, with a triangular cross-section, base towards the scleral spur
- *Scleral spur*: firm fibrous projection from the sclera, with Schlemm's canal at its base and the longitudinal portion of the ciliary muscle inserting into its posterior surface.
- *Schlemm's canal*: circumferential septate drain, with an inner wall of endothelium containing giant vacuoles and an outer wall obliquely punctuated by collector channels that drain into the episcleral veins.
- *Ciliary body*: comprises the ciliary muscle and ciliary epithelium, arranged anatomically as the pars plana and pars plicata (containing the ciliary processes). Contraction of the ciliary muscle permits accommodation and increases trabecular outflow. The ciliary epithelium is a cuboidal bilayer arranged apex to apex with numerous gap junctions. The inner layer is non-pigmented, with high metabolic activity, and posteriorly is continuous with the neural retina. The outer layer is pigmented and posteriorly is continuous with the RPE.

Physiology

Aqueous production

Aqueous humour is a clear, colourless, plasma-like BSS produced by the ciliary body. It is a structurally supportive medium, providing nutrients to the lens and cornea. It differs from plasma in having lower glucose (80% of plasma levels), low protein (assuming an intact blood aqueous barrier), and high ascorbate. It is formed at about 2.5 microlitre/min by a combination of active secretion (70%), ultrafiltration (20%), and osmosis (10%). Active secretion is complex, involving the maintenance of a transepithelial potential by the Na^+K^+ pump, ion transport by symports and antiports (including the important $Na^+/K^+/2Cl^-$ symport), calcium- and voltage-gated ion channels, and carbonic anhydrase.

Aqueous outflow
While the trabecular route is the major outflow, the uveoscleral contribution may be as much as 30%.

Trabecular (conventional) route
Most aqueous humour leaves the eye by this passive pressure-sensitive route. About 75% of outflow resistance is due to the trabecular meshwork itself, with the major component being the outermost (juxtacanalicular) portion of the trabecular meshwork. This comprises several layers of endothelial cells embedded in ground substance which appears to act as a filter, which is continually cleaned by endothelial cell phagocytosis. Onward transport into Schlemm's canal is achieved by pressure-dependent transcellular channels (seen as giant vacuoles of fluid crossing the endothelium) and paracellular pores. Aqueous is then transported via collector channels to the episcleral veins and on to the general venous circulation.

Uveoscleral (unconventional) route
The aqueous passes across the iris root and ciliary body into the supraciliary and suprachoroidal spaces, from where it escapes via the choroidal circulation.

IOP

$$\text{Flow in} = \text{Flow out} = C\,(\text{IOP} - Pv) + U$$

Where C is the pressure-sensitive outflow facility (via trabecular meshwork), U is the pressure-independent outflow (via uveoscleral route), and Pv is the episcleral venous pressure. Typical values are:

$$2.5\ \mu L/\text{min} = 0.3\ \mu L/\text{min/mmHg}\,(16 - 9\text{mmHg}) + 0.4\ \mu L/\text{min}$$

Variation in IOP
Within the population
Normal IOP within the population is generally taken to be: mean IOP ± 2 SD = 16 ± 2 (2.5), i.e. a range of 11–21mmHg. However, there is a positive skew to this distribution.

Within the individual
Mean diurnal variation is up to 5mmHg in normals but can be up to 10–15mmHg in POAG. IOP tends to peak in the morning in most individuals. Posture, pulse pressure, respiration, extremes of BP, exercise, and season also have an effect. The effect of posture on IOP may have significant clinical impact, with some studies showing glaucoma progression to be more strongly associated with supine (vs sitting) IOP and to correlate with the magnitude of the increase in IOP caused by posture. It has been suggested that some patients with glaucoma may be prone to nocturnal IOP spikes.

Glaucoma: assessment

Over 1 million sight tests are performed each year in the UK. Of these, about 60,000 people are referred to ophthalmologists for assessment of possible glaucoma (see Tables 10.1–10.3). Of these, about one-third will be diagnosed with glaucoma, one-third with OHT, and one-third will be discharged. At initial consultation, consider: (1) evidence for glaucoma vs normal variant or alternative pathology (see Table 10.3), (2) evidence for underlying cause (i.e. type of glaucoma), (3) factors that may influence treatment. Be cautious of interpreting any one abnormality in isolation, e.g. apparent field defects may be artefactual and disappear with repeated testing due to the ' learning effect' (see Box 10.1).

> **Box 10.1 Significant glaucomatous field loss**
>
> The European Glaucoma Society recommends that the following abnormalities be regarded as significant:
> * Abnormal glaucoma hemifield test.
> * Three abnormal points at p <5% level, one of which should be at p <1% level and none of which should be contiguous with the blind spot.
> * Corrected PSD <5% if the VF is otherwise normal, *provided that* they are confirmed on two consecutive tests *and* there is no other retinal or neurological disease affecting the VF.

Table 10.1 An approach to assessing possible glaucoma

Visual symptoms	Asymptomatic, haloes, ache, precipitants (dim light, reading, exercise), subjective loss of vision/field
POH	Previous surgery (incl. refractive) or trauma, concurrent eye disease, refractive error, amblyopia
PMH	Diabetes, hypertension, ischaemic heart disease (IHD), asthma/COPD, transient ischaemic attack (TIA)/CVA, thyroid disease, chronic obstructive sleep apnoea, peripheral and central vasospasm (Raynaud's phenomenon, migraine), anaemia
FH	Family members with glaucoma (age of onset) and their outcome (e.g. any glaucoma-related blindness)
Dx	Current/previous topical medications, current drugs (interactions), systemic β-blockers, current/previous use of steroids (any route)
Ax	Allergies or relevant drug contraindications
VA	Best corrected (distance and near acuity)
Visual function	Check for RAPD, colour vision (Ishihara plates)
Cornea	Pigment deposition (Krukenberg spindle), KPs, guttata, pachymetry
AC	Peripheral (van Herrick)/central AC depth, cells, pigment
Gonioscopy	Angle configuration, iris approach, abnormal pigmentation, PAS, NVA, angle recession
Tonometry	IOP (Goldmann applanation tonometry (GAT))—measure in two meridia in high corneal astigmatism
Iris	Transillumination defects (mid-peripheral/focal/sectorial), PXF, heterochromia, iris stromal hypoplasia, neovascularization of the iris (NVI), iris nodules, configuration (plateau, convex, concave)
Lens	Cataract (phacomorphic/phacolytic), phacodonesis, subluxation, ACIOL
Optic disc	Size, vertical C/D ratio, colour (pallor—diffuse/segmental), optic disc asymmetry, NRR (contour, notches, haemorrhages), pits, colobomata, optic disc drusen
Disc vessels	Baring, bayonetting, trifurcation (optic disc drusen), shunt vessels
Peripapillary area	Haemorrhages, PPA, pigmentation, RNFL defects
Fundus	Chorioretinal scarring, retinoschisis, retinal detachment (can cause field loss), maculopathy, previous CRVO/branch retinal vein occlusion (BRVO)

Table 10.2 The 'glaucoma triad'

Evidence for glaucoma	Features
Raised IOP	>21mmHg
Abnormal disc	C/D ratio asymmetry
	Large C/D ratio for disc size
	NRR notch/thinning (ISNT rule)
	Disc haemorrhage
	Vessel bayoneting/nasally displaced
	PPA (B-zone)
VF defect	Nasal step
	Paracentral scotoma
	Arcuate scotoma
	Altitudinal scotoma
	Residual temporal or central island of vision

'ISNT rule' describes the normal contour of the disc rim, being thickest inferiorly, thinner superiorly, then nasally, and thinnest temporally. This rule often fails to apply when the optic discs have an anomalous configuration. IOP does not need to be >21mmHg to develop glaucomatous optic neuropathy. Anomalous optic discs are difficult to assess.

Table 10.3 A short differential diagnosis of the 'glaucoma triad'

IOP	Discs	VF	Consider
Raised IOP	Normal	Normal	OHT
	Borderline	Normal	Glaucoma suspect/pre-perimetric glaucoma
	Borderline	Consistent defect	Highly suspicious: treat as glaucoma
	Abnormal	Consistent defect	Glaucoma
Normal IOP	Normal	Normal	Normal
	Borderline	Normal	Physiological cupping
	Stable abnormality	Stable defect	Congenital disc anomaly
			Previous optic disc insult
	Evolving abnormality	Evolving defect	Normal-tension glaucoma (NTG)
			Other optic neuropathy

Ocular hypertension

OHT describes an IOP >21mmHg (representing 2 SD above the population mean) in the presence of a healthy OD and normal VF. This population is positively skewed, with 5–7% of those aged >40 having an IOP >21mmHg. In the absence of glaucomatous damage, it is difficult to differentiate those in whom such an IOP is physiological from those in whom it is pathological (i.e. will 'convert' to POAG) (see Box 10.2 for devices to measure IOP).

Risk of 'conversion' to POAG

In the Ocular Hypertension Treatment Study (OHTS), the 'conversion rate' was found to be 9.5% over 5y (untreated). If treated with topical medication (to reduce IOP by >20% and to achieve ≤24mmHg), this 'conversion rate' was reduced to 4.4%.

Risk factors (and their hazard ratios, HR) demonstrated in the OHTS trial include:[1]

- *Older age*: HR 1.2 per decade.
- *Higher IOP*: HR 1.1 per mmHg.
- *Larger C/D ratio*: HR 1.2 per 0.1.
- *Greater pattern SD*: HR 1.3 per 0.2dB.
- *Thinner CCT*: HR 1.7 per 40 micron.

Thinner CCT may lead to underestimation of IOP, such that the measured IOP may be less than the true IOP. Other possible risk factors include African American ethnicity, FH, myopia, and other suspicious disc/peripapillary changes.

Who to treat?

There is considerable variation in practice. Some practitioners treat all >21mmHg. Consider treating:

- *Isolated OHT*: if IOP >27mmHg.
- *OHT and suspicious disc*: if IOP >21mmHg.
- *OHT and thin cornea*: if IOP >21mmHg.

Relatively thin corneas (CCT <555 microns) were associated with a 3-fold risk of 'conversion' to POAG vs thick corneas (>588 microns). Some practitioners use pachymeter routinely and 'correct' the IOP for corneal thickness. One estimate is that, for every 20 microns that the CCT is >550 microns, the IOP is under-read by 1mmHg; interestingly, this calculation reclassifies many NTG patients as high-tension POAG and OHT patients as normals. There is not a close linear relationship between CCT and IOP, so caution should be used when interpreting corrective algorithms.

Other factors that may suggest a lower threshold for treatment include:

- OHT and only eye.
- OHT and CRVO or AION in either eye.
- OHT and FH of glaucoma (especially of blinding disease).

Monitoring

For those not requiring treatment, follow up 6–12mo (IOP, disc appearance), and perform perimetry every 6–12mo.

For those requiring treatment, follow up as per POAG (see ➲ Primary open-angle glaucoma, p. 354).

Box 10.2 Devices used to measure IOP

Measurement of IOP may be affected by CCT, corneal hysteresis (a measure of structural rigidity), corneal astigmatism, and axial length. Different methods of measuring IOP are variably affected by these factors. As the accurate estimation of IOP is fundamental to the management of glaucoma, it is important to appreciate the limitations of the devices in common usage.

- GAT (Haag-Streit, Bern, Switzerland): the ubiquitous slit-lamp mounted contact applanation device; it is calibrated for measuring IOP in subjects with an average CCT and is significantly affected by deviations in CCT.
- Reichert Ocular Response Analyser (ORA; Reichert Ophthalmic Instruments, Buffalo, USA): automated non-contact device that scans the central cornea during deformation by an air-pulse and estimates the IOP both from the applanation point achieved during deformation and during recovery. The average of these two points—known as the Goldmann-correlated IOP value—is indicated as IOPg. A more sophisticated estimate—the corneal compensated IOP (IOPcc)—takes into account the difference between the two applanation values, which indicates the corneal hysteresis and reflects the structural rigidity of the cornea.
- Pascal dynamic contour tonometer (Swiss Microtechnology AG, Bern, Switzerland): a slit-lamp mounted digital device that provides a direct transcorneal measurement of diastolic IOP; it also measures ocular pulse amplitude, enabling an estimate of systolic IOP. It is less affected by CCT than GAT.
- TonoPen XL (Reichert Ophthalmic Instruments, Buffalo, USA): a portable contact instrument that estimates the IOP, based on the Mackay–Marg principle. It displays the average of multiple independent readings. Like GAT, it is affected by CCT but is less affected by corneal curvature and can be useful in irregular corneas.
- ICare tonometer (Icare Finland, Espoo, Finland): a portable contact instrument that is the only contact device not to require topical anaesthesia. Like GAT and the TonoPen, it is affected by CCT but is less affected by corneal curvature and can be useful in irregular corneas and those who do not tolerate other contact methods.

1. Gordon MO et al. The Ocular Hypertension Treatment Study: baseline factors that predict the risk of primary open-angle glaucoma Am J Ophthalmol 2004;138:684–5.

Primary open-angle glaucoma

This is an adult-onset optic neuropathy, with glaucomatous optic disc and/ or VF changes, open angles, and no other underlying disease (cf. secondary open-angle glaucomas). The term is usually reserved for those with 'high-tension' glaucoma, i.e. IOP >21mmHg (cf. normal-tension glaucoma). Although it is present in 1% of the population, up to 50% of cases may be undiagnosed.

Risk factors

- *Age*: increasing age (uncommon <40y).
- *Ethnicity*: African-Caribbean—more frequent, younger onset, more severe.
- *FH*: first-degree relative confers 1 in 8 risk; higher in siblings.
- *Steroid-induced IOP elevation*: more common in POAG and those with FH of POAG.
- *Other possible risk factors*: include vascular disease (e.g. diabetes and hypertension) and myopia (the disc is said to be more vulnerable due to the scleral canal morphology).

Clinical features

- Usually asymptomatic (rarely, eye ache and haloes—transient corneal oedema if ↑↑ IOP).
- IOP >21mmHg, often with high diurnal variability.
- *Disc changes*: C/D asymmetry, high C/D for disc size, vertical elongation of the cup, NRR notch/thinning (does not follow 'ISNT' rule; see Table 10.2), disc haemorrhage, vessel bayonetting/nasally displaced, PPA (β-zone). β-zone PPA describes choroidal atrophy immediately adjacent to the disc; it may correspond to areas of retinal ganglion cell loss and VF defects. α-zone PPA is more peripheral, irregularly pigmented, and less specific for glaucoma.
- *VF defects*: (1) focal defects respecting the horizontal meridian, including nasal step, baring of the blind spot, paracentral scotomas, arcuate defects, and altitudinal defects; (2) generalized depression.

Treatment

- *Counselling*: see Box 10.3.
- *Medical*: topical—prostaglandin analogue, β-blocker, α2-agonist, carbonic anhydrase inhibitor. All have contraindications and side effects. Some of these topical therapies are also available in preservative-free formulations for those patients who are allergic to, or have developed toxicity to, the preservatives.
- *Laser trabeculoplasty (argon (ALT)/selective (SLT))*: may be appropriate first-line treatment for those who are frail or in whom adherence is likely to be an issue; it is most effective in those with moderate trabecular pigmentation. IOP control fails with time (sometimes rapidly), with 50% failure rate at 5y.

- *Trabeculectomy* (± augmented): may be appropriate 1° treatment for patients who have advanced disease and need low target IOPs, are drop-intolerant or are at high risk of progression. Trabeculectomy with anti-scarring MMC is the gold standard surgical intervention and is most often used after failure of maximal tolerated medical therapy (MTMT) (see ➲ Filtration surgery: trabeculectomy, p. 392). In resistant cases, consider:
  - Shunt procedures (e.g. Baerveldt, Molteno, Ahmed, or other tubes); destructive procedures to the ciliary body (diode laser cycloablation, cyclocryotherapy) (see ➲ Laser procedures in glaucoma, p. 388).

Box 10.3 An approach to the medical treatment of POAG

(1) Counsel patient
Nature and natural history of condition; implications for driving; effect of drops; important side effects; importance of compliance; probability of lifetime treatment; that they will not notice any day-to-day benefit.

(2) Define target IOP
Usually ≥20% reduction initially; target IOP should be lower if there is already advanced damage, disease continues to progress, or other risk factors are present.

(3) Select drug
First line, consider: prostaglandin agonist or β-blocker. Note contraindications.

(4) Teach how to administer drops (incl. nasolacrimal occlusion)

(5) Review treatment (e.g. 6wk later)
- *Effects*: is there significant IOP reduction, and has the target IOP been reached? Some advocate a treatment trial of one eye so that therapeutic efficacy can be gauged against the other eye (which controls for diurnal variation).
- *Side effects*: local (e.g. allergic) and systemic (e.g. lethargy, dizziness, wheeze, etc.).

(6) Decide re further treatment
- If no significant reduction in IOP → stop drop, and try another first-line agent; check compliance.
- If significant reduction but target IOP not met → augment with another agent (another first-line drug or second-line such as topical carbonic anhydrase inhibitor).
- If target IOP achieved → continue; review (e.g. 3mo).
- If target IOP achieved BUT disc or field continues to progress, then target may need to be lowered. Consider other risk factors such as pressure spikes (may need IOP phasing), systemic hypotension, or poor compliance.

Normal-tension glaucoma

NTG is generally regarded as a subcategory of POAG, although clinical cases often have a distinct phenotype. It has been suggested that local vascular dysregulation at the optic disc may be an important factor in the pathogenesis of this disease. Patients with NTG may also have evidence of central (migraine) or peripheral (Raynaud's phenomenon) vascular dysregulation and low BP.

Risk factors
- *Age*: more common in the elderly, but up to one-third may be <50y.
- *Ethinicity*: more common in Japan.
- *Sex*: possible ♀ preponderance.

Clinical features
- Usually asymptomatic.
- IOP <21mmHg.
- *OD changes*: as for POAG, although disc haemorrhages and acquired pits may be more common and the cup may be larger and shallower (saucerization).
- *VF defects*: as for POAG, although: (1) focal defects are more often in the superior hemifield (especially superonasal) and are said to be deeper, steeper, and closer to fixation; (2) generalized depression is less marked than in high-tension POAG.

Differential diagnosis and investigations
- *POAG*: perform pachymetry (permits estimation for potential 'under-reading' of IOP (see ➲ Ocular hypertension, p. 352)) and IOP phasing to assess IOP range. IOP phasing constitutes regular IOP checks (e.g. 1-hourly) over an extended period of the day (e.g. 0800–1800h).
- *2° glaucoma*: clinical assessment.
- *PACG*: clinical assessment (especially gonioscopy).
- *Compressive optic neuropathy*: consider fine-cut MRI of the anterior visual pathway (optic nerves/tracts/chiasm) with gadolinium enhancement if the clinical picture is not typical of glaucoma. In particular, be alert to neuropathology if: positive visual symptoms, unexplained VA reduction, reduced colour vision, RAPD, optic disc pallor, VF defect observing the vertical midline, or mismatch between optic disc and VF defect.
- *Chronic obstructive sleep apnoea (COSA)*.
- *Congenital anomaly of the optic disc (e.g. coloboma)*.
- *Other optic neuropathies*: consider sending blood for FBC, B12, folate, ESR, VDRL, TPHA, ACE, ANA, ANCA, CRP, Leber's hereditary optic neuropathy (LHON); CXR (see Table 16.3).
- *Nocturnal hypotension*: consider 24h ambulatory BP monitoring, especially if on topical or systemic β-blockers or on other anti-hypertensive drugs.

Who to treat?

The Collaborative Normal Tension Glaucoma study[2] demonstrated that, considering the group as a whole, an IOP reduction by >30% slows the rate of field loss but that, even without treatment, 50% of NTG patients actually show no progression of field defects at 5y.[3] Risk factors for progression were:

- ♀ sex.
- Migraine.
- Disc haemorrhage at diagnosis.

Treatment

Generally, as for POAG, although some clinicians emphasize the role of optic nerve head perfusion and the possible role of nocturnal dips in BP. This may be confirmed on 24h ambulatory BP monitoring. On this basis, consider using prostaglandin analogues (better IOP control at night), rather than non-selective β-blockers (may reduce blood flow at night), and, for treatment of systemic hypertension, β-blockers may be avoided in favour of calcium channel blockers. It is optimal to work with a physician to optimize 24h BP control and avoid nocturnal hypotension. Treat contributory causes, e.g. COSA (refer to respiratory physician for sleep study and continuous positive airway pressure (CPAP)), anaemia, and folate/B12 deficiency.

2. Collaborative Normal Tension Glaucoma Study Group. Comparison of glaucomatous progression between untreated patients with normal-tension glaucoma and patients with therapeutically reduced intraocular pressures. *Am J Ophthalmol* 1998;**126**:487–97.

3. Collaborative Normal Tension Glaucoma Study Group. The effectiveness of intraocular pressure reduction in the treatment of normal tension glaucoma. *Am J Ophthalmol* 1998;**126**:498–505.

Primary angle-closure glaucoma

PACG is a significant cause of blindness worldwide. It is present in about 0.1% of the general population over 40y old but up to 1.5% of the Chinese population over 50. Acute primary angle closure (APAC) is an ophthalmic emergency. The terminology surrounding this condition has been reassessed by a consensus panel of glaucoma experts in the light of epidemiological studies[4] and is outlined under ➲ Terminology, p. 358.

Risk factors

Epidemiological

- *Age*: >40y old; mean age of diagnosis ± 60y.
- ♀ sex.
- *Ethnicity*: Chinese, South East Asians, Inuit.

Anatomical

Pupil block mechanism

- Narrow angle, shallow AC, relatively anterior iris–lens diaphragm, large lens (older, cataract), small corneal diameter, short axial length (usually hypermetropic); risk increases with increasing lens thickness to axial length ratio.
- In pupillary block, apposition of the iris to the lens impedes aqueous flow from PC to AC, causing relative build-up of pressure behind the iris, anterior bowing of the peripheral iris, and subsequent angle closure.

Plateau iris mechanism

- Plateau iris configuration (relatively anterior ciliary body that apposes the peripheral iris to the trabeculum; AC depth normal centrally, shallow peripherally with flat iris plane).
- Mild forms of plateau iris configuration are vulnerable to pupil block, but 'higher' plateau configurations may result in plateau iris syndrome where the peripheral iris bunches up and blocks the trabeculum directly. This means that angle closure can occur despite a patent PI.

Terminology

The following hierarchy has been suggested:

(1) Anatomically narrow drainage angle (ANDA): defined on gonioscopy.
(2) Iridotrabecular contact (ITC): defined on gonioscopy.
(3) Primary angle closure (PAC): ITC with ↑IOP or peripheral anterior synechiae (PAS) or symptoms suggestive of episodes of acute PAC.
(4) Acute primary angle closure (APAC): ITC with acute symptomatic ↑↑IOP.
(5) Primary angle closure glaucoma (PACG): PAC with glaucomatous damage (changes in the optic disc and VF).

Acute primary angle closure (APAC)

Clinical features
- Pain (periocular, headache, abdominal), blurred vision, haloes, nausea, vomiting.
- *Ipsilateral*: red eye, raised IOP (usually 50–80mmHg), corneal oedema, angle closed, fixed semi-dilated pupil; glaucomflecken; contralateral angle narrow; bilateral shallow AC.

Differential diagnosis
- *Consider*: 2° angle closure (e.g. phacomorphic, inflammatory, neovascular) or acute glaucoma syndromes such as Posner–Schlossman syndrome or PDS (see Table 10.4).

Treatment
- As per Box 10.4.

PAC

Clinical features
- Narrow angles with ITC and one or more of: ↑IOP, PAS, or symptoms suggestive of episodes of APAC.

Treatment
- Treat with 'prophylactic' Nd-YAG PIs.

Primary angle closure glaucoma (PACG)

This may occur due to: (1) synechial closure, which is either asymptomatic ('creeping') or follows episodes of acute/subacute angle closure, or (2) a POAG-like mechanism but in the context of narrow angles.

Clinical features
- As for PAC with evidence of glaucomatous optic neuropathy (characteristic optic disc and VF changes (see ➔ Glaucoma: assessment, p. 348).

Treatment
- Treat with Nd-YAG PIs (although beware IOP spike if extensive PAS); medical treatment (as for POAG) and surgical therapy (consider lens extraction and/or trabeculectomy, but note ↑risk of aqueous misdirection syndrome), as required.

4. Foster PJ et al. The definition and classification of glaucoma in prevalence surveys. *Br J Ophthalmol* 2002;**86**:238–42.

Acute primary angle closure

Acute primary angle closure (APAC) is an ophthalmic emergency requiring urgent treatment to prevent irreversible optic nerve damage. The clinical features and differential diagnosis are outlined earlier (see ➲ Primary angle-closure glaucoma, p. 358). An approach to treatment is given in Box 10.4. See Table 10.4 for glaucoma syndromes presenting acutely.

Box 10.4 An approach to the treatment of **APAC**

Immediate

- Systemic: acetazolamide 500mg IV stat (then 250mg PO 4×/d).
- Ipsilateral eye:
  - β-blocker (e.g. timolol 0.5% stat, then 2×/d).
  - Sympathomimetic (e.g. apraclonidine 1% stat).
  - Steroid (e.g. prednisolone 1% stat, then q 30–60min).
  - Pilocarpine 2% (once IOP <50mmHg, e.g. twice in first hour, then 4×/d).
- Admit patient.
- *Consider*: corneal indentation with a 4-mirror goniolens may help relieve pupil block; lying the patient supine may allow the lens to fall back away from the iris; analgesics and anti-emetics may be necessary.
- Pilocarpine 1% is often given to the contralateral eye while awaiting Nd-YAG PI (although some glaucoma specialists advise against this due to a risk of inducing reverse pupil block). In either case, the priority is for prompt bilateral PIs.

Intermediate

- Check IOP hourly until adequate control.
- If IOP not improving: consider systemic hyperosmotics (e.g. glycerol PO 1g/kg of 50% solution in lemon juice or mannitol 20% solution IV 1–1.5g/kg).
- If IOP still not improving: consider acute Nd-YAG PI (can use topical glycerin to temporarily reduce corneal oedema).
- If IOP still not improving:
  - Review the diagnosis (e.g. could this be aqueous misdirection syndrome with a patent PI?).
  - Consider repeating Nd-YAG PI or proceeding to surgical PI, argon laser iridoplasty, paracentesis, cyclodiode photocoagulation, or emergency cataract extraction/trabeculectomy.

Definitive

- Bilateral Nd-YAG or surgical PI.

NB Some eyes may develop chronic ↑IOP, either from synechial closure or from a POAG-like mechanism, and will require long-term medical ± surgical treatment.

Table 10.4 Glaucoma syndromes that may present acutely with symptomatic ↑IOP (selected)

Glaucoma type	Critical features	Additional features
Closed angle		
Primary angle closure	Closed angle, shallow AC; fixed mid-dilated pupil; iris bombé	Corneal oedema; contralateral angle narrow; may have plateau iris. Short axial length
Angle pulled shut (anterior pathology)		
Neovascular	Rubeosis ± synechial angle closure zipped shut	Signs of underlying pathology, e.g. diabetes, CRVO, carotid artery occlusive disease
Inflammatory closed angle	Synechial angle closure with PAS. Angle zipped shut by PAS	Signs of uveitis. Systemic disease
Angle pushed shut (posterior pathology)		
Phacomorphic	Ipsilateral intumescent lens	Appositional closure; contralateral open angle. High lens thickness:axial length ratio
Lens dislocation	Poor lenticular support permits anterior dislocation	Abnormalities of zonules or lens size. Systemic disease (e.g. Marfan's syndrome)
Aqueous misdirection	Shallow AC despite patent PI; no iris bombé	Usually post-surgery in short axial length eyes
Choroidal pathology	Choroidal detachment, haemorrhage, or effusion	Recent history of surgery/extensive laser. Evidence of nanophthalmos or uveal effusion syndrome

(Continued)

Table 10.4 (Cont.)

Glaucoma type	Critical features	Additional features
Open angle		
Inflammatory open angle	Elevated IOP with significant flare/cells; open angle	Other signs of cause, e.g. uveitis, trauma, surgery
Steroid-induced	↑IOP associated with steroid use (but may be lag of days or weeks)	Signs of underlying pathology, e.g. uveitis
Posner–Schlossman syndrome	Recurrent unilateral IOP spikes in fairly quiet, white eye	Corneal oedema
Pigmentary	Mid-peripheral spoke-like transillumination (TI) defects; trabecular pigmentation	Pigment in AC, on cornea, lens, and/or iris; ♂ myopes; 20–45y; post-exercise IOP spikes
Red cell	Hyphaema	Corneal blood staining
Ghost cell	Vitreous haemorrhage; bleached erythrocytes in AC	Posterior segment bleeding point (PVD, retinal tear, new vessels on disc (NVD), new vessels elsewhere (NVE), CNV)
Phacolytic	Lens protein in AC with (hyper)mature cataract	AC cells + flare, open angle ± clumps of macrophages. Refractile protein crystals in AC
Lens particle	Retained lens fragment in AC post-surgery/trauma	AC inflammation
Intraocular tumour	Posterior segment tumour	± cataract; mass seen on US

Pseudoexfoliation syndrome

PXF is a common, but easily missed, cause of 2° glaucoma. The term was originally chosen to distinguish it from 'true' exfoliation syndrome, in which heat or infrared radiation caused damage to the lens capsule (e.g. in glass blowers). Confusingly, this distinction has become blurred, with PXF increasingly being referred to as exfoliation syndrome.

PXF is a systemic condition in which a whitish dandruff-like material is deposited over the anterior segment of the eye and other organs such as skin, heart, lungs, kidneys, and meninges. Although its exact nature is unclear, it appears to include abnormal elastic microfibrils, BM material, and glycosaminoglycans. A number of small studies have suggested an association with cardiovascular and cerebrovascular disease, possibly via elevation of plasma homocysteine levels. In some parts of Scandinavia, PXF is present in up to 20% of the general population and up to 90% of the glaucoma population. It has been strongly associated with a single nucleotide polymorphism of the lysyl oxidase-like 1 (*LOXL1*) gene (Chr 15q24.1).

Risk factors

- *Age*: >40y old; increases with age.
- ♀ sex.
- *Ethinicity*: North European (Finnish, Icelandic); Mediterranean (Cretan); possibly any population in which it is carefully looked for.

Clinical features

- Dandruff-like material on pupillary border and anterior lens capsule (centrally and peripherally with a clear intermediate zone), peripupillary transillumination defects, poor mydriasis, iridodonesis/phacodonesis (**NB** Risk of zonulodialysis during cataract surgery), pigment in the AC, pigment and pseudoexfoliative material on the endothelium.
- *Gonioscopy*: irregular pigment deposition in the trabeculum and anterior to Schwalbe's line (Sampaolesi's line), PXF material in the angle; angle is usually open but may be narrow.

PXF glaucoma (glaucoma capsulare)

Glaucoma occurs in up to 25% of patients with PXF (i.e. up to 10-fold increased risk). Although the disease presents similarly to POAG, the disease course is more severe, with poorer response to medication and more frequent need for surgery.

Mechanism of glaucoma

- *Open angle*: deposition of PXF material and pigment in the trabecular meshwork.
- *Narrow angle (rare)*: weak zonules with anterior movement of the lens–iris diaphragm; PS.

Clinical features
- Features of PXF (see ⮕ Clinical features, p. 364), ↑IOP, disc changes, and field defects as for POAG (see ⮕ Primary open-angle glaucoma, p. 354).

Treatment of PXF glaucoma (open-angle type)
- *Medical*: as for POAG, but generally less effective; greater role for miotics (e.g. pilocarpine).
- *ALT*: particularly effective early on; >50% failure rate by 5y.
- *SLT*: similar efficacy to ALT but less destructive and repeatable.
- *Trabeculectomy*: higher complication rate but similar overall success to trabeculectomy in POAG.

Pigment dispersion syndrome

This describes the release of pigment from the mid-peripheral posterior surface of the iris, from where it is distributed around the anterior segment. Pigment release is thought to occur as a result of posterior bowing of the mid-peripheral iris rubbing against the zonules. This unusual iris configuration may be due to 'reverse pupil block' in which there is a transient ↑IOP in the AC relative to the PC; this is supported by an observed improvement when treated with miotics or Nd-YAG PIs. PDS is inherited as an AD trait (Chr 7q36), with a possible second locus on Chr 18q; the exact gene(s) have not yet been identified. See Table 10.5 for chronic glaucoma syndromes. See Table 10.4 for syndromes that typically present in an acute/subacute manner.

Risk factors
- *Myopia*.
- *Age*: 20–40.
- ♂ sex.
- *Ethnicity*: Caucasian.

Clinical features
- Pigment on the corneal endothelium (sometimes in a vertical line—Krukenberg spindle), pigment elsewhere (e.g. in the AC, posterior lens capsule—Zentmeyer's line), mid-peripheral spoke-like transillumination defects; increased rate of lattice degeneration (so need regular checks of peripheral retina).
- *Gonioscopy*: open angle, concave peripheral iris, 360° homogeneous pigmentation of the trabeculum, and pigment may be anterior to Schwalbe's line inferiorly.

Pigmentary glaucoma

Glaucoma may develop in 33–50% of patients with PDS.

Clinical features
- Usually asymptomatic, but blurred vision, haloes, and red eye(s) may occur after acute pigment shedding following mydriasis or exercise.
- ↑IOP ± corneal oedema (if acute); features of PDS (see ➲ Clinical features, p. 366); disc changes and VF defects as for POAG (see ➲ Primary open-angle glaucoma, p. 354).

Treatment
- *Topical*: as for POAG; miotics have theoretical benefits (minimize iridozonular contact) but tend to be poorly tolerated in this age group and carry a small risk of inducing retinal detachment (myopia, lattice degeneration).
- *ALT*: particularly effective early on; >50% failure rate by 5y.
- *SLT*: similar efficacy to ALT but less destructive and repeatable. SLT should be performed with caution in cases of PDS, as high post-laser IOP spikes have been reported.
- *Trabeculectomy*: similar success rate to surgery in POAG, but increased risk of hypotensive maculopathy (especially if augmented with antifibrotic agents).
- *PI*: controversial; theoretical benefits in cases with marked reverse pupillary block in early stages of disease—no clear trial data to support routine use of PI.

Table 10.5 Chronic glaucoma syndromes (selected)

Glaucoma type	Critical features	Additional features
Open angle		
Primary open angle	↑IOP; disc cupping; VF defect; normal open angle	Other glaucomatous disc changes
Normal tension	Normal IOP; disc cupping; VF defect; normal open angle	Other glaucomatous disc changes
PXF	Dandruff-like material on pupil margin and lens surface	Unevenly pigmented trabeculum; peripupillary TI defects; corneal endotheliopathy
Pigmentary	Mid-peripheral spoke-like TI defects; heavy trabecular pigmentation	Pigment in AC, on cornea, lens, iris, ♂ myopes aged 20–45y
Steroid-induced	↑IOP associated with steroid use (but may be lag of days or weeks)	Signs of underlying pathology, e.g. uveitis, eczema
Angle recession	Recessed iris	Other signs of trauma
↑*episcleral venous pressure*	Engorged episcleral vein(s)	Vascular abnormalities according to underlying pathology
Intraocular tumour	Posterior segment tumour	Cataract; mass seen on US
Schwartz–Matsuo syndrome	Rhegmatogenous retinal detachment (RRD)	Mild AC 'inflammation'
Closed angle		
Chronic angle closure	PAS	May have had subacute attacks of angle closure—ischaemic iris damage

(Continued)

Table 10.5 (*Cont.*)

Glaucoma type	Critical features	Additional features
Angle pulled shut (anterior pathology)		
Neovascular	Rubeosis ± synechial closure	Signs of underlying pathology, e.g. diabetes, CRVO, CAOD
Inflammatory closed angle	Intermittent synechial closure	Signs of uveitis, seclusio pupillae
ICE syndrome	Abnormal endothelial growth over angle	Iris distortion/atrophy; corneal hammered metal appearance
Epithelial downgrowth	Epithelial downgrowth through wound to spread over angle and cornea	Surgical/traumatic wound, previous leaking wound
Angle pushed shut (posterior pathology)		
Phacomorphic	Ipsilateral intumescent lens	Appositional closure; contralateral open angle
Aqueous misdirection	Shallow AC despite patent PI; no iris bombé	Usually post-surgery in hypermetropic/short axial length eyes

Other glaucoma syndromes, which may also present in an insidious manner, include inflammatory open angle, red cell, ghost cell, phacolytic, Posner–Schlossman syndrome (all open angle), and surgically induced angle closure (tight scleral buckle, PK). See Table 10.4 for syndromes that typically present in an acute/subacute manner.

Neovascular glaucoma

Posterior segment ischaemia drives neovascularization of the iris and drainage angle, leading to a fibrovascular membrane. Initially, this overlies the trabecular meshwork so that the angle appears open, but, with time, PAS form and the membrane contracts to cause complete synechial angle closure. Ischaemic CRVO and diabetes each account for about a third of the cases of NVG. The advent of anti-VEGF therapies is an exciting new development in the management of NVG.

Causes

Include:
- Ischaemic CRVO (common); risk of progression to NVG is 50%.
- Diabetic retinopathy (common); risk of NVG highest in PDR.
- *Other vascular disorders:* OIS, CRAO, BRVO.
- *Other retinal disease:* chronic retinal detachment, sickle cell retinopathy.
- Retinal or choroidal tumours.

Clinical features

- Pain is often a feature and may be severe; predisposing condition may be known or may be suggested by the history (e.g. sudden loss of vision several months previously in cases of CRVO and NVG).
- *Iris rubeosis:* abnormal/non-radial vessels at pupil sphincter margin; ↑IOP; AC flare/cells, hyphaema; ectropion uvea; conjunctival injection and corneal oedema if acute ↑IOP or decompensating; disc changes and field loss as for POAG (see ➤ Primary open-angle glaucoma, p. 354).
- *Gonioscopy:* abnormal vessels in the angle; fibrovascular membrane overlying the trabeculum (open-angle type) or membrane + synechial angle closure (angle-closure type).

Investigation (to determine cause)

- Dilated fundoscopy in all cases ± FFA.
- *Carotid Doppler US:* if no retinal pathology or asymmetric diabetic retinopathy.
- *B-scan US:* if poor fundal view (cataract may be associated with chronic retinal pathology such as tumours, detachment, inflammation).

Treatment

- Treatment of NVG has often been challenging and unsatisfactory but is undergoing a positive transformation with the advent of anti-VEGF therapies.

Of underlying cause

For example:
- PRP for retinal ischaemia.
- Retinal reattachment for retinal detachment.
- Carotid endarterectomy for suitable carotid artery stenosis.
- Exacerbating factors, e.g. anaemia, hyperviscosity.

Of neovascularization

- PRP to decrease retinal ischaemic drive long term. Sometimes there will be no fundal view, and anti-VEGF therapy can be administered to temporize. Vitrectomy/endolaser photocoagulation ± cataract extraction may be considered, depending on *visual prognosis*.
- Anti-VEGF therapies have been shown to have a significant impact on neovascularization and improve survival of drainage surgery. Small retrospective studies using intravitreal bevacizumab have shown regression of neovascularization and ↓IOP, both when used alone[5] or in combination with PRP.[6]

Of ↑IOP and inflammation

- Cycloplegic (e.g. atropine 1% 2×/d) + frequent topical steroids (e.g. prednisolone acetate 1% 1–4-hourly) + ocular hypotensive agents, as for POAG.
- If medical treatment fails, consider trabeculectomy (augmented), tube-shunt procedures, or cyclodestruction (e.g. cyclodiode), depending on *visual prognosis*.

Of pain

- Cycloplegia (atropine).
- Lubricants for sick corneal epithelium (keep high index of suspicion for microbial keratitis).
- If the eye is blind and painful, consider retrobulbar alcohol or chlorpromazine, or evisceration/enucleation.

5. Wakabayashi T *et al.* Intravitreal bevacizumab to treat iris neovascularization and neovascular glaucoma secondary to ischemic retinal diseases in 41 consecutive cases. *Ophthalmology* 2008;**115**:1571–80.

6. Ehlers JP *et al.* Combination intravitreal bevacizumab/panretinal photocoagulation versus panretinal photocoagulation alone in the treatment of neovascular glaucoma. *Retina* 2008;**28**:696–702.

Inflammatory glaucoma: general

Raised IOP in the context of intraocular inflammation is a common clinical problem. The challenge is to elucidate the time course (acute vs chronic ↑IOP), the state of the angle (open vs appositional closure vs synechial closure), and the underlying mechanism of elevated IOP.

Therapy may be made difficult due to marked fluctuations in IOP (ciliary body shutdown → IOP↓, trabeculitis → IOP↑) and concerns over whether the treatment could be making things worse (steroid-induced glaucoma).

Open-angle type

Acute

- *Mechanism*: acute trabeculitis (particularly with HSV, VZV), trabecular meshwork blockage.

Clinical features

- ↑IOP; open angle; signs of uveitis ± keratitis; IOP returns to normal after acute episode of inflammation.

Treatment

- *Of inflammatory process*: treatment of underlying cause may be sufficient (e.g. topical steroids and cycloplegic for acute anterior uveitis (AAU); see ➔ Acute anterior uveitis, p. 422).
- *Of ↑IOP*: if features of concern (e.g. IOP >27mmHg; sustained ↑IOP; vulnerable optic disc) consider topical (e.g. β-blocker, carbonic anhydrase inhibitor) or systemic (e.g. acetazolamide) medication for as long as required.

Chronic

- *Mechanism*: trabecular scarring; chronic trabeculitis.

Clinical features

- ↑IOP; open angle; no active inflammation but may have signs of previous episodes; ± disc changes or field defects (see ➔ Glaucoma: assessment, p. 348). Always transilluminate the iris to detect diffuse or sectorial iris atrophy.

Treatment

- *Medical*: as for POAG; some clinicians may avoid prostaglandin agonists.
- If medical treatment fails, consider trabeculectomy (poorer results than for POAG but improves if augmented with antifibrotic therapy or tube procedure). However, to improve outcome of the operation, tight control of inflammation must first be achieved.
- If surgical treatment fails, consider cyclodestruction (e.g. cyclodiode), but significant risk of phthisis.

Steroid-induced glaucoma

Although related to the treatment, rather than the underlying disease process, this is an important differential diagnosis of inflammatory glaucoma. Raised IOP due to steroids requires a reduction in the potency and frequency of topical corticosteroids (± use of steroid-sparing agents), whereas, if it is due to uncontrolled inflammation, the steroid dose may need to be increased. The steroid-induced IOP elevation may be dose-dependent.

Angle-closure type

With seclusio pupillae

- *Mechanism*: 360° posterior synechiae (seclusio pupillae) blocks anterior flow of aqueous humour, causing iris bombé and appositional angle closure.

Clinical features

- ↑IOP; seclusio pupillae; iris bombé; shallow AC; angle closure (appositional); signs of previous inflammatory episodes.

Treatment

- *Of inflammatory process*: minimize PS formation by rapid and effective treatment of anterior uveitis (consider subconjunctival Betnesol® and mydricaine, if required).
- *Of ↑IOP*: Nd-YAG PI—PI should be larger (or multiple) than is necessary for acute angle-closure glaucoma (AACG) (**NB** AC will be shallow, so watch out for the corneal endothelium), and surgical PI may be necessary if Nd-YAG PI closes. Consider topical (e.g. β-blocker, carbonic anhydrase inhibitor) or systemic (e.g. acetazolamide) medication as a temporary measure or for as long as required.

With synechial closure

- *Mechanism*: PAS may lead to angle closure; risk of synechial closure is increased in presence of granulomatous inflammation and possibly pre-existing narrow angles.

Clinical features

- ↑IOP, shallow AC, PAS with angle closure, signs of previous inflammatory episodes.

Treatment

- *Medical*: as for POAG, but some clinicians would advise caution with prostaglandin agonists.
- If medical treatment fails, consider trabeculectomy (augmented) or tube-shunt procedures (increased risk of post-operative hypotony).
- If surgical treatment fails, consider cyclodestruction (e.g. cyclodiode), but significant risk of phthisis.
- Ensure patent PI in all angle-closure cases.

Inflammatory glaucoma: syndromes

Posner–Schlossman syndrome

This is a syndrome of recurrent unilateral episodes of painless high IOP occurring in a 'white' eye. It typically affects young ♂. The cause is not known; acute trabeculitis has been postulated, possibly 2° to HSV.

Clinical features
- Blurring of vision, haloes, painless.
- ↑IOP (40–80mmHg), white eye, minimal flare, occasional cells/KPs, no synechiae (PS or PAS), open angle.

Treatment
- *Of inflammatory process*: topical steroid (e.g. dexamethasone 0.1% 4×/d).
- *Of ↑IOP*: consider topical (e.g. β-blocker, α2-agonist, carbonic anhydrase inhibitor) or systemic (e.g. acetazolamide), according to IOP level.

NB Chronic recurrent inflammatory episodes may lead to severe angle damage.

Fuchs' heterochromic uveitis (*syn* Fuchs'
heterochromic cyclitis)

Fuchs' heterochromic uveitis (see ➒ Anterior uveitis syndromes (1), p. 426) is a syndrome of mild chronic anterior uveitis, iris heterochromia, and cataract—may be complicated by glaucoma in 10–30% cases.

It typically affects young adults, and there is no sex bias. It is unilateral in >90% cases. Recent studies have shown strong association with the rubella virus.

Clinical features
- ↓VA due to cataract; floaters; often asymptomatic.
- White eye, white stellate KPs over whole corneal endothelium, mild flare, few cells, iris atrophy (washed out, moth-eaten), transillumination defects, abnormal iris vessels, iris heterochromia ('becomes bluer'; more obvious if observed in natural light), iris nodules, cataract (posterior cortical/subcapsular), vitritis, ↑IOP.
- *Gonioscopy*: open angle; ± twig-like neovascularization of the angle (NVA).

Treatment
- *Of inflammatory process*: not usually necessary.
- *Of ↑IOP*: treat as for POAG (see ➒ Primary open-angle glaucoma p. 354).

Lens-related glaucoma

Lens-related glaucoma may result from abnormalities of lens size, lens position, release of lens protein (mature cataract/trauma/surgery), and/or the consequent inflammatory response.

Phacomorphic glaucoma

- *Mechanism*: the enlarging lens causes pupil block and anterior bowing of the iris, with 2° angle closure. In an eye of normal axial length, this occurs 2° to an intumescent cataractous lens; in a short eye, this may result simply from the normal increase in lens size with age.

Clinical features

- ↑IOP, shallow AC, fixed semi-dilated pupil, swollen cataractous lens.
- Ipsilateral closed angle (appositional; sigma sign may be seen on indentation gonioscopy).
- Contralateral angle may be open with deep AC (in contrast to PACG); however, this helpful sign may not be present if contralateral eye also has significant cataract.

Treatment

- *Medical* (topical and systemic): as for PACG.
- Nd-YAG PI to reverse pupil block component.
- Early cataract extraction is the definitive treatment—needs an experienced surgeon.

Phacolytic glaucoma

- *Mechanism*: the hypermature cataract loses soluble lens proteins through the anterior capsule, causing trabecular obstruction and subsequent 2° open-angle glaucoma.

Clinical features

- ↑IOP, lens protein in a deep AC (may form a pseudohypopyon), hypermature/mature cataract, open angle (with lens protein); AC tap reveals lens protein and foamy macrophages.

Treatment

- *Medical*: topical (e.g. β-blocker, α2-agonist, carbonic anhydrase inhibitor) or systemic (e.g. acetazolamide) agents, as required; consider topical steroids for associated inflammation.
- Early cataract extraction—needs experienced surgeon.

Phacoanaphylactic uveitis

- *Mechanism*: this is an inflammatory reaction to lens protein, usually following traumatic capsular rupture or post-operative retention of lens material (when it must be distinguished from endophthalmitis). This insult may also cause sensitization such that lens protein exposure in the contralateral eye (surgery, hyper/mature cataract) may be associated with an aggressive response.

Clinical features

- Recent trauma/surgery, exposed lens protein, AC flare + cells ± hypopyon, KPs, synechiae (PS + PAS), angle usually open (but ± PAS); IOP may be high, normal, or low.

Treatment

- *Of inflammatory process*: topical steroid (e.g. dexamethasone 0.1% hourly) and surgical removal of any retained lens fragments.
- *Of ↑IOP*: medical—topical (e.g. β-blocker, α2-agonist, carbonic anhydrase inhibitor) or systemic (e.g. acetazolamide) agents, as required.
- *For contralateral cataract*: consider removal by intracapsular cataract extraction (ICCE) to reduce lens protein exposure.

Glaucoma 2° to lens subluxation/dislocation

- *Mechanism*: pupil block by anterior lens subluxation or complete dislocation into the AC; there may also be a coincident angle abnormality (e.g. Marfan's syndrome).

Clinical features

- ↑IOP, subluxed/dislocated lens ± corneal oedema (if acute or lenticulo-corneal touch); lenticular astigmatism and variable refraction.

Treatment

- *Positional*: dilate and lie patient supine (to encourage posterior movement of lens), and constrict (to keep lens safely behind pupil); long-term miotic therapy may be needed, unless the lens dislocates safely into the vitreous.
- *Early lens extraction*: if positional measures fail, if complete dislocation into the AC, if cataract, or if recurrent problem. Often best dealt with by a vitreoretinal approach.

Other secondary open-angle glaucoma

Steroid-induced

Exogenous, and occasionally endogenous, steroids may decrease outflow facility, leading to ↑IOP after a few days or weeks. In the normal population, 5% will have an IOP increase of >15mmHg and 30% will have an increase of 6–15mmHg if given topical steroids for up to 6wk. POAG patients are often particularly sensitive to this steroid effect.

Possible mechanisms include prostaglandin inhibition (e.g. PGF2A) and structural changes in the extracellular matrix (glycosaminoglycans) and trabecular meshwork (cross-linking of actins). A history of steroid administration should be specifically asked for, as patients may not volunteer use of steroid-containing anabolics, skin or haemorrhoid creams, inhaled steroids, or episodic courses of oral steroids (e.g. for exacerbations of asthma/COPD).

Treatment Ideally decrease frequency/potency or stop steroid (± steroid-sparing agent) to normalize IOP—liaise with prescribing physician. If corticosteroids essential and IOP still elevated, then treat as POAG (see ➲ Primary open-angle glaucoma, p. 354).

Red cell glaucoma

Hyphaema (usually traumatic) leads to blockage of the trabecular meshwork by red blood cells. In 10% of cases, a rebleed may occur, usually at about 5d post-injury. Patients with sickle cell disease/trait do worse and are harder to treat (e.g. sickling may be worsened by the acidosis from carbonic anhydrase inhibitors).

Treatment
- *Of hyphaema*: strict bed rest, topical steroid (e.g. dexamethasone 0.1% 6×/d), mydriatic/cycloplegic (e.g. atropine 1% 2×/d) (see ➲ Hyphaema, p. 128).
- *Of IOP*: topical (e.g. β-blocker, α2-agonist, carbonic anhydrase inhibitor) or systemic (e.g. acetazolamide) agents, as required.
  - *Surgical*: AC paracentesis ± AC washout. In rare refractory cases, trabeculectomy may be needed.

Ghost cell glaucoma

Vitreous haemorrhage leads to blockage of the trabecular meshwork by degenerate red blood cells, usually 2–4wk after the haemorrhage. These cells, which may be seen in the AC and the angle, are tan-coloured, having lost haemoglobin.

Treatment Medical treatment (as for POAG, see ➲ Primary open-angle glaucoma, p. 354) is usually sufficient. If this fails, consider AC washout + vitrectomy to remove persistent vitreous haemorrhage.

Angle recession glaucoma

Blunt trauma may cause angle recession and associated trabecular damage. Traumatic angle recession carries a 10% risk of glaucoma at 10y, the risk increasing with extent of recession. Look for asymmetry of AC depth, pupil, and angle.

- *Screening*: periodic IOP check (e.g. 3mo, 6mo, yearly), if known angle recession.
- *Treatment*: as for POAG (see ⊃ Primary open-angle glaucoma, p. 354).

Raised episcleral venous pressure

Aqueous drainage is reduced as episcleral venous pressure increases (see ⊃ Anatomy and physiology, p. 346). This may occur as a result of vascular abnormalities in the orbit (Sturge–Weber syndrome, orbital varices), cavernous sinus (AV fistulae), or superior vena cava (SVC; SVC obstruction). Episcleral venous pressure manifests as unilateral/bilateral engorged episcleral veins, chemosis, proptosis, with blood in Schlemm's canal on gonioscopy.

Treatment Primarily directed at the underlying pathology, although medical, and occasionally surgical, lowering of IOP may be necessary.

Tumours

Tumours may cause ↑IOP via open-angle mechanisms (clogging or infiltration of trabecular meshwork with tumour cells) or, for larger posterior segment tumours, rubeosis (2° to ischaemia) or 2° angle closure (anterior displacement of lens–iris diaphragm).

Suspect in atypical unilateral glaucoma; if poor view of posterior segment (usually due to cataract), a B-scan US is essential. About 20% of malignant melanoma is associated with ↑IOP.

Treatment Directed by the underlying tumour, although ↑IOP itself suggests a poor prognosis.

Schwartz–Matsuo syndrome

This is the uncommon association of anterior segment inflammation (mild) and ↑IOP (with an open angle) arising from an RRD. The photoreceptor outer segments gain access to aqueous humour from subretinal space and obstruct the trabecular meshwork. It is discussed further (see ⊃ Anterior uveitis syndromes (1), p. 426). The ↑IOP and anterior uveitis may be treated medically in the interim but tend to resolve rapidly with surgical repair of the retinal detachment.

Other secondary closed-angle glaucoma

Iridoschisis

Bilateral splitting and atrophy of anterior iris leaf is associated with ↑IOP, usually 2° to angle closure (due to pupil block), but sometimes due to debris blocking the trabecular meshwork (open angle). It is uncommon and usually occurs in the elderly.

Treatment
- Angle-closure type with Nd-YAG PI.
- Open-angle type, as for POAG (see ➔ Primary open-angle glaucoma, p. 354).

Iridocorneal endothelial (ICE)

A unilateral condition in which abnormal corneal endothelium migrates across the angle, the trabecular meshwork, and the anterior iris, so causing significant anterior segment distortion. ICE syndrome is rare, usually occurs in 20–40y old ♀, and carries a 50% risk of glaucoma. HSV has been proposed as a causative agent.

Three overlapping syndromes are described: Chandler syndrome (predominantly corneal), essential iris atrophy (predominantly iris changes), and iris naevus (Cogan–Reese) syndrome (appearance of a diffuse naevus or pigmented nodules, which probably represent protrusions of iris stroma).

Clinical features
- Unilateral pain, blurred vision.
- Unilateral fine corneal guttata ('beaten metal'), corneal oedema. (±↑IOP), iris atrophy corectopia (displaced pupil), pseudopolycoria (accessory pupil).
- *Gonioscopy*: broad-based PAS that may insert anterior to Schwalbe's line.

Investigation
- Consider specular microscopy to demonstrate endothelial changes.

Treatment
- Medical (e.g. β-blocker, α2-agonist, carbonic anhydrase inhibitor, prostaglandin agonist), surgery (trabeculectomy ± augmented or tube procedures), or cyclodestruction, as required.

Posterior polymorphous dystrophy (PPD)

A bilateral condition in which abnormal corneal endothelium may form extensive iridocorneal adhesions, with angle closure. Clinically, it may appear similar to ICE syndrome but is dominantly inherited, bilateral, and usually detectable in childhood (although may only be symptomatic later). PPD carries a 15% risk of glaucoma. Treat glaucoma as for POAG (see ➔ Primary open-angle glaucoma, p. 354).

Epithelial downgrowth

A deranged healing response in which trauma or surgery (poorly constructed or leaking wound, vitreous incarceration) allows epithelium to proliferate down through the wound and onto the endothelial surface. Once free of its normal environment, it may proliferate unchecked across the corneal endothelium and angle, so causing glaucoma in a similar manner to ICE syndrome.

Treatment is very difficult: lower IOP as for POAG; intracameral antifibrotic agents (e.g. 5-FU) and extensive surgical excision have been used. Prognosis for vision is poor.

Fuchs' endothelial dystrophy

In Fuchs' endothelial dystrophy (see ⭢ Corneal dystrophies: posterior, p. 256), oedema of the peripheral cornea may cause 2° angle closure, especially in at-risk eyes with pre-existing shallow ACs.

Iatrogenic glaucoma

Aqueous misdirection syndrome

(*syn* malignant glaucoma, ciliary block, ciliolenticular block)

Mechanism

It is thought that posterior misdirection of aqueous into the vitreous causes anterior displacement of vitreous, ciliary processes, and lens/PCIOL with 2° angle closure.

Risk factors

- Short axial length, chronic angle closure, previous acute angle closure, nanophthalmos, uveal effusion syndrome.
- Post-procedure: surgery (trabeculectomy, tube procedures, cataract extraction, peripheral iridectomy); laser (Nd-YAG PI).
- Miotic therapy (rare).

Clinical features

- Often ↓VA due to acute ↑/very high IOP or significant myopic shift; may be asymptomatic.
- ↑IOP (may be normal initially), shallow/flat AC, no pupil block (so no iris bombé and occurs despite a patent PI), no choroidal/suprachoroidal cause (detachment/haemorrhage).

Treatment

- Ensure that a patent PI is present (repeat Nd-YAG PI, if necessary).
- Dilate (atropine 1% 3×/d + phenylephrine 2.5% 4×/d).
- *Systemic* ↓*IOP*: acetazolamide 500mg IV stat (then 250mg PO 4×/d) ± mannitol/glycerol.
- *Topical* ↓*IOP*: β-blocker (e.g. timolol 0.5% stat, then 2×/d) + sympathomimetic (e.g. apraclonidine 1% stat, then 3×/d).

If medical treatment fails, consider:

Laser

- YAG disruption of anterior vitreous face (if aphakic/pseudophakic, perform posterior capsulotomy/hyaloidotomy; if phakic, a hyaloidotomy can be attempted through the patent PI).
- Argon laser to the ciliary processes (through the patent PI; relieves block by causing shrinkage of the processes).
- Trans-scleral cyclodiode photocoagulation of the ciliary body (in one quadrant) may also be successful in breaking the acute attack.[7]

Surgery

- The aim in surgery is to achieve adequate posterior–anterior communication to re-establish aqueous humour flow, for which the key surgical step is peripheral zonulo-hyaloidectomy.
- *If phakic*: cataract extraction (phacoemulsification or ECCE), posterior capsulotomy, and anterior vitrectomy; cataract surgery in these situation can be facilitated by preliminary pars plana vitreous debulking as part of a vitrectomy–phacoemulsification–vitrectomy procedure.[8]
- *If aphakic/pseudophakic*: pars plana vitrectomy and posterior capsulotomy.

Post-cataract surgery

Acute post-operative ↑IOP may be due to retained viscoelastic, lens fragments, or inflammation. A single dose of acetazolamide SR 250mg may be used prophylactically against the risk of an early post-operative pressure spike. Less commonly, glaucoma may arise due to suprachoroidal haemorrhage, phacolysis, phacoanaphylaxis (see ➋ Lens-related glaucoma, p. 376), Amsler haemorrhage in Fuchs' heterochronic uveitis (see ➋ Inflammatory glaucoma: syndromes, p. 374), epithelial downgrowth (see ➋ Other secondary closed-angle glaucoma, p. 380) syndrome, aqueous misdirection, or the UGH syndrome.

Post-vitreoretinal surgery

- *With intraocular gases*: acute post-operative ↑IOP is usually due to expansion/overfill of SF6 or C3F8. *Treatment*: decide according to IOP and half-life of gas, but usually short-term medical treatment sufficient (e.g. acetazolamide SR 250mg 2×/d for 5d); or else remove some of the gas.
- *With scleral buckles*: 2° angle closure may occur due to ciliary body swelling and choroidal detachment (possibly due to pressure on the vortex veins). *Treatment*: usually resolves spontaneously; treat medically in the interim.
- *With silicone oil*: oil in the AC blocking the trabecular meshwork (and possibly other mechanisms) may cause an ↑IOP, presenting from days to months after surgery. *Treatment*: sometimes resolves spontaneously; treat medically in the interim; consider cyclodestruction if persists. **NB** Early removal of oil (<6mo) may ↓IOP. After this period, removal of oil makes little difference due to incorporation of oil by macrophages.
- *Vitrectomy*: may facilitate ghost cell glaucoma (see ➋ Other secondary open-angle glaucoma, p. 378) and increase the risk of rubeosis in PDR.

7. Stumpf TH *et al*. Transscleral cyclodiode laser photocoagulation in the treatment of aqueous misdirection syndrome. *Ophthalmology* 2008;**115**:2058–61.

8. Sharma A *et al*. Vitrectomy–phacoemulsification–vitrectomy for the management of aqueous misdirection syndromes in phakic eyes. *Ophthalmology* 2006;**113**:1968–73.

Pharmacology of IOP-lowering agents

See Table 10.6 for pharmacological groups.

Prostaglandin analogues

These analogues of PGF2α increase uveoscleral outflow.

- *Ocular side effects: common*—conjunctival hyperaemia, increased pigmentation of iris (and sometimes lid skin), thickening and lengthening of lashes, loss of orbital fat; *rare*—uveitis, CMO, reactivation of herpetic kerato-uveitis.
- *Contraindications*: may be associated with CMO after complicated cataract surgery (possibly active uveitis).

β-blockers

These reduce aqueous production, probably by acting on β-receptors on the non-pigmented ciliary epithelium and vasoconstriction of the arterioles supplying ciliary processes.

- *Ocular side effects*: uncommon; allergic blepharoconjunctivitis, punctate keratitis.
- *Contraindications*: asthma/COPD (bronchospasm may occur, even with selective β1 agents), heart block, bradycardia, or cardiac failure. Try to avoid in nursing mothers, as it is secreted in breast milk.
- *Drug interactions*: concurrent use of cardiac-directed Ca^{2+} antagonists, such as verapamil, may compound bradycardia, heart block, and hypotension.

Carbonic anhydrase inhibitors

These reduce aqueous production by inhibiting carbonic anhydrase isoenzyme II (and hence bicarbonate production) in the non-pigmented ciliary epithelium.

- *Ocular side effects*: common; burning, tearing, allergic blepharoconjunctivitis (up to 10%).
- *Contraindications*: sulfonamide sensitivity; renal failure, liver failure (systemic acetazolamide).
- *Drug interactions*: K^+ losing diuretics (e.g. thiazide) may cause profound hypokalaemia if used concurrently with acetazolamide. K^+ supplementation is not usually required for acetazolamide used alone.

Sympathomimetics

The highly α2-selective brimonidine is well tolerated, and apraclonidine (α1 + α2) is useful for short-term use, e.g. after laser iridotomy. Non-selective sympathomimetics, such as adrenaline (epinephrine), dipivefrine, and the adrenergic neurone blocker guanethidine are now seldom used due to their frequent side effects.

- *Ocular side effects: common*—allergic blepharoconjunctivitis (up to 15% for brimonidine, 30% for apraclonidine); *older agents*—scarring, mydriasis, adrenochrome deposits; *uncommon*—CMO in aphakia (possibly pseudophakia).
- *Contraindications*: heart block, bradycardia.
- *Drug interactions*: monoamine oxidase inhibitors.

Miotics (parasympathomimetics)

Muscarinic receptor agonism leads to ciliary muscle contraction, which pulls on the scleral spur to open the trabecular meshwork. Pilocarpine is used first line in narrow-angle glaucoma; sometimes still used in POAG. May be useful in pigmentary glaucomas, aphakic glaucoma, and some 2° glaucomas (e.g. post-PK).

- *Ocular side effects*: fluctuating myopia, miosis (constricted VF, reduced night vision).
- *Contraindications*: inflammatory or aqueous misdirection/malignant glaucoma.

Table 10.6 Pharmacological groups

Group	Mechanism	Advantages	Systemic side effects	Examples
Topical				
Prostaglandin analogues	Increase uveoscleral outflow	↓IOP by 30% Well-tolerated	Bronchospasm (rare)	Latanoprost 0.005% Travaprost 0.004% Bimatoprost 0.03% + 0.01% (preser vative-free available) Tafluprost 0.015% (preservative-free)
β-blocker	Decrease aqueous production	20y follow-up ↓IOP by ± 25% Well tolerated (in most cases)	Bronchospasm Bradycardia Heart block Hypotension Glucose intolerance Lethargy Depression Impotence	*Non-selective:* Timolol 0.25% +0.5% (available preservative-free) Carteolol 1% + 2% (has intrinsic sympathomimetic activity) Levobunolol 0.5% (available preservative-free) *β1-selective:* Betaxolol 0.25% + 0.5%
Carbonic anhydrase inhibitors	Decrease aqueous production	↓IOP by ± 20%	Metallic taste See list below (for systemic)	Brinzolamide 1% Dorzolamide 2%
α2-agonists	Decrease aqueous production Increase uveoscleral outflow	↓IOP by ± 20%	Bradycardia Hypotension Insomnia Irritability GI disturbance	Brimonidine 0.2% Apraclonidine 0.5% + 1% (1% is preservative-free)
Miotics	Increase trabecular outflow	↓IOP by ± 30%+	Sweating Sialorrhoea Nausea Headache Bradycardia	Pilocarpine 0.5%–4% (available preservative-free)

(Continued)

Table 10.6 (Cont.)

Group	Mechanism	Advantages	Systemic side effects	Examples
Systemic				
Carbonic anhydrase inhibitor	Decrease aqueous production Acidosis may cause hypotension	↓IOP by ≤65%	Lethargy Depression Anorexia Hypokalaemia Renal calculi Blood dyscrasia	Acetazolamide
Hyper-osmotic agents	Creates an osmotic gradient	Rapidly ↓IOP (onset 30min)	Hypertension Vomiting Cardiac failure MI Hyperglycaemia (mannitol) Urinary retention	Mannitol (IV) Glycerol (PO)

Laser procedures in glaucoma

Laser procedures have a vital part in the treatment of many forms of glaucoma. Directions on how to carry out a number of these procedures are given in Chapter 24, as indicated.

Nd-YAG peripheral iridotomy

Essence

Nd-YAG laser photodisruption causes a full-thickness hole through the iris, permitting flow of aqueous humour from PC to AC.

Indication

- *Treatment*: angle closure with pupil block—may be acute/subacute/chronic, 1°/2°.
- *Prophylaxis*: occludable narrow angles (including fellow eye in angle closure).

Complications

- Bleeding, inflammation, raised IOP, corneal burns (caution with shallow AC), glare, and optical aberrations.

ALT

Essence

Argon laser photocoagulation of the angle structures, resulting in reduction of IOP. The actual mechanism is debated, whether 'mechanical' (focal tissue contraction/scarring causes opening up of the trabecular meshwork and widening of Schlemm's canal), 'biological' (induced inflammatory cytokines trigger a cascade which upregulates MMPs, altering the extracellular matrix), or 'repopulative' (trabecular epithelial cells are stimulated to divide and migrate into burn sites from healthy adjacent sites).

Indication

- Open-angle glaucoma with pigmented trabeculum—commonly POAG/PXF glaucoma/PDS glaucoma.
- Medical and surgical options undesirable or ineffective.

Complications

- Bleeding, inflammation (usually mild), PAS, IOP spike may increase failure rate of subsequent trabeculectomy.
- Failure occurs at a rate of 6–10%/y and is often sudden.[9] Long-term follow-up is necessary.

SLT

Essence

An alternative to ALT, SLT uses a Q-switched frequency-doubled Nd-YAG laser to selectively target pigmented cells and to minimize damage to angle structures (cf. ALT).[10]

Indication

- As for ALT.

Complications

- Similar to ALT; a transient, subclinical, reversible corneal endotheliopathy is often seen in the early stages after SLT.
- Failure rate is similar to ALT.[10]

Argon laser peripheral iridoplasty (ALPI)

Essence

A ring of argon laser burns causes cicatricial contraction of the peripheral iris stroma to tighten the iris and widen the angular approach.

Indication

- Plateau iris syndrome (procedure of choice).
- APAC (uncommon indication but may be used where unresponsive to medical therapy and Nd-YAG PI has failed or is technically difficult).[11]

Complications

- Inflammation (usually mild), IOP spike, corneal burns.

Trans-scleral diode laser cyclophotocoagulation (*syn* 'cyclodiode')

Essence

Selective destruction of the ciliary body achieved with either a diode or, less commonly, a Nd-YAG laser.

Indication

- Intractable ↑IOP (e.g. in rubeotic or synechial angle closure) where other treatment modalities have failed or are contraindicated (e.g. where the patient is too systemically unwell to tolerate surgery).
- Refractory acute angle closure.[12]
- Temporizing measure prior to trabeculectomy; gentle titrated diode laser cycloablation can be used in eyes with good visual potential.

Complications

- Anterior inflammation (may get hypopyon with NVG), hypotony, haemorrhage, scleral thinning, perforation, cataract, lens subluxation, phthisis, and sympathetic endophthalmitis.

Endodiode laser photocoagulation (*syn* 'endoscopic cyclophotocoagulation', ECP)

Essence

Direct photocoagulation of the ciliary processes with an endolaser using endoscopic visualization. ECP is much easier technically if performed in a pseudophakic eye than a phakic eye; may be performed as a combined procedure (with phacoemulsification).

Indication

- As for trans-scleral diode laser cyclophotocoagulation.

Complications

- Inflammation, CMO, cataract (if phakic), endophthalmitis, suprachoroidal haemorrhage, retinal detachment, hypotony, phthisis.

9. Spaeth GL *et al.* Argon laser trabeculoplasty controls one third of progressive uncontrolled open angle glaucoma for 5 years. *Arch Ophthalmol* 1992;**110**:491–4.

10. Damji KF *et al.* Selective laser trabeculoplasty vs argon laser trabeculoplasty: a randomized controlled trial. *Br J Ophthalmol* 2006;**90**:1490–4.

11. Ritch R *et al.* Argon laser peripheral iridoplasty. *Ophthalmic Surg Lasers* 1996;**27**:289–300.

12. Manna A *et al.* Cyclodiode laser in the treatment of acute angle closure. *Eye (Lond)* 2012;**26**:742–5.

Surgery for glaucoma

Glaucoma surgery includes iris procedures (surgical iridectomy), angle procedures (goniotomy, trabeculotomy), filtration procedures (trabeculectomy, deep sclerectomy), minimally invasive glaucoma surgery (MIGS), and setons (tube drainage surgery). In adult glaucoma, the commonest operation and gold standard is trabeculectomy with/without augmentation. Augmentation with antifibrotics is indicated according to risk of fibrosis and filtration failure. Artificial drainage tubes (or setons) require considerable experience and are generally reserved for resistant cases.

Surgical iridectomy and surgical cyclodialysis have become less common since the advent of YAG laser PI and cyclodiode. Goniotomy and trabeculotomy are generally restricted to congenital glaucoma (see ➜ Glaucoma in children, pp. 800–2) (see Table 10.7 for common surgical procedures).

Table 10.7 Common surgical procedures in glaucoma

Procedure	Mechanism	Indication
Iris procedures		
PI	Relieves pupil block	Laser PI not possible (patient cooperation, thick iris, poor view, e.g. persistent oedema)
Angle procedures		
Goniotomy	Opens the abnormal angle (probably)	1° congenital glaucoma (1° trabecular meshwork dysgenesis)
Trabeculotomy	Opens Schlemm's canal directly to AC	Congenital glaucoma, including 1° congenital glaucoma and anterior segment dysgenesis
Filtration procedures (penetrating)		
Trabeculectomy	Forms new drainage channel from AC to sub-Tenon's space	Has a place in most chronic glaucomas (adult and paediatric)
Augmented trabeculectomy	Trabeculectomy with antifibrotic agent to reduce scarring	Standard trabeculectomy has failed/would be likely to fail
Artificial drainage tubes	Silicone tube from AC to episcleral explant	Augmented trabeculectomy has failed/would be likely to fail
Filtration procedures (non-penetrating)		
Deep sclerectomy	Exposes the trabecular meshwork and removes the internal wall of Schlemm's canal	Alternative to penetrating filtration procedures
Viscocanalostomy	As above + viscoelastic injected to open up Schlemm's canal	Alternative to penetrating filtration procedures

Filtration surgery: trabeculectomy

Indication
- *When to operate*: may be first line if high risk of progression or patient aims to be 'drop-free'; more commonly reserved when medical therapy is proving inadequate.
- *Which operation*: assess risks of operation failure (e.g. from scarring) against the increased risk of complications in augmented trabeculectomy or tube procedures (see Table 10.8 and Table 10.9).

Method (standard trabeculectomy with fornix-based flap described)
- *Consent*: explain what the operation does and possible complications, including failure, hypotony, infection, haemorrhage, and reduced vision.
- *Preoperative*: consider preoperative steroid treatment for 10d pre-op to help reduce post-op scarring, and apraclonidine 1% immediately pre-op to reduce intra-op bleeding.
- *Preparation*: with 5% povidone iodine and drape.
- *Place traction suture*: either corneal (avascular, but care re cheese wiring or penetration) or superior rectus (risk of haematoma).
- *Form conjunctival flap*: incise at limbus with 6–8mm arc.
- *Form scleral flap (rectangular/trapezoidal)*: incise the outline of the flap to a depth of 50% scleral thickness, before anterior lamellar dissection, to free the posterior and lateral aspects of the flap. Pre-placed scleral flap 'releasable' sutures give maximal control.
- *Place a paracentesis*: oblique in the temporal cornea.
- *Form sclerostomy*: make a perpendicular incision at the sclerolimbal junction to form the anterior margin of the sclerostomy. Complete sclerostomy posteriorly by removing a block of sclerolimbal tissue with the punch (e.g. Khaw or Kelly punch) or blade/scissors (e.g. Vannas).
- *Perform peripheral iridectomy*: this should be broad-based but short and peripheral. This is primarily to prevent iris blockage of the trabeculectomy, although it will also relieve any coincident pupil block.
- *Suture scleral flap*: sutures can either be fixed, releasable (leave access via a corneal groove), or adjustable (can be loosened by massaging posterior aspect of scleral flap). Assess opening pressure of scleral flap by injecting BSS via the paracentesis.
- Close conjunctiva and Tenon's layers together securely to prevent retraction and consequent leak. This can be achieved with two lateral purse-string sutures and central mattress sutures.
- *Post-operative*: subconjunctival steroid (e.g. betamethasone) and antibiotic (e.g. cefuroxime).

Post-procedure
- Topical antibiotic (e.g. chloramphenicol 0.5% 4×/d) and steroid (e.g. prednisolone acetate 1% 2-hourly initially, tapering down over 2mo; in eyes at high risk of failure, taper steroid over 3–4mo).
- Review at 1d and 1wk, then according to need.

Fixed, releasable, and adjustable sutures

Optimal bleb drainage is not always achieved. Post-operatively, bleb drainage may be increased by removing or loosening selected scleral sutures. The technique depends on the suture type used:
- *Fixed sutures*: if the suture can be visualized through Tenon's layer, it may be released by argon laser suture lysis.
- *Releasable sutures*: these are tied with a slip-knot and loop into a corneal groove to permit access; they can be released at the slit-lamp without disturbing the conjunctival flap.
- *Adjustable sutures*: these can be loosened by massaging the posterior aspect of the scleral flap at the slit-lamp.

Table 10.8 Choice of filtration procedure

Procedure	Indication
Trabeculectomy	
Standard	Low risk of scarring
	Low risk of failure from other causes
Augmented trabeculectomy	
5-FU (50mg/mL) or MMC (0.2mg/mL)	Moderate risk of scarring
	Planned combined trabeculectomy/cataract surgery
	Previous surgery involving the conjunctiva (not trabeculectomy)
MMC (0.4mg/mL)	High risk of scarring
	Previous failed trabeculectomy
	Chronic inflammation (conjunctival or intraocular)
	High-risk glaucoma (including uveitic, traumatic)
Seton procedures	
Baerveldt, Molteno, and Ahmed	Previous failed augmented trabeculectomy
	Multiple further operations likely to be necessary
	Inadequate healthy conjunctiva for trabeculectomy
	High-risk glaucoma (including traumatic, aphakic, neovascular, aniridia, cellular overgrowth, e.g. ICE, epithelial downgrowth syndrome)

Table 10.9 Comparison of fornix vs limbal-based flaps for trabeculectomy

	Fornix-based	Limbal-based
Operative	Easier	Access can be difficult
	Faster	Slower
	Good sclerostomy exposure	Adequate sclerostomy exposure
Use of antifibrotics	Take care to avoid wound margin	Relatively safe
Post-operative manipulation	Easier	More difficult
Post-operative	More conjunctival wound leaks	Fewer conjunctival wound leaks
	Less posterior scarring	More posterior scarring 'ring of steel'

Filtration surgery: antifibrotics

The control of post-op wound healing is critical to the success of glaucoma filtration surgery. Antifibrotics, such as 5-FU and MMC, permit the surgeon to modulate the fibrosis and scarring that may 'close off' an otherwise satisfactory trabeculectomy.

As this fibrotic response will vary between patients, the use of antifibrotics is titrated according to the predicted risk of scarring (see Table 10.8). They should not be used indiscriminately, as they may cause significant side effects (see Box 10.5).

Agents

- *5-FU:* inhibits DNA synthesis and RNA function; usual dose 50mg/mL.
- *MMC:* alkylates DNA, inhibits DNA and RNA synthesis; usual dose 0.2–0.4mg/mL.

Indications

- *Moderate risk of scarring:* 5-FU (50mg/mL) or MMC (0.2mg/mL)
- *High risk of scarring:* MMC (0.4mg/mL).
- If very high risk or failed augmented trabeculectomy, consider a seton procedure (see Table 10.8).

Risk factors for scarring

- *Age:* <40.
- *Ethinicity:* African-Caribbean, Indian subcontinent.
- *Previous surgery involving conjunctiva:* includes trabeculectomy, cataract surgery with scleral tunnel, vitreoretinal surgery.
- *Glaucoma type:* neovascular, aphakic, inflammatory, traumatic.
- *Chronic inflammation:* chronic conjunctivitis, uveitis.
- *Topical treatment:* risk of failure increases with the number of topical medications (and duration).

Intraoperative use (As part of trabeculectomy; see ➋ Filtration surgery: trabeculectomy, p. 392)

- Select agent and concentration (50mg/mL 5-FU; 0.2–0.4mg/mL MMC) according to patient risk of fibrosis and risk of complications.
- *Prepare sponges:* sponges need to be cut to size and then soaked in the antifibrotic of choice; polyvinyl alcohol sponges are the sponge of choice, as they disintegrate less than those made of methyl cellulose, leaving less fibrogenic debris and causing less FB giant cell reactions.
- During trabeculectomy, place sponge under the conjunctival/Tenon's flap into the sub-Tenon's space for appropriate duration (5min for 5-FU; 2–5min for MMC); avoid contact with cornea and conjunctival wound edge; ensure no intraocular administration.
- Remove sponges; all cytotoxics/used sponges require safe disposal separate to clinical waste.
- Irrigate eye well.

Post-operative use
- Select agent (usually 5-FU).
- Using a small calibre needle (29–30G) on a 1mL syringe, administer antifibrotic as posteriorly as possible, adjacent to, *but not into*, the bleb.
- The usual dose is 5mg of 5-FU (usually 0.1mL of 50mg/mL 5-FU); MMC is occasionally used (at a dose of 0.02mg), but there are concerns over its potential toxicity.

Box 10.5 Potential complications of antifibrotics
- Corneal epithelial erosions.
- Corneal endothelial decompensation.
- Limbal stem cell failure.
- Wound leak.
- Bleb leak.
- Hypotony.
- Scleritis.
- Cataract.
- Blebitis.
- Endophthalmitis.

Filtration surgery: complications of penetrating procedures (1)

Intraoperative complications

- *Conjunctival flap damage*: may get persistent leak, especially if exposed to antifibrotics, buttonholes, especially if previous surgery.
- *Scleral flap damage*: may not close in controlled manner.
- *Bleeding*: may be conjunctival, scleral, from the iris, or, most seriously, suprachoroidal.
- *Vitreous loss*: increased risk with posterior sclerostomy.
- *Wound leak*: from damaged conjunctiva or inadequate closure.

Early post-operative complications

Shallow AC

Examination ± US should identify the reason for a shallow AC (see Table 10.10). If the AC is very shallow, it may not be possible to see if the PI is patent or not (see Table 10.10 for diagnosis).

Specific treatment will depend on the underlying cause, but, in general, when there is a risk of corneal decompensation from lenticulo-corneal touch, urgent measures are required to reform the AC (e.g. with bss, viscoelastic, or gas).

Low IOP/hypotony

- IOP <6mmHg is associated with flat AC, choroidal detachment, suprachoroidal haemorrhage, hypotonous maculopathy, and corneal oedema.
- *General treatment*: intensive potent topical steroids + cycloplegic-mydriatic (atropine 1% tds); stop IOP-lowering agents; consider surgery (reform AC ± drain choroidal effusions) if corneal decompensation from lens touch (absolute indication) or 'kissing' choroidal detachments.

Wound leak

In milder cases, where antifibrotics have not been used, resolution is likely within 48h; in the interim, a BCL may be applied, and topical steroids may be temporarily stopped. However, more severe wound leaks (particularly with antifibrotics) usually require surgical resuturing.

Ciliary body shutdown

This rare complication is associated with post-operative inflammation, requiring treatment with systemic and topical corticosteroids. The AC should be reformed with viscoelastic.

Overfiltration

In clinically significant early hypotony with maculopathy, it is necessary to expedite surgical intervention to explore and resuture the scleral flap so that it provides adequate resistance to aqueous outflow.

Table 10.10 Differential diagnosis of shallow AC after trabeculectomy

	IOP	Seidel	PI	Bleb
Wound leak	Low	+	Patent	Poor/flat
Ciliary body shutdown	Low	–	Patent	Poor/flat
Overfiltration	Low	–	Patent	Extensive
Pupil block	High	–	Non-patent	Flat
Malignant glaucoma	High	–	Patent	Flat
Suprachoroidal haemorrhage	Variable	–	Patent	Variable

High IOP

- *Pupil block*: PI is either incomplete or blocked by inflammatory debris:
  - Perform a new Nd-YAG PI (or complete old iridectomy); then topical mydriatic-cycloplegic + steroids.
- *Malignant glaucoma*: aqueous misdirection may occur, especially in short eyes (see ➲ Iatrogenic glaucoma, p. 382). There are rare forms of aqueous misdirection in which IOP can be normal.
- *Filtration failure:* obstruction of the sclerostomy and scleral flap may be internal (incarceration of iris, ciliary processes, or vitreous), scleral (fibrin, blood), or external (tight scleral flap sutures).

Infection

Isolated blebitis

Presents as a painful red eye, often with discharge and photophobia; the bleb is milky with loculations of pus, conjunctival injection (especially around the bleb), and increasing IOP ± AC activity (cells/flare ± hypopyon).

- *Identify organism*: swab bleb ± AC tap.
- Treat with intensive fortified topical antibiotics (e.g. ofloxacin and penicillin hourly) and systemic antibiotic (e.g. ciprofloxacin 750mg 2×/d); adjust according to response and organism identified (commonly, staphylococci if early, and streptococci and haemophili if late); consider addition of topical steroids after 24h. A mydriatic-cycloplegic agent can help reduce pain and inflammation.
- Early and frequent review to determine if further intervention, including vitreous biopsy/intravitreal antibiotics, indicated.

Endophthalmitis

- Clinical features as for blebitis, but more severe, ↓VA, and vitritis.
- Investigate and treat as for other post-operative endophthalmitis (see ➲ Post-operative endophthalmitis, p. 336). However, endophthalmitis occurring after trabeculectomy tends to run a more aggressive course with a worse prognosis than after cataract surgery.

Visual loss

'Wipe-out' of the remaining field may occur in the presence of a vulnerable optic nerve (associated with ↑IOP, hypotony, or systemic hypotension), or hypotonous changes may lead to reduced acuity (e.g. from maculopathy). Avoid adrenergic agents in local anaesthetic mixtures, and minimize periods of systemic hypotension in GA.

Filtration surgery: complications of penetrating procedures (2)

Late post-operative complications

- *Filtration failure*: subconjunctival fibrosis ('ring of steel'), especially with limbal-based flaps, may lead to a poorly filtering encapsulated bleb (tense localized dome). Treat with bleb needling revision + subconjunctival antifibrotic (usually 5-FU) and post-procedure topical steroids/antibiotics.
- *Leaky bleb*: sweaty or leaky blebs are more common in augmented or non-guarded filtration surgery. If small leak, low risk of infection, and not hypotonous, then may be monitored initially. Otherwise consider BCL, autologous blood injection, compression sutures, or bleb revision surgery.
- *Infection*: blebitis/endophthalmitis (see ➡ Filtration surgery: complications of penetrating procedures (1), p. 398; and also ➡ Post-operative endophthalmitis, p. 336).
- *Visual loss*: post-operative lens opacities probably account for most of the post-operative drop in acuity—cataract surgery carries a 10–30% risk of subsequent bleb failure; astigmatism.
- *Ptosis*: often resolves spontaneously; more common with superior rectus traction sutures (rather than corneal) and in revision surgery where conjunctiva has been mobilized from superior fornix.

Non-penetrating glaucoma surgery

Non-penetrating glaucoma surgery (NPGS) describes a group of techniques in which improved aqueous drainage is achieved surgically without penetrating into the AC at the time of initial surgery. Controversy continues regarding their long-term success rate, partly due to the long learning curve associated with these challenging techniques. It is likely that, in experienced hands, NPGS with augmentation can achieve similar long-term success to that seen with penetrating glaucoma surgery, but final IOPs are often higher than after augmented trabeculectomy surgery. Although NPGS has a lower rate of early hypotony after surgery, serious complications, including severe hypotony, endophthalmitis, and suprachoroidal haemorrhage, have all been described with NPGS.

Deep sclerectomy

Mechanism

Deep sclerectomy is effectively a form of guarded filtration (such as trabeculectomy) but with the rate of drainage being controlled at the level of the trabecular meshwork/Descemet's membrane, rather than at the scleral flap.

Outline

Deep sclerectomy involves the formation of conjunctival and superficial scleral flaps, followed by a deep (90% depth) scleral flap to expose Schlemm's canal. Schlemm's canal is then deroofed and its endothelium and juxtacanalicular trabecular meshwork peeled off to improve drainage. Part of the deep scleral flap is then excised to form the deep sclerectomy space. At this stage, antifibrotics may be applied and an implant may be inserted. The conjunctival flap is then closed.

Variations

- Antifibrotics: in high-risk cases, antifibrotic agents are sometimes applied to the deep scleral flap to reduce intrascleral scarring. Although no benefit was demonstrated with 5-FU, some small studies have shown improved IOP control with use of MMC.[13]
- Implants: implants may be inserted into the deep scleral space to maintain the space during healing and effectively form an 'intrascleral bleb'. Implants may either be absorbable (e.g. Aquaflow or SKGel) or non-absorbable (e.g. T Flux). Implant use is associated with better IOP control than deep sclerectomy alone: 69% vs 39% achieving IOP <21mmHg off medication at 4y.[14,15]
- Goniopuncture: Nd-YAG goniopuncture is usually used as a 2° procedure where sufficient IOP control has not been achieved by the surgical procedure alone; this effectively converts it to a penetrating procedure. In one longer study, goniopuncture was performed in about half of all cases. Sight-threatening complications, such as hypotony, have been reported after goniopuncture.

Complications

Moderate hypotony (with a deep AC) is to be expected and may transiently affect vision. Causes of high IOP include: (1) inadequate dissection of the trabecular meshwork/Descemet's membrane (treated with Nd-YAG goniopuncture); (2) rupture of the trabecular meshwork/Descemet's membrane by mild ocular trauma (e.g. rubbing, Valsalva manoeuvre), causing iris prolapse and blockage of the drainage site (requires revision of the drainage site and conversion to a conventional trabeculectomy); (3) PAS formation blocking the drainage site (may be reversible with laser iridoplasty). Very rarely, detachment of Descemet's membrane may occur. All complications seen with penetrating surgery have been reported with deep sclerectomy.

Viscocanalostomy

Mechanism

Viscocanalostomy is proposed to work by increasing aqueous flow into Schlemm's canal; there is, however, little evidence to support this.

Outline

The procedure is similar to deep sclerectomy with the creation of conjunctival, superficial scleral, and deep scleral flaps, and deroofing of Schlemm's canal. However, the key feature is that Schlemm's canal is then opened with a viscoelastic, which, it is argued, directly improves drainage by this route. The superficial scleral flap is tightly sutured to minimize filtration into the sub-Tenon's space, encouraging drainage into Schlemm's canal.

Variations

- Antifibrotics and implants: as with deep scleretomy, both antifibrotics and implants may be used in viscocanalostomy.

Complications

Complications are similar to that seen with deep sclerectomy. Detachment of Descemet's membrane (occurring at the time of injection of viscoelastic) occurs more commonly than in deep sclerectomy but is still uncommon.

13. Kozobolis VP *et al.* Primary deep sclerectomy versus primary deep sclerectomy with the use of mitomycin C in primary open angle glaucoma. *J Glaucoma* 2002;**11**:287–93.

14. Shaarawy T *et al.* Deep sclerectomy in one eye vs deep sclerectomy with collagen implant in the contralateral eye of the same patient: long-term follow-up. *Eye* 2005;**19**:298–302.

15. Shaarawy T *et al.* Long-term results of deep sclerectomy with collagen implant. *J Cataract Refract Surg* 2004;**30**:1225–31.

Micro-invasive glaucoma surgery

Over the past decade, there has been an increasing number of MIGS devices being developed in an attempt to improve the safety profile of glaucoma surgery. However, IOP reduction achieved with the use of these devices are less than IOP reduction achieved with trabeculectomy. Therefore, at present, their role in the management of advanced disease has not been defined.

Ex-Press glaucoma filtration device

This small stainless steel minishunt drains aqueous fluid from the AC into the subconjunctival space and is used in conjunction with standard trabeculectomy surgery.

Canaloplasty

Canaloplasty is performed by passing a 9-0 or 10-0 prolene suture through 360° of Schlemm's canal with the aid of a microcatheter and viscoelastic to dilate the canal. The procedure involves the construction of a deep sclerectomy-type flap to enable Schlemm's canal to be accessed.

iStent

This small transtrabecular titanium stent drains aqueous fluid from the AC into Schlemm's canal. The device is placed through a 2.8mm clear corneal incision with the aid of a gonioscopy lens and is inserted in the inferonasal quadrant of the angle via an introducer. Immediate blood reflux from the canal of Schlemm through the stent's snorkel is a positive sign. The iStent can be inserted at the time of phaco cataract surgery or into pseudophakic or phakic eyes. The role of the iStent in advanced glaucoma has not yet been defined.

Trabectome

This thermal cautery device ablates a 2- to 4-clock-hour segment of trabecular meshwork and Schlemm's canal under direct visualization with a gonioscopy lens. The principle is to connect the AC directly with the collector channels in the canal of Schlemm. The trabectome can be used at the time of cataract surgery or in phakic or pseudophakic eyes. The role of this technology is still being evaluated in advanced glaucoma.

CyPass Micro-Stent

This supraciliary microstent is implanted through a 1.5mm clear corneal incision and is designed to increase uveoscleral outflow by draining aqueous from the AC into the suprachoroidal space. The device is inserted over a micro-guidewire which creates a small cyclodialysis cleft.

Solx Gold Shunt

This small Solx Gold Shunt is placed into the supraciliary space through a 3mm incision to increase uveoscleral outflow, again aiming to facilitate direct access of aqueous from the AC to the suprachoroidal space. All current supraciliary microstents may develop fibrosis around the device, leading to failure.

Other microshunt devices

Several other microshunts are currently under development and evaluation. The Hydrus Microstent functions as an intracanalicular scaffold inside Schlemm's canal and is inserted during cataract surgery. It is made of a biocompatible alloy. The Aquesys system utilizes an *ab interno* approach to access the subconjunctival space. A flexible permanent gelatin implant is inserted through a clear corneal incision.

Uveitis

Anatomy and physiology

Uveitis describes intraocular inflammation both of the uveal tract itself and of neighbouring structures (e.g. retina, vitreous, optic nerve). Uveitis is relatively common, with an incidence of around 15 new cases per 100,000 population/y and acute presentations (often recurrences) making a significant contribution to the emergency ophthalmic workload.

Anatomy

The uveal tract comprises the iris, ciliary body, and choroid.

Iris

This is the most anterior part of the uveal tract. It extends from its relatively thin root in the AC angle to the pupil. It is divided by the collarette into the central pupillary zone and the peripheral ciliary zone. The anterior surface is of connective tissue with an incomplete 'border layer' overlying the stroma which contains the vessels, nerves, and sphincter pupillae. The sphincter pupillae is a ring of true smooth muscle supplied by the short ciliary nerves (III) under parasympathetic control. The posterior surface comprises an epithelial bilayer. The anterior layer of this is lightly pigmented and contains the radial myoepithelial processes of the dilator pupillae which extend from the iris root. These are supplied by two long ciliary nerves (Va) under sympathetic control. The anterior layer is continuous with the pigmented outer layer of the ciliary body. The posterior epithelial layer is cuboidal, densely pigmented, and is continuous with the non-pigmented inner layer of the ciliary body.

Ciliary body

This comprises the ciliary muscle and ciliary epithelium, arranged anatomically as the pars plana and pars plicata (containing the ciliary processes). The ciliary epithelium is a cuboidal bilayer arranged apex to apex with numerous gap junctions. The inner layer is non-pigmented, with high metabolic activity, and posteriorly is continuous with the neural retina. The outer layer is pigmented and posteriorly is continuous with the RPE.

Choroid

This is a vascular layer extending from the ora serrata (where it is 0.1mm thick) to the optic disc (0.3mm thick). From the inside out, it comprises Bruch's membrane (RPE BM, collagen, elastin, collagen, choriocapillaris BM), the choriocapillaris (capillary layer), the stroma (medium-sized vessels in Sattler's layer, large vessels in Haller's layer), and the suprachoroid (a potential space).

Physiology

Iris

Pupillary functions include light regulation, depth of focus, and minimizing optical aberrations. The iris also maintains the blood–aqueous barrier (tight junctions between iris capillary endothelial cells) and contributes to aqueous circulation and outflow (uveoscleral route). In inflammation, there is breakdown of the blood–aqueous-barrier, leading to flare and cells in the AC.

Ciliary body

The non-pigmented layer contributes to the blood–aqueous barrier (tight junctions between non-pigmented epithelial cells). The non-pigmented and pigmented layers together are responsible for aqueous humour production. Contraction of the ciliary muscle permits accommodation and increases trabecular outflow. The ciliary body also contributes to the uveoscleral outflow route.

Choroid

With 85% of the ocular blood flow (cf. <5% for the retina), the choroid provides effective supply of oxygen/nutrients, removal of waste products, and heat dissipation. It may also have a significant role in ocular immunity.

Classification of uveitis (1)

The classification of uveitis may be anatomical (see Table 11.1), clinical, pathological, or aetiological, and all of these may be useful in defining a uveitis entity. Anatomical classification has been formalized by the International Uveitis Study Group (IUSG) and amended by the SUN group (2005). Anterior uveitis accounts for the majority of uveitis in Western populations; a much smaller proportion is made up of posterior, intermediate, and panuveitis.

Anatomical classification

Table 11.1 Anatomical classification of uveitis[*]

Type	1° site of inflammation	Includes
Anterior uveitis	AC	Iritis
		Iridocyclitis
		Anterior cyclitis
Intermediate uveitis	Vitreous	Pars planitis
		Posterior cyclitis
		Hyalitis
Posterior uveitis	Retina or choroid	Focal, multifocal, or diffuse choroiditis
		Chorioretinitis
		Retinochoroiditis
		Retinitis
		Neuroretinitis
Panuveitis	AC, vitreous and retina, or choroid	

[*] Jabs DA *et al.* Standardization of Uveitis Nomenclature (SUN) for reporting clinical data. *Am J Ophthalmol* 2005;**140**:509–16.

Clinical classification

The most recent clinical classification of uveitis is outlined in Table 11.2. Clinical behaviour may be further described in terms of onset, duration, and course of uveitis (see Table 11.3).

Pathological classification

Pathological classification separates granulomatous and non-granulomatous uveitis. The term 'granulomatous' is sometimes used in the clinical context to describe uveitis with large, greasy 'mutton fat' KPs (macrophages) and iris nodules (which may include Koeppe and Busacca nodules). However, this is strictly a histological term and is not accurate as a clinical descriptor. Indeed, this clinical picture may be seen in diseases with non-granulomatous histopathology, and true granulomatous diseases may present with 'non-granulomatous' uveitis.

Aetiological classification

An aetiological classification helps define the cause, context, and treatment options for the disease, but, in many patients, a 'true' aetiology is not found.

Table 11.2 IUSG clinical classification of uveitis[*]

Group	Subgroup
Infectious	Bacterial
	Viral
	Fungal
	Parasitic
	Others
Non-infectious	Known systemic association
	No known systemic association
Masquerade	Neoplastic
	Non-neoplastic

[*] Deschenes J et al.; International Uveitis Study Group. International Uveitis Study Group (IUSG): clinical classification of uveitis. *Ocul Immunol Inflamm* 2008;**16**:1–2.

Table 11.3 Descriptors of uveitis[*]

Type	Descriptor	Definition
Onset	Sudden	
	Insidious	
Duration	Limited	≤3mo
	Persistent	>3mo
Course	Acute	Sudden onset + limited duration
	Recurrent	Repeated episodes; inactive periods ≥3mo off treatment
	Chronic	Persistent; relapse in <3mo off treatment

[*] Jabs DA et al. Standardization of Uveitis Nomenclature (SUN) for reporting clinical data. *Am J Ophthalmol* 2005;**140**:509–16.

Classification of uveitis (2)

See Table 11.4 for differential diagnosis of uveitis by anatomical type.

Table 11.4 Differential diagnosis of uveitis by anatomical location (selected)

Anterior	Idiopathic
	HLA-B27 group
	Juvenile idiopathic arthritis (JIA)
	Fuchs' heterochromic uveitis (FHU)
	Sarcoidosis
	Syphilis
	Posner–Schlossman
Intermediate	Idiopathic (pars planitis and non-pars planitis types)
	MS
	Sarcoidosis
	IBD
	Lyme disease

Table 11.4 (*Cont.*)

Posterior	Retinitis	Focal	Idiopathic
			Toxoplasma
			Onchocerciasis
			Cysticercosis
			Masquerade
		Multifocal	Idiopathic
			Syphilis
			HSV
			VZV
			Cytomegalovirus (CMV)
			Sarcoidosis
			Masquerade
			Candidiasis
	Choroiditis	Focal	Idiopathic
			Toxocariasis
			TB
			Masquerade
		Multifocal	Idiopathic
			Histoplasmosis/presumed ocular histoplasmosis syndrome (POHS)
			Sympathetic ophthalmia
			VKH
			Sarcoidosis
			Serpiginous
			Birdshot
			Masquerade
			Multiple evanescent white dot syndrome (MEWDS)
Pan			Idiopathic
			Sarcoidosis
			Behçet's disease
			VKH
			Infective endophthalmitis
			Syphilis

Uveitis: assessment

All patients require a detailed history (ophthalmic and general) and a thorough ophthalmic examination, including dilated fundoscopy of both eyes. In some cases, a systemic examination may also be necessary (see Table 11.5). For example, an apparently classic AAU may have posterior segment involvement (notably CMO), may be 2° to more posterior disease (e.g. toxoplasma retinochoroiditis), or may be part of a panuveitis (e.g. sarcoid) and have systemic involvement.

Table 11.5 An approach to assessing uveitis

Symptoms	Anterior: photophobia, redness, watering, pain, ↓VA; may be asymptomatic
	Intermediate: floaters, photopsia, ↓VA
	Posterior: ↓VA, photopsia, floaters, scotomata
POH	Previous episodes and investigations; surgery/trauma
PMH	Arthropathies (e.g. ankylosing spondylitis), chronic infections (e.g. HSV, TB), systemic inflammation (e.g. sarcoid, Behçet's disease)
Systems review	Detailed review of all systems
FH	Family members with uveitis or related diseases
SH	Travel/residence abroad, pets, IV drugs, sexual history
Dx	Including any systemic immunosuppression
Ax	Allergies or relevant drug contraindications
VA	Best corrected/pinhole; near
Visual function	Check for RAPD, colour vision
Conjunctiva	Circumcorneal injection
Cornea	Band keratopathy, KPs (distribution, size, pigment)
AC	Flare/cells, fibrin, hypopyon
Gonioscopy	PAS (consider if ↑IOP)
Iris	Transillumination defects/sectoral atrophy, miosis, PS, heterochromia, Koeppe or Busacca nodules
Lens	Cataract, aphakia/pseudophakia
Tonometry	
Dilated fundoscopy	(Non-contact handheld lens ± indirect/indenting)
Vitreous	Haze, cells, snowballs, opacities, subhyaloid precipitates (KP-like but on posterior vitreous face)
Optic disc	Disc swelling, glaucomatous changes, atrophy
Vessels	Inflammation (sheathing, leakage), ischaemia/occlusion (BRAO, B/CRVO, retinal oedema)
Retina	CMO, uni-/multifocal retinitis (blurred white lesions may progress to necrosis, atrophy, or pigmentation)
Choroid	Uni-/multifocal choroiditis (deeper yellow-white lesions) ± associated ERD

Grading of activity

Grading of AC cells and flare is easy and a useful indicator of disease activity. Activity within the vitreous is harder to assess—quantification of vitreous cells is of limited use due to their persistence; degree of vitreous haze is a more useful indicator (see Table 11.6).

Table 11.6 Grading of AC flare,[*] AC cells,[*] and vitreous haze[†]

Flare	
Grade	Description
0	None
1+	Faint
2+	Moderate (iris + lens clear)
3+	Marked (iris + lens hazy)
4+	Intense (fibrin or plastic aqueous)
Cells	
Grade	Number of cells counted with 1mm × 1mm slit
0	<1
0.5+	1–5
1+	6–15
2+	16–25
3+	26–50
4+	>50
Vitreous haze	
Grade	Clarity of posterior pole
0	None
0.5+	Trace (slight blurring of the optic disc margin ± loss of the nerve fibre layer reflex)
1	Mild blurring of optic disc and retinal vessels
2	Significant blurring of the optic disc and retinal vessels but still visible
3	Optic disc visible with blurred borders; no retinal vessels visible
4	Optic disc not visible

[*] Jabs DA et al. Standardization of Uveitis Nomenclature (SUN) for reporting clinical data. *Am J Ophthalmol* 2005;**140**:509–16.

[†] Nussenblatt RB et al. Standardization of vitreal inflammatory activity in intermediate and posterior uveitis. *Ophthalmology* 1985;**92**:467–71.

Uveitis: systemic review

See Table 11.7 for a systemic review of uveitis.

Table 11.7 Systemic review (not exhaustive) which may provide clues to underlying disease

System	Symptom	Associated disease
CVS	Chest pain—pericarditis	TB, RA, SLE
	Chest pain—myocarditis	Syphilis
	Palpitations	Sarcoidosis, ankylosing spondylitis, syphilis, RA, SLE, HIV
	Oedema—cardiac failure	TB, sarcoidosis, syphilis, RA, SLE, HIV
	Oedema—inferior vena cava (IVC) obstruction	Behçet's disease
RS	Cough	TB, sarcoidosis, GPA, HIV, toxocariasis
	Haemoptysis	TB, GPA, HIV, RA, SLE, sarcoidosis
	Stridor	Relapsing polychondritis
	Chest pain—pleuritic	Sarcoidosis, TB, GPA, SLE, RA, lymphoma, HIV
	Shortness of breath	Sarcoidosis, TB, GPA, SLE, RA, HIV
GI	Diarrhoea	IBD, Behçet's, HIV
	Blood/mucus in stools	IBD, Behçet's, HIV
	Jaundice	IBD (with cholangitis or hepatitis) toxoplasmosis, HIV
GU	Dysuria/discharge	Reiter's, syphilis, TB
	Haematuria	GPA, IgA nephropathy, tubulointerstitial nephritis and uveitis (TINU), SLE, TB
	Genital ulcers	Behçet's, syphilis, HLA-B27-related disease
	Testicular pain	Behçet's, HLA-B27-related disease
ENT	Deafness/tinnitus	VKH, sympathetic ophthalmia, GPA
	Earlobe pain/swelling	Relapsing polychondritis
	Oral ulcers	Behçet's, HSV, HLA-B27-related disease, SLE
	Sinus problems	GPA
	Recurrent epistaxis	GPA

Table 11.7 (*Cont.*)

System	Symptom	Associated disease
Musculoskeletal	Joint pain/swelling/stiffness	HLA-B27-related arthropathies, JIA, sarcoidosis, RA, SLE, Behçet's, relapsing polychondritis, GPA, Lyme
	Lower back pain	HLA-B27-related arthropathies, TB
Skin	Rash—erythema nodosum	Sarcoidosis, Behçet's, TB, IBD
	Rash—vesicular	HSV, VZV
	Rash—other	Psoriasis, syphilis, Lyme, SLE, Behçet's, Reiter's, JIA, TB
	Photosensitivity	SLE
	Vitiligo	SLE, VKH, sympathetic ophthalmia, leprosy
	Alopecia	SLE, VKH
	Raynaud's phenomenon	SLE, RA
CNS	Headaches	Sarcoidosis, VKH, Behçet's, TB, SLE, lymphoma
	Collapse or fits	Sarcoidosis, VKH, Behçet's, SLE, HIV, toxoplasmosis, lymphoma
	Weakness	MS, sarcoidosis, Behçet's, HIV, leprosy, syphilis, toxoplasmosis, lymphoma
	Numbness/tingling	MS, sarcoidosis, Behçet's, HIV, leprosy, lymphoma
	Loss of balance	MS, sarcoidosis, Behçet's, VKH, HIV, syphilis, lymphoma
	Speech problems	MS, sarcoidosis, Behçet's, HIV, lymphoma
	Behaviour change	VKH, sarcoidosis, Behçet's, SLE, GPA, HIV, TB, syphilis, lymphoma
General	Fever/night sweats	JIA, lymphoma, VKH, SLE, RA, IBD, sarcoidosis, Kawasaki
	Swollen glands	Sarcoidosis, lymphoma, HIV, JIA, TB, RA, syphilis, toxoplasmosis

Uveitis: investigations

When to investigate

Ideally, one would perform the minimum number of investigations to gain the maximum amount of information. The usefulness of the test will depend on the pre-test probability of the diagnosis and the specificity and sensitivity of the test (see ➲ Investigations, p. 1022). Consider also the potential morbidity of certain tests (e.g. in FFA or vitreous biopsy). In general, investigations may be performed for:

- *Diagnosis*: by identifying causative or associated systemic disease; by identifying a definite aetiology (e.g. an organism).
- *Management*: monitoring disease activity/complications (e.g. OCT for macular oedema); monitoring potential side effects of treatment (e.g. blood tests for some immunosuppressants).

Role of investigations in diagnosis

The aetiology of most uveitis is unknown, although an autoimmune/auto-inflammatory cause is often proposed. In many cases, a careful history and examination provides the majority, if not all, of the information needed for diagnosis. Some uveitis syndromes, like FHU, Behçet's, toxoplasmosis, are often diagnosed purely on clinical grounds. Investigations are helpful in identifying uveitis of infective origin (e.g. TB, syphilis, herpes viral uveitides, etc.) or systemic disease (e.g. lymphoma, sarcoidosis, demyelination). The role of some investigations is controversial, e.g. when to test HLA-B27 status.

Role of investigations in management

Monitoring disease

This is almost entirely by clinical examination; however, in certain situations, investigations may be helpful (see Table 11.8). For example:

- *OCT*: extremely useful in establishing macular causes of worsening vision, particularly where clinical diagnosis is difficult due to imperfect visualization or pre-existing macular disease (e.g. ERM, CMO, macular hole, vitreomacular traction); this has largely replaced FFA for this purpose.
- *FFA*: particularly helpful in assessing retinal vascular involvement (leakage, ischaemia), neovascularization, and optic disc leakage.
- *ICG*: choroidal disease (birdshot, sarcoidosis, VKH).
- *EDTs*: required for monitoring birdshot retinochoroidopathy.
- *VFs*: for monitoring optic nerve damage either due to disease or associated ↑IOP.

Monitoring therapies

Regular BP, weight, BM, and urinalysis are recommended for patients on systemic corticosteroids. Blood tests (e.g. FBC, U+E, LFT) are necessary for some of the other immunosuppresive agents.

Table 11.8 Suggested investigations in diagnosis of uveitis types

	Investigation	Consider
Baseline	FBC	
	ESR	
	Syphilis serology	Syphilis
	ANA (in children)	
	Urinalysis	TINU (protein), diabetes (glucose)
	CXR	TB, sarcoidosis
Selective	ACE	Sarcoidosis
	ANCA	GPA (PR3)
	Toxoplasma serology	Toxoplasmosis
	Toxocara ELISA	Toxocariasis
	Borrelia serology	Lyme disease
	HLA-B27	B27-associated disease
	HLA-A29	Birdshot chorioretinopathy
	Mantoux test	TB (reactive), sarcoidosis (anergic)
	FFA and ICG	
	Electrophysiology	
	B-scan US	
	High-resolution CT thorax	Sarcoidosis
	MRI head scan	Demyelination, sarcoidosis, lymphoma
	Gallium scan	Sarcoidosis
	Lumbar puncture (LP)	Demyelination, lymphoma
	Conjunctival biopsy	Sarcoidosis
	PCR of intraocular fluid	Infection
	Vitreous biopsy	Infection, lymphoma
	Choroidal biopsy	Lymphoma

Uveitis: complications and treatment

Complications

The main complications of intraocular inflammation are: cataract, CMO, and glaucomatous optic neuropathy. These may occur in isolation but often in combination. Other complications include: band keratopathy, vitreous debris/vitritis, retinal detachment, non-glaucomatous optic neuropathy, CNV, macular scar, macular hole, ERM, retinal scars, subretinal fibrosis.

Treatment

Treatment of non-infectious uveitis may be medical or surgical, or a combination of both. Medical therapy is primarily corticosteroid and can be given topically, periocularly, intravitreally, and systemically. Systemic immunosuppressants (and biologics) may need to be added in resistant, sight-threatening cases. The use of anti-VEGF agents, such as intravitreal bevacizumab, may play a role in the treatment of CNV and macular oedema. 2° ↑IOP is normally treated with the many topical therapies that are now available, and they may need to be given in combination. Although topical prostaglandin analogues have been implicated in causing uveitis and CMO, they are not contraindicated in uveitis patients. Surgery includes cataract, glaucoma, and vitreoretinal procedures.

See Box 11.1 for an approach to performing a diagnostic paracentesis.

Box 11.1 An approach to performing a diagnostic paracentesis (aqueous humour 'tap')

A number of techniques are used, based on patient position, preferred instruments, and location. Either a 27G fixed-needle tuberculin syringe or a 1mL syringe with a fine-bore (27–30G) needle is commonly used. The purpose-designed O'Rourke pipette is no longer being manufactured. We describe one common approach here.

Pre-procedure

- *Consent*: explain what the procedure involves and the potential risks (a survey of 560 consecutive diagnostic paracenteses noted only one serious complication (traumatic cataract)), but advise of potential sight-threatening risks, including endophthalmitis;[*] explain the importance of keeping their eye still, and give them a target to fix on.
- Instil topical local anaesthetic (e.g. oxybuprocaine).
- Instil 5% povidone iodine into the conjunctival sac; the povidone iodine is drawn up into an empty Minims® container for ease of administration.
- Position the patient at the slit-lamp so that they are comfortable with their head securely against the head-band and chin against the chin-rest.
- Instruct the patient to look straight ahead at a defined target.
- A lid speculum is not usually required; the upper lid and eyelashes may be held out of the way by an assistant.
- Wash hands and don sterile gloves.
- Ensure the syringe plunger is moving smoothly.
- Insert the needle (attached to the syringe) at the paralimbal clear cornea in a plane above and parallel to the iris, with the bevel of the needle facing forward, until the whole bevel penetrated the cornea.
- Under direct vision, hold the syringe between the thumb and middle fingers, and use the index finger to pull the plunger to aspirate OR ask an experienced assistant to carefully and slowly withdraw the plunger whilst updating you of the volume withdrawn.
- Stop withdrawal and remove needle if the AC starts to shallow or if sufficient AqH has been withdrawn (e.g. 100–150 microlitres). Depending on the starting depth of the AC and phakic status of the patient, the amount of AqH that can be safely withdrawn is usually 50–150 microlitres.

Post-procedure

- Instil a topical antibiotic (e.g. chloramphenicol 0.5%) immediately and 4×/d for 3d post-procedure.
- Send AqH for analysis (commonly for PCR), and ensure safety of sample and staff (particular care is required if a fixed-needle syringe has been used).
- Examine 20min post-procedure to check that the AC is formed and that there is no leak.

[*] Trivedi D *et al*. Safety profile of anterior chamber paracentesis performed at the slit lamp. *Clin Experiment Ophthalmol* 2011;39:725–8.

Acute anterior uveitis

Anterior uveitis accounts for around 75–90% of all cases of uveitis. It represents a wide spectrum of disease—it may be isolated, part of a panuveitis, or part of a systemic disease.

Idiopathic AAU

In around 50% of patients with AAU, it occurs in isolation (i.e. HLA-B27-negative with no underlying systemic disease). It affects any age (biphasic peaking at 30 and 60y) and both sexes equally. It is almost always unilateral but may affect both eyes sequentially. Recurrences are common; rarely, it may become persistent.

Clinical features
- Pain, photophobia, redness, blurred vision.
- Circumlimbal injection, KPs (especially inferior), AC flare/cells, PS, anterior vitreous cells (spill-over).

Treatment
- Frequent potent topical steroid (e.g. dexamethasone 0.1% or prednisolone acetate 1% up to every 30min initially, titrating according to disease), and
- Dilate (e.g. cyclopentolate 1% 3×/d; atropine 1% 3×/d in severe cases); this may be the only chance to break the synechiae; if poor dilation, consider subconjunctival Mydricaine No 2 (procaine/atropine/adrenaline); subconjunctival betamethasone may also be necessary. Apart from breaking PS, pupil dilation also helps relieve ciliary spasm and reduces pain. Local heat may also encourage pupil dilation e.g. hot glove.

NB If not responding after 48h of half-hourly drops, may require expert advice (e.g. consideration of oral steroids).

HLA-B27-associated AAU

Up to 50% of patients with AAU are HLA-B27-positive (cf. 8% in the general population). B27-related disease peaks at 30y of age, is commoner in ♂, and is associated with a positive FH. It may be associated with ankylosing spondylitis, Reiter's disease, and, less commonly, psoriasis or IBD. It is almost always unilateral but may affect both eyes sequentially ('flip-flop'); rarely may become persistent. Inflammation is often more severe and recurrences more frequent than in idiopathic AAU (see Table 11.9).

Clinical features
- Pain, photophobia, redness, blurred vision.
- Anterior segment inflammation may be severe: circumlimbal injection, KPs (especially inferior), AC flare/cells/fibrin (fibrin is a key feature in HLA-B27-associated uveitis) ± hypopyon, PS, anterior vitreous cells. A number of weeks after presentation when the anterior uveitis has responded to treatment and the eye is white, some patients present with reduced vision due to CMO.

Treatment
- As for idiopathic AAU.

Other causes

Although the vast majority of AAU is idiopathic or HLA-B27-related, it is important to be keep an open mind. 'Atypical' features may suggest an alternative diagnosis requiring different treatment. Important differential diagnoses include:

Herpes viral group (HSV, VZV, CMV) anterior uveitis

Consider if: associated with ↑IOP, recurrence soon after stopping treatment, unilateral, with patchy/sector iris atrophy/transillumination defects resulting in semi-dilated/irregular pupil (unusual for CMV) ± reduced corneal sensation (check before putting in the drops prior to tonometry) ± evidence of active/previous keratitis (see ➔ Viral uveitis (1), p. 446).

Posner–Schlossman syndrome

Consider if: ↑IOP (40–80mmHg), white eye, few KPs, minimal flare, occasional AC cells, no synechiae (PS or PAS), open angle (see ➔ Posner–Schlossman syndrome, p. 426).

Systemic disease

AAU is associated with a number of systemic diseases, some of which may be undiagnosed at the time of presentation. For example, a fibrinous uveitis in a middle-aged adult may be the first presentation of their diabetes and may imply poor glycaemic control. Systemic diseases to consider include: diabetes, sarcoidosis, vascular disease (e.g. carotid artery stenosis), and renal disease (e.g. TINU, IgA nephropathy).

Table 11.9 Comparison of HLA-B27-positive vs negative AAU

	HLA-B27 positive	HLA-B27 negative
Age at onset (y)	32–35	39–48
Gender	♂:♀ 1.5–2.5:1	1:1
Eye involvement	Unilateral 48–59% Alternating 29–36%	Bilateral 21–64%
Pattern of uveitis	Acute in 80–87%	Chronic in 43–61%
Recurrence	Frequent	Uncommon
KP	Mutton fat KP in 0–3%	Mutton fat KP in 17–46%
Fibrin in AC	25–56%	0–10%
Hypopyon	12–15%	0–2%
Associated systemic disease	48–84%	1–13%
FH	Yes	No
PS	40.4%	18.7%
Cataract	12.9%	13.6%
OHT	11.4%	11.4%
Glaucoma	4.4%	6.6%
CMO	11.7%	1.0%

Table published in Albert & Jakobiec's Principles and Practice of Ophthalmology (Third Edition) by Albert and Miller, p 1139. Copyright Elsevier; reproduced by kind permission.

Uveitis with seronegative spondyloarthropathies

Spondyloarthropathy describes a group of interrelated inflammatory arthropathies affecting the synovium and extra-articular sites. The spondyloarthropathies include the following conditions: ankylosing spondylitis, reactive arthritis, IBD-related arthritis, juvenile spondyloarthropathies, and psoriatic arthritis. Clinical manifestations include inflammatory back pain, enthesitis (inflammation of the entheses where tendons or ligaments insert into the bone), dactylitis (inflammation of an entire digit), uveitis, and usually an asymmetrical arthritis that affects lower limbs. Based on a systematic review, which included nearly 30,000 patients, the mean prevalence of uveitis in spondyloarthropathies has been estimated at 33% overall, with AAU being the most common type seen. There is a strong association with HLA-B27.[1]

HLA-B27 is a type I major histocompatibility complex (MHC; Chr 6) molecule, a cell surface polypeptide involved in presenting antigen to the immune system. There are 24 subtypes of HLA-B27, encoded by 26 different alleles. Subtypes vary by ethnic origin, and some are more highly associated with inflammatory disease, notably HLA-B*2705 (the ancestral type), B*2702 (more common in Caucasians), and B*2704 (more common in Orientals). HLA-B27 is present in 8% of the general population but is seen in up to 50% of patients with AAU.[2]

Ankylosing spondylitis

Ankylosing spondylitis is a chronic spondyloarthropathy, predominantly affecting the spine and sacroiliac joints. More common in ♂, it usually presents in early adulthood. Of those with ankylosing spondylitis: 95% are HLA-B27 positive; 25% will develop anterior uveitis; of these, 80% will have involvement of both eyes, but nearly always sequentially.

Clinical features

- *Ophthalmic*: AAU; unilateral but may affect both eyes sequentially ('flip-flop'); rarely may become persistent.
- *Systemic*: axial arthritis, sacroiliitis, kyphosis, stiffness, enthesitis, aortic regurgitation.

Treatment

- *Ophthalmic*: as for idiopathic AAU (see ➲ Idiopathic AAU, p. 422).
- *Systemic*: investigation and treatment by rheumatologist. This may include lumbar spinal X-ray (bamboo spine; sacroiliitis) and HLA-B27 status; treatment may include oral NSAIDs; physiotherapy.

Reiter's syndrome (reactive arthritis)

Reiter's syndrome describes a reactive arthritis, urethritis (or cervicitis), and conjunctivitis occurring after a sexually transmitted or dysenteric infection.[3] Candidates include *Chlamydia*, *Yersinia*, *Salmonella*, and *Shigella*. Of those with Reiter's syndrome: 70% are HLA-B27 positive; 50% will develop conjunctivitis, and 12% anterior uveitis.

Clinical features

- *Ophthalmic*: bilateral mucopurulent conjunctivitis; AAU; keratitis (punctate epitheliopathy, subepithelial infiltrates).

- *Systemic*: oligoarthritis (typically knees, ankles, sacroiliac joints), enthesitis (incl. plantar fasciitis), aphthous oral ulcers, circinate balanitis, keratoderma blenorrhagica (scaling skin rash on the soles).

Treatment
- *Ophthalmic*: conjunctivitis—self-limiting; AAU—as described previously.
- *Systemic*: investigation and treatment by rheumatologist.

IBD

Of those with ulcerative colitis (UC) and Crohn's disease, around 5% will develop anterior uveitis.[4]

Clinical features
- *Ophthalmic*: AAU; rarely epi-/scleritis or retinal vasculitis.
- *Systemic*: gut inflammation (patchy, transmural, anywhere from mouth to anus in Crohn's; continuous, superficial, colorectal in UC), cholangitis, chronic active hepatitis, arthritis (oligo- or ankylosing spondylitis-like), rash (erythema nodosum, pyoderma gangrenosum).

Treatment
- *Ophthalmic*: as for idiopathic AAU (see ➲ Idiopathic AAU, p. 422).
- *Systemic*: investigation and treatment by gastroenterologist.

Psoriatic arthritis

Of those with psoriasis: 10% will develop psoriatic arthritis, and, of these, 10% will develop anterior uveitis.[5]

Clinical features
- *Ophthalmic*: conjunctivitis; AAU; rarely keratitis (peripheral corneal infiltrates).
- *Systemic*: salmon-pink lesions with silvery scaling which may be in isolated plaques (more common on extensor, rather than flexor, surfaces) or as a pustular rash (soles and palms or, more seriously, generalized); nail changes (pitting, onycholysis, oil-drop); arthritis may be axial (ankylosing spondylitis-like), oligoarthritis (Reiter's-like), distal interphalangeal joints (osteoarthritis-like) with nail changes, symmetrical peripheral arthropathy (RA-like), or arthritis mutilans.

Treatment
- *Ophthalmic*: the conjunctivitis is self-limiting; treat anterior uveitis as for idiopathic AAU (see ➲ Idiopathic AAU, p. 422).
- *Systemic*: investigation and treatment by dermatologist and rheumatologist.

1. Zeboulon N et al. Prevalence and characteristics of uveitis in the spondyloarthropathies: a systematic literature review. *Ann Rheum Dis* 2008;**67**:955.

2. Tay-Kearney ML et al. Clinical features and associated systemic diseases of HLA-B27 uveitis. *Am J Ophthalmol* 1996;**121**:47.

3. Leirisalo-Repo M. Reactive arthritis. *Scand J Rheumatol* 2005;**34**:251.

4. Cury DB et al. Ocular manifestations in a community-based cohort of patients with inflammatory bowel disease. *Inflamm Bowel Dis* 2010;**16**:1393.

5. Rehal B et al. Ocular psoriasis. *J Am Acad Dermatol* 2011;**65**:1202.

Anterior uveitis syndromes (1)

Fuchs' Heterochromic Uveitis (FHU, syn Fuchs' heterochromic cyclitis)

This is an uncommon, 'chronic', 'non-granulomatous' anterior uveitis of unknown cause, although rubella virus has now been implicated. It typically affects young adults, and there is no gender bias. It is unilateral in about 90%.

Clinical features
- Floaters, glare; ↓VA due to cataract ± vitreous opacities; may be asymptomatic.
- White eye, white stellate KPs over whole corneal endothelium, mild flare, few cells, iris atrophy (washed out, moth-eaten), transillumination defects (not sectoral), abnormal iris vessels, iris heterochromia with the affected eye appearing 'bluer', heterochromia difficult to assess in brown irides, iris nodules (Koeppe > Busacca) are frequently seen; absence of PS; posterior subcapsular cataract in about 80%; vitreous opacities are common; ↑IOP in 10–15% leading to 2° glaucoma in some cases; occasional iris crystals.
- *Gonioscopy*: open angle; ± twig-like NVA; these may lead to hyphaema in response to paracentesis, e.g. at surgery (Amsler haemorrhage).

Treatment
- *Of inflammatory process*: not usually necessary as topical corticosteroid appears ineffective, and mydriatic unnecessary as PS do not form.
- *Of cataract*: conventional phakoemulsification but with careful post-operative control of inflammation. Corticosteroid prophylaxis is not normally required prior to surgery. Excellent visual outcome, with 90% patients achieving 6/9 vision. A large Amsler haemorrhage at surgery may result in a poorer visual outcome and ↑IOP.
- *Of ↑IOP*: treat as for POAG (see ➡ Primary open-angle glaucoma, p. 354), but may require augmented drainage surgery/tube.

Posner–Schlossman syndrome

This is an inflammatory glaucoma syndrome characterized by recurrent unilateral episodes of very high IOP with only mild AC activity. It typically affects young ♂. The suggested aetiology is of acute trabeculitis, perhaps 2° to herpesvirus, e.g. HSV.

Clinical features
- Blurring of vision, haloes, painless.
- ↑IOP (40–80mmHg), white eye, few KPs, minimal flare, occasional AC cells, no synechiae (PS or PAS), open angle.

Treatment
- *Of inflammatory process*: topical steroid (e.g. dexamethasone 0.1% or prednisolone acetate 1% 4×/d initially, titrating according to disease).
- *Of ↑IOP*: consider topical (e.g. β-blocker, α-agonist, carbonic anhydrase inhibitor, prostaglandin analogue) or systemic (e.g. acetazolamide), according to IOP level.

Anterior segment ischaemia

This is an uncommon, but important, cause of anterior uveitis, particularly in the elderly.

Clinical features
- Dull ache, usually unilateral.
- AC significant flare/moderate cells, sluggish pupil; if part of ocular ischaemic syndrome (OIS), there may also be dilated irregular retinal veins (not tortuous), attenuated retinal arterioles, mid-peripheral retinal haemorrhages, rubeosis, and posterior segment neovascularization.

Investigate for carotid artery stenosis with carotid Doppler US, and refer to vascular surgeon, if indicated.

Schwartz syndrome

This is the uncommon association of anterior segment inflammation (mild) and ↑IOP (with an open angle) arising from an RRD. Detachments most commonly associated with this syndrome were large in area (and macula-off), flat in height, and long in duration. Postulated mechanisms include mechanical blockage by photoreceptor outer segments and trabeculitis. Refer to a vitreoretinal team for assessment and repair (see ➲ Rhegmatogenous retinal detachment, pp. 486–8). The ↑IOP and anterior uveitis may be treated medically in the interim but tend to resolve rapidly with surgical repair.

Anterior uveitis syndromes (2)

TINU

This is the rare association of tubulointerstitial nephritis (often presenting as acute renal failure) and uveitis. It typically affects young ♀ (median age 15; ♀:♂ 3:1) but can occur at almost any age. It is commonly idiopathic but may be associated with drugs (NSAIDs, penicillin, furosemide) or infection (streptococci, staphylococci, etc.).

Clinical features

- *Uveitis*: usually anterior (80%), bilateral (77%), and most often presents after the systemic disease (65%); uveitis may recur or follow a persistent course in over 50%. Ocular complications include PS, ↑IOP, and cataract.
- *Renal disease*: usually recovers, but chronic renal impairment occurs in 11%, with dialysis being required in 4%.

Investigations

- *Serum*: ↑creatinine, ↑ESR.
- *Urine*: proteinuria, haematuria, ↑β2-microglobulin levels, sterile pyuria.
- *Renal biopsy*: required for definitive diagnosis; shows oedema in the renal interstitium, with predominantly mononuclear infiltrate of activated T-cells, plasma cells, and histiocytes. The glomerular and vascular structures are relatively unaffected.

Treatment

- The renal disease is commonly treated with systemic steroids; the uveitis may be treated as for idiopathic AAU.

IgA nephropathy

This is a relatively common renal disease of children and young adults, in which recurrent micro- or macroscopic haematuria may be related to respiratory tract infections. In some patients, episodes are associated with an anterior uveitis, which may be treated as for idiopathic AAU.

Kawasaki disease

This is an uncommon acute vasculitis of children, defined as fever (≥5d) with four of the following five criteria: conjunctival injection, rash, desquamation of extremities, cervical lymphadenopathy, and mucosal changes (pharyngeal injection, cracked red lips, strawberry tongue). An anterior uveitis is common in the first week of illness; rarely, disc oedema and dilated retinal vessels are seen. Most seriously, cardiac abnormalities (notably coronary artery aneurysms) occur in 20%.

Uveitis with juvenile idiopathic arthritis

JIA is the commonest chronic rheumatic disease of childhood. It is a heterogeneous group of disorders characterized by a chronic inflammatory arthritis. One or more joints are affected with swelling or limited joint range and pain on movement for at least 6wk, with the age at onset being <16y. JIA is more common in ♀ than ♂. The incidence is 5–18 per 100,000, with prevalence of ~1 per 1,000 children, although the prevalence may be higher, as many children may be undiagnosed or incorrectly diagnosed. JIA is classified using the International League of Associations of Rheumatologists (ILAR) classification (see Box 11.2). The prevalence of uveitis in JIA overall is ~8–30%, but, in young oligoarticular onset group (i.e. arthritis in which up to four joints are involved), it may be as high as 45–57%.[6]

Risk factors for uveitis are: young age at diagnosis, ♀ sex, ANA positivity, and the subtype of JIA, in particular, the persistent and extended oligoarthritis groups. **NB** Although JIA-associated uveitis is more common in girls, the rate of complications and visual loss is higher in boys.[7]

Classification

> **Box 11.2 Classification of JIA (ILAR)**
>
> - Systemic arthritis.
> - Oligoarthritis—persistent.
> - Oligoarthritis—extended.
> - Polyarthritis—RF negative.
> - Polyarthritis—RF positive.
> - Psoriatic arthritis.
> - Enthesitis-related arthritis.
> - Undifferentiated arthritis.

Clinical features

Ophthalmic

- Asymptomatic; rarely floaters; ↓VA from cataract.
- White eye, band keratopathy, small KPs, AC cells/flare, PA, cataract, 2° glaucoma, vitritis, CMO; other complications include hypotony that may lead to phthisis bulbi.

NB In long-standing uveitis, chronic breakdown of the blood–aqueous barrier leads to persistent flare; AC cells are therefore a better guide than flare to disease activity.

Screening (See Table 11.10)

Principles

(1) *Initial screening examination*: uveitis often starts soon after onset of arthritis but may also start before the arthritis. *The initial screening examination is therefore a clinical priority and should occur as soon as possible and no later than 6wk from referral.*

(2) *Symptomatic patients* or patients suspected of cataracts or synechiae should be seen within *1wk* of referral.

Table 11.10 Summary of follow-up for JIA (*Guidelines for screening for uveitis in JIA* by the Royal College of Ophthalmologists and the British Society for Paediatric and Adolescent Rheumatology, 2006)

First screening: within 6wk of referral

Subsequent screening:
Every 2mo from onset of arthritis for 6mo
Then every 3–4mo for duration listed:

Duration of screening

Disease type/ANA status	Age of onset (y)	Duration (y)
Oligoarticular, psoriatic, and enthesitis-related, irrespective of ANA status	<3	8
	3–4	6
	5–8	3
	9–10	1
Polyarticular, ANA+	<6	5
	6–9	2
Polyarticular, ANA–	<7	5

Alternatively, all these groups may be screened until 11–12y old. Older patients (>11y) should be screened for 1y.

Treatment

- *Of uveitis*: refer to a tertiary referral centre for advice about specific immunosuppression if: (1) complications are present at onset or (2) if the disease is active after 2y of topical treatment. Management of complex cases is optimized in tertiary centres with joint clinics between a paediatric rheumatologist and specialist ophthalmologist. Treatment options include topical steroid eye drop, mydriatics, sub-Tenon injections of steroids, orbital floor injections, occasionally systemic steroids (IVMP pulses or oral prednisolone), and increasingly with weekly methotrexate. Ciclosporin, mycophenolate, and anti-TNF agents (infliximab, adalimumab) may also be considered.
- *Of ↑IOP*: initially topical therapy, but up to two-thirds may require surgery (commonly an augmented trabeculectomy or a tube procedure).
- *Of cataract*: aim to defer until the eye has been quiet for a minimum of 3mo, although weigh against the risk of amblyopia in younger children; there is considerable debate over surgery, including whether to implant a lens or leave aphakic.
- *Of band keratopathy*: chelation with EDTA or excimer phototherapeutic keratectomy.

6. BenEzra D et al. Uveitis and juvenile idiopathic arthritis: a cohort study. *Clin Ophthalmol* 2007;**1**:513–18.

7. Kalinina AV et al. Male gender as a risk factor for complications in uveitis associated with juvenile idiopathic arthritis. *Am J Ophthalmol* 2010;**149**:994–9.

Intermediate uveitis

The term intermediate uveitis refers to uveitis where the vitreous is the major site of inflammation The term pars planitis may be used where there is snowbank or snowball formation occurring in the absence of an associated infection or systemic disease (i.e. idiopathic).

Intermediate uveitis accounts for around 10% of all cases of uveitis. It is bimodal, being commonest in young adults, but with a second peak in the middle-aged/elderly. ♂ and ♀ are equally affected. It is bilateral in 80% but is often asymmetric.

Clinical features

- Floaters, ↓VA (may indicate macular oedema); may be asymptomatic.
- Vitritis (cells, 'snowballs'), exudation at the ora serrata ('snowbanking', commonly inferior but can be 360°), peripheral periphlebitis, rarely vitreous haemorrhage; some AC activity is common.
- *Complications*: CMO, cataract, 2° glaucoma, cyclitic membrane, tractional retinal detachment (TRD), retinal tears, vitreomacular traction, ERM, retinal neovascularization, retinoschisis.

Investigation

- Consider FBC, U+E, ESR, VDRL, TPHA, urinalysis, CXR for all patients; further investigation should be directed by clinical indication (see Table 11.11). OCT or FFA may be helpful to confirm CMO.

Treatment

- *Observation*: if no CMO and VA >6/12, then monitor only.
- *Medical therapy*:
  - *Topical*: if significant AC activity, control with topical corticosteroids and mydriatics (e.g. cyclopentolate 1% 1–2×/d).
  - Periocular/intraocular/systemic therapy is required if CMO or visually disabling floaters; consider periocular or intraocular treatments where unilateral or very asymmetric disease (or if cannot tolerate systemic therapy).
  - *Periocular*: corticosteroid (e.g. orbital floor/sub-Tenon's methylprednisolone/triamcinolone 40mg); risk of ↑IOP.
  - *Intravitreal*: intravitreal triamcinolone 2–4mg is well established but unlicensed. Sustained-release devices include Retisert® (0.59mg fluocinolone acetonide; estimated release 0.5 micrograms/d), with a number of studies showing significant reductions in the number of inflammatory episodes and decreased reliance on systemic corticosteroids or other immunomodulatory therapies (Fluocinolone Acetonide Uveitis Study Group; Multicentre Uveitis Steroid Treatment)[8]. Ozurdex® (0.7mg dexamethasone) also has evidence of benefit and is licensed for non-infectious posterior segment uveitis (HURON study).[9] Iluvien® (0.23mg fluocinolone acetonide; estimated release 0.2 micrograms/d) is currently being evaluated. All intravitreal corticosteroids are associated with a risk of ↑IOP, cataract, and endophthalmitis; ↑IOP appeared to be particularly common with Retisert®, but we currently lack equivalent long-term data on the newer steroid delivery systems.

- *Systemic*: corticosteroids (e.g. prednisolone initially 1mg/kg/d and titrating down or, in severe cases, pulsed methylprednisolone 500–1,000mg three doses daily or alternate days) ± other immunosuppresives (e.g. methotrexate, mycophenolate, azathioprine, ciclosporin) normally reserved for bilateral or resistant disease, or failure to get oral corticosteroid dose to <10mg/d, or intolerable corticosteroid side effects. There may be a role for anti-TNF (infliximab, adalimumab) in more resistant cases (contraindicated in patients with MS).
- Surgical therapy:
  - *Vitrectomy*: indications include vitreous opacities, CMO, vitreomacular traction, ERM, retinal detachment. It may be combined with phacoemulsification and IOL implant for visually disabling cataract. Often intravitreal triamcinolone 4mg is given at the end of surgery, provided there are no contraindications (e.g. known steroid-induced rise in IOP).
  - Cataract surgery is frequently required.
  - Glaucoma surgery may be needed if there is a failure of medical therapy for IOP control.

Table 11.11 Associations of intermediate uveitis

Group	Cause	Consider
1° ocular	Idiopathic/pars planitis	After exclusion of other associations
2° systemic	MS	MRI brain, LP
	Sarcoid	ACE, Ca, CXR, CT thorax
	IBD	Bowel studies, biopsy
	CNS/intraocular lymphoma	MRI brain, LP
2° infective	Toxocara	Serology
	Lyme disease	Serology
	HTLV-1	Serology

8. Multicentre Uveitis Study Treatment (MUST) Trial Research Group *et al.* Randomized comparison of systemic anti-inflammatory therapy versus fluocinolone acetnoide implant for intermediate, posterior, and panuveitis: the mulitcenter uveitis steroid treatment trial. *Ophthalmology* 2011;**118**:1916–26.

9. Lowder C *et al.* Dexamethasone intravitreal implant for noninfectious intermediate or posterior uveitis. *Arch Ophthalmol* 2011;**129**:545–53.

Retinal vasculitis

Retinal vasculitis comprises inflammation of the retinal vasculature. It may be a 1° ocular disease or 2° to either infection or systemic disease.

Clinical features

- ↓VA, floaters, positive scotomata; may be asymptomatic if peripheral.
- Perivascular sheathing of arteries, veins, or capillaries; retinal haemorrhages; vitritis; disc swelling, CMO.
- *Complications*: B/CRVO, neovascularization, vitreous haemorrhage, ischaemic maculopathy, TRD.

Investigations

- *FFA*: vessel wall staining, vascular leakage, skip lesions, widespread capillary leakage, new vessel leakage, disc leakage, petalloid macular leakage, enlarged focal avascular zone (FAZ) (ischaemia), vascular occlusion, capillary 'dropout'.
- Consider FBC, U+E, ESR, VDRL, TPHA, ANA, ANCA, urinalysis, CXR for all patients; further investigation should be directed by clinical indication (see Table 11.12 and Table 11.13).

Treatment

Where possible, the underlying disease is treated, e.g. with antibiotics for infective cases, e.g. TB. Treatment options are similar to that used for intermediate uveitis (see ➌ Intermediate uveitis, p. 432). In most instances, immunosuppression is required. Corticosteroids are first line and may be periocular, PO (e.g. prednisolone 1–2mg/kg), IV (e.g. pulsed methylprednisolone 500–1,000mg three doses daily or alternate days), or intraocular (intravitreal triamcinolone or fluocinolone acetonide intravitreal sustained-release device). Ciclosporin and azathioprine tend to be used second line, although methotrexate, mycophenolate, tacrolimus, sirolimus, anti-TNF, e.g. infliximab/adalimumab, and interferon alfa (mainly in Behçet's) and cyclophosphamide (mainly in GPA) also have their place.

Table 11.12 Causes of retinal vasculitis

Group	Cause	Consider
1° ocular	Intermediate uveitis	Urine, blood glucose
	Birdshot chorioretinopathy	EDTs
	Eales' disease	PPD skin test, CXR
	VKH	
	Sympathetic ophthalmia	
2° infective	CMV	PCR
	HSV	PCR
	VZV	PCR
	HTLV-1	Serology
	HIV	Serology, CD4 count, PCR
	Toxoplasmosis	Serology
	TB	PPD skin test, IGRA, CXR
	Lyme disease	Serology
	Cat-scratch disease	Serology, PCR
	Syphilis	Serology (VDRL, TPHA)
	Whipple's disease	PCR
2° systemic	Leukaemia	FBC, LP, bone marrow
	Lymphoma	MRI brain, LP
	SLE	ANA, dsDNA
	Behçet's disease	Pathergy
	Sarcoidosis	ACE, Ca, CXR, HRCT thorax
	GPA	c-ANCA (PR3)
	PAN	p-ANCA, tissue biopsy
	Churg–Strauss syndrome	p-ANCA, CXR, tissue biopsy
	Antiphospholipid syndrome	Anticardiolipin antibodies

Table 11.13 Diagnostic pointers in retinal vasculitis

Clinical feature	Possible cause of vasculitis
Arteritis	ARN (HSV, VZV), systemic vasculitis (inc Churg-Strauss syndrome, SLE, PAN, cryoglobulinaemia), IRVAN syndrome
RVO	Behçet's disease, sarcoidosis, SLE
RPE changes	TB, sarcoidosis, lymphoma
Capillary closure	TB, MS, sarcoidosis

Sarcoidosis (1)

This relatively common granulomatous multisystem disorder may be life-threatening. The eye is affected in up to 25% of patients. Of these, anterior uveitis occurs in 60%; posterior segment disease occurs in 25% of patients. Sarcoidosis affects up to 0.1% of the population, being higher in ♀ and with peaks in the third and sixth decades. It is commoner in African-Caribbeans, Irish, and Scandinavians.

The cause of sarcoidosis is unknown; there is PCR evidence for several agents (including atypical mycobacteria) that may trigger the disease in susceptible individuals. The Th1 response predominates in typical sarcoid granulomata, although it appears that a transition to the Th2 response underlies progressive pulmonary fibrosis.

The presentation may be acute or insidious. An acute presentation, typically with erythema nodosum and bihilar lymphadenopathy (BHL), has a better prognosis. The course tends to be self-limiting, although steroids may hasten recovery. An insidious presentation is more commonly followed by a relentless progression to pulmonary fibrosis.

Classification

Recently, a number of diagnostic criteria have been proposed for intraocular sarcoidosis (see Table 11.14).

Clinical features

Ophthalmic

- *Anterior uveitis* (2/3 are persistent, 1/3 acute; unilateral or bilateral; 'granulomatous'): circumlimbal injection, mutton fat KPs, AC flare/cells, PS, vitreous cells; iris granulomas and nodules.
- *Intermediate uveitis*: vitreous cells, snowballs, snowbanking.
- *Posterior uveitis*: CMO (commonest cause of ↓VA), periphlebitis (± patchy sheathing ± 'candle wax dripping'), occluded vessels (especially BRVO), neovascularization, choroidal/retinal/preretinal nodules (probably granulomata), pigment epithelial changes, disc swelling (from inflammatory papillitis, optic nerve granuloma, or papilloedema 2° to CNS disease). Peripheral multifocal chorioretinitis (small punched-out atrophic spots) are highly suggestive of sarcoidosis.
- *Complications*: cataract, glaucoma (↑risk with duration of active disease), CNV.

Systemic

- *RS*: often asymptomatic despite CXR changes, dry cough, dyspnoea; BHL, parenchymal disease.
- *CVS*: pericarditis, cardiomyopathy, conduction defects, cardiac failure, cor pulmonale.
- *Skin*: erythema nodosum (red, tender, elevated lesions typically on the shins; commonest in younger ♀); cutaneous granulomata (non-tender, nodules/papules/macules, almost anywhere, including the lids); lupus pernio (uncommon, bluish plaque, typically on the face/ears).
- *Joints*: arthritis (commoner in acute sarcoid); bone cysts (usually in the digits).

- *Glands*: swelling of any of lacrimal, salivary, parotid, and submaxillary glands, lymphadenopathy, hepatosplenomegaly.
- *CNS* (neurosarcoidosis, commoner in patients with posterior uveitis): cranial nerve palsies (most commonly VIIn; can be bilateral), peripheral neuropathy, myopathy, aseptic meningoencephalitis (typically basal leptomeninges); CNS granuloma may mimic a tumour; optic nerve involvement may present as an atypical optic neuritis.

Table 11.14 Proposed diagnostic criteria for intraocular sarcoidosis*

Four levels of certainty are recommended where other possible causes (notably tuberculous uveitis) have been excluded:

Definite ocular sarcoidosis	Biopsy-supported diagnosis with a compatible uveitis
Presumed ocular sarcoidosis	Biopsy not done; presence of BHL with a compatible uveitis
Probable ocular sarcoidosis	Biopsy not done and BHL negative, presence of three of the suggestive intraocular signs, and two positive investigational tests
Possible ocular sarcoidosis	Biopsy negative, four of the suggestive intraocular signs, and two of the investigations are positive

* Herbort CP et al. International criteria for the diagnosis of ocular sarcoidosis: results of the first international Workshop on Ocular Sarcoidosis (IWOS). *Ocul Immunol Inflamm* 2009;**17**:160–9.

Sarcoidosis (2)

Investigations

The diagnosis is essentially clinical but may be supported by investigations such as serum ACE (angiotensin-converting enzyme), imaging, and ideally typical histology. In some cases, it may be difficult to distinguish neurosarcoidosis from MS.

- *Serum ACE* (commonly elevated in active sarcoid due to synthesis by activated macrophages; 'false positives' (see Box 11.3)), serum Ca^{2+} (less commonly elevated).
- *CXR*: abnormal in >90% with ocular sarcoid—stage 0 (normal); stage 1 (BHL only); stage 2 (BHL + parenchymal disease); stage 3 (parenchymal disease only).
- *HRCT thorax*: high sensitivity and specificity; particularly useful in those with normal CXR.
- *MRI brain/optic nerves* (ideally fat-suppressed, gadolinium-enhanced, T1) and LP in suspected neurosarcoid.
- *Gallium-67 scan*: typical uptake pattern is lacrimal and parotid glands (panda appearance) or mediastinum (lambda sign).
- *PET-CT scan*: although traditionally used to detect cancers, PET (positron emission tomography) captures images of minuscule changes in the body's metabolism caused by the growth of abnormal cells, while CT images simultaneously allows the exact location, size, and shape of the diseased tissue to be pinpointed. Essentially, small lesions (e.g. lymph nodes) are detected with PET and then precisely located with CT.
- *Biopsy*: transbronchial, endobronchial, or conjunctival biopsy may reveal the typical non-caseating granulomata of whorls of epithelioid cells surrounding multinucleate giant cells. Bronchoalveolar lavage (BAL) may show lymphocytosis with high CD4+/CD8+ ratio, but low specificity.
- *FFA*: include ischaemia (hypofluoroescence), leakage from periphlebitis, new vessels, CMO (hyperfluorescence).
- *ICG*: choroidal stromal vasculitis, early lobular hypofluorescence, late hyperfluorescence (focal or diffuse).

Box 11.3 **Differential diagnosis of elevated serum ACE**
- Child (peaks at 13y of age, adult level by 18y).
- Sarcoidosis.
- Mycobacterial infection (including leprosy and TB).
- Certain chronic lung diseases (including berylliosis, silicosis, farmer's lung, histoplasmosis, lymphangiomyomatosis).
- Gaucher's disease.

Treatment

Of ophthalmic disease:

- *Anterior segment inflammation*: as for idiopathic AAU (see ➲ Idiopathic AAU, p. 422).
- *Posterior segment inflammation*: as for intermediate uveitis (see ➲ Intermediate uveitis, p. 432).
- *Cataract*: conventional surgery but with tight control of inflammation.
- *Glaucoma*: medical ± surgical (augmented trabeculectomy).
- *CNV*: medical treatment, laser, PDT, or surgery. There may be a role for intravitreal anti-VEGF therapy.

Sarcoidosis syndromes

- *Heerfordt's syndrome* (uveoparotid fever): parotid/submandibular gland enlargement, VIIn palsy, uveitis.
- *Löfgren's syndrome*: fever, erythema nodosum, BHL.
- *Mickulicz's syndrome*: diffuse swelling of lacrimal/salivary glands (most commonly due to sarcoidosis).

Behçet's disease

Possibly first recognized by Hippocrates, the modern description of this disease dates from the Greek Adamantiades and the Turk Behçet. It is an idiopathic, chronic multisystem disease characterized by recurrent episodes of acute inflammation. The commonest ophthalmic presentation is of a sight-threatening panuveitis and retinal vasculitis.

Prevalence is highest along the traditional Silk Route, peaking in Turkey where up to 0.4% of the population may be affected. It typically affects young adults. There is some geographical variation of risk factors, including gender, FH (more significant in Middle Eastern countries), and the HLA-B51 allele (more significant in Japan, with a relative risk of 6.7).

Clinical features

Ophthalmic

- *Anterior uveitis*: acute anterior non-granulomatous uveitis, typically with hypopyon.
- *Posterior uveitis*: vitiritis, macular oedema, retinal infiltrates/ haemorrhage/oedema, occlusive periphlebitis ± BRVO/CRVO), neovascularization ± vitreous haemorrhage/TRD, diffuse capillary leakage.
- *Complications*: cataract, glaucoma, end-stage disease (optic atrophy, retinal atrophy with attenuated vessels; often blind).

Systemic

- *Oral ulceration* (aphthous or scarring).
- *GU* (genital ulceration).
- *Skin lesions*: erythema nodosum, pseudofolliculitis, papulopustules, acneiform rash.
- *Joints* arthritis (mono/poly).
- *Vascular*: thromboses (venous > arterial), including superficial thrombophlebitis, SVC/IVC obstruction.
- *GI*: nausea, vomiting, abdominal pain, bloody diarrhoea.
- *CNS*: meningoencephalitis, sinus thrombosis ± intracranial hypertension, cranial or peripheral neuropathies, focal CNS signs.

Investigations

- There are no laboratory tests to diagnose Behçet's disease, but there are classification criteria (see Table 11.15).
- *Positive pathergy test*: sterile pustule appearing 24–48h after oblique insertion of 20G needle.
- *MRI/MRV brain*: if neurological features.

Treatment

- Liaise with physician; systemic corticosteroids (e.g. initially 1–2mg/kg/d prednisolone PO); IV (e.g. pulsed methylprednisolone 500–1000mg three doses daily or alternate days); for an acute flare, consider adding steroid-sparing agents (immunosuppressants), including ciclosporin, azathioprine, and anti-TNF therapies (e.g. infliximab or adalimumab), or interferon alfa.

Table 11.15 Criteria for classification of Behçet's disease (International Study Group for Behçet's Disease[*][†]

	Diagnostic (classification) criteria
Must have:	• Recurrent oral ulceration (minor, major, or herpetiform) ≥3× in 12mo
Plus two of:	• Recurrent genital ulceration (aphthous or scarring)
	• Eye lesions: uveitis (anterior, posterior, or cells in the vitreous) or retinal vasculitis
	• Skin lesions: erythema nodosum, pseudofolliculitis, or papulopustular lesions; or acneiform rash (in post-adolescent patient not on corticosteroids)
	• Positive pathergy test

[*] International Study Group for Behçet's Disease. Criteria for diagnosis of Behçet's disease. *Lancet* 1990;**335**:1078–80.

[†] International Study Group for Behçet's Disease. Evaluation of diagnostic ('classification') criteria in Behçet's disease—towards internationally agreed criteria. *Br J Rheumatol* 1992;**31**:299–308.

Vogt–Koyanagi–Harada disease

VKH is a multisystem inflammatory disease affecting the eyes (bilateral granulomatous panuveitis), ears, brain, skin, and hair. It is thought to be a T-cell-mediated autoimmune disease directed against melanocyte antigen(s). Prevalence is higher in darker skinned races, including Asians, native Americans, Hispanics, and those from the Middle and Far East. It is commonest in women in their third and fourth decades but may occur in either sex at any age. It is associated with HLA-DR4, notably HLA-DRB1*0405 which recognizes various melanocyte proteins. VKH may arise after cutaneous injury, presumably via liberation of melanocyte antigens.

Clinical features

There is often a prodrome of fever, meningism, and auditory symptoms for a few days, before blurring/profound visual loss from the uveitis develops (see Table 11.16).

Ophthalmic
- *Anterior uveitis*: bilateral granulomatous anterior uveitis, PS, iris nodules, AC shallowing.
- *Posterior uveitis*: multifocal choroditis, multifocal detachments of sensory retina, ERD, choroidal depigmentation 'sunset glow fundus'), Dalen–Fuchs nodules (peripheral yellow-white choroidal granulomas), subretinal fibrosis.
- *Complications*: cataract, glaucoma, CNV membrane.

Systemic
- *Cutaneous*: late features—vitiligo, alopecia, poliosis.
- *Auditory*: tinnitus, deafness, vertigo.
- *Neurological*: sterile meningitis (headache, neck stiffness), encephalitis, (convulsions, altered consciousness), cranial neuropathies (including ocular motility disturbance).

Investigations

- *FFA*: focal areas of delay in choroidal perfusion, multifocal areas of pinpoint leakage, large placoid areas of hyperfluorescence, pooling within subretinal fluid (SRF), and optic nerve staining.
- *US*: low to medium reflective diffuse choroidal thickening.
- *LP* (not always required): lymphocytic pleocytosis.

Treatment

Liaise with physician; start high-dose systemic corticosteroids (e.g. 1–2mg/kg/d prednisolone PO or methylprednisolone 1g/d IV for 3d); for resistant or recurrent disease, consider adding steroid-sparing agents (immunosuppressants) such as methotrexate, azathioprine, mycophenolate and ciclosporin.

Table 11.16 Revised diagnostic criteria for VKH disease (AUS criteria)*

1		No history of penetrating ocular trauma or surgery preceding initial onset of uveitis
2		No clinical or laboratory evidence suggestive of other ocular disease entities
3		Bilateral ocular involvement:
	a	● Early:
		(1) Diffuse choroiditis (focal SRF or bullous serous retinal detachments)
		(2) If fundus findings equivocal, then there must be characteristic FFA findings AND diffuse choroidal thickening (in the absence of posterior scleritis on US)
	b	● Late:
		(1) History suggestive of prior presence of early features AND two or more of:
		(2) Ocular depigmentation (Sunset glow fundus or Sugiura sign)
		(3a) Nummular chorioretinal depigmented scars
		(3b) RPE clumping/migration
		(3c) Recurrent or chronic anterior uveitis
4		Neurological/auditory findings:
	a	● Meningismus (malaise, fever, headache, nausea, abdominal pain, neck/back stiffness)
	b	● Tinnitus
	c	● CSF pleocytosis
5		Integumentary findings (not preceding ocular/CNS disease):
	a	● Alopecia
	b	● Poliosis
	c	● Vitiligo

Complete VKH requires all criteria (1 to 5).

Incomplete VKH requires criteria 1 to 3 AND either 4 or 5.

Probable VKH (isolated ocular disease) requires criteria 1 to 3.

* Read RW et al. Revised diagnostic criteria for Vogt–Koyanagi–Harada disease: report of an international committee on nomenclature. *Am J Ophthalmol* 2001;**131**:647.

Sympathetic ophthalmia

Sympathetic ophthalmia is a rare bilateral granulomatous panuveitis which bears remarkable parallels to VKH but differs in being causally related to antecedent trauma or surgery. Although this response to injury can occur within a few days or over 60y later, it usually arises between 1 and 12mo after injury. It appears to be a T-cell-mediated response to an ocular antigen, presumably liberated during the initial insult. It occurs in 0.1% cases of penetrating ocular trauma and in 0.01% cases of routine vitrectomy. In one prospective study (BOSU), the commonest cause of sympathetic ophthalmia was ocular (particularly vitreoretinal) surgery.[10]

Clinical features

Ophthalmic

- *Anterior*: bilateral granulomatous anterior uveitis with mutton fat KPs, PS.
- *Posterior*: vitritis, choroidal infiltration, Dalen–Fuchs nodules, macular oedema, ERD; the exciting eye may be phthsical.
- *Complications*: cataract, 2° glaucoma, end-stage disease (optic atrophy, chorioretinal scarring).

Systemic

- As for VKH, but systemic involvement less common.

Prevention

After trauma, there is a short window of opportunity (~10d), in which enucleation would almost certainly prevent sympathetic ophthalmia. This may be the best option for blind painful eyes with no hope of useful vision. However, for the many traumatized eyes with visual potential, there is now a strong trend to preserve the eye where possible.

Treatment

Once inflammation has developed, the role of enucleation of the exciting eye is controversial; some suggest that it may favourably modify the disease if performed within 2wk of symptoms.

- *Immunosuppression: start* with high-dose systemic corticosteroids (e.g. 1–2mg/kg/d prednisolone PO or methylprednisolone 1g/d IV for 3d); for resistant/recurrent disease or unacceptable steroid side effects, consider adding steroid-sparing agents such as methotrexate, azathioprine, ciclosporin, mycophenolate. With aggressive treatment, around 60% may achieve >6/15 in the sympathizing eye.[11]

10. Kilmartin DJ *et al.* Prospective surveillance of sympathetic ophthalmia in the UK and Republic of Ireland. *Br J Ophthalmol* 2000;**84**:259–63.

11. Galor A *et al.* Sympathetic ophthalmia: incidence of ocular complications and vision loss in the sympathizing eye. *Am J Ophthalmol* 2009;**148**:704–10.

Viral uveitis (1)

HSV

HSV1 (very rarely HSV2) may cause an anterior uveitis which is usually associated with keratitis but may be isolated.

Clinical features
- *Anterior*: unilateral persistent anterior uveitis with KPs, PS, and patchy iris atrophy (with transillumination defects); semi-dilated pupil ± corneal scarring/keratitis/↓corneal sensation (see ➔ Herpes simplex keratitis, p. 232); the uveitis may be 'granulomatous'.
- Glaucoma is common (2° to trabeculitis or blockage by inflammatory debris).
- *Posterior* (rare): healthy individuals may get ARN (see ➔ ARN, p. 448); those with disseminated HSV or HSV encephalitis may get an occlusive vasculitis (usually bilateral), with relatively few haemorrhages but commonly complicated by retinal detachment.

Treatment
- If keratitis, then antiviral cover generally required (see ➔ Herpes simplex keratitis, p. 232).
- *For isolated anterior uveitis*: titrate topical steroids, according to inflammation, and taper very slowly (frequency/potency), as highly steroid-sensitive and relapses are common; cycloplegia.
- For frequent recurrences, consider long-term oral antiviral prophylaxis.

VZV

1° VZV infection (chickenpox) commonly causes a widespread vesicular rash which may be associated with keratitis (superficial, disciform, or stromal), mild anterior uveitis, and, very occasionally, necrotizing retinitis. Reactivation (shingles) usually occurs in the elderly or immunosuppressed and frequently affects Va (ophthalmic branch), known as HZO. Of this group, up to 40% have anterior uveitis, with an increased risk if the nasociliary branch is involved (Hutchinson sign: vesicles at side of nose). Typical ocular inflammation (e.g. disciform keratitis with anterior uveitis) may also occur without the rash (HZO sine herpete).

Clinical features
- *Anterior*: unilateral anterior uveitis with KPs, PS, and segmental iris atrophy, (with transillumination defects) ± conjunctivitis, keratitis, epi-/scleritis; the uveitis may be 'granulomatous'.
- Glaucoma is common (up to 40%).
- *Posterior*: ARN or PORN may develop (see ➔ Viral uveitis (2), p. 448).

Treatment
- *For isolated anterior uveitis*: titrate topical steroids, according to inflammation, and taper very slowly (frequency/potency) as highly steroid-sensitive and relapses are common with steroid withdrawal; cycloplegia.
- For HZO, see ➔ Herpes zoster ophthalmicus, p. 236.

CMV

CMV anterior uveitis occurs in immunocompetent individuals and, in recent years, has been increasingly recognized as a cause of hypertensive uveitis. CMV retinitis is the leading cause of visual loss in AIDS but may also occur in patients who are immunosuppressed due to therapy (e.g. associated with organ transplants) or other disease (e.g. lymphoma). HIV and non-HIV-associated infections behave fairly similarly, both being dependent on the degree of immune system suppression/recovery.

Clinical features

- Anterior uveitis: unilateral, usually with ↑IOP; there may be no obvious iris atrophy (cf. HSV, VZV).
  - *Treatment*: often challenging but may respond to oral valganciclovir. IOP control may also be difficult.
- Corneal endotheliitis (more common in the Far East): corneal involvement ranges from small areas of focal endotheliitis (may be coin-shaped) to diffuse bullous keratopathy, stromal corneal oedema, KPs (variable appearance), AC inflammation usually mild with no PS ± diffuse iris atrophy, ↑IOP.
- Posterior: CMV retinitis (see ➲ HIV-associated disease: posterior segment, p. 454).

Treatment

- *For anterior uveitis or corneal endotheliitis*: oral valganciclovir.

Viral uveitis (2)

ARN

This rare syndrome of necrotizing retinitis is caused by VZV, HSV1, and HSV2 infection (children). It may occur in the immunocompromised and healthy individuals of any age. In the National UK ARN Survey 2001–2, there were 31 cases (22 ♂, 9 ♀; aged 13–85y, mean 54), of which 28 cases (90.3%) were unilateral. VZV was the commonest cause (identified in ten patients), followed by HSV1 (five patients) HSV2 (four patients). Based on this study, the incidence of ARN in the UK is ~1 case per 1.6 to 2.0 million population/y.

Clinical findings
- Usually unilateral ↓VA, floaters, discomfort.
- Predominantly peripheral disease comprising occlusive arteritis, full-thickness peripheral necrotizing retinitis (well demarcated, spread circumferentially), marked vitritis ± AC activity.
- *Complications*: retinal detachment (in up to 75%; rhegmatogenous or tractional), ischaemic optic neuropathy.
- *Prognosis*: second eye involvement occurs in around 30% (may occur simultaneously to several years later).

Investigations
- AC tap ± vitreous biopsy with PCR to identify viral DNA.

Treatment
- *For all patients*: antiviral (e.g. aciclovir IV dose 10mg/kg 3×/d for 2wk, then PO 400–800mg 5×/d dose for 6–12wk); consider systemic corticosteroids (vs inflammation), aspirin (vs arterial occlusion), barrier laser photocoagulation (vs retinal breaks), but no clear evidence. Retinal detachment repair is challenging due to the necrotic retina and number of breaks; vitrectomy with silicone oil injection is most commonly used. Alternative treatments include valaciclovir (a prodrug of aciclovir)1–2g 3×/d orally for 6–8wk and intravitreal foscarnet 2.4mg/0.1mL as initial treatment.
- *If immunosuppressed*: consider lifelong antiviral treatment.

Progressive outer retinal necrosis

This very rare devastating necrotizing retinitis is caused by VZV infection in the context of immunosuppression (usually HIV with CD4+ T-cell counts <50/mm^3).

Clinical findings
- Uni-/bilateral, painless, rapid ↓VA.
- Rapidly coalescing white areas of outer retinal necrosis (often central as well as peripheral) but with minimal vasculitis, retinitis, or vitritis (cf. ARN; see Table 11.17).

Treatment

This should be coordinated between an ophthalmologist with experience in HIV ocular disease and an HIV physician. Options include IV ganciclovir or foscarnet with additional intravitreal ganciclovir. The prognosis is very poor, partly due to the extremely high rate of retinal detachment.

Table 11.17 Diagnostic criteria for ARN and PORN[*]

	ARN	PORN
Appearance	One or more foci of full-thickness retinal necrosis with discrete borders	Multiple foci of deep retinal opacification which may be confluent
Location	Peripheral retina (usually adjacent/outside temporal arcades)	Peripheral retina Macular involvement
Progression	Rapid (but usually responds to treatment)	Extremely rapid
Direction	Circumferential	No consistent direction
Vessels	Occlusive vasculopathy (arterial)	No vascular inflammation
Inflammation	Prominent AC and vitreous inflammation	Minimal or none
Suggestive features	Optic neuropathy/atrophy Scleritis Pain	Perivenular clearing of retinal opacification

[*] Engstrom RE Jr et al. The progressive outer retinal necrosis syndrome. A variant of necrotizing herpetic retinopathy in patients with AIDS. *Ophthalmology* 1994;**101**:1488–502.

Viral uveitis (3)

West Nile virus (WNV) infection

The WNV is an enveloped single-stranded RNA flavivirus. The virus is widely distributed in Africa, Europe, Australia, and Asia, and, since 1999, it has spread rapidly throughout the Western hemisphere, including the USA, Canada, Mexico, and the Caribbean and into parts of Central and South America. WNV infection is a zoonotic disease, most often transmitted to human by an infected *Culex* mosquito vector, with wild birds serving as its reservoir. The incubation period of WNV ranges from 3 to 14d.

Clinical features
Systemic disease
- In humans, most (80%) are apparently asymptomatic, and, of the 20% of people who are symptomatic, most have a self-limited febrile illness.

Ocular disease
- Asymptomatic or mild ↓VA.
- Most (80%) patients develop a bilateral (rarely unilateral) multifocal chorioretinitis; the chorioretinal lesions usually develop early in the course of disease, with most (65%) lesions classed as already being inactive at presentation; commonly associated with a mild/moderate vitritis.
- Diabetes mellitus appears to be a potential risk factor.

Investigations
This requires a high index of suspicion and specific laboratory testing.
- *Serum ± CSF*: WNV-specific IgM antibody.

Treatment
At present, there is no proven treatment for WNV infection. In cases of severe systemic disease, intensive supportive therapy is indicated.

Chikungunya virus infection

Chikungunya virus is an arthropod-borne alphavirus in the family *Togaviridae*. It has three distinct genotypes, the East African, West African, and Asian, maintained in monkeys and wildlife population. Epidemics are sustained by human–mosquito–human transmission by several mosquito species. The incubation period is 2–5d, and the disease manifests 48h after a mosquito bite.

Clinical features
Systemic disease
It is usually a self-limiting febrile illness, lasting for few days to weeks, often associated with arthralgia/arthritis, skin rash, low back pain; most patients recover without consequence.

Ocular disease
- Anterior uveitis: unilateral or bilateral; typically diffuse fine KPs, with ↑IOP similar to herpetic disease; conjunctivitis and keratitis also reported.
- Posterior uveitis: unilateral or bilateral; ↓VA, ↓colour vision, central or centrocecal scotoma, and peripheral field defects; retinitis (retinal haemorrhages, oedema, vasculitis similar to herpetic retinitis), choroiditis, neuroretinitis, and optic neuritis.

Investigations
- FBC (leucopenia, lymphocytosis, mild thrombocytopenia); ↑ESR and ↑CRP.
- *Virus isolation*: RT-PCR for the virus-amplifying fragment of *E-2* gene.
- *Serology*: Chikungunya-specific IgM antibody; and/or fourfold increase in Chikungunya-specific IgG in acute and convalescent sera.

Treatment
- For the systemic disease, treatment is mainly symptomatic, including rest, NSAIDs, and paracetamol.
- Topical steroid, dilation, and ocular hypotensives.
- For the retinitis, some have given oral aciclovir and steroid.

Other viruses

Other common viruses that may cause an anterior or posterior uveitis include measles (with subacute sclerosing panencephalitis, SSPE), mumps, rubella, EBV, CMV, and HTLV-1.

SSPE

A rare neurodegenerative syndrome following measles infection; exhibits a retinitis with focal pigmentary changes in the fovea ± papilloedema or optic atrophy.

Human T-lymphotropic virus type 1 (HTLV-1)

This RNA retrovirus, common in Japan and parts of Africa, causes leukaemia and tropical spastic paraparesis; it may cause uveitis in isolation (usually intermediate) or 2° to leukaemia (usually posterior with retinal vasculitis ±2° infection, e.g. CMV).

HIV-associated disease: anterior segment

HIV (HIV-1 and 2) is an RNA retrovirus which infects CD4+ T-cells, causing AIDS. Worldwide, around 40 million people are infected with HIV,
with around 5 million new infections and 3 million deaths/y (WHO data
for 2003). Most infected people live in developing countries (notably
sub-Saharan Africa) and under socio-economic deprivation. Transmission
may be via infected blood or other bodily fluids. Major risk factors include
unprotected sexual intercourse, IV drug abuse, blood transfusion, and
maternal infection (vertical transmission).

The main markers of disease are CD4 level and viral load. The CD4 level
is a good indicator of HIV-induced immunocompromise and correlates with
susceptibility to infections (see Table 11.18 and Table 11.19). The viral load
(i.e. RNA copies/mL) correlates with risk of progression.

Prognosis is greatly improved with highly active antiretroviral therapy
(HAART). This regimen involves using at least three antiretroviral drugs,
usually two nucleoside reverse transcriptase inhibitors and either a protease
inhibitor or a non-nucleoside reverse transcriptase inhibitor. Management
of eye disease should be coordinated between an ophthalmologist with
experience in HIV and an HIV physician.

Conjunctival microvasculopathy

Microvascular abnormalities of the conjunctiva are common. The mechanism is unclear. Irregular calibre vessels are seen which may be in a cork-
screw pattern. Conjunctival microvasculopathy may be associated with
abnormalities of the retinal microvasculature.

Keratouveitis

- *VZV keratouveitis* is common in HIV, with or without the typical
  dermatomal rash of HZO. The features include a moderate anterior
  uveitis, ↑IOP, and iris atrophy. Treatment is with systemic antiviral (e.g.
  aciclovir or famciclovir) (see ➜ Herpes zoster ophthalmicus, p. 236).
- *HSV keratouveitis* is less common, with probably equal prevalence to
  the general population. In HIV patients, however, it tends to be limbal,
  more severe, with more recurrences, and dendrites may be larger and
  less defined. Treatment is with topical ± systemic antiviral (e.g. aciclovir)
  (see ➜ Herpes simplex keratitis, p. 232).
- *Microsporidial keratouveitis* presents with bilateral irritation and
  photophobia, punctate keratopathy, often with a follicular conjunctivitis
  and/or an anterior uveitis.

Anterior uveitis

Anterior uveitis is seen in over half of all patients with HIV. VZV and HSV
tend to cause relatively mild inflammation (often with ↑IOP and iris atrophy). However, posterior uveitis, associated with toxoplasma or syphilis,
may also cause significant AC inflammation. Uveitis may also be caused
by concurrent therapy, notably rifabutin (anti-atypical mycobacteria) and
cidofivir (anti-CMV).

Table 11.18 Ophthalmic complications of HIV infection

	Infective	Tumour	Other
Adnexae	HZO Molluscum contagiosum Preseptal cellulitis	Kaposi's sarcomaSCC	Conjunctival microvasculopathy
Orbit	Orbital cellulitis	Non-Hodgkin's lymphoma	
Anterior segment	Viral keratitis *(VZV, HSV)* Bacterial keratitis *(S. aureus, S. epidermidis, P. aeruginosa)* Protozoan keratitis *(microsporidia)*		Conjunctival microvasculopathy Vortex keratopathy (antivirals, atovaquone) Dry eye Anterior uveitis
Posterior segment	CMV retinitis VZV retinitis *(incl. PORN, ARN)* HSV retinitis *(incl. ARN)* Toxoplasma retinochoroiditis Syphilis retinitis Pneumocystis choroiditis Cryptococcus choroiditis Tuberculous choroiditis	Ocular-CNS non-Hodgkin lymphoma	Retinal microvasculopathy Ischaemic maculopathy Immune recovery uveitis
Neuro-ophthalmic	Cerebral toxoplasmosis Cryptococcal meningitis Neurosyphilis Progressive multifocal leukoencephalopathy	Ocular-CNS non-Hodgkin's lymphoma	Optic neuritis Optic atrophy Ocular motility disorders

Table 11.19 CD4 level and typical diseases relevant to the eye

CD4 count (cells/mm³)	Ocular disease
250–500	HZO TB
150–250	Lymphoma Kaposi's sarcoma
50–150	Pneumocystosis Toxoplasmosis Microsporidiosis VZV retinitis
<50	CMV retinitis

HIV-associated disease: posterior segment

This may affect up to 40% of patients with AIDS, but usually only when CD4 <50/mm^3. Since the advent of HAART, there has been a dramatic reduction in CMV retinitis.

Clinical features
- Floaters, ↓VA, and/or field loss.
- *Anterior*: AC inflammation (± distinctive stellate KPs) is usually mild or absent (depending on degree of immunosuppression).
- *Posterior*: vitritis (usually mild/absent) with retinitis which may be:
  - *Haemorrhagic retinitis*: haemorrhage and necrosis, with loss of fundal details ('pizza pie' appearance).
  - *Granular retinitis*: relatively indolent, with minimal haemorrhage and no vascular sheathing.
  - *Perivascular retinitis*: 'frosted branch angiitis' which spreads along the course of the retinal vessels.

Complications include retinal detachment (up to 30%), retinal atrophy, and optic nerve disease (5%).

Treatment
- *HAART*: sustaining a CD4 count >50/mm^3 is effective prophylaxis against CMV retinitis. Late introduction of HAART to patients with CMV retinitis is still likely to induce an immune recovery; in such patients, anti-CMV treatments are required at least until immune recovery occurs.
- *Specific anti-CMV treatment*: this involves 'induction' and 'maintenance' therapy. Commonly used agents include systemic antiviral (e.g. valganciclovir, ganciclovir, foscarnet, or cidofivir), intravitreal implants (ganciclovir) or injections (ganciclovir and/or foscarnet), or a combination. Lifelong maintenance treatment is recommended for all patients without immune recovery.

This is decreasing in frequency due to the toxoplasmacidal effect of pro-phylactic agents actually intended to eliminate *Pneumocystis*-related lung disease. Ocular toxoplasmosis in HIV is more severe, often multifocal (even bilateral), associated with moderate/severe anterior uveitis and vitritis, and is commonly associated with neuro-toxoplasmosis. In contrast to the immunocompetent situation, it always requires treatment (and should not be given with corticosteroids (see Ⓩ Toxoplasmosis, p. 462)).

Pneumocystis carinii **choroiditis**

This is relatively uncommon, particularly amongst those on systemic prophylaxis for *Pneumocystis carinii* pneumonia (co-trimoxazole), as opposed to inhalational (pentamidine). The choroiditis is often bilateral, comprises yellow choroidal patches of 1/4 to 2DD in size around the posterior pole, with minimal vitritis. It is often asymptomatic. Treatment is with systemic co-trimoxazole or pentamidine.

Cryptococcus choroiditis

This rare condition is usually associated with cryptococcal meningitis and may be associated with an optic neuropathy or papilloedema. It is characterized by multifocal off-white choroidal lesions, occasionally with a retinitis or endophthalmitis. Treatment is with a systemic antifungal (e.g. amphotericin or fluconazole).

Immune recovery uveitis

Eyes with inactive CMV retinitis may show a paradoxical worsening of inflammation as T-cell recovery takes place. Presentation includes moderate/severe vitritis, TRD, CMO, and retinal neovascularization.

Syphilis choroiditis/chorioretinitis

Co-infection with syphilis may occur due to sexual transmission. Syphilis may cause protean ocular and systemic manifestations (see ➲ Syphilis, p. 460).

HIV microvasculopathy

Around 75% of HIV-infected individuals develop microvascular abnormalities of the retina and/or conjunctiva (see ➲ HIV-associated disease: anterior segment, p. 452). It is not clear if this is due to HIV-induced thrombotic tendency, an immune phenomenon, or a direct result of HIV infection of the vessels.

Retinal microvasculopathy

In the retina, there may be tortuosity of the vessels with cotton wool spots (CWS), telangiectasia, intraretinal haemorrhages, and venous or arterial occlusions.

Mycobacterial disease (1)

TB

Worldwide >1 billion people are infected by *Mycobacterium tuberculosis*, a facultative intracellular bacterium. TB (1° or post-1°) develops in around 10%, and, of these, ocular disease develops in around 1%. Widespread chronic inflammation develops with characteristic caseating granulomata. This immune reaction, or occasionally direct ocular penetration, may lead to uveitis. Ocular TB may be difficult to diagnose due to its protean manifestations and the frequent absence of any systemic or radiological evidence of respiratory disease.

Clinical features
Ophthalmic
- *External*: lid abscess, conjunctival infiltration/nodules, phlyctenulosis, scleritis (usually anterior necrotizing), interstitial keratitis.
- *Anterior*: typically granulomatous anterior uveitis with mutton fat KPs, iris granulomata, PS, but can be non-granulomatous.
- *Posterior*: vitritis, vasculitis (periphlebitis ± B/CRVO ± ischaemia), macular oedema, choroidal granulomata (usually multifocal around the posterior pole ± inflammatory retinal detachment), serpiginous choroidopathy; optic neuropathy; Eales' disease (retinal vasculitis with neovascularization and high risk of vitreous haemorrhage, typically in young ♂).

Systemic
- *RS*: pneumonia, pleural effusion, fibrosis.
- *GI*: ileocaecal (may obstruct), peritoneum (ascites).
- *GU*: sterile pyuria, epididymitis, salpingitis + infertility (in ♂).
- *CNS*: meningitis, CNS tuberculoma (may mimic tumour).
- *Skeletal*: arthritis, osteomyelitis.
- *Skin*: lupus vulgaris.
- *CVS*: constrictive pericarditis, pericardial effusion.
- *Adrenal*: hypoadrenalism (Addison's disease).
- *LN*: lymphadenopathy, scrofula.

Investigation
- *Microbiology*: sputum, early morning urine (acid-fast bacillus, stains with Ziehl–Neelsen stain).
- *CXR*: classically apical infiltrates or cavitation; also consolidation, pleural effusion, hilar lymphadenopathy; normal in 50% of cases of ocular TB.
- *Tuberculin skin test (TST)*: standard testing involves intradermal injection of 0.1mL of 1:1,000 strength tuberculin PPD (i.e. 10 tuberculin units) and measuring the induration 72h later. Interpret with caution (see Box 11.4), since the response can be very variable with up to 17% false negatives and bacille Calmette–Guérin (BCG) vaccination inducing 'false' positives (but usually only if within 5y). A 1:10,000 strength tuberculin PPD may be used if active TB is suspected, since an intense reaction may become necrotic.
- *IGRA*: see Box 11.5.

Box 11.4 Interpretation of Mantoux testing (CDC recommendations 2005)

- For *high-risk* individuals (immunosuppressed, contacts of active TB, typical CXR changes), the test is considered positive if induration ≥5mm.
- For *moderate risk* (e.g. health workers, those with chronic disease, children, immigrants from endemic areas), induration must be ≥10mm.
- For *low risk*, the test is only considered positive if induration ≥15mm.

Box 11.5 IGRA, e.g. QuantiFERON-TB Gold (QFT-G), T-SPOT (type of ELISpot assay)

Advantages

This measures the release of interferon after stimulation *in vitro* by *Mycobacterium tuberculosis* antigens. The main advantages of this assay vs TST is:

- Lack of cross-reaction with BCG and most non-tuberculous mycobacteria.
- No need for patient to return for test reading in 48–72h.

Specificity and sensitivity

In the immunocompromised host and in paediatric populations, studies suggest that the QFT-G correlates better with the risk of TB than the TST, but data remain inconclusive. It is more specific than the TST because it is not confounded by prior BCG vaccination. In active TB, it has similar sensitivity to the TST. Current cross-sectional evidence suggests that, for the diagnosis of latent TB infection (LTBI), the sensitivity is similar to TST.

Treatment

Standard unsupervised treatment

If patient compliance is likely to be good, treatment is unsupervised with a daily regimen, usually using combination tablets, such as Rifater®, to increase convenience. Initial 2mo of rifampicin, isoniazid, pyrazinamide, ethambutol. Continuation 4mo of rifampicin and isoniazid only.

Supervised and extended treatment

Otherwise directly observed therapy (DOT) is instituted, with higher doses of the same drugs given three times/wk. Treatment may be prolonged to 9mo if immunosuppressed or disseminated disease.

Additional treatment

For ocular complications, such as CMO, retinal vasculitis, and persistent inflammation, consider oral corticosteroids but only if on effective anti-TB treatment.

Monitoring

U+E and LFT should be checked before starting treatment with rifampicin, isoniazid, and pyrazinamide. VA should be checked before starting treatment with ethambutol and the patient advised to report any visual disturbance (↓VA, ↓colour vision, ↓VF).

Mycobacterial disease (2)

Leprosy (Hansen's disease)

Worldwide, around 15 million people have leprosy, of whom about two-thirds are in Asia. The spectrum of leprosy is cased by the interaction of the obligate intracellular bacterium *Mycobacterium leprae* with the host's immune system. A poor cell-mediated immune response leads to the lepromatous form which is generalized and commonly affects the eyes. A strong response leads to tuberculoid leprosy which is more localized and rarely affects the eye.

Clinical features

Ophthalmic

- *External*: madarosis, trichiasis, lagophthalmos (VIIn palsy), conjunctivitis, epi-/scleritis, keratitis (neuropathic/exposure/2° infection).
- *Anterior*: anterior uveitis usually persistent, less commonly AAU; 'iris pearls' at the pupil margin which may enlarge and drop into the AC, iris atrophy, miosis.

Systemic

- *Tuberculoid*: thickened/tender nerves associated with hypopigmented anaesthetic patches and muscle atrophy.
- *Lepromatous*: nerve changes less marked but widespread infiltration, including skin, ears, nose (saddle nose), face (leonine appearance), larynx (hoarse voice).

Investigation and treatment

This should include skin/nasal mucosa smears for non-cultivable acid-fast bacilli. Systemic treatment should be coordinated by a specialist centre with multidisciplinary support. Treatment of eye disease is usually with topical steroids.

Spirochaetal and other bacterial uveitis

Syphilis

The spirochaete *Treponema pallidum* is usually transmitted by sexual contact or transplacentally. Acquired syphilis is divided into 1°, 2°, and tertiary stages. Congenital syphilis may be divided into early (equivalent to acquired 2° stage) and late (equivalent to acquired third stage).

Clinical features

(See Table 11.20 and Table 11.21.)

Anterior uveitis

This is the commonest ocular feature of both 2° and tertiary syphilis.
- Granulomatous or non-granulomatous; variable severity; ± roseolae (vascular fronds on the iris); ± iris atrophy; nodules on the iris/iridocorneal angle occur in tertiary disease only.

Posterior uveitis

This may be uni- or bilateral, uni- or multifocal, and choroiditis or chorioretinitis.
- Yellow plaque-like lesions with overlying vitritis ± serous retinal detachment. Resolution of the lesions results in a pigmentary retinopathy.

Investigation

(See Table 11.22.)
- *Non-treponemal serology*: venereal disease research laboratory (VDRL) tests disease activity; it may become negative in later disease syphilis. Rapid plasma reagin (RPR) is a simple test used in screening.
- *Treponemal serology*: fluorescent treponemal antibody absorption (FTA-ABS) and haemagglutination tests (TPHA) test previous or current infection. They do not distinguish from other treponematoses (e.g. yaws).
- Dark ground microscopy of chancre/mucocutaneous lesion.
- *LP*: consider if active ocular disease, suspected neurosyphilis, or HIV. CSF typically shows raised protein, pleocytosis, and positive VDRL.
- *HIV test*: co-infection is increasingly observed.

Treatment

Management of syphilitic eye disease should be in conjunction with a GU physician. Treatment requires high-dose penicillin, with an extended regimen for late latent and tertiary syphilis. Benzathine benzylpenicillin is now the preferred preparation for syphilis in the UK (unlicensed indication). Spirochaete death may transiently worsen inflammation (Jarisch–Herxheimer reaction). Consider topical steroids for interstitial keratitis and anterior uveitis. Systemic steroids must be used with caution but have a role in sight-threatening posterior uveitis or scleritis.

Other bacteria

Other bacteria which may cause uveitis include the spirochaetes *Borrelia burdorferi* (Lyme disease) and *Leptospira interrogans* (leptospirosis, including Weil's disease), the Gram-positive bacillus *Tropheryma whippelii* (Whipple's disease), and the Gram-negative bacilli *Bartonella henselae* (cat-scratch disease) and *Brucella* (brucellosis).

Table 11.20 Ophthalmic complications of syphilis

Adnexae	Gummata	Madarosis
Anterior segment	Conjunctival chancre Papillary conjunctivitis Epi-/scleritis	Interstitial keratitis Anterior uveitis
Posterior segment	Multi-/unifocal choroiditis/chorioretinitis	Neuroretinitis Retinal vasculitis
Neuro-ophthalmic	Argyll Robertson pupils Papilloedema Retrobulbar neuritis	Perioptic neuritis Ocular motility disorders VF defects

Table 11.21 Stages of syphilis

Stage	Main features
Congenital	
Early <2y of age	Mucocutaneous rash; periostitis and osteochondritis Chorioretinitis and retinal vasculitis producing the characteristic salt-and-pepper fundus
Late >2y of age	Saddle nose, frontal bossing, sabre shins, Hutchinson's teeth Interstitial keratitis
Acquired	
1° from 2wk post-infection	Painless ulcer (chancre), with regional lymphadenopathy, appears 2–6wk post-infection and resolves within a further 6wk
2° from 8wk post-infection	Diffuse maculopapular rash (including palms/soles), often with generalized lymphadenopathy, malaise, and fever Anterior or posterior uveitis
Tertiary from 5y post-infection	Around one-third progress to this stage. Aortitis may cause aortic regurgitation and dissection. Neurosyphilis may cause meningitis, CNS vasculitis, and parenchymatous degeneration, resulting in the syndromes of tabes dorsalis and generalized paresis of the insane (GPI) Anterior or posterior uveitis; interstitial keratitis

Table 11.22 Serological tests for syphilis

	1°		2°	Tertiary	Treated
	Early	Late			
VDRL	−/+	+	+	+	− or low +
Titre	Rising titre		Titre α activity	Titre may wane	Falling titre
FTA-ABS	+	+	+	+	+
TPHA	−/+	+	+	+	+

False-positive VDRL may occur in other conditions, including EBV, mycoplasma, autoimmune disease, chronic liver disease, and malignancy.

Protozoan uveitis

Toxoplasmosis

The protozoan *Toxoplasma gondii* is an obligate intracellular parasite which is estimated to infect up to 50% of the world's population. Lifetime risk of ocular toxoplasmosis is around 18/100,000 in the UK, but up to 20 times this level in West Africa.

Epidemiology

Prevalence and incidence of ocular symptoms after infection depend on socio-economic factors and the circulating parasite genotypes. Ocular toxoplasmosis is more common in South America, Central America, and the Caribbean and parts of tropical Africa, as compared to Europe and Northern America, and is quite rare in China. Ocular disease in South America is more severe than in other continents due to the presence of extremely virulent genotypes of the parasite.

Drinking untreated water is considered the major source of *Toxoplasma* infection in developing countries vs eating raw/undercooked meat/products in more developed countries. Acquired infection is now a more important source of ocular toxoplasmosis than congenital infection, and so prevention should be directed toward the whole population.

The definitive host is the cat; livestock and humans are only intermediate hosts. Oocysts are excreted in cat faeces which are ingested by humans/livestock in which they may become encysted (bradyzoite) or actively proliferate (tachyzoite). Human infection arises from contact with cat faeces/contaminated soil, ingestion of undercooked meat (bradyzoites), contaminated water, or transplacentally. Vertical transmission rate (transplacental) increases from 15% in the first trimester to 60% in the third trimester; disease severity is, however, much greater if acquired in early pregnancy.

Clinical features

Ophthalmic

Affects both eyes in 40%, but, if simultaneously active, suspect immunocompromise:

- Asymptomatic finding, floaters, ↓VA.
- Vitritis (may have 'vitreous precipitates' akin to KPs on posterior surface of PVD), retinitis (white, fluffy area when active; becomes circumscribed and pigmented as it heals; atrophic scar with pigmented border when inactive; satellite lesions adjacent to old scars commonly seen); retinal vasculitis (periphlebitis); may have an anterior uveitis often with ↑IOP.
- *Other presentations include*: scleritis, punctate outer retinitis (with quiet vitreous), large lesions (especially in the elderly), endophthalmitis-like, neuroretinitis, serous retinal detachments, pigmentary retinopathy.
- *Complications*: cataract, glaucoma, CNV membrane.

Systemic

- *Congenital*: the impact of transplacental infection is greatest early in pregnancy; complications include hydrocephalus, cerebral calcification, hepatosplenomegaly, retinochoroiditis (more commonly bilateral and affecting the macula).
- *Acquired*: if immunocompetent, is usually asymptomatic but may have fever and lymphadenopathy; if immunocompromised (usually HIV-positive patients), may have life-threatening disease, including encephalitis, intracerebral cysts, hepatitis, myocarditis.

Investigation

This is essentially a clinical diagnosis. Interpret positive serological tests with caution. Many of the adult population are positive for anti-*Toxoplasma* IgG; however, IgM antibodies do suggest acquired infection, and negative serology in undiluted serum makes the diagnosis unlikely. PCR of intraocular samples may also be used.

Treatment

Box 11.6 Indications for treatment

- Lesions involving disc, macula, or papillomacular bundle.
- Lesions threatening a major vessel.
- Marked vitritis.
- Any lesion in an immunocompromised patient.

A recent systematic review showed no level 1 evidence to support the efficacy of routine antibiotic or corticosteroid treatment for acute *Toxoplasma* retinochoroiditis in immunocompetent patients.[12] There is level 2 evidence suggesting that long-term prophylactic treatment may reduce recurrences in chronic relapsing disease. Nevertheless, generally accepted indications for treatment are outlined in Box 11.6.

- *Systemic*: ≥4wk of prednisolone AND co-trimoxazole OR clindamycin/sulfadiazine OR pyrimethamine/sulfadiazine/folinic acid (weekly FBC required) OR atovaquone. Steroids must not be used without effective anti-toxoplasmosis therapy and should not be given if immunosuppressed. For maternal infection acquired during pregnancy, use spiramycin (named-patient basis) to reduce transplacental spread. Atovaquone may theoretically reduce recurrences, as it is active against bradyzoites as well as tachyzoites. Azithromycin is used in some centres.

Prognosis

In immunocompetent patients, the disease is self-limiting and hence does not require treatment unless sight-threatening. Recurrence is common; mean number of recurrences is two, but a wide range is seen.

Pregnancy

Education is key (see Table 11.23). Some countries perform serial antenatal serological screening to detect active toxoplasmosis in order to permit early initiation of treatment. Treat maternal infection acquired during pregnancy with spiramycin.

Table 11.23 Toxoplasmosis and pregnancy

Advice	Wash all fruit/vegetables
	Avoid unpasteurized goat's milk
	Cook all meat thoroughly
	Avoid handling cat litter (or use rubber gloves)
Risk of transmission	15–60% risk if acquired during pregnancy
	No risk otherwise (even if recurrence of active disease during pregnancy)

Microsporidiosis

Microsporidia are protozoan obligate intracellular parasites, of which four genera may cause the human disease microsporidiosis. This is usually seen in the immunosuppressed (notably in AIDS) where it may present as chronic diarrhoea, respiratory infection, or keratoconjunctivitis. Microsporidial keratoconjunctivitis presents with bilateral irritation and photophobia, punctate keratopathy, often with a follicular conjunctivitis and/or an anterior uveitis.

12. Kim SJ et al. Interventions for Toxoplasma retinochoroiditis. *Ophthalmology* 2013;**120**:371–8.

Nematodal uveitis

Toxocariasis

The ascarid *Toxocara canis* is one of the commonest of all nematode infections and is a significant cause of visual loss worldwide. The definitive hosts are puppies (or kittens for the less common *T. catis*). Ova excreted in faeces are inadvertently ingested by humans in whom they develop into larvae. The larvae invade the gut wall and spread haematogenously throughout the body, notably to the liver, lung, brain, heart (visceral larva migrans), or the eye (ocular toxocariasis). Larval death causes an intense inflammatory reaction. Infection by *Toxocara* usually occurs <3y of age, although some ocular disease may not present until adulthood.

Clinical features

Ophthalmic

Ocular toxocariasis is unilateral. Presentation may vary with age:
- *Diffuse chronic endophthalmitis (age 2–9y)*: ↓VA + floaters; white eye with chronic anterior uveitis, PS, vitritis, snowbanking, macular oedema, ERD; complications include TRD, cyclitic membrane, cataract, hypotony.
- *Posterior pole granuloma (age 6–14y)*: ↓VA; yellow-white granuloma 1–2DD at the macula/papillomacular bundle with retinal traction and vitreous bands.
- *Peripheral granuloma (age 6–adult)*: usually asymptomatic until significant traction; yellow-white granuloma anterior to the equator with vitreous bands; traction may cause macula heterotopia or retinal detachment (tractional or rhegmatogenous).
- *Less common presentations include*: isolated anterior uveitis, intermediate uveitis, optic papillitis, and vitreous abscess.

Systemic (visceral larva migrans)

Usually <4y of age.
- Fever, pneumonitis + bronchospasm, hepatosplenomegaly, fits, myocarditis, death (rare); eosinophilia.

Investigation

This is essentially a clinical diagnosis, although ELISA for serum antibodies may be supportive, and B-scan US may help differentiate from other diagnoses.

Treatment

- *Ocular toxocariasis*: systemic or periocular steroids titrated according to disease severity; antihelminthics (e.g. thiabendazole) are of limited use; consider vitrectomy to clear debris, relieve traction, and to repair retinal detachments.

Diffuse unilateral subacute neuroretinitis (DUSN)

An increasingly recognized cause of posterior uveitis in young people, in which a solitary nematode persists in the subretinal space for years, causing progressive damage. Two unknown nematodes may cause the syndrome. They have different sizes (0.5mm and 1–2mm) and occur in different geographical distributions. Signs include a unilateral vitritis, optic disc swelling, deep retinal grey-white lesions, and sometimes the worm itself. Treatment is difficult. If directly visualized, the worm may be killed by argon laser; if not, use antihelminthics (e.g. thiabendazole). Steroids suppress inflammation but do not alter outcome.

Onchocerciasis

Worldwide onchocerciasis (river blindness) affects around 20 million people, causing visual impairment in 10%. The filarial nematode *Onchocerca volvulus* is spread between humans (definitive host) by bites of the Simulium blackfly (vector). Having entered the subcutaneous tissue, the larvae mature into adult worms (up to 80cm long) and mate to produce microfilariae within large subcutaneous nodules. The microfilariae then spread to nearby tissues which may include the eye. The Simulium breed in areas of fast-flowing water which also tend to be those regions which are most fertile and heavily farmed.

Ocular disease from the microfilariae includes sclerosing keratitis (with an opaque 'apron' over the inferior cornea), chorioretinitis, sclerosis of the retinal vessels, optic neuritis, and optic atrophy. Microfilariae may best be seen in the AC after face down posturing. Histology may be obtained from skin nodules.

Treatment was traditionally with diethylcarbamazine (which induces the severely itchy Mazzotti reaction) but has now been replaced with ivermectin.

Fungal uveitis

Candidiasis

Candida albicans is a higher fungus of the class *Blastomycetes*. It is yeast-like (i.e. reproduces by budding) and imperfect (i.e. no sexual stage has yet been identified). It is often a commensal of skin, mouth, and vagina, but opportunistic systemic infection may arise from haematogenous spread, notably in IV drug abuse, indwelling venous catheters, and immunosuppression (see Box 11.7). Uveitis in an IV drug abuser should be considered fungal until proven otherwise.

Clinical features
- *Risk group*: IV drug abuse, indwelling catheters (haemodialysis, parenteral nutrition), immunosuppression (AIDS, steroids, cytotoxics, long-term antibiotics), systemic debilitation (malignancy).
- ↓VA, floaters, pain; often bilateral.
- Multifocal retinitis (yellow-white fluffy lesions ≥1DD in size) ± vitritis (colonies appear as 'cotton balls' which may be joined together forming a 'string of pearls') ± anterior uveitis.
- *Complications*: retinal necrosis, TRD.

Investigation and treatment
- *Vitrectomy* (send whole vitrectomy cassette) for microscopy/culture to confirm diagnosis.
- *Intravitreal antifungals* (e.g. 5 micrograms amphotericin).
- *Systemic antifungals*: liaise with microbiologist/infectious disease specialist; oral fluconazole (usually 400mg initially, then 200mg 2×/d) ± flucytosine is generally effective; consider IV amphotericin (dose according to preparation) for known systemic involvement or resistant cases; duration of treatment is usually ≥4wk.
- Review frequently; admission may be helpful, especially if poor compliance likely or IV treatment necessary.

Aspergillosis

Aspergillus may occasionally cause an endogenous endophthalmitis similar to *Candida*. It generally occurs in those with chronic pulmonary disease who are severely immunosuppressed. It is more aggressive than candidal infection, with pain and rapid visual loss being marked. A confluent yellowish infiltrate is seen in the subretinal space which progresses to a subretinal hypopyon. Other features include intraretinal haemorrhages, dense vitritis, and AC hypopyon. Treatment is similar to *Candida* but usually requires IV Amphotericin. Final VA is usually <6/60.

Histoplasmosis and POHS

Histoplasma capsulatum is a higher dimorphic fungus which grows as a yeast at 37°C and as a mycelium in soil. It is endemic in southern Europe, southern USA, central America, and Asia. Ocular disease from direct infection of the globe is rare, usually occurs in the very young or the immunosuppressed, and may involve posterior/panuveitis or endophthalmitis. Treatment is with ketoconazole or amphotericin.

More commonly, *H. capsulatum* is invoked as the possible agent underlying POHS, albeit via an abnormal immune response. The evidence for *H. capsulatum* being the causative agent is, however, inconclusive. Epidemiology indicates that, while there is correlation between regions of high prevalence of *H. capsulatum* and POHS, an apparently identical syndrome is seen in non-endemic areas (such as the UK, northern Europe, and northern USA). It is most common in the fourth decade. It is usually bilateral but sequential, with a mean interval of 4y between onset of symptoms in each eye.

Clinical features
- Well-demarcated atrophic choroidal scars (≤1DD) around posterior pole/mid-periphery ('histo' spots); PPA; peripheral linear atrophic streaks; no significant vitritis.
- *Complications*: CNV (type 2); this is often the presenting feature of otherwise asymptomatic disease.

Investigation and treatment
Diagnosis is clinical, but FFA is required if CNV suspected. Antifungals have no benefit. Active lesions at the macula are often treated with immunosuppression (commonly corticosteroids). CNV are commonly treated with anti-VEGF therapies, although previously both argon laser, PDT, and surgical removal have all been used.[13]

Box 11.7 **Infections in the immunosuppressed: key points**

Which patients?
- HIV-positive.
- Post-transplantation (stem cell/solid organ).
- Therapeutic immunosuppression for systemic disease, e.g.
    - SLE.
    - RA.
    - GPA.

Which organisms?
- HIV—depends on CD4 count (see Table 11.19), but commonly CMV, toxoplasmosis (beware atypical presentations), syphilis, TB.
- Post-transplantation—commonly CMV or fungi.
- Therapeutic immunosuppression for systemic disease—commonly CMV, toxoplasma (beware atypical presentations); occasionally fungi.

13. Ramaiya KJ et al. Ranibizumab vs PDT for POHS. *Ophthalmic Surg Lasers Imaging Retina* 2013;44:17–21.

White dot syndromes (1)

See Table 11.24 for summary.

Acute posterior multifocal placoid pigment epitheliopathy (APMPPE)

This is an uncommon condition of young adults which is usually bilateral and may be preceded by a flu-like illness.

Clinical features
- Acute ↓VA sequentially in both eyes (usually after a few days interval).
- Post-equatorial placoid lesions of the RPE (initially creamy-white but fade over weeks, leaving irregular pigmentary changes), mild vitritis.

Investigations
- *FFA*: early dense hypofluorescence and late hyperfluorescence of lesions (classically described as 'block early and stain late').
- *ICG*: hypofluorescence of placoid areas.

Treatment
Spontaneous recovery within 2–3mo, so treatment is not usually indicated. Careful monitoring is important, as it may be difficult to distinguish APMPPE from the early stages of serpiginous choroidopathy.

Serpiginous choroidopathy

This is a rare, bilateral condition of the middle-aged that may superficially resemble APMPPE but has a much worse prognosis. TB should be excluded in all patients, as a serpiginous choroidopathy is a well-recognized clinical manifestation of TB; syphilis can also cause a similar picture.

Clinical features
- ↓VA but often asymptomatic until macular involvement.
- Serpiginous (pseudopodial) or geographic lesions at the level of the RPE/inner choroid (greyish-yellow, typically spread centrifugally from the disc but may 'skip', becomes atrophic over months with irregular depigmentation/pigmentation), mild vitritis.
- *Complications*: extensive subretinal scarring, CNV membrane (≤30%).

Investigations and treatment
- *FFA*: early dense hypofluorescence and late staining of lesions; inactive lesions may be hyperfluorescent due to atrophy.
- *ICG*: hypofluorescence of lesions.
- Corticosteroids/other immunosuppressives are commonly used in the acute phase, although there is no clear evidence of benefit. CNV membranes may be treated by laser, PDT, or surgery. There may be a role for intravitreal anti-VEGF therapy.

Table 11.24 Summary of white dot syndromes

Syndrome	Age	Sex	Laterality	Vitritis	Lesion size	Prognosis
PIC	20–40	♀ > ♂	Bilateral	–	1/10DD	Guarded
POHS	20–50	♂=♀	Bilateral	–	1/3DD	Guarded
MEWDS	20–40	♀ > ♂	Unilateral	+	1/5DD	Good
APMPPE	20–40	♂=♀	Bilateral	+	1DD	Good
Serpiginous choroidopathy	30–60	♂=♀	Bilateral	+		Poor
Birdshot chorioretinopathy	23–79	♀ > ♂	Bilateral	++	1/4–1/2DD	Guarded
Multifocal choroiditis with panuveitis (MCP)	30–60	♀ > ♂	Bilateral	++	1/10DD	Guarded

Birdshot chorioretinopathy

This is an uncommon bilateral condition of unknown aetiology, usually occurring in middle-aged Caucasian adults with a slight ♀ preponderance. Over 95% are HLA-A29 positive.

Clinical features
- ↓VA, ↓colour vision, floaters, nyctylopia.
- Oval, cream-coloured lesions radiating from the optic disc to the equator, associated with large choroidal vessels; become atrophic (but not normally pigmented), moderate vitritis, vasculitis, CMO.
- *Complications*: CNV membrane, optic atrophy.

Investigations
- *HLA testing*: HLA-A29 positive in >95%. If HLA-A29 negative, consider sarcoid as a differential since this can give a similar picture.[14]
- VFs.
- *FFA*: hyperfluorescence of the optic disc, retinal vessel leakage ± CMO; profuse leakage from choroidal circulation may mask spots (i.e. spots may be more visible on clinical examination than on FFA).
- *ICG*: hypofluorescent spots; inactive lesions remain hypofluorescent, whereas active lesions show late isofluorescence (i.e. become less obvious).
- *ERG*: ↓b-wave amplitude and latency, disease progression may be assessed using the 30Hz flicker implicit time; EOG: ↓Arden index. This is one condition in which electrodiagnostic results play a key role in directing treatment.[15]

Treatment
- The benefit of treatment in this condition is not well established. Common practice is to treat any CMO with 'rescue' corticosteroids and maintain on long-term immunosuppressants.

14. Brézin AP *et al.* HLA-A29 and birdshot chorioretinopathy. *Ocul Immunol Inflamm* 2011;**19**:397–400.

15. Holder GE *et al.* Electrophysiological characterization and monitoring in the management of birdshot chorioretinopathy. *Br J Ophthalmol* 2005;**89**:709–18.

White dot syndromes (2)

Multifocal choroiditis with panuveitis (MCP) and punctate inner choroidopathy (PIC)

These are uncommon bilateral conditions with some similarities to POHS. Both are commoner in women, but PIC tends to affect a younger age group. A viral aetiology has been suggested. Whether these represent separate conditions or a spectrum of disease is still a matter of debate.[16]

Clinical features

- ↓VA, scotomata, photopsia.
- *MCP*: choroidal lesions (grey, peripheral + posterior polar), vitritis, anterior uveitis, CMO, subretinal fibrosis, CNV membrane.
- *PIC*: 'quiet' eye (no vitritis) with lesions at the level of the inner choroid/retina (initially yellow-white but become atrophic pigmented scars similar to POHS; posterior polar), serous retinal detachment, CNV membrane.

Investigations and treatment

- *FFA*: early hypofluorescence and late hyperfluorescence (staining) of lesions.
- *ICG*: hypofluorescent lesions (often more numerous than visible clinically).
- *OCT*: may track progression of PIC lesions.[17]

If CNV: intravitreal anti-VEGF therapy is commonly used, although intravitreal corticosteroids and PDT may also have a role.[18]

The benefit of immunosuppression in this condition is not well established and is particularly difficult to judge in PIC where typical measures of active inflammation are lacking. Common practice in MCP is to treat any CMO with 'rescue' corticosteroids and maintain on long-term immunosuppressants.

Multiple evanescent white dot syndrome (MEWDS)

This is a rare unilateral condition, typically of young women, which may be preceded by a flu-like illness.

Clinical features

- Acute ↓VA, scotomata ± photopsia, transient RAPD sometimes present.
- Small white dots at level of outer retina/RPE, tiny orange-white dots at the fovea (this 'foveal granularity' is nearly pathognomonic), mild vitritis.

Investigations and treatment

- *FFA*: each white dot consists of punctate hyperfluorescent spots in a 'wreath-like' cluster, with late staining; disc leakage and retinal capillary leakage.
- *ICG*: multiple hypofluorescent dots which become confluent around the optic disc.
- *ERG*: ↓a-wave.

Spontaneous recovery within 2–3mo, so treatment is not usually indicated.

Acute zonal occult outer retinopathy (AZOOR)

This may form part of a spectrum of disease comprising MEWDS, MCP, PIC, and the acute idiopathic blind spot enlargement syndrome (AIBES). It is an uncommon condition affecting one or both eyes, typically in myopic young/middle-aged women after a flu-like illness.

Clinical features

- Acute scotomata, worse in bright light; photopsia.
- Acutely may have mild vitritis; later may have zonal atrophy/irregular pigmentation (RP-like).

Investigations and treatment

- *ERG*: variably abnormal in a patchy distribution and often asymmetric.
- Immunosuppression is common during the acute phase but is of no proven benefit.

16. Spaide RF *et al.* Redefining multifocal choroiditis and panuveitis and punctate inner choridopathy through multimodal imaging. *Retina* 2013;**33**:1315–24.

17. Zhang X *et al.* Spectral-domain OCT findings at each stage of punctate inner choroidopathy. *Ophthalmology* 2013;**120**:2678–83.

18. Rouvas A *et al.* Intravitreal ranibizumab for the treatment of inflammatory choroidal neovascularization. *Retina* 2011;**31**:871–9.

Vitreoretinal

Anatomy and physiology

Anatomy

Vitreous

The vitreous makes up 80% of ocular volume or about 4.0mL. It is a transparent gel, of which 99% is water. The remainder consists of hyaluronic acid and collagen (types II, IX, and a V/XI hybrid).

Collagen fibrils connect the vitreous to the retinal internal limiting membrane.

The vitreous base is a 3–4mm wide zone overlying the ora serrata.

Retina

See **➜** Anatomy and physiology (1), p. 516.

The retina is a transparent light-transforming laminated structure, comprising photoreceptors, interneurones, and ganglion cells overlying the RPE.

Superficial retinal vessels form four major arcades over the surface of the retina. Within the suprachoroidal space are the long posterior ciliary nerves and arteries that can be seen peripherally at 3 and 9 o'clock. Similarly, the vortex ampullae (which drain into the vortex veins) may be seen in all four diagonal quadrants just anterior to the equator.

Vitreoretinal adhesions

- *Normal attachments* are strongest at the disc, the fovea, and, in particular, the ora serrata/vitreous base that remains adherent, even when PVD is otherwise complete.
- *Abnormal attachments* include areas of lattice degeneration (posterior border), white-without-pressure, congenital cystic tufts, pigment clumps, and condensations around vessels.

Physiology

Forces of attachment

The retinal position is maintained by hydrostatic forces and, to a lesser extent, by the adhesion of the interphotoreceptor matrix. The hydrostatic forces are both active (the RPE pump) and passive (the osmotic gradient).

Forces of detachment

Vitreoretinal traction may be dynamic (due to eye movement) or static (due purely to vitreoretinal interaction, e.g. diabetic fibrovascular proliferation). The direction of static forces may be tangential, bridging, or anteroposterior. Gravitational forces are probably a significant factor in superior breaks.

Vitreous liquefaction

The ageing vitreous becomes progressively liquefied (synersis), resulting in optically empty fluid-filled spaces (lacunae) and a reduction in the shock-absorbing capacity of the vitreous.

Liquefaction occurs earlier in myopia, trauma, inflammation, and many collagen and connective tissue disorders. A break in the cortical vitreous permits vitreal fluid to flow through into the retrohyaloid space, causing separation and collapse of the remaining vitreous (PVD).

Retinal detachment: assessment

Retinal detachment is a relatively common sight-threatening condition, with an incidence of about 1/10,000/y (see Tables 12.1–12.3).

Rhegmatogenous retinal detachment (RRD)

This is usually an ophthalmic emergency, notably in the presence of a U-shaped tear and where the macula is still 'on' (i.e. attached) (see ⬧ Rhegmatogenous retinal detachment (1), p. 486).

It is the commonest form of retinal detachment and usually arises when PVD causes a break in the retina, although some RRD arise without PVD (e.g. with round holes or with dialysis).

Untreated, it almost always leads to a blind eye but, with appropriate early treatment, may have an excellent outcome.

Table 12.1 An approach to assessing retinal detachments

Visual symptoms	Asymptomatic; flashes, floaters, distortion, 'curtain' field defect, ↓VA
POH	Refractive error (myopia), surgery (e.g. complicated cataract extraction), laser treatment, trauma
PMH	Connective tissue syndromes (e.g. Stickler), diabetes, anaesthetic history
FH	Retinal problems/detachments, connective tissue syndromes
SH	Driver; occupation
Dx	Anti-thrombotic and anti-coagulant use
Ax	Allergies or relevant drug contraindications
VA	Best corrected/pinhole
Pupils	RAPD (if extensive retinal detachment)
Cornea	Clarity (for surgery)
AC	Cells/flare (mild activity is common)
Lens	Cataract
Tonometry	IOP may be low, normal, or high
Vitreous	Haemorrhage, pigment ('tobacco dust', Shafer's sign)
Fundus	Retinal detachment: location, extent, age (atrophy, intraretinal cysts, pigment demarcation lines), proliferative vitreoretinopathy (vitreous haze, retinal stiffness, retinal folds); retinal break(s): location, associated degeneration
Macula	On, threatened, or off
Other eye	Degenerations, breaks, other disease

Indirect fundoscopy with scleral indentation to the ora serrata of both eyes.

Tractional retinal detachment (TRD) and exudative retinal detachment (ERD)

In these, there are usually no causative breaks in the retina; it is either pulled (tractional) or pushed (exudative) from position.

- Tractional detachments (see ➲ Tractional retinal detachment, p. 490) tend to be slowly progressive but may be static for long periods.
- Exudative detachments (see ➲ Exudative retinal detachment, p. 491) may fluctuate according to the underlying disease process.

Table 12.2 Differentiating features of retinal detachments

	RRD	ERD	TRD
Vitreous	Pigment ± blood	No pigment ± inflammatory cells	No pigment
Fluid	Fairly static	Dependent shifting fluid	Little fluid, non-shifting
Shape	Convex corrugated	Convex smooth	Concave
Retinal features	Break(s) ± degeneration	Normal or features of underlying disease	Preretinal fibrosis

Table 12.3 Differentiating features of RRD vs retinoschisis

	RRD	Retinoschisis
Dome	Convex corrugated	Convex smooth
Laterality	Unilateral	Usually bilateral
Field defect	Relative	Absolute
Chronic changes	Demarcation line	No demarcation line
Breaks	Present	Absent or small inner leaf holes
Response to laser	No uptake	Good uptake

Peripheral retinal degenerations

Almost all eyes have some abnormality of the peripheral retina. Only about 1 in 40 of the population develop any form of retinal break. Identification of different types of peripheral retinal degeneration permits risk stratification and selective treatment of those lesions that are likely to progress (see Table 12.4).

It is important to appreciate that prophylactic laser treatment may carry the risk of *causing* retinal breaks.[1]

Lattice degeneration

Lattice degeneration is present in about 6% of the normal population but 30% of all RRDs. It is more common in myopes and connective tissue syndromes (e.g. Stickler).

- Areas of retinal thinning with criss-cross white lines ± small round holes within the lesion; typically circumferential but may be radial (more common in Stickler).
- Retinal tears may occur at posterior margin and at the ends of areas of lattice (due to strong vitreous adhesion) → retinal detachment.
- Clinical retinal detachment occurs in only 1% of patients with lattice degeneration.[2] Prophylactic laser treatment is not usually performed in asymptomatic eyes, unless the fellow eye has previously had a detachment.

Snailtrack degeneration

- Snailtrack degeneration is relatively common in myopes and may be an early form of lattice degeneration.[3]
- Long circumferential areas of retinal thinning with a glistening appearance ± large round holes.
- Large round holes within the lesion may lead to retinal detachment.

Peripheral cystoid degeneration

- Peripheral cystoid degeneration increases with age to become almost universal.
- Close-packed tiny cystic spaces at the outer plexiform/inner nuclear level ± retinoschisis.

Retinoschisis (degenerative type)

- Retinoschisis is present in about 5% of the normal population but is more common in hypermetropes. It is usually bilateral. It is asymptomatic, unless posterior extension causes a significant field defect.
- Splitting of retina usually at outer plexiform/inner nuclear level leads to inner leaf ballooning into the vitreous cavity; usually inferotemporal and arising in areas of peripheral cystoid degeneration.
- Rarely, a combination of small inner leaf holes and the less common larger outer leaf breaks may lead to retinal detachment.

White without pressure

- This is fairly common in young and heavily pigmented patients. It represents the vitreoretinal interface and is probably of no significance.
- Whitened ring of retina just posterior to the ora and underlying the vitreous base.

Snowflake degeneration

- Snowflake degeneration may represent vitreous attachments to retinal Müller cells. It is probably of no significance; rare familial cases probably reflect a different process.
- Diffuse frosted appearance with white dots.

Pavingstone degeneration

- Pavingstone degeneration is common with increasing age and myopia.
- Irregular patches of absent RPE and choriocapillaris, forming windows to the large choroidal vessels and sclera ± mild retinal thinning.

Cobblestone degeneration

- Cobblestone degeneration is commoner with increasing age and is of no significance.
- Small drusen-like bodies with pigment ring at level of Bruch's membrane.

Reticular pigmentary degeneration (honeycomb pigmentation)

- Reticular pigmentary degeneration is commoner with increasing age and is of no significance.
- Honeycomb pattern of peripheral pigmentation.

Meridional folds

- Meridional folds do not increase risk of retinal detachment, but, in cases of detachment, the hole(s) may be closely related to these folds.
- Small radial fold of retina in axis of dentate process ± small hole at base.

Retinal tufts

- Retinal tufts are common lesions and often associated with holes; however, they are usually within the vitreous base and thus of no significance.
- White inward projections of retina due to abnormal traction ± small holes.

Table 12.4 Peripheral retinal degenerations

Moderate risk	Low risk	Minimal risk
Lattice	Peripheral cystoid degeneration	Pavingstone degeneration
Snailtrack	Retinoschisis	Cobblestone degeneration
	White without pressure	Reticular pigmentary degeneration
	Snowflake degeneration	
	Meridional folds	
	Retinal tufts	

1. Chauhan DS et al. Failure of prophylactic retinopexy in fellow eyes without a posterior vitreous detachment. Arch Ophthalmol 2006;**124**:968–71.

2. Byer NE. Long-term natural history of lattice degeneration of the retina. Ophthalmology 1989;**96**:1396–402.

3. Shukla M et al. A possible relationship between lattice and snail track degenerations of the retina. Am J Ophthalmol 1981;**92**:482–5.

Retinal breaks

Around 2.5% of the population have an identifiable full-thickness retinal defect (break). As progression to retinal detachment is rare and retinopexy (laser or cryotherapy) is not without risk, attempts have been made to identify and treat only the high-risk group. High risk may be a function of the type of break (e.g. fresh symptomatic U-tear associated with acute PVD), the eye (e.g. high myopia), events in the contralateral eye (e.g. giant retinal tear), or the patient as a whole (e.g. Stickler syndrome) (see Table 12.5 and Table 12.6).

Retinal hole

This is a full-thickness retinal defect due to atrophy without vitreoretinal traction. It may be associated with peripheral retinal degeneration, e.g. lattice or snailtrack. An operculated hole is used to denote a hole caused by PVD where the operculum has avulsed and is now free-floating within the vitreous.

Retinal tear

This is a full-thickness U-shaped defect due to PVD. It is associated with abnormal vitreous adhesions, e.g. lattice degeneration. Ongoing vitreoretinal traction at flap apex causes progression to RRD in at least one-third of cases.

Giant retinal tear

A giant retinal tear is a tear of >3 clock-hours in extent. They are normally located in the peripheral retina at the posterior border of the vitreous base. They are associated with PVD, distinguishing a giant retinal tear from a retinal dialysis. The vitreous remains attached to the anterior retinal remnant. They are associated with systemic disease (e.g. Marfan's syndrome and Stickler syndrome), trauma, and high myopia. They can become bilateral in 16.5%, with retinal breaks noted in the fellow eyes of 60% of cases.[4] A Cochrane review looking at prophylactic treatment for giant retinal tears in 2012 did not find any studies that met the inclusion criteria for the review.

Dialysis

This is a full-thickness circumferential disinsertion of the retina from the ora serrata. It may arise spontaneously or after trauma. It is not related to PVD and usually progresses slowly as the vitreous is attached. It is usually inferotemporal, but post-trauma cases may be superonasal.

Treatment of retinal breaks

- Treatment is controversial. Common practice is that all U-tears (especially if symptomatic) should be treated, usually with laser photocoagulation or, less commonly, cryotherapy. Asymptomatic small round holes are commonly not treated. Dialyses are treated with scleral buckling if there is associated retinal detachment or with laser/cryotherapy if no/limited retinal detachment.

- Fellow eye treatment is also controversial. In giant retinal tear, the fellow eye is often treated, e.g. with 360° cryotherapy or laser.[5] In a case of simple RRD, lattice in the fellow eye is often not treated, unless there is an additional risk factor, e.g. high myopia, aphakia, etc.
- A 'retinal detachment warning' should be given in all cases, i.e. advise to seek urgent ophthalmic review if further episodes of new floaters, flashes, a 'curtain' field defect, or drop in vision.

Table 12.5 Risk factors for RRD according to type of break

High risk	Low risk
Giant retinal tear in the other eye	Asymptomatic small round holes
U-tear, large hole, or dialysis	Breaks within the vitreous base

Table 12.6 Risk factors for RRD according to other ocular and systemic features

Ocular	General	Trauma (blunt/penetrating) surgery
	Refractive	Myopia
	Lenticular	Aphakia
		Pseudophakia (especially complicated surgery, e.g. vitreous loss)
		Posterior capsulotomy
	Retinal	Lattice degeneration
		Retinoschisis
		Retinal necrosis (CMV, ARN/PORN)
	Other eye	Previous contralateral retinal detachment (especially giant retinal tear)
Systemic		Stickler syndrome
		Marfan's syndrome
		Ehlers–Danlos syndrome

4. Freeman HM. Fellow eyes of non-traumatic giant retinal breaks. In: Ryan SJ (ed.) *Retina* (Volume 3). St. Louis: Mosby; 2001. pp.2366–70.

5. Wolfensberger TJ *et al.* Prophylactic 360° cryotherapy in fellow eyes of patients with spontaneous giant retinal tears. *Ophthalmology* 2003;**110**:1175–7.

Posterior vitreous detachment

With age, the vitreous becomes progressively liquefied (syneresis). This results in optically empty spaces (lacunae) and a reduction in its shock-absorbing capability. The liquefaction process occurs earlier in myopia, trauma, inflammation, and many disorders of collagen and connective tissue. When a break in the cortical vitreous occurs, vitreal fluid can flow through into the retrohyaloid space to cause separation of the vitreous and retina, with collapse of the remaining vitreous—PVD.

It is of significance because: (1) it is very common; (2) it may be associated with a retinal tear in 10% cases; and (3) the symptoms are similar to retinal detachment.

Clinical features

- Flashes (usually an arc of white light in the temporal field of view), floaters (usually a ring or cobwebs; move or 'wobble' with ocular movement; the less common shower of black specks suggests haemorrhage and is more often associated with a retinal tear).
- *Vitreous*: Weiss ring (indicates detachment at the optic disc), visible 'wrinkly' posterior hyaloid face; occasionally haemorrhage.
- *Complications*: retinal break(s), vitreous haemorrhage, retinal detachment.

NB It is critical to achieve a complete fundal examination using 360° scleral indentation to rule out any associated retinal breaks. Remember in eyes with retinal breaks, there is >1 break in 50% cases.

Treatment

- *Uncomplicated PVD:* reassure, but give 'retinal detachment warning', i.e. advise to seek urgent ophthalmic review if further episodes of new floaters, flashes, a 'curtain' field defect, or drop in vision
- *PVD complicated by vitreous haemorrhage:* clear visualization of whole retina to the ora serrata is necessary to rule out breaks/early RRD; if not possible, then use B-scan US (see Table 12.7); follow up frequently as an outpatient until haemorrhage has cleared.

NB US can miss retinal tears: a large fundus-obscuring haemorrhage in a high-risk eye is best treated by early vitrectomy.

- *PVD complicated by retinal tear:* treat, e.g. by laser photocoagulation (focal argon retinopexy).

Table 12.7 Ultrasonic features of vitreoretinal pathology

PVD	Faintly reflective posterior hyaloid face may appear incomplete, except on eye movement
	Eye movement induces staccato movement with 1s after-movement
	Low reflectivity on A-scan
	No blood demonstrated on colour flow mapping
RRD	Highly reflective irregular convex membrane
	Eye movement induces undulating after-movement (unless PVR)
	High reflectivity on A-scan Single peak on A-scan
	Blood demonstrated on colour flow mapping
TRD	Highly reflective membrane tented into vitreous Eye movement induces no after-movement of membrane
	Blood demonstrated on colour flow mapping
Choroidal detachment	Highly reflective regular dome-shaped membrane Attached to the vortex ampulla/vein
	Blood demonstrated on colour flow mapping, both in retina (6–8cm/s) and choroid (8–10cm/s) Twin peak on A-scan
Vitreous haemorrhage	Reflective particulate matter within the vitreous space (indistinguishable from vitritis)
	A subhyaloid haemorrhage will show an elevated posterior vitreous face with delayed movement on ocular motility
	More detailed examination can usually distinguish the underlying cause, e.g. RRD, CNV, PDR, or C/BRVO

Rhegmatogenous retinal detachment (1)

RRD is usually an ophthalmic emergency. Untreated, it usually progresses to blindness and even phthisis. However, with appropriate early treatment, it may have an excellent outcome. It is the commonest form of retinal detachment, with an incidence of 1/10,000/y.

RRD occurs when vitreous liquefaction and a break in the retina allow fluid to enter the subretinal space and separate the neural retina from the RPE (see Box 12.1 and Table 12.8 and Table 12.9).

Clinical features

- Flashes (usually temporal, more noticeable in dim conditions), floaters (distinct, e.g. Weiss ring, or particulate, e.g. blood), 'curtain' type field defect, ↓VA (suggests macula involvement).
- *Vitreous*: PVD + vitreal pigment ('tobacco dust') ± blood. These are more obvious on vitreous movement: ask the patient to look up and down while at the slit-lamp.
- *Retinal break(s)*: usually U-tear (occasionally giant, i.e. >3 clock-hours); sometimes large round holes or dialysis. The upper temporal quadrant is the commonest location (60%). Identifying the 1° break may be assisted by considering the effect of gravity on the SRF (see Box 12.1, modified from Lincoff's rules).[6] However, multiple breaks are common, and meticulous view of the whole peripheral retina is essential.
- *Retinal detachment*: unilateral corrugated convex dome of retina and loss of RPE markings; usually peripheral (SRF extends to ora serrata) but occasionally posterior polar if 2° to a macular or other posterior hole.
- *Chronic changes*: retinal thinning, demarcation lines from 3mo, intraretinal cysts from 1y; some develop proliferative vitreoretinopathy. May also have RAPD (if extensive detachment), relative field defect, ↓IOP (but may be normal or ↑ (Schwartz syndrome)), and mild AC activity.

RRD associated with round holes or dialysis

These are not associated with a PVD and so do not get associated symptoms of flashes and floaters; these RRD are therefore usually picked up as an asymptomatic finding or when macular involvement causes ↓VA.

Box 12.1 Locating the 1° retinal break[*]

In superior retinal detachments[*]

- For superonasal or superotemporal detachments, the break is usually near the superior border of the detachment.
- For symmetric superior detachments crossing the vertical meridian (i.e. superonasal and superotemporal), the break is usually near 12 o'clock.

In inferior retinal detachments

- For inferior detachments, the break is usually on the side with most fluid (i.e. the higher fluid level) BUT:
  - It may be quite inferior (i.e. not related to the superior border), and
  - Slower fluid accumulation means that non-midline breaks may still result in symmetrical inferior detachments.
- For bullous inferior detachments, the 1° break is above the horizontal meridian, sometimes at the apex of a peripheral track of detached retina.

[*] Lincoff H et al. Finding the hole. Arch Ophthalmol 1971;**85**:565–69.

Table 12.8 Features of a chronic retinal detachment

Retinal thinning
Demarcation lines ('high tide marks')
Intraretinal cysts
Proliferative vitreoretinopathy

Table 12.9 Proliferative vitreoretinopathy

Type	A		Vitreous haze/pigment
			Pigment on inner retina
	B		Retinal wrinkling + stiffness
	C		Rigid retinal folds ('starfolds')
Subtypes of C			
Location	Pre-equatorial		Anterior
	Post-equatorial		Posterior
Extent	1–12		Number of clock-hours
Contraction	Type 1		Focal
	Type 2		Diffuse
	Type 3		Subretinal
	Type 4		Circumferential
	Type 5		Anterior

6. Lincoff H et al. Finding the hole. Arch Ophthalmol 1971;**85**:565–69.

Rhegmatogenous retinal detachment (2)

Investigation
- *Consider US*: if unable to adequately visualize (e.g. dense cataract or haemorrhage).
- *B-scan US*: highly reflective irregular convex membrane; eye movement induces undulating after-movement (unless PVR).
- *A-scan US*: single highly reflective spike.

Treatment
Urgent vitreoretinal referral
- Macula-on detachments with a U-tear should be referred urgently.
- Once the macula has detached, there is some evidence that surgery within 7–10d has the same visual outcome.[7,8]

Preoperative posturing
- *Posture so that dependent fluid moves away from macula*: it is mainly useful for upper bullous detachments and giant retinal tears (position so tear is unfolded).
- Traditional posturing for superior detachments would usually involve being flat on one's back, with ipsilateral cheek to pillow for temporal detachments (i.e. right cheek for right eye) and contralateral cheek to pillow for nasal detachments (i.e. left cheek for right eye).
- Posturing is not of use in RRD associated with round holes or a dialysis.

Surgery
Scleral buckling and vitrectomy have advantages in different contexts. Vitrectomy is now the more commonly used procedure (about 80% cases), but there is considerable inter-surgeon variation.
- *Scleral buckling* (see ➜ Scleral buckling procedures, p. 506): suitable for most simple RRD and procedure of choice if no pre-existing PVD; segmental (single breaks or multiple breaks within 1 clock-hour) vs encircling (more extensive breaks).
- *Pneumatic retinopexy* (see ➜ Pneumatic retinopexy, p. 504): has a lower success rate of 66%[9] and is thus better utilized in carefully selected cases of localized shallow detachments with small superior breaks 1 clock-hour apart between 11 and 1 o'clock.
- *Vitrectomy* (see ➜ Vitrectomy: outline, p. 508): indicated for retinal detachments with posterior retinal breaks, giant retinal tears, proliferative vitreoretinopathy, but also increasingly used for bullous retinal detachments of all types, including those with high-risk features (e.g. aphakia/pseudophakia).
- *Combined vitrectomy and scleral buckling procedure*: indicated for inferior retinal breaks, multiple small breaks at the ora serrata, and traumatic retinal detachment.

7. Ross WH *et al.* Visual recovery in macula-off rhegmatogenous retinal detachments. *Ophthalmology* 1998;**105**:2149–53.

8. Hassan TS *et al.* The effect of duration of macular detachment on results after the scleral buckle repair of primary, macula-off retinal detachments. *Ophthalmology* 2002;**109**:146–52.

9. Fabian ID *et al.* Pneumatic retinopexy for the repair of primary rhegmatogenous retinal detachment: a 10 year retrospective analysis. *JAMA Ophthalmol* 2013;**131**:166–71.

Tractional retinal detachment

TRD (see Table 12.10) is uncommon. It arises due to a combination of contracting retinal membranes, abnormal vitreoretinal adhesions, and vitreous changes. It is usually seen in the context of diseases that induce a fibrovascular response, e.g. diabetes.

Clinical features

- Often asymptomatic; distortion (if macular involvement).
- *Retinal detachment*: concave tenting of retina that is immobile and usually shallow ± macular ectopia (drag); slowly progressive.
- May also have relative field defect, metamorphopsia on Amsler grid, ↓VA, and evidence of underlying disease process (e.g. diabetic retinopathy).
- *Complications*: may detach the macula or may develop a break to become a rapidly progressive combined tractional RRD.

Treatment

Surgery is difficult and thus often deferred until the macula is threatened or detached. It usually requires removal of tractional forces by vitrectomy and membrane peel, or delamination followed by tamponade with either a long-acting gas or oil, if needed (retinal break).

Surgery for TRD is based on the underlying cause. Vitrectomy with delamination, segmentation, membrane dissection is the mainstay of treatment, particularly when the tractional detachment is 2° to PDR. The adjuvant use of anti-VEGF, such as bevacizumab, reduces haemorrhages. Peroperative use of triamcinolone and bimanual techniques improve the accuracy of membrane dissection, reducing the incidence of iatrogenic retinal breaks.

Outcomes of vitrectomy for non-clearing vitreous haemorrhages have improved with advances such as the use of wide-angled viewing systems, endolaser, and use of anti-VEGF. Patients should be considered for vitrectomy earlier to prevent visual morbidity due to retinal dysfunction.

Table 12.10 Causes of TRD (selected)

PDR
ROP
Sickle cell retinopathy
Familial exudative vitreoretinopathy (FEVR)
Vitreomacular traction syndrome
Incontinentia pigmenti
Retinal dysplasia

Exudative retinal detachment

Exudative (serous) retinal detachment (ERD) is relatively rare. It arises from damage to the outer blood–retinal barrier, allowing fluid to access the sub-retinal space and separate retina from RPE (see Table 12.11).

Clinical features

- Distortion and ↓VA (if macula involved), which may fluctuate; relative field defect; floaters (if vitritis).
- *Retinal detachment*: smooth convex dome that may be shallow or bullous; in bullous ERDs, the fluid moves rapidly to the most dependent position ('shifting fluid'); the fluid may be clear or cloudy (lipid-rich); no vitreous pigment, PVD, retinal breaks, or evidence of traction.
- May also have irregular pigmentation of previously detached areas and evidence of underlying disease (e.g. abnormal Coats' vessels).

Investigation and treatment

- All patients require a full ophthalmic and systemic examination, BP, and urinalysis.
- Consider B-scan US, especially if posterior scleritis suspected.
- Surgery is very rarely indicated, and treatment is directed towards the underlying disease process.

Table 12.11 Common causes of ERD

Congenital		Nanophthalmos (→2° uveal effusion syndrome)
		Mucopolysaccharidoses (II and VI)
		FEVR
Acquired	Vascular	Exudative AMD
		Coats' disease
		Central serous chorioretinopathy
		Vasculitis
		Malignant hypertension
		Pre-eclampsia
	Tumours	Choroidal tumours
	Inflammatory	Posterior uveitis (notably VKH syndrome, sympathetic ophthalmia)
		Posterior scleritis
		Post-operative inflammation
		Extensive PRP
		Orbital cellulitis
		Idiopathic orbital inflammatory disease

Retinoschisis

Retinoschisis is, by definition, a splitting of the retina. Degenerative retinoschisis is common, being present in about 5% of the normal adult population.

Degenerative retinoschisis

Degenerative retinoschisis (see Table 12.12) is more common in hypermetropes and is usually bilateral.

In typical senile retinoschisis, the split is at the outer plexiform/inner nuclear level. In the less common reticular type, the split is at the nerve fibre layer (i.e. as occurs in XL juvenile retinoschisis; see ➔ X-linked juvenile retinoschisis, p. 494).

Clinical features

- Asymptomatic (unless very posterior extension); absolute field defect.
- *Retinoschisis*: split retina with inner leaf ballooning into the vitreous cavity; usually inferotemporal; arises in areas of peripheral cystoid degeneration; scleral indentation may cause outer leaf to whiten, sometimes with a reticular appearance.
- *'T-bar test'*: using the indirect ophthalmoscope, project a T-shape using the head of a scleral indenter onto the retinoschisis. The patient will be unable to see the T-shape due to the absolute scotoma caused by the retinoschisis.

Complications

- Inner leaf breaks (small/round) and/or outer leaf breaks (less common; large with rolled edges).
- *Retinal detachment*: either low-risk limited type (outer leaf break only, with fluid from the schisis cavity causing local retinal elevation) or high-risk rhegmatogenous type (inner and outer leaf breaks, with full-thickness retinal elevation beyond area of schisis).

Investigations

This is essentially a clinical diagnosis, but laser take-up by the posterior leaf or OCT findings can differentiate from retinal detachment.

Treatment

No treatment is necessary unless complicated by retinal detachment.

X-linked juvenile retinoschisis

This rare condition is seen in ♂ and may present in childhood with maculopathy. It results in retinal splitting at the nerve fibre layer (cf. typical degenerative retinoschisis). Visual prognosis is poor. (See ➔ X-linked juvenile retinoschisis, p. 494.)

Table 12.12 Differentiating retinoschisis from chronic RRD

	Retinoschisis	RRD
Vitreous	Clear	Pigment ± blood
Dome	Convex smooth	Convex corrugated
Laterality	Usually bilateral	Unilateral
Field defect	Absolute	Relative
Signs of chronicity	No demarcation line	Demarcation line
Breaks	Absent or small inner leaf holes	Present
Response to laser	Good uptake	No uptake

Hereditary vitreoretinal degenerations

These are rare inherited conditions characterized by premature degeneration of vitreous and retina.

Interestingly, the 1° abnormality may be vitreal with 2° retinal changes (e.g. Stickler syndrome) or retinal with 2° vitreous abnormalities (e.g. XL juvenile retinoschisis).

Stickler syndrome

This condition arises from abnormalities in type II collagen (*COL2A1*, Chr 12q13 and Chr 11q13.2) and type XI collagen (*COL11A1*, Chr 1p21) and is AD with complete penetrance but variable expressivity.

Also known as hereditary arthro-ophthalmopathy, it is the commonest of this group of conditions and the commonest cause of inherited RRD.

Clinical features

- High myopia, optically empty vitreous, perivascular pigmentary changes (lattice-like).
- COL2A1 has membranous remnants in the vitreous cavity, whilst COL11A1 has beaded vitreous remnants.[10]
- *Complications*: retinal tears, giant retinal tears, retinal detachments, cataract (comma-shaped cortical opacities), ectopia lentis, glaucoma (open-angle).
- *Systemic*: epiphyseal dysplasia → degeneration of large joints, cleft palate, bifid uvula, mid-facial flattening, Pierre–Robin sequence, sensorineural deafness, mitral valve prolapse.

Investigations and treatment

- Essentially a clinical diagnosis, although molecular genetic testing allows the ophthalmologist to distinguish ocular from non-ocular variants. This allows prophylaxis to be given at a younger age
- Consider annual dilated fundoscopy
- Unfortunately, retinal detachments are common (up to 70%) and carry a poor prognosis with a high prevalence of giant retinal tears.
- Prophylactic retinopexy reduces the retinal detachment rate to 8%.[11]
- Multidisciplinary care may include genetic counselling.
- Treat myopia early to prevent amblyopia.

X-linked juvenile retinoschisis

This rare condition appears to arise from abnormalities in an intercellular adhesion molecule (located on Xp22), which results in retinal splitting at the nerve fibre layer.

It is seen in ♂ and may present in early childhood with maculopathy. Visual prognosis is poor.

Clinical features
- Foveal schisis with spoke-like folds separating cystoid spaces (superficially resembles CMO but no leakage on FFA); later non-specific atrophy; peripheral retinal schisis ± inner leaf breaks (may coalesce to leave free-floating retinal vessels).
- *Complications*: vitreous haemorrhage, retinal detachment.

Investigations
- This is essentially a clinical diagnosis.
- Scotopic ERG shows selective loss of b-wave and oscillatory potentials.
- *VF*: absolute VF loss in schitic areas.

Treatment
Prophylactic treatment of X-linked juvenile retinoschisis is highly controversial and may cause retinal detachment.[12]

Goldmann–Favre syndrome

This very rare condition is similar to juvenile retinoschisis but is AR, with more marked peripheral abnormalities (RP-like changes with whitened retinal vessels).

FEVR

This rare condition usually shows AD inheritance (Chr 11q).

Clinical features
- Abrupt cessation of peripheral retinal vessels at the equator (more marked temporally), vitreous bands in the periphery.
- *Complications*: neovascularization, subretinal exudation (akin to Coats' disease), macular ectopia (akin to ROP), retinal detachment.

Other hereditary vitreoretinal degenerations

These include Wagner syndrome, erosive vitreoretinopathy, Knobloch syndrome, AD neovascular inflammatory vitreoretinopathy, and AD vitreoretinochoroidopathy.

10. Richards AJ et al. Variation in the vitreous phenotype of Stickler syndrome can be caused by different amino acid substitutions in the X position of the type II collagen Gly-X-Y triple helix. *Am J Hum Genet* 2000;**67**:1083–94.

11. Ang A et al. Retinal detachment and prophylaxis in Type 1 Stickler syndrome. *Ophthalmology* 2008;**115**:164–8.

12. Kellner U et al. X-linded congenital retinoschisis. *Graefes Arch Clin Exp Ophthalmol* 1990;**228**:432-7.

Choroidal detachments and uveal effusion syndrome

Choroidal detachments

Choroidal detachments (see Table 12.13 and Table 12.14) are usually seen in the context of acute hypotony, e.g. after glaucoma filtration surgery or cyclodestructive procedures. They are usually easily distinguished from retinal detachments.

Clinical features
- Smooth convex dome(s) of normal/slightly dark retinal colour.
- Arises from extreme periphery (may include ciliary body, and ora serrata becomes easily visible) but posterior extension limited by vortex vein adhesions to the scleral canals.
- Choroidal detachments may touch ('kissing choroidals'), causing retinal adhesion and retinal detachment.

Treatment
- Management is either by observation (e.g. if this reflects an appropriate post-trabeculectomy fall in IOP) or by treating the underlying disease process.
- Choroidal haemorrhage may require surgical drainage, although this may be best left until the blood has liquefied.

Uveal effusion syndrome

This is a rare syndrome of the choroid and ciliary body, causing ERD, thought to arise from impaired posterior segment drainage usually associated with scleral thickening.

Idiopathic uveal effusion syndrome usually affects healthy adult men. It is sometimes divided into three types:
- Nanophthalmic eyes (type 1).
- Non-nanophthalmic eyes with clinically abnormal sclera (type 2).
- Non-nanophthalmic eyes with clinically normal sclera (type 3).

Nanophthalmos and the presence of clinically detectable thickened/rigid sclera are a good predictor both for histologically abnormal sclera and of a good response to surgery.[13]

Clinical features
- Combined choroidal detachments and ERD.

Treatment
- *Surgery*: scleral windows (± application of MMC) may decompress the vortex veins.

Table 12.13 RRD vs choroidal detachment

	RRD	Choroidal detachment
Colour	Pale	Darker/normal colour
Dome	Convex corrugated	Convex smooth
Breaks	Present	Absent
Ora serrata	Visible with indentation	Easily visible
Maximal extent	*Anterior*: ora serrata	*Anterior*: ciliary body
	Posterior: unlimited	*Posterior*: vortex veins

Table 12.14 Common causes of choroidal detachment

Effusion	Hypotony
	Extensive PRP
	Extensive cryotherapy
	Posterior uveitis
	Uveal effusion syndrome
	Nanophthalmos
Haemorrhage	Intra-operative
	Trauma
	Spontaneous

13. Uyama M et al. Uveal effusion syndrome: clinical features, surgical treatment, histological examination of the sclera and pathophysiology. *Ophthalmology* 2000;**107**:441–9.

Epiretinal membranes

Common synonyms for the disease reflect its appearance (macular pucker, cellophane maculopathy) and uncertain pathogenesis (premacular fibrosis, idiopathic premacular gliosis).

The condition is more common with increasing age (present in 6% of those over 50y), in ♀, and after retinal insults (see Box 12.2).

The membranes are fibrocellular and avascular and are thought to arise from the proliferation of retinal glial cells that have migrated through defects in the internal limiting membrane (ILM); such defects probably arise most commonly during PVD.

Clinical features

- Asymptomatic, metamorphopsia, ↓VA.
- Membrane may be transparent (look for glistening light reflex), translucent, or white; retinal striae; vessels may be tortuous, straightened, or obscured; pseudohole.

NB The features are well demonstrated on red-free light.

- *Complications*: fovea ectopia; tractional macular detachment; CMO; intra-/preretinal haemorrhages.

Investigations

- *OCT*: not essential, but confirms diagnosis (may differentiate pseudo- vs true hole) and useful to compare pre- and post-operative status.
- *FFA*: seldom used now due to advent of OCT, but nicely demonstrates vascular abnormalities and any associated CMO.

Treatment

- *Indications*: severely symptomatic membranes; ensure that macular function is not limited by an additional underlying pathology (e.g. ischaemia due to a vein occlusion).
- *Surgery*: vitrectomy/membrane peel; some surgeons assist visualization by staining with various dyes, e.g. trypan blue, indocyanine green, ILM blue, membrane dual and brilliant blue G. Due to concerns about retinal toxicity, the risks and benefits of using dyes as an adjuvant stain should be assessed on a case by case basis.
- A double stain technique to peel ERM and ILM has reduced the recurrence rate of ERM by removing the ILM that acts as a scaffold for proliferating cells.[14]
- *Complications*: include cataract (up to 70% rate of significant nuclear sclerosis within 2y), retinal tears/detachment, retinal toxicity from dyes, worsened acuity (up to 15%), and symptomatic recurrence (5%).

Prognosis

- The disease is fairly stable, with over 75% patients showing no further reduction in VA after diagnosis.
- With surgery, 60–85% patients show visual improvement (≥2 Snellen lines).
- Poor prognostic features are duration of symptoms before surgery, underlying macular pathology, and lower preoperative acuity (but may still show significant improvement).

Box 12.2 Causes of ERMs

- Idiopathic.
- Retinal detachment surgery.
- Cryotherapy.
- Photocoagulation.
- Trauma (blunt or penetrating).
- Posterior uveitis.
- Persistent vitreous haemorrhage.
- Retinal vascular disease (e.g. BRVO).

14. Shimada H *et al*. Double staining with brilliant blue G and double peeling for epiretinal membrane. *Ophthalmology* 2009;**116**:1370–6.

Macular hole

The incidence of macular hole is about 1/10,000/y; it is more common in women (2:1 ♀:♂) and has a mean age of onset of 65y.

In some cases, a predisposing pathological condition is identified. In the remaining 'idiopathic' cases, abnormal vitreomacular traction may be observed clinically and with OCT. Release of this traction by vitrectomy ± removal of tangential traction by ILM peeling appears to underlie the success of surgery in treating this condition (see Box 12.3 for causes).

Staging

The developing idiopathic age-related macular hole may initially be asymptomatic but can cause a progressive distortion of vision and a drop in acuity to ~6/120. Worsening acuity approximately correlates with the pathological stages described by Gass.

Clinical features

- *Stage 1*: no sensory retinal defect:
  - a: small yellow foveolar spot ± loss of foveal contour.
  - b: yellow foveolar ring.
- *Stage 2*: small (100–400 microns) full-thickness sensory retinal defect.
- *Stage 3*: larger (≥401 microns) full-thickness sensory retinal defect with cuff of SRF ± yellow deposits in base of hole.
- *Stage 4*: as for stage 3 but with complete vitreous separation.
- Watzke–Allen test (thin beam of light projected across the hole is seen to be thinned centrally or 'broken') may help differentiate from pseudo- or lamellar holes.

Investigations

- *OCT*: may assist diagnosis and staging where required. Advances in OCT interpretation have led to the recognition that the preoperative base diameter, as measured by OCT, has one of the strongest associations with anatomical and visual outcome.[15]
- *FFA*: not usually indicated but usually shows a window defect.

Treatment

- Refer to vitreoretinal surgeon; the chance of successful surgery is highest if performed within 6mo and halves if surgery delayed by >1y.[16]
- *Medical*: enzymatic vitreolysis, using ocriplasmin, has been shown to relieve vitreomacular traction in 26.5% of eyes and to close stages 1 and 2 macular holes in 40.6% of eyes.[17]
- *Surgery*: vitrectomy, ILM peel, and gas is the standard recognized procedure. Face-down posturing and adjunctive agents, such as autologous serum/platelets, can improve success rates with larger holes (>400 microns) or recurrent holes.
- The use of vital dyes can facilitate visualization of the ILM and help achieve complete atraumatic peeling of the ILM.
- *Complications*: include cataracts (50% rate of significant nuclear sclerosis within 2y), retinal tears/detachment (about 1%), failure (anatomical up to 10%; visual up to 20%), late re-opening of hole (5%), and endophthalmitis.

Prognosis

- Stage 1 holes spontaneously resolve in 50%.
- *Without surgery*: stage 2 holes almost always progress, resulting in final VA of about 6/120.
- *With surgery*: early stage 2 holes show anatomical closure in >90% and visual success (≥2 Snellen lines) in 80%.
- If there is a PVD in the fellow eye, the risk of a macular hole is <1% over 5y. If there is no PVD in the fellow eye, the risk is about 10–20% over 5y.[18]

Box 12.3 Causes of macular holes

- Idiopathic.
- Trauma.
- CMO.
- ERM/vitreomacular traction syndrome.
- RRD.
- Laser injury.
- Pathological myopia (with posterior staphyloma).
- Hypertension.
- Diabetic retinopathy.

15. Ullrich S *et al*. Macular hole size as a prognostic factor in macular hole surgery. *Br J Ophthalmol* 2002;**86**:390–3.

16. Jaycock PD *et al*. Outcomes of macular hole surgery: implications for surgical management and clinical governance. *Eye* 2005;**19**:879–84.

17. Stalmans P *et al*. Enzymatic vitreolysis with ocriplasmin for vitreomacular traction and macular holes. *N Engl J Med* 2012;**367**:606–15.

18. Ezra E *et al*. Incidence of idiopathic full-thickness macular holes in fellow eyes. A 5-year prospective natural history study. *Ophthalmology* 1998;**105**:353–9.

Laser retinopexy and cryopexy for retinal tears

Laser retinopexy (slit-lamp or indirect delivery systems)

Mechanism

Laser light is absorbed by target tissue generating heat and causing local protein denaturation (photocoagulation), adhering the neural retina to the RPE. Green light is mainly absorbed by melanin and haemoglobin (Hb).

Indication

- Retinal break with risk of progression to RRD (usually U-tears) and without excessive SRF.
- Equatorial and post-equatorial lesions can be reached with slit-lamp delivery system; more anterior lesions require indirect laser with indentation or cryotherapy.

Method

- *Consent*: explain what the procedure does, likely success rate (about 80%), and possible complications, including need for retreatment (about 20%), detachment despite treatment (9%, half of which are from a different break).
- *Ensure maximal dilation* (e.g. tropicamide 1% + phenylephrine 2.5%) and topical anaesthesia (e.g. oxybuprocaine 0.4%).

Slit-lamp

- *Set laser* (varies according to model): commonly, spot size of 500 microns, duration 0.1s, and low initial power, e.g. 100mW.
- *Position CL* (usually a wide field lens, e.g. Transequator or the 3-mirror; both require coupling agent).
- *Focus and fire laser* to generate 2–3 rings of confluent grey-white burns (adjust power appropriately).

Indirect ophthalmoscope

- *Set laser* (varies according to model): commonly, duration 0.1s and low power, e.g. 100mW.
- *Insert speculum*, and coat cornea with hypromellose (hydroxypropyl-methylcellulose) or ensure regular irrigation to maintain clarity.
- While *viewing* with indirect ophthalmoscope, gently indent to clearly visualize lesion.
- *Focus and fire laser* to generate 2–3 rings of confluent grey-white burns (adjust power appropriately). If the anterior portion of the tear is still out of reach or not visible, then a laser barricade up to the ora may suffice.

Complications

- Intra-operative: retinal/vitreous haemorrhage.
- Post-operative: failure resulting in retinal detachment, ERM formation, CMO.

Cryopexy

Mechanism

Freezing causes local protein denaturation, adhering the neural retina to the RPE.

Indications

- Retinal break with risk of progression to RRD (usually U-tears) and without excessive SRF.
- Cryotherapy is most suitable for pre-equatorial lesions. It has advantages over laser retinopexy, where there is a small pupil or media opacity, but may induce more PVR.

Methods

- *Consent*: explain what the procedure does, likely success rate, and possible complications, including failure/need for retreatment, discomfort, inflammation, and retinal/choroidal detachment.
- *Ensure maximal dilation* (e.g. tropicamide 1% + phenylephrine 2.5%)
- *Give local anaesthesia* (e.g. by subconjunctival injection, as this preserves mobility).
- *Insert speculum*, and coat cornea with hydroxypropylmethylcellulose or ensure regular irrigation to maintain clarity.
- While *viewing* with indirect ophthalmoscope, gently indent with the cryoprobe to clearly visualize lesion.
- *Surround* the break with a single continuous ring of applications. The duration of each application should be just long enough for the retina to whiten. The probe should not be removed until thawing has occurred.
- *Post-procedure*: consider mild topical steroid/antibiotic combination (e.g. Betnesol-N® 4×/d for 1wk).

Complications

- Intra-operative: retinal/vitreous haemorrhage.
- Post-operative: inflammation, failure resulting in retinal detachment, ERM formation.

Pneumatic retinopexy

Pneumatic retinopexy for superior retinal breaks

Mechanism

The aim of a pneumatic retinopexy is to use an intraocular tamponade agent to seal a superior retinal break. Direct apposition of the tamponade agent to the break closes the break for a sufficient duration to allow retinopexy to take effect. This then allows SRF to be absorbed via the RPE pump mechanism.

Indications

- Simple RRD where there is a single superior break located between 11 o'clock and 1 o'clock and where the extent of detachment is sufficiently small to allow the buoyancy of the bubble to be effective.
- In patients who are unfit for surgery but able to posture upright.

Methods

- *Consent*: explain that this is a minor procedure with a need for post-operative posturing. Explain the risks of a repeat procedure, infection, haemorrhage, and raised IOP. However, patients should be aware that final VA does not seem to be affected if a repeat procedure is required.
- *Ensure maximal dilation* (e.g. tropicamide 1% + phenylephrine 2.5%).
- *Examine* the eye, and localize the break.
- *Mark* the break, and ensure that there is a single break or a collection of breaks very close together that will be tamponaded by the gas bubble at full expansion.
- *Perform cryotherapy or retinopexy* to the break.
- *Perform paracentesis* before or after gas insertion.
- *Inject the gas* of your choice (0.3mL of C3F8 or 0.4mL of SF6). Ensure that you get one large and complete gas bubble.
- *Instruct* patient about posturing.
- *Post-procedure*: consider mild topical steroid/antibiotic combination (e.g. Betnesol-N® 4×/d for 1wk).

Complications

- *Intra-operative*: acutely raised IOP, haemorrhage, and subconjunctival gas.
- *Post-operative*: new or missed breaks, subretinal gas, delayed absorption of SRF, cataract formation, and endophthalmitis.

Prognosis

Though initial results appear lower (75.5%) than for scleral buckling (85–88%), the final anatomic and functional results are similar at around 97%.[19] Careful case selection has been shown to improve 1° success rates.

19. Holz ER et al. View 3: the case for pneumatic retinopexy. Br J Ophthalmol 2003;**87**:787–9.

Scleral buckling procedures

Scleral buckling

Mechanism

It is suggested that the buckle closes the break by multiple mechanisms, including moving the RPE closer to the retina and moving the retina closer to the posterior vitreous cortex. It is postulated that these may reduce flow through the break (including the amount of fluid pumped through during eye movements) and relieve vitreous traction on flap tears.

Indications

- *Most simple RRD and dialyses*: procedure of choice in situations where there is no pre-existing PVD, as a vitrectomy would require the induction of a PVD during surgery (hazardous manoeuvre).
- *Segmental buckles*: for single breaks or multiple breaks within 1 clock-hour.
- *Encircling bands*: traditionally for extensive/multiple breaks or breaks in the presence of high-risk features (e.g. aphakia/pseudophakia, etc.); however, the majority of these would now have a vitrectomy (and no local buckle or encirclement).

Methods

- *Consent*: explain what the operation does and possible complications, including failure, diplopia, refractive change, inflammation, infection, haemorrhage, explant extrusion, and worsened vision.

Perform appropriate conjunctival peritomy

- *Inspect sclera* for thinning and anomalous vortex veins; place traction sutures around selected rectus muscles to assist positioning.
- *Identify break* by indirect ophthalmoscope and indentation, using the cryoprobe (or one of a number of instruments specifically designed for this purpose).
- *Apply cryopexy* to all breaks. Each application should last just long enough for the retina to whiten; the probe should not be removed until thawing has occurred. Mark the external position of the break on the sclera, using indentation and a marker pen.
- *Select buckle size*: this should cover double the width of the retinal tear; position so that it extends from ora serrata to cover the posterior lip of the break.
- *Place partial-thickness 5-0 non-absorbable sutures*, using a spatulated needle. These are usually mattress-type sutures and are placed at least 1mm away from the buckle on either side (NB Wider separation of sutures may result in a higher buckle. The number of sutures depends on the size of explant).
- *Tighten sutures*. NB Tighter sutures results in a higher buckle, but over-tightening can result in scleral 'cheese wiring'.
- *Confirm buckle position* is correct and that arterial perfusion of the optic nerve is unaffected.
- *Close conjunctiva* (e.g. with 7-0 absorbable suture).

Complications
- *Intra-operative*: scleral perforation, SRF drainage problems (retinal incarceration, choroidal/subretinal haemorrhage).
- *Post-operative*: infection, glaucoma, extrusion, choroidal effusion/detachment, ERM, CMO, diplopia, refractive change.

Prognosis
Anatomical success >90%, but only about 50% achieve a VA of 6/18 (macula-off detachments).

Options

Choice of buckle (See Table 12.15)

Table 12.15 Buckle options

Material	Solid silicone rubber vs silicone sponge
Orientation	Radial vs circumferential segmental vs encircling
Size	Wide range available (and can be cut to size)

Drainage procedures
- Trans-scleral drainage of SRF, with a 27–30G needle or 5-0 spatulated needle, is done in an area of deep SRF, preferably below the level of the macula and in the bed of the scleral explant. Doing this whilst maintaining the IOP elevated (e.g. by digital pressure on the globe) reduces risk of haemorrhage. It is not commonly done, as most buckling procedures can succeed without this manoeuvre.
- Drainage of SRF is sometimes combined with the injection of intravitreal air in the DACE (drain–air–cryotherapy–explant) procedure.

Vitrectomy: outline

Vitrectomy

Mechanism

Vitrectomy removes dynamic tractional forces exerted on the retina by the vitreous; static tractional forces arising from membranes/fibrovascular proliferation can be removed at the same time.

Vitrectomy also allows surgical access to the retina to permit drainage of SRF, removal of intraocular membranes, removal of retained lens fragments, and insertion of tamponade agents. Transconjunctival sutureless 23 and 25G vitrectomy systems are gaining in popularity over 20G systems in most developed countries.

Advantages of smaller gauge surgery

- Reduced operating time.
- Improved patient comfort (smaller incisions/no sutures).
- Reduced post-operative inflammation.
- More rapid visual recovery.

Disadvantages

- Increased risk of hypotony.
- Increased rate of cataract, compared to scleral buckling surgery.

Indications

Retinal detachments

- *RRD*: traditionally reserved for those with posterior retinal breaks, giant retinal tears, proliferative vitreoretinopathy, or media opacity; now usage widened to include most bullous detachments and detachments associated with aphakia/pseudophakia (or other higher-risk features).
- *TRD.*

Other

- *Diagnostic*: e.g. biopsy for endophthalmitis, lymphoma.
- *Pharmacological*: e.g. administration of antibiotics, steroids.
- *Macular pathology*: macular holes, ERMs.
- *Trauma*: e.g. removal of FB.
- *Persistent media opacity*: vitreous haemorrhage, inflammatory debris, floaters (severe).
- *Complications of cataract surgery*: dropped nucleus, dislocated IOL.

Method

- *Consent*: explain what the operation does, the presence of a post-operative gas bubble, the importance of posturing, and possible complications, including failure, inflammation, infection, haemorrhage, and worsened vision.
- *Insert three entry site sleeved cannulas 4mm (phakic) or 3.5mm (aphakic/pseudophakic) behind the limbus, placed inferotemporally, superotemporally, and superonasally.*

- *Secure the infusion cannula* to the inferotemporal cannula. The infusion is used both to maintain the globe (so permitting aspiration) and can be used to increase pressure if intraocular bleeding occurs. It is important to visualize the tip of the infusion port before turning on the infusion.
- *Insert the light-pipe and then the vitrector* through the two superior cannulae under visualization (CL or indirect microscope system with inverter).
- *Vitrectomy*: of the posterior vitreous face and extending out to the periphery.
- *Replace the infusion fluid with a tamponade agent, if required* (usually gas, sometimes oil for complicated cases).
- *Remove the cannulae, and assess wound for leak (should self-seal).*
- *Post-operative care*: if intraocular gas tamponade used, advise re posturing; warn against air travel and the use of nitrous oxide (anaesthetic agent) until the intraocular gas resorbed.

Complications

- *Intra-operative*: retinal breaks (posterior, peripheral), choroidal haemorrhage, lens touch.
- *Post-operative*: retinal breaks/RRD, cataract, glaucoma, inflammation, endophthalmitis (1/2,000), hypotony, corneal decompensation, sympathetic ophthalmia (0.01% of routine vitrectomy).
- *Tamponade gas-associated*: ↑IOP, posterior subcapsular 'feathering' of the lens (usually temporary), anterior IOL movement (if pseudophakic).
- *Silicone oil-associated*: ↑IOP, hyperoleum ('inverse hypopyon'), adherence to silicone IOL, oil keratopathy (if oil in AC), peri-oil fibrosis, cataract, emulsification, and 2° glaucoma.

Prognosis

Anatomical success for simple RRD ~90%; chance of anatomical success rises with repeated procedures.

Vitrectomy: heavy liquids and tamponade agents

Perfluorocarbon ('heavy') liquids

Indications May be useful in:
- Repositioning of giant retinal tears.
- Flattening PVR-associated retina.
- Floating up dislocated lens fragments or IOLs.
- Assisting haemostasis.

Agents
Perfluoro-*n*-octane is the most commonly used agent, perfluorodecalin is also used.

Tamponade

Indications
- *Simple retinal detachment*: consider air or SF6/air mix.
- *Complicated retinal detachment* (e.g. PVR, giant retinal tear, multiple recurrences): consider C3F8/air mix, silicone oil, or 'heavy' silicone oil. Overall, silicone oil and C3F8 are similarly effective in PVR, although silicone oil is associated with better final VA in anterior disease, does not require post-operative posturing, and allows easier intra-operative and immediate post-operative visualization. 'Heavy' silicone oils are denser than water and so allow tamponade of the inferior retina. They may be useful when there are inferior breaks or an inferior retinectomy, especially with PVR.
- Where vitrectomy has been performed for indications other than retinal detachment, there may be no need for tamponade.

Agents (See Table 12.16 and Table 12.17)

Table 12.16 Common gaseous tamponade agents

Agent	Symbol	Expansion if 100%	Non-expansile concentration (mixed with air) (%)	Duration (wk)
Air	Air	Nil	100	≤1
Sulfur hexafluoride	SF6	× 2	20	1–2
Perfluoro-ethane	C2F6	× 3	16	4–6
Perfluoro-propane	C3F8	× 4	12	8–10

Table 12.17 Common fluid tamponade agents

Agent	Symbol	Density (specfic gravity, g/mL)	Viscosity (cs)	Maximum permitted duration
Balanced salt solution	BSS	1		
Perfluorocarbon liquid (heavy liquid)	PFCL	2	Dependent on particular molecule (mostly low)	Intra-operative use only
Silicone oil	Si oil	0.97	1,000 or 5,000	Ideally 3–6mo, but can be used long-term
Combined SFA and Si oil	Densiron	1.06	1,387	Ideally <6wk as prone to emulsification
	Oxane-HD	1.02	3,300	

Complications
- ↑IOP (may be related to overfill), posterior subcapsular 'feathering' of the lens, anterior IOL movement (if pseudophakic).

Posturing
- Post-operative posturing by the patient aims to achieve effective tamponade of the break by the gas bubble and to keep the gas bubble away from the crystalline lens.
- Posturing should start as soon as possible (same day of surgery) for as much of each day as possible (commonly 50min in every hour, and adopt appropriate sleeping posture), and continue for 1–2wk (some variation according to tamponade agent).
- The posture required will depend on the location of the break but aims to move the break as superiorly as possible.
- Advise against flying or the use of nitrous oxide anaesthetic agents until the gas bubble has resolved—these situations can result in blindness due to expansion of the gas bubble and subsequent ↑IOP.

Advances in retinal surgery

Gene therapy for retinal diseases

The eye has been shown to be a good target for gene therapy, using vectors (either viral or non-viral) to deliver therapeutic interventions safely to the retina. This promising advance aims to administer molecular treatments to the retina in an attempt to cure retinal diseases with a genetic basis.[20]

Genetic conditions that can suitably be targeted require a relatively intact photoreceptor and RPE morphology to allow treatment to work prior to any long-lasting structural damage occurring.[21]

Mechanism

A solution of vectors containing the target molecule is introduced into the subretinal space by performing a pars plana vitrectomy and injecting the therapeutic agent through a retinotomy.

Complications

- Intraocular haemorrhage.
- Infection.
- Cataract.
- Iatrogenic retinal breaks.
- Unplanned retinal detachments.

Clinical trials

Ongoing studies include:

- Recombinant adeno-associated virus (rAAV)-mediated gene therapy for severe early-onset degeneration due to defects in the *RPE65* gene that causes LCA. Early results from this work show good tolerability of the treatment, with some improvement in visual function.
- rAAV-mediated gene therapy to assess the safety, tolerability, and therapeutic benefit of *REP1* gene that causes choroideraemia.
- rAAV-mediated gene therapy to assess the safety and tolerability of the genetic code for the antiangiogenic protein sFLT01 (a fusion of VEGF and PIGF) in neovascular AMD.
- Other registered studies include rAAV-MERTK for RP associated with MERTK mutations.

Retinal prosthesis

Prosthetic retinal implants aim to harness the remaining neural activity in the remainder of retinal cells in degenerative retinal diseases. This approach is potentially useful in eye pathology where there is a healthy anterior segment and a relatively intact optic nerve.

Mechanism

In order to employ the neural cells in the retina, an external camera or, less commonly, an intraocular device is used to detect and capture light-based images, which are then processed and converted to an electrical signal. A retinal prosthesis (chip/electrode) is used to stimulate any remaining retinal neurones, bypassing destroyed photoreceptors.[22]

There are a number of stimulating electrodes currently being investigated by clinical trials. These electrodes have been placed in various anatomic locations: epiretinally, subretinally, in the suprachoroidal space, and inside the optic nerve.[23]

Each of these systems has its advantages and disadvantages. The VA demonstrated in early participants has been poor; however, some of the trials have demonstrated the ability of participants to read using their retinal prosthesis. The main area of hope appears to be the ability to improve mobility and orientation for some blind people.

20. Sundaram V et al. Retinal dystrophies and gene therapy. Eur J Pediatr 2011;**171**:757–65.

21. Lipinski DM et al. Clinical applications of retinal gene therapy. Prog Retin Eye Res 2013;**32**:22–47.

22. Ong JM et al. The bionic eye: a review. Clin Experiment Ophthalmol 2011;**40**:6–17.

23. Weiland JD et al. Retinal prostheses: current clinical results and future needs. Ophthalmology 2011;**118**:2227–37.

Chapter 13

Medical retina

Anatomy and physiology (1)

The retina is a remarkable modification of the embryonic forebrain that gathers light, codes the information as an electrical signal (transduces), and transmits it via the optic nerve to the processing areas of the brain.

Embryologically, it is derived from the optic vesicle (neuroectoderm), with an outer wall that becomes the RPE, a potential space (the subretinal space), and an inner wall that becomes the neural retina.

Neural retina

This is a thin (150–400 microns) layer of transparent neural tissue, continuous with the non-pigmented layer of the ciliary body anteriorly. The retina comprises photoreceptors (rods, cones), integrators (bipolar, horizontal, amacrine, ganglion cells), an output pathway (nerve fibre layer), and support cells (Müller cells). On histological examination, the retina is typically divided into ten layers: in particular, three layers predominantly containing nuclei (outer/inner nuclear layers and ganglion cell layer) and two layers predominantly containing synaptic connections (outer and inner plexiform layers).

In normal states, the retina contains relatively little extracellular space, with Müller cells acting as the 'scaffolding' for the neural and vascular elements. The basal lamina of their inner cell processes make up the ILM, while their posterior cell processes connect to the photoreceptors, forming the external limiting membrane (ELM). The ILM provides an anchor for the collagen framework of the vitreous. The ELM may act as a partial barrier to the passage of large molecules in either direction (e.g. protecting the retinal extracellular space in cases of SRF build-up).

The central retina (macula lutea) is defined histologically by a multilayered ganglion cell layer (i.e. >1 cell thick) and approximates to a 5,500 microns oval, centred on the fovea and bordered by the temporal arcades. When removed from the underlying choroid (as in gross dissection of a post-mortem eye), it appears yellowish due to xanthophyll pigments (lutein and zeaxanthin). The macula is further divided into perifovea (1,500 microns wide band, defined by six layers of bipolar cells), parafovea (500 microns wide band, defined by 7–11 layers of bipolar cells), and fovea (1,500 microns diameter circular depression). The fovea comprises a rim, a 22° slope, and a central floor the foveola (350 microns diameter, 150 microns thin). The umbo is the very centre of the foveola (150 microns diameter), with maximal cone density equating to highest acuity. In most normal eyes, a foveal light reflex may be seen to directly overlie the umbo; in younger eyes, a larger oval light reflex may be seen at the inner retinal surface, roughly corresponding to the foveal margins.

RPE

RPE is a continuous hexagonal monolayer of epithelial cells that extends anteriorly from the margins of the optic nerve to the ora serrata where it is continuous with the pigmented layer of the ciliary body. The apices form microvilli that envelop the photoreceptor outer segments. Near the apices, adjacent RPE cells are joined by numerous tight junctions to form the outer blood–retinal barrier. The base of the RPE is crenellated (to increase surface area) and mitochondrion-rich.

The RPE is highly pigmented with melanin, particularly in the central macular area. This melanin pigment, in combination with melanin in the choroid, impairs visualization of the underlying choroidal vasculature (especially in highly pigmented ethnic groups). The RPE becomes less pigmented with age, making the choroidal vessels more evident and often imparting a 'tessellated' or 'tigroid' appearance to the fundus.

Bruch's membrane

Bruch's membrane is the sheet-like condensation of the innermost layer of the choroid, consisting of five layers and 2–4 microns in thickness. The BM of the RPE forms the inner layer of Bruch's membrane. A central layer of elastic tissue is then covered by collagenous layers on its inner and outer aspect. The fifth and outer layer of Bruch's membrane is the basement membrane of the choriocapillaris. Changes in the composition and thickness of Bruch's membrane, particularly with ageing, are key to the development of CNV and other macular disease.

Choroid

The choroid is a largely vascular structure, surrounded by an elastic network in a net-like manner. The short posterior ciliary arteries pierce and run through the sclera, forming an outer layer of large choroidal vessels (Haller's layer), with medium-sized branches giving rise to the middle stromal layer of the choroid (Sattler's layer) and terminal arterioles giving rise to an internal layer of capillary vessels (choriocapillaris). The choroidal stroma also contains numerous cells, including melanocytes, fibrocytes, and immune cells, such as macrophages, and is densely innervated.

Sclera

The sclera is a largely avascular structure, consisting mainly of compact, interlacing bundles of collagen with small quantities of elastic tissue. Between the choroid and sclera is a thin 'lamina fusca,' consisting of closely packed lamellae of collagen fibres connecting the sclera and choroid; this potential 'suprachoroidal space' may become distended with blood or fluid.

Anatomy and physiology (2)

Physiology

Retinal blood supply

The neural retina has a dual blood supply derived from branches of the ophthalmic artery, including the central retinal artery (which provides the retinal circulation) and the posterior ciliary arteries (which provide the choroidal circulation).

Anatomically, the retinal circulation supports the inner two-thirds of the retina, whereas the choroidal circulation supports the outer third; the watershed is at the outer plexiform layer.

The retinal circulation comprises a small part of ocular blood flow (5%), but with a high level of oxygen extraction (40% AV difference), contrasting with figures of 85% and 5% for the choroidal circulation. In the retinal circulation, the arterial branches lie in the nerve fibre layer but give rise both to an inner capillary network (ganglion cell layer) and an outer capillary network (inner nuclear layer). However, there are no capillaries in the central 500 microns the foveal avascular zone.

The outer blood–retinal barrier is formed by the tight junctions of the RPE cells, whereas the inner is formed by the non-fenestrated endothelium of the retinal capillaries.

Neural retina

Photoreceptors

Each human eye contains about 120 million rods and 6.5 million cones. The rods subserve peripheral and low-light (scotopic) vision, whereas the cones permit normal (photopic), central, and colour vision.

The rods reach their highest density at 20° from the fovea, in contrast to blue cones which are densest in the perifovea, and red and green cones which are densest (up to 385,000/mm^2) at the umbo.

Light perception is mediated in the outer segments of the photoreceptors by a group of G protein receptors called opsins (rhodopsin in rods, iodopsins in cones), which are bound to a vitamin A-derived chromophore 11 *cis* retinal. These transmembrane photopigment molecules undergo *cis–trans* isomerization on absorption of a photon of light (495nm for rods, 440–450nm for blue, 535–555nm for green, and 570–590nm for red cones).

Activation of a single photopigment molecule starts a chemical phototransduction cascade (transducin activates phosphodiesterase which, in turn, hydrolyses cyclic guanosine monophosphate (cGMP), with 100-fold amplification at every stage.

Falling cGMP levels cause closure of Na channels, with photoreceptor hyperpolarization. The resting potential is then restored by the action of recoverin, which activates guanylate cyclase to cGMP and reopens Na channels.

Bipolar and amacrine cells

Rods synapse with 'on' bipolar cells which, in turn, synapse with amacrine and ganglion cells. Cones synapse with 'on' and 'off' bipolar cells which, in turn, synapse with 'on' and 'off' ganglion cells.

Negative feedback is provided by the laterally interacting horizontal cells (between photoreceptors) and amacrine cells (between bipolar cells and ganglion cells). This contributes to the centre-surround phenomenon exhibited by ganglion cells, in which they are activated by stimulation in the centre of their receptive field but inhibited by stimulation of the surround.

Ganglion cells

Ganglion cell representation is maximal at the fovea where the cone:ganglion cell ratio approaches 1:1.

The ganglion cells can be divided into two main populations.

- The parvocellular system subserves fine VA and colour. These ganglion cells are mainly foveal, have small receptive fields, and show spectral sensitivity.
- The magnocellular system subserves motion detection and coarser form vision. These ganglion cells are mainly peripheral, have larger receptive fields, have high luminance and contrast (but no spectral) sensitivity, and are very sensitive to motion. This division is preserved, both in the lateral geniculate nucleus (LGN) (layers 1–2 magnocellular, 3–6 parvocellular) and the visual cortex.

RPE

The RPE is vital to the normal function of the neural retina. Functions include:

- The maintenance of the outer blood–retinal barrier and retinal adhesion.
- Storage of metabolites and vitamin A.
- Nutrient supply to the photoreceptors.
- Absorption of scattered light (by melanosomes).
- Production and recycling of photopigments.
- Phagocytosis of photoreceptor discs (each sheds >100 discs/d).

Age-related macular degeneration (1)

AMD is the leading cause of blindness for the 'over 50s' in the Western world. Its prevalence increases with age. One study found visually significant disease (VA ≤6/9) in about 1% for 55–65y, 6% for 65–75y, and 20% for >75y.[1] Numerous classification systems exist; the Age-Related Eye Disease Study (AREDS) classification system is commonly used (see Table 13.1).

Other risk factors include smoking, gender (♀ > ♂), ethnic origin (white Caucasian high risk), diet, CVS risk, and hypermetropia. The possible role of cataract surgery in accelerating progression of AMD is controversial, with conflicting reports in the world literature. Several genetic loci have been associated with AMD, including major loci in the complement factor H (*CFH*) gene on Chr 1q32 and the ARMS2/HTRA1 locus on the Chr 10q26 gene cluster, and other complement pathway-related genes.

Non-neovascular (dry) AMD

Accounting for 90% of AMD, this tends to lead to gradual, but potentially significant, reduction in central vision. It is characterized by drusen (hard or soft) and RPE changes (focal hyperpigmentation or atrophy).

Histology

There is loss of the RPE/photoreceptor layers, thinning of the outer plexiform layer, thickening of Bruch's membrane, and atrophy of choriocapillaris exposing the larger choroidal vessels to view. Drusen are PAS-positive amorphous deposits, lying between the RPE membrane and the inner collagenous layer of Bruch's membrane; they may become calcified.

Clinical features

- ↓VA, metamorphopsia, scotomas; usually gradual in onset.
- Hard drusen (small <63 microns, well-defined, of limited significance), soft drusen (larger, pale yellow, poorly defined, tendency to coalesce and form 'confluent drusen,' increased risk of CNV), RPE focal hyperpigmentation, RPE atrophy ('geographic atrophy' if well demarcated and with visibility of the underlying choroidal vessels).

Investigation

- *FFA*: is not usually necessary. In patients with non-specific visual complaints or examination findings, OCT may be used to screen for signs of CNV (e.g. intraretinal and subretinal fluid).
- *Drusen*: on OCT, small and intermediate drusen appear as discrete areas of RPE elevation with variable reflectivity, while larger drusen are seen as dome-shaped areas of RPE elevation with underlying hyporeflectivity.
- *RPE hyperpigmentation*: on OCT, pigment clumping and migration may be seen as discrete foci of hyperreflectivity with underlying shadowing, most commonly located in the outer retina and overlying drusen.
- *Geographic atrophy*: atrophic changes are most clearly seen on FAF where they appear as areas of markedly decreased autofluorescence. On OCT, atrophic changes appear as areas of sharply demarcated choroidal hyperreflectivity due to loss of the overlying RPE. 'Outer retinal tubulations', ovoid hyporeflective spaces with hyperreflective borders in the outer nuclear layer, may also be seen (rosettes of degenerating photoreceptors seen in advanced atrophy and/or disciform scars).

Table 13.1 AREDS classification of AMD*

Classification	Clinical findings
Category 1: no AMD	None or a few small drusen (<63 microns in diameter)
Category 2: early AMD	Any or all of the following: multiple small drusen; few intermediate drusen (63–124 microns in diameter); RPE abnormalities
Category 3: intermediate AMD	Any or all of the following: extensive intermediate drusen; at least one large drusen (≥125 microns in diameter, roughly equivalent to width of a retinal vein at the rim of the optic disc); geographic atrophy not involving the fovea
Category 4: advanced AMD	Geographic atrophy involving the fovea or any features of neovascular AMD

* Age-Related Eye Disease Study Research Group. Risk factors associated with age-related macular degeneration: a case-control study in the age-related eye disease study: Age-Related Eye Disease Study Report Number 3. *Ophthalmology* 2000;**107**:2224–32.

Treatment
- *Supportive*: counselling and linking to support group/social services.
- *Refraction*: with increased near-add; low-vision aid assessment/provision often best arranged in a dedicated low vision clinic.
- *Registration*: should be offered, as it may improve access to services.
- *Amsler grid*: regular use of an Amsler grid allows the patient to detect new or progressive metamorphopsia, prompting them to seek ophthalmic review.
- *Lifestyle changes:* smoking cessation. Increased intake of food rich in macular carotenoids (e.g. spinach, cabbage, broccoli) and in omega-3 fatty acids (e.g. oily fish such as salmon, mackerel, anchovies, sardines).
- *Vitamin supplementation*: in AREDS, vitamin supplements containing high-dose antioxidants and minerals (vitamins C and E, β-carotene, and zinc) delayed AMD progression from intermediate to advanced stages (particularly those in category 4 with neovascular AMD already in one eye). β-carotene may lead to an increased incidence of lung cancer in former smokers; the results of AREDS2 suggest that lutein + zeaxanthin may be an appropriate carotenoid substitute. Numerous supplements are commercially available, including: Bausch & Lomb's, PreserVision® (AREDS and AREDS2 formulations), Alcon's, I-Caps®.

1.   Owen CG *et al.* The estimated prevalence and incidence of late stage age related macular degeneration in the UK. *Br J Ophthalmol* 2012;**96**:752–6.

Age-related macular degeneration (2)

Neovascular (wet) AMD

Although much less common, neovascular AMD leads to rapid and severe loss of vision. Nearly 40,000 new cases of wet AMD are estimated to occur each year in the UK,[2] accounting for up to 90% of blind registration due to AMD.

In the last decade, exciting advances in the treatment of wet AMD with anti-VEGF therapies have been made. Recent population-based data suggest that legal blindness attributable to wet AMD will be significantly reduced in many countries through the use of these agents.[3]

Histology

New capillaries grow from the choriocapillaris though Bruch's membrane and proliferate in the sub-RPE (type I neovascularization) and/or subretinal space (type 2 neovascularization). There may be associated haemorrhage, exudation, serous retinal detachment, PED, or scar formation. Type I CNV is commoner in AMD; type 2 is commoner in younger patients (e.g. with POHS).

AMD variants

Although wet AMD is predominantly a disorder of the choroidal vasculature, the retinal circulation may also be involved in 10–15% of patients, a variant termed retinal angiomatous proliferation (RAP). These lesions have recently been termed type III neovascularization to denote intraretinal vascular complexes that arise from both deep retinal capillaries and the choroid.

Polypoidal choroidal vasculopathy (PCV), originally described as a distinct disease entity, is now thought to be a variant of wet AMD, characterized by polypoidal dilatation of the choroidal vasculature with serosanguineous PEDs. PCV is the most common presentation of wet AMD in populations of Asian or African descent but also occurs in Caucasians.

CNV lesions may also sometimes develop, contiguous with the optic disc, so-called peripapillary CNV, or in the retinal periphery. The natural history of such lesions is variable.

Clinical features

- ↓VA, metamorphopsia, scotoma; may be sudden in onset.
- A grey membrane is sometimes visible; more commonly, it is deduced from associated signs, including subretinal (red) or sub-RPE (grey) haemorrhage, subretinal/sub-RPE exudation, retinal or pigment epithelial detachment, CMO, or subretinal fibrosis (disciform scar).
- RAP lesions should be suspected in eyes with parafoveal intraretinal haemorrhage, associated PED, and circinate exudate. An adjacent retinal vessel is sometimes seen to 'dive' into the outer retina ('right-angled').
- RPE tears ('rips') may sometimes occur in eyes with serous PED and appear as areas of atrophy adjacent to areas of marked hyperpigmentation (corresponding to rolled-up RPE once located in the atrophic area).

Investigations

- Urgent FFA is vital for diagnosis and assessment for treatment (see Fig. 13.1 and Fig. 13.2). ICG should also be performed where there is a clinical suspicion of PCV.
- OCT is now central to detection and long-term monitoring of wet AMD; signs of disease activity on OCT include presence of intraretinal or subretinal fluid, as well as increases in sub-RPE fluid.[4]

- *Type 2 ('classic') CNV*: on FFA, appears as early well-demarcated lacy hyperfluorescence with progressive leakage. On OCT, appears as hyperreflective material in the subretinal space.
- *Type 1 ('occult') CNV*: on FFA, appears as fibrovascular PED (irregular elevation with stippled hyperfluorescence at 1–2min post-injection) or as late leakage of undetermined source (poorly demarcated hyperfluorescence 5–10min post-injection). On OCT, appears as irregular broad elevation of the RPE, with separation from the underlying Bruch's membrane.
- *Type 3 ("RAP) CNV*: on FFA, shows a similar appearance to a small area of classic CNV, with early hyperfluorescence and progressive leakage (although the exact appearance may vary, depending on its stage of evolution). On OCT, RAP lesions typically appear as serous or fibrovascular PED with overlying CMO.
- *PCV*: on ICG, a branching vascular network may be seen on early frames, with hyperfluorescence of polyps in late frames. On OCT, the branching vascular network appears as a shallow elevation of the RPE, while the polypoidal lesions appear as sharper protuberances. Serosanguineous detachments of the RPE are seen as multiple, large, dome-shaped elevations of the RPE. On enhanced depth imaging (EDI)-OCT, the choroid is often markedly thickened, with dilatation of large choroidal vessels (in contrast to wet AMD where the choroid is usually thinned).

Treatment

Supportive: offer counselling, refraction, registration, Amsler grid, and encourage lifestyle changes as for non-neovascular AMD.

Anti-VEGF therapies

Intravitreal anti-VEGF therapy has become the treatment of choice for all subfoveal CNV lesions types (see ➔ Anti-vascular endothelial growth factor therapy, p. 528–530)

PDT

Although anti-VEGF therapy is the preferred strategy for the treatment of CNV, PDT remains an option in those for whom anti-VEGF therapy is contraindicated or in those who do not wish to have repeated intravitreal injections. Anti-VEGF monotherapy appears to result in superior visual outcomes to approaches combining anti-VEGF and PDT. However, in patients with PCV, such a combination approach may be more effective than anti-VEGF monotherapy for inducing polyp regression.

Laser photocoagulation

Focal laser photocoagulation is not commonly performed but may still be of benefit in cases of extrafoveal/peripapillary CNV or in eyes with extrafoveal polyps 2° to PCV. Laser may obviate the need for repeated intravitreal injections; however, treatment results in a localized scotoma and recurrence is common.

2. Owen CG *et al.* The estimated prevalence and incidence of late stage age related macular degeneration in the UK. *Br J Ophthalmol* 2012;**96**:752–6.

3. Bloch SB *et al.* Incidence of legal blindness from age-related macular degeneration in Denmark: year 2000 to 2010. *Am J Ophthalmol* 2012;**153**:209–13.e2.

4. Keane PA *et al.* Evaluation of age-related macular degeneration with optical coherence tomography. *Surv Ophthalmol* 2012;**57**:389–414.

Age-related macular degeneration (3)

Role of FFA in diagnosis of wet AMD

FFA should be performed to assess all eyes suspected of wet AMD, except where precluded by allergy or other systemic considerations. In particular, FFA allows assessment of CNV location and classification (see Fig. 13.1 and Fig. 13.2).

Determination of CNV location is critical; for well-demarcated lesions located extrafoveally, the use of laser photocoagulation may allow the patient to avoid the need for monthly intravitreal injections over an extended follow-up period.

Consideration of angiographic lesion classification is also important when determining whether to initiate treatment. In lesions classified as 'occult' on FFA, the decision to treat can often be deferred if there is no evidence of recent disease progression; many such lesions remain quiescent for extended time periods.

FFA may also be useful for the exclusion of other macular disease that can mimic the features of neovascular AMD such as retinal macroaneurysms resulting in submacular haemorrhage, central serous chorioretinopathy resulting in subretinal and sub-RPE fluid, and pattern dystrophies where there is progressive staining of vitelliform-like material.

FFA can also assist in the diagnosis of conditions where CNV is present but due to aetiologies other than AMD (see Table 13.2) Non-AMD CNV may respond differently to anti-VEGF blockade (e.g. requiring fewer treatments) and, in some cases, may benefit from supplementary treatment (e.g. systemic immunosuppression for inflammatory CNV).

Table 13.2 Common causes of CNV

Degenerative	AMD
	Pathological myopia (lacquer crack)
	Angioid streaks
Trauma	Choroidal rupture
	Laser
Inflammation	POHS
	Multifocal choroiditis
	Serpiginous choroidopathy
	Birdshot retinochoroidopathy
	Punctate inner choroidopathy
	VKH
Dystrophies	Best's disease
Other	Chorioretinal scar (any cause)
	Tumour
Idiopathic	

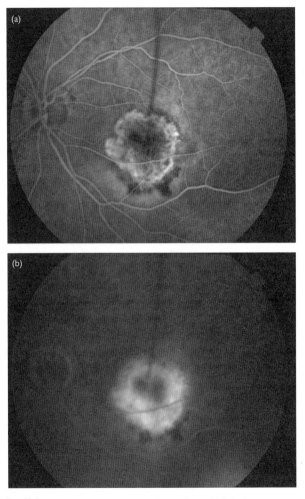

Fig. 13.1 FFA of classic choroidal neovascular membrane. (a) Early phase: well-demarcated lacy hyperfluorescence. (b) Late phase: progressive leakage.

Age-related macular degeneration (4)

Calculating risk of developing advanced AMD

The AREDS observed a number of factors to be predictive of developing advanced AMD. This can be used to predict a patient's risk of developing advanced AMD (CNV or geographic atrophy of the fovea) as follows: assign to *each eye* one risk factor for the presence of large drusen (>125 microns) and one risk factor for pigment abnormality, and sum the risk factors (i.e. 0–4 scale).

Where advanced AMD has already developed in one eye, the risk of developing AMD in the second eye can be estimated as follows: the presence of advanced AMD in the affected eye counts as two risk factors, and this is added to any risk factors present in the second eye.

The 5y risk is then estimated as per Table 13.3.

Table 13.3 Predicting risk of developing advanced AMD[*]

Number of factors	5y risk (%)
0	0.5
1	3
2	12
3	25
4	50

[*] Ferris FL et al. Age-Related Eye Disease Study (AREDS) Research Group. A simplified severity scale for age-related macular degeneration: AREDS Report No. 18. *Arch Ophthalmol* 2005;**123**:1570–4.

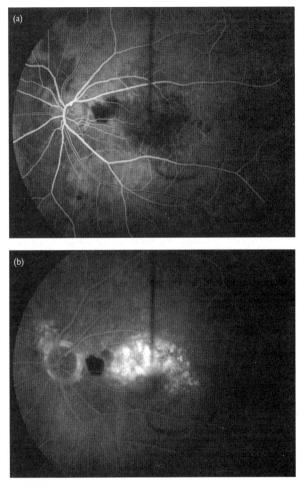

Fig. 13.2 FFA of occult choroidal neovascular membrane. (a) Early phase: stippled hyperfluorescence usually maximal at 1–2min, masking by blood adjacent to disc; (b) Late phase: progressive leakage.

Anti-vascular endothelial growth factor therapy: outline

VEGF-A (also referred to as VEGF) is a secreted protein that induces developmental and pathological angiogenesis, vascular permeability, and inflammation. Anti-VEGF therapies reduce vascular hyperpermeability, leading to resolution of intraretinal and subretinal fluid and restoration of normal retinal architecture. Anti-VEGF therapies also halt progression of pathologic neovascularization, if present.

Mechanism

Currently, there are three licensed drugs: pegaptanib, ranibizumab, and aflibercept. The off-label use of bevacizumab is also common practice.

- *Pegaptanib* is a pegylated aptamer that functions as a selective VEGF inhibitor (VEGF-165 isoform). It is less effective than other anti-VEGF therapies and is no longer in widespread use.
- *Ranibizumab* is a humanized monoclonal antibody fragment that binds all isoforms of VEGF-A.
- *Bevacizumab* is derived from the same humanized monoclonal antibody as ranibizumab.
- *Aflibercept* is a 'fusion' protein that acts as a decoy receptor. Aflibercept binds VEGF-A with higher affinity than ranibizumab or bevacizumab and is also distinguished by its ability to bind placental growth factors 1 and 2.

Evidence for anti-VEGF therapy in wet AMD

Ranibizumab 0.5mg/0.05mL

The efficacy of ranibizumab in patients with wet AMD was first demonstrated by the MARINA and ANCHOR trials.[5,6] ~33% of patients receiving monthly injections of ranibizumab 0.5mg demonstrated moderate visual gain (defined as ≥15 letters gained), while ~95% avoided moderate visual loss (defined as ≥15 letters gained).

Bevacizumab 1.25mg/0.05mL

The CATT and IVAN studies demonstrated that bevacizumab was similar in efficacy to ranibizumab but that OCT-guided 'as-required' retreatment regimens resulted in less gain in VA, whether instituted at enrolment or after 1y of monthly treatment.[7,8,9]

Aflibercept 2mg/0.05mL

The efficacy of aflibercept was demonstrated in the VIEW 1 and VIEW 2 studies.[10] ~30% of patients receiving aflibercept 2mg every 4wk for 3mo, and then every 8wk, gained ≥15 letters, while ~95% avoided ≥15 letters loss.

Evidence for anti-VEGF therapy in diabetic macular oedema

Ranibizumab 0.5mg/0.05mL (licensed dose in EU); 0.3mg/0.05mL (USA)

The efficacy of ranibizumab in patients with diabetic macular oedema (DMO) was demonstrated by multiple studies, including the RISE and RIDE trials.[11] In RISE, 44.8% of patients receiving monthly injections of ranibizumab 0.3mg gained ≥15 letters (compared to 18.1% receiving sham). In RIDE, 33.6% of patients receiving monthly injections of ranibizumab 0.3mg gained ≥15 letters (compared to 12.3% receiving sham). For both studies, macular laser was available in both treatment and control groups—ranibizumab-treated patients required significantly fewer such procedures.

Evidence for anti-VEGF therapy in RVO

Ranibizumab 0.5mg/0.05mL

The efficacy of ranibizumab in treatment of CRVO and BRVO was demonstrated in the CRUISE and BRAVO studies, respectively.[12],[13] In CRUISE, 47.5% of patients receiving monthly injections of ranibizumab 0.5mg gained ≥15 letters (compared to 16.9% receiving sham). In BRAVO, 61.1% of patients receiving monthly injections of ranibizumab 0.5mg gained ≥15 letters (compared to 28.8% receiving sham).

Aflibercept 2mg/0.05mL

The efficacy of aflibercept in treatment of CRVO was demonstrated in the COPERNICUS and GALILEO studies.[14] Treatment with aflibercept led to ≥15 letters gained in 55.3% (COPERNICUS) and 60.2% (GALILEO) of patients.

NICE guidelines

In 2008, NICE (UK) issued guidance for the use of ranibizumab/pegaptanib in wet AMD (and for aflibercept in 2013).
- Treatment with ranibizumab was recommended if eye to be treated has:
  - Best corrected VA between 6/12 and 6/96.
  - No permanent structural damage to the central fovea.
  - Lesion size ≤12 disc areas in greatest linear dimension.
  - Evidence of recent disease progression.
- Pegaptanib was not recommended for treatment of wet AMD.

In 2013, NICE recommended ranibizumab as a treatment for DMO.
- Treatment with ranibizumab was recommended if eye to be treated has:
  - A central retinal thickness of 400 microns or more at the start of treatment.
  - The manufacturer provides the medication with the discount agreed in a revised patient access scheme.

5. Rosenfeld PJ et al. Ranibizumab for neovascular age-related macular degeneration. N Engl J Med 2006;355:1419–31.

6. Brown DM et al. Ranibizumab versus verteporfin for neovascular age-related macular degeneration. N Engl J Med 2006;355:1432–44.

7. CATT Research Group et al. Ranibizumab and bevacizumab for neovascular age-related macular degeneration. N Engl J Med 2011;364:1897–908.

8. IVAN Study Group et al. Ranibizumab versus bevacizumab to treat neovascular age-macular degeneration: one-year findings from the IVAN randomized trial. Ophthalmology 2012;119:1399–411.

9. CATT Research Group et al. Ranibizumab and bevacizumab for treatment of neovascular age-related macular degeneration: two-year results. Ophthalmology 2012;119:1388–98.

10. Heier JS et al. Intravitreal aflibercept (VEGF trap-eye) in wet age-related macular degeneration. Ophthalmology 2012;119:2537–48.

11. Nguyen QD et al. Ranibizumab for diabetic macular edema: results from 2 phase III randomized trials: RISE and RIDE. Ophthalmology 2012;119:789–801.

12. Brown DM et al. Sustained benefits from ranibizumab for macular edema following branch retinal vein occlusion: 12-month outcomes of a phase III study. Ophthalmology 2011;118:1594–602.

13. Campochiaro PA et al. Sustained benefits from ranibizumab for macular edema following central retinal vein occlusion: twelve-month outcomes of a phase III study. Ophthalmology 2011;118:2041–9.

14. Brown DM et al. Intravitreal aflibercept injection for macular edema secondary to central retinal vein occlusion: 1-year results from the Phase 3 COPERNICUS Study. Am J Ophthalmol 2013;155:429–37.

Anti-vascular endothelial growth factor therapy: in practice

Intravitreal injection of anti-VEGF therapies

In advance

- *Discuss procedure and take informed consent*: explain purpose (to maintain current vision and potentially improve acuity), risks, and that multiple injections may be required (see Box 13.1).
- Additionally, if using bevacizumab, it should be explained that this drug is not licensed and that licensed alternatives exist for AMD.

Intravitreal injections[15]

Setting

Intravitreal injections may be given in theatre or a dedicated clean room in outpatients that meets stringent conditions such as being enclosed, free from interruptions, good illumination, washable floor, and non-particulate ceiling (i.e. dust-free). Full gowning is not necessary, but hands should be washed and sterile gloves worn.

Preparation

- Confirm consent and correct eye to be injected; measure IOP; ensure adequate dilation; instil topical anaesthesia.
- Set up equipment trolley, and ensure all treatments (including post-injection antibiotics) are available.

Procedure

- Wash hands, and don sterile gloves.
- Instil topical anaesthetic.
- Instil 5% povidone iodine on to the ocular surface; clean periocular area with povidone iodine; drape and insert lid speculum.
- Consider whether supplementation of anaesthesia is necessary: subconjunctival or sub-Tenon's (e.g. lidocaine 1%).
- Prepare syringe/needle/drug immediately prior to injection, and ensure any air in the syringe/needle is expelled prior to injection; maintain aseptic technique throughout.
- Note injection site; this should be 3.0–3.5mm (aphakic/pseudophakic) or 3.5–4mm (phakic) posterior to limbus in either superotemporal or inferotemporal quadrants.
- Insert needle (27–30G; 1/2–5/8in long) perpendicularly, aiming towards the centre of the globe.
- Inject indicated volume of anti-VEGF (ranibizumab 0.05mL; bevacizumab 0.05mL; aflibercept 0.05mL); carefully remove needle; a sterile cotton-tipped applicator can be used as counterpressure and to prevent any reflux.
- Instil topical antibiotic (e.g. chloramphenicol 0.5%); for immediate post-injection, a preservative-free preparation is recommended.

Post-injection
- Test gross VA.
- Check for central retinal artery patency (may not be necessary if acuity satisfactory).
- Check IOP (in practice, this is now often omitted unless specific concern).

Follow-up
- Topical antibiotics (e.g. chloramphenicol 0.5% 4×/d) for ≥3d.
- Review in clinic according to retreatment regimen.
- Signs of disease activity in wet AMD include:
  - Deterioration in VA.
  - Evidence of CNV leakage on fluorescein angiography.
  - Abnormal retinal thickness on OCT, with evidence of intraretinal, subretinal, or sub-RPE fluid.
  - Presence/recurrence of intraretinal or subretinal haemorrhage.

Box 13.1 Summary of patient advice regarding intravitreal injections

Potential side effects/complications
- Endophthalmitis <0.1%.
- Retinal detachment.
- Lens damage/cataract.
- Raised IOP.
- Conjunctival haemorrhage.
- Vitreous floaters.
- Intraocular inflammation.
- Eye pain.
- Visual loss.

Contraindications
- Allergy to any of the components.
- Ocular and periocular infections.

Advice to patient
- Endophthalmitis warning symptoms should be explained.
- Advise that floaters post-procedure are to be expected.

15. Amoaku W *et al. Royal College of Ophthalmologists Guidelines for intravitreal injections procedure.* (2009). Available at: ℘ http://www.rcophth.ac.uk/core/core_picker/download.asp?id=167&filetitle=Guidelines+for+Intravitreal+Injections+Procedure+2009

Photodynamic therapy

PDT describes the laser stimulation of a photoactivated dye that results in the destruction of CNV. This technique aims to selectively destroy the membrane while minimizing damage to adjacent structures.

Indications

The commonest indication has been for AMD, but it has also been used for other CNVs, e.g. in myopia, inflammatory membranes, etc. Its role as a single agent in the treatment of CNV has now been largely replaced by anti-VEGF therapies, but it appears to be finding a new therapeutic niche in diseases such as central serous chorioretinopathy, PCV, and in treatment of certain ocular tumours (e.g. choroidal haemangiomas).

Mechanism

Verteporfin is a photoactivated dye that binds to lipoproteins and becomes concentrated in the proliferating vascular bed of the CNV. Laser light of 689nm wavelength is directed onto the CNV, activating the dye. The standard energy level used for tumours or AMD/polypoidal lesions (600mW/$cm^2 \times 83s = 50J/cm^2$) is too low to cause thermal damage but is sufficient to activate the dye that catalyses the formation of the free radical 'singlet oxygen'. This causes local endothelial cell death and occlusion of the blood supply to the CNV.

PDT in practice

In advance

- Discuss procedure, and take informed consent (see Box 13.2).

On the day

- Calculate spot size (greatest linear diameter + 1,000 microns).
- Confirm consent: purpose, risks (see Box 13.2).
- Ensure safety precautions (hat, long sleeves, sunglasses, resuscitation equipment available).
- IV cannula in large vein (e.g. antecubital fossa).
- Reconstitute 15mg powder with 7mL water for injections to produce a 2mg/mL solution, then dilute requisite dose (6mg/m^2 BSA) with glucose 5% to a final volume of 30mL, and give over 10min. Check laser is functioning before starting infusion, and check set-up parameter.
- At 15min since start of infusion, start 83s of laser (689nm, variable spot size, 600mW/cm^2).
- For CSR, small RCTs suggest benefit from either standard, half dose(3mg/m^2) delivered over 8min and treatment at 10min after infusion start, or reduced fluence (300mW/cm^2).

Follow-up

Review with FFA (+ ICG for polypoidal lesion) *and OCT* at 12wk for neovascular AMD at 12wk. If recurrent leakage occurs, PDT may be performed up to 4×/y. If severe ↓VA of ≥4 lines within 1wk of treatment, do not retreat, unless VA returns to pre-treatment level.

Box 13.2 Summary of patient advice regarding PDT

Side effects
- Injection site reactions: inflammation, leakage, hypersensitivity.
- Back pain: 2%.
- Transient visual disturbances.
- Significant visual loss: up to 4%.

Contraindications
- Liver failure.
- Porphyria.
- Allergy to any of the components.

Advice to patient
For 48h post-PDT, avoid direct sunlight and bright lights (including sun-lamps, halogen, or strip-lights, and undraped windows). If it is necessary to go outside during daylight hours (e.g. returning from PDT clinic), wear wide-brimmed hat, sunglasses, long-sleeved shirt, trousers, and socks.

Evidence for PDT in subfoveal choroidal neovascular membrane due to AMD

Predominantly classic choroidal neovascular membrane (includes classic with no occult)
- Treatment benefit demonstrated in the TAP (the Treatment of AMD with Photodynamic therapy) study:
  - *TAP1*: <15 letters lost in 67% vs 39% at 1y (p <0.001).
  - *TAP2*: <15 letters lost in 59% vs 31% at 2y (p <0.001).

Minimally classic choroidal neovascular membrane
- No robust evidence of benefit.

100% occult choroidal neovascular membrane
- Questionable benefit in subanalysis of VIP Study. Negative outcome in VIO Study. No robust evidence of benefit.

Evidence for PDT in subfoveal choroidal neovascular membrane due to myopia
- Treatment benefit overall at 1y but not significant at 2y.
- *VIP1*: <8 letters lost in 72% vs 44% at 1y (p <0.01) and in 51% vs 36% at 2y (p= 0.11). Emerging evidence suggests a superiority of ranibizumab over PDT for this indication.

NICE guidelines
Although, in 2006, NICE (UK) made recommendations for the use of PDT in the treatment of classic subfoveal CNV, the 2008 NICE (UK) guidance for ranibizumab and 2013 guidance for aflibercept have resulted in anti-VEGF being first-line indication for CNV 2° to AMD.

Diabetic eye disease: general

Diabetes mellitus is estimated to affect 246 million people worldwide, and, by 2030, it is estimated this will rise to over 552 million.[16] It is the commonest cause of blindness in the working population, being associated with a 20-fold increase in blindness.

WHO divides diabetes into type 1 (insulin-dependent) and type 2 (non-insulin-dependent).

- Type 1 is typically of juvenile onset and is characterized by insulin deficiency.
- Type 2 is typically of adult/elderly onset and is characterized by insulin resistance.

Clinical features

Systemic disease

Presentation

- *Type 1*: acutely with diabetic ketoacidosis or subacutely with weight loss, polyuria, polydipsia, fatigue.
- *Type 2*: incidental finding (may have long asymptomatic period); or symptoms of weight loss, polyuria, polydipsia, fatigue; or complications.

Systemic complications

- *Macrovascular*: MI (3–5× risk), peripheral vascular disease, stroke (>2× risk).
- *Microvascular*: nephropathy, neuropathy.

Ophthalmic

- *Retinopathy and sequelae*: risk varies according to type of disease (1 vs 2), duration of disease, glycaemic control, hypertension, hypercholesterolaemia, nephropathy, pregnancy, and possibly intraocular surgery.
  - In type 1 diabetes, retinopathy is rare at diagnosis but present in over 90% after 15y.
  - In type 2 disease, retinopathy is present in 20% at diagnosis but only rises to 60% after 15y.
- *Diabetic maculopathy* is the main cause for severe sight loss, rather than proliferative retinopathy.
- *Cataract*: occurs at a younger age and progress more quickly. Often poor dilatation of pupils. Increased risk of PCO and endophthalmitis post-surgery.
- *Other*: numerous ocular conditions occur more frequently in diabetes, including dry eye, decreased corneal sensation, decreased corneal healing with risk of recurrent erosions, anterior uveitis, rubeosis, neovascular glaucoma (NVG), ocular ischaemic syndrome (OIS), papillitis, AION, orbital infection, and cranial nerve palsies.

Diagnosis

- Venous fasting plasma glucose ≥7mmol/L.
- Oral glucose tolerance test (usually performed by physician) with a 2h value of >11.1mmol/L.

Diabetes Control and Complications Trial (DCCT)

For type 1 disease, the DCCT demonstrated that tight control (HbA1c 7.2% vs 9%) was associated with 76% reduction in retinopathy, 60% reduction in neuropathy, and 54% reduction in nephropathy.[17]

The DCCT also provided evidence for 'early worsening' of diabetic retinopathy, following initiation of intensive glycaemic control (i.e. in the first 3–12mo following initiation). This finding was more common and more sight-threatening in patients with more severe retinopathy and/or very poor glycaemic control.

UK Prospective Diabetic Study (UKPDS)

For type 2 disease, UKPDS demonstrated that tight control (HbA1c 7% vs 7.9%) was associated with 25% reduction in microvascular disease. Additionally, tight BP control (144/82 vs 155/87) was associated with 37% reduction in microvascular disease and 32% reduction in diabetes-related deaths.[18]

In both DCCT and UKPDS, extended periods of good glycaemic control also demonstrated 'metabolic memory' or 'legacy effect', with beneficial effects on retinopathy, even after regression of glycaemic control.

Action to Control Cardiovascular Risk in Diabetes (ACCORD)

For type 2 disease, the ACCORD study evaluated very intensive glycaemic control (targeting HbA1c <6%) vs standard control (targeting HbA1c 7–7.9%).[19] The glycaemia trial, along with studies evaluating control of BP and lipids, was halted early because of an increased rate of death from all causes in participants treated with intensive control.

16. International Diabetes Federation. *IDF Diabetes Atlas, 6th edition.* (2013). Brussels: International Diabetes Federation. Available at: ℘ http://www.idf.org/diabetesatlas

17. The Diabetes Control and Complications Trial Research Group. The effect of intensive treatment of diabetes on the development and progression of long-term complications in insulin-dependent diabetes mellitus. *N Engl J Med* 1993;**329**:977–86.

18. United Kingdom Prospective Diabetes Study Group. Intensive blood-glucose control with sulphonylureas or insulin compared with conventional treatment and risk of complications in patients with type 2 diabetes (UKPDS 33). *Lancet* 1998;**352**:837–53.

19. ACCORD Study Group et al. Effects of medical therapies on retinopathy progression in type 2 diabetes. *N Engl J Med* 2010;**363**:233–44.

Diabetic eye disease: assessment

When assessing the diabetic patient, the ophthalmologist aims to: (1) assess risk factors for eye disease (and to a lesser extent other systemic complications); (2) ensure modifiable risk factors are treated; (3) detect and grade eye disease; and (4) institute ophthalmic treatment where necessary (see Tables 13.4–13.6).

Table 13.4 An approach to assessing diabetic eye disease

Visual symptoms	Asymptomatic; ↓VA, distortion, floaters
POH	Previous diabetic eye complications; laser treatment; surgery; concurrent eye disease
PMH	Diabetes: age of diagnosis, type and duration, 'who looks after your diabetes?', 'what is your long-range diabetes test result/HbA1c?'; hypertension: 'how often is it checked?', hypercholesterolaemia, smoking; pregnancy; IHD, cerebrovascular disease, peripheral vascular disease, nephropathy, neuropathy
SH	Driver; occupation
Dx	Treatment for diabetes (diet, oral hypoglycaemics (ask about pioglitazone), insulin types, and frequency), hypertension, hypercholesterolaemia; aspirin/antiplatelet agents; warfarin
Ax	Allergies or relevant drug contraindications
VA	Best corrected/pinhole/near
Cornea	Tear film
Iris	Rubeosis
Lens	Cataract
Tonometry	
Vitreous	Haemorrhage, asteroid hyalosis
Fundus	Retinopathy (microaneurysms, haemorrhages, exudates, IRMAs, venous beading, venous loops, neovascularization), maculopathy (fluid, exudates, retinal thickening), TRD/RRD, arterial/venous occlusion, ocular ischaemia
Disc	New vessels, papillitis, AION

Table 13.5 Definitions in diabetic eye disease

Retinopathy[*]	
Background (low risk)	Microaneurysms, small haemorrhages, hard exudates, occasional CWS
Pre-proliferative (high risk)	IRMAs, venous beading/loops, clusters of large blot haemorrhages, multiple CWS
Proliferative	
NVD	New vessels at the disc or within 1DD of the disc ('*high-risk*': NVD >1/3 disc area or any NVD with vitreous or preretinal haemorrhage)
NVE	New vessels elsewhere in the retina ('*high-risk*': NVE >1/2 disc area with vitreous or preretinal haemorrhage)
Maculopathy	
Focal	Well-circumscribed areas of leakage, with oedema and full/part rings of exudates often surrounding a microaneurysm
Diffuse	Generalized leakage with oedema
Ischaemic	↓VA with relatively normal clinical appearance, but macular ischaemia on FFA
Mixed	Combination, e.g. of diffuse and ischaemic
Clinically significant macular oedema (CSMO)	• Retinal thickening at or within 500 microns of the centre of the macula • Hard exudates at or within 500 microns of the centre of the macula if associated with adjacent retinal thickening • Retinal thickening of >1 disc area, any part of which is within 1DD of the centre of the macula.

[*] The alternative Airlie House classification (as used in the ETDRS) includes the following categories of non-proliferative diabetic retinopathy (NPDR):
- Mild NPDR: at least one microaneurysm.
- Moderate NPDR: severe retinal haemorrhages in at least one quadrant; or CWS, venous beading, or IRMA definitely present.
- Severe NPDR: severe retinal haemorrhages in four quadrants; or venous beading in two quadrants; or extensive IRMA in one quadrant.
- Very severe NPDR: any two of the features of severe NPDR.

Effectively, background retinopathy corresponds to mild NPDR, whereas pre-proliferative retinopathy would include the range from moderate to very severe non-proliferative retinopathy.

The international (AAO) classification has similarities to a simplified form of the Airlie House criteria. A summary of the equivalence of the different classification systems may be found in the Royal College of Ophthalmologists Diabetic Retinopathy Guidelines 2012 at: ℘ http://www.rcophth.ac.uk

Table 13.6 An approach to diabetic eye disease*

Retinopathy	
None/background	Discharge to community screening service for annual review; if significant systemic disease, consider review at 9–12mo by hospital eye service
Pre-proliferative	Observe 4–6-monthly (consider early PRP in select cases, e.g. in only eye where first eye lost to PDR or prior to cataract surgery)
Proliferative (active)	PRP (1–2 sessions × ≥1,000 × 200–500 microns × 0.1s)—wherever possible, this should occur on the same day or within 2wk; evolving role for anti-VEGF therapies. In young patients with type 1 diabetes, PRP should be delivered over 3–4 sessions, as increased risk of macular oedema post-PRP if excess burns applied in single session
Proliferative (regressed)	Observe 4–6-monthly (signs of decreased neovascularization activity include: regression of vessels ± fibrosis, resolution of retinal haemorrhages, decreases in retinal vessel dilatation and tortuosity)
Proliferative with coexisting DMO	For 'high-risk' cases, consider combined macular laser and PRP (with completion of PRP over three sessions, rather than 1–2). For 'low-risk' cases, it may be possible to perform macular laser initially, with PRP at subsequent follow-up. Anti-VEGF therapies may be of particular use in this context, although practice guidelines are still evolving
Maculopathy	
Focal leakage	Focal laser photocoagulation (n × 50–100 microns × 0.08–0.1s); review at 3–4mo
Diffuse leakage	Grid laser photocoagulation (n × 100–200 microns × 0.1s); review at 3–4mo
Ischaemic	FFA to confirm diagnosis; observation may be appropriate if significant ischaemia and/or no response to previous laser
Persistent maculopathy	Anti-VEGF therapies (ranibizumab approved by NICE for cases with central retinal thickness >400 microns); intravitreal iluvien in pseudophakic eyes; consider vitrectomy if vitreomacular traction
Rubeosis	
Rubeosis + clear media	Urgent PRP × anti-VEGF therapies

(Continued)

Table 13.6 (*Cont.*)

Rubeosis + vitreous haemorrhage	Vitrectomy + endolaser
Rubeotic glaucoma	Urgent PRP/anti-VEGF therapies ↓IOP with topical medication/cyclodiode/augmented trabeculectomy/tubes
Vitreous haemorrhage	
No view of fundus	US to ensure retina flat + review 2–4-weekly until adequate view
Adequate view	Ensure retina flat + PRP
Persistent	Vitrectomy + endolaser + anti-VEGF therapies

* See also Royal College of Ophthalmologists. *Diabetic retinopathy guidelines.* (2012). Available at: ℘ http://www.rcophth.ac.uk/core/core_picker/download.asp?id=1789&filetitle=Diabetic+Retinopathy+Guidelines+2012+%28minor+update+July+2013%29

Diabetic eye disease: management

Treatment: systemic

Glycaemic control

- A personalized target should be set, usually HbA1c 6.5–7.5% (48–58mmol/mol); set less strict targets in patients with established cardiovascular disease and in older subjects.
- *For type 1 disease*: insulin regimens include: (1) twice daily premixed insulins and (2) ultra-fast or soluble insulins with each meal and long-acting insulin at night.
- *For type 2 disease*: start with diet, followed by metformin and then a sulfonylurea if not overweight (e.g. gliclazide or glibenclamide); a DPP-4 inhibitor or a glitazone (e.g. pioglitazone) may be used as an alternative or in combination; pioglitazone has been associated with the development of DMO; insulin may be required.

BP control

- Aim for systolic ≤130mmHg in those with established retinopathy and/or nephropathy (in those without retinopathy, usually aim for <140mmHg).
- Encourage regular monitoring of BP (including at home, if possible).
- Effective anti-hypertensives include ACE inhibitors (usually first line in type 2 diabetes), angiotensin II receptor (AIIR) antagonists, β-blockers, or thiazide diuretics.

Cholesterol control

- Aim for lipid lowering if >30% 10y risk of coronary heart disease (current recommendations, although ideally treat all with risk >15%). This can be calculated from the Framingham equation or the Joint British Societies nomogram (see *BNF*).
- A statin is the drug of choice; consider adding fenofibrate to a statin for non-proliferative retinopathy in type 2 diabetes (evidence for benefit in the ACCORD eye study).[20]

Support renal function

- Microalbuminuria is indicative of early nephropathy and is associated with increased risk of macrovascular complications.
- ACE inhibitors or AIIR antagonists are preferred.

Lifestyle

- *Smoking cessation*: smoking greatly increases macrovascular disease, and strategies to assist the patient 'give-up' should be explored.
- *Weight control*: mainly in type 2 disease, particularly if BMI >25.
- *Exercise >30min/d*: ↓weight, ↓BP, ↑insulin sensitivity, improves lipid profile.

Pregnancy

- Progression of retinopathy is a significant, but relatively low, risk in pregnancy.
- Pregnant women with pre-existing diabetes should be offered retinal assessment following their first antenatal clinic appointment (i.e. first trimester, typically 8–12wk). If normal, further assessment should be in the third trimester, typically 28wk or, if retinopathy present, an additional assessment should occur in the second trimester, typically 16–20wk. Post-partum follow-up also required.

20. ACCORD Study Group *et al*. Effects of medical therapies on retinopathy progression in type 2 diabetes. *N Engl J Med* 2010;**363**:233–44.

Diabetic eye disease: screening

What is screening?

Screening is the systematic testing of a population (or subgroup) for signs of asymptomatic or ignored disease.

Screening for diabetic eye disease

The classification systems for diabetic retinopathy range from the very detailed Airlie House system (generally for use in trials) to the dichotomous non-proliferative vs proliferative division. In terms of clinical management, the traditional background/pre-proliferative/proliferative grading system is the most familiar to 1° care physicians and optometrists and has been adopted by the National Screening Committee (UK).

Although screening may be by dilated fundoscopy, quality assurance can be more readily achieved where there is a photographic record. Hence a national programme of digital photographic screening is underway. Photography could potentially be performed by mobile units, by selected 1°/2° care units, or by community optometrists. Grading of the photographs could be performed by the same units (if approved) or the photographs could be sent to an approved centre. The UK National Screening Committee guidelines undergo regular revision and are available at ℘ http://diabeticeye.screening.nhs.uk (see Table 13.7).

Appropriate referral to the hospital eye service

- *Pre-proliferative retinopathy (R2)*: referral to hospital eye service (HES) (target ≤13wk).
- *Proliferative retinopathy (R3)*: fast-track referral (target ≤2wk)
- *Maculopathy fulfilling screening guidelines (M1)*: referral to HES (target ≤13wk).
- *Time between listing once seen in eye clinic and photocoagulation if new screen (P1)*: proliferative retinopathy (R3) ≤2wk, maculopathy target ≤10wk.
- *Unclassifiable (U)*: referral to HES.

NB The NHS Diabetic Eye Screening Programme in England only operates an annual screening programme, and patients should therefore only be discharged to screening if at sufficiently low risk to receive 12-monthly photographic assessments.

Table 13.17 National screening committee recommendations for grading and management of retinopathy

Retinopathy	R0	None		Annual screening
	R1	Background	Microaneurysm(s)	Annual screening
			Retinal haemorrhage(s)	Inform diabetes care team
			Venous loop	
			Any exudate in presence of other non-referable DR features	
			Any CWS in presence of other non-referable DR features	
	R2	Pre-proliferative	Venous beading	Refer to HES
			Venous reduplication	
			IRMA	
			Multiple deep, round or blot haemorrhages	
	R3a	Proliferative (active)	New vessels on disc (NVD)	Fast-track referral to HES
			New vessels elsewhere (NVE)	
			Pre-retinal or vitreous haemorrhage	
			Pre-retinal fibrosis ± tractional retinal detachment	
	R3s	Proliferative (stable post treatment)	Evidence of peripheral retinal laser AND stable retina from photo-graph taken at or shortly after discharge from HES	
Maculopathy	M0		No maculopathy	Annual screening
	M1		Exudate within 1 DD of the centre of the fovea	Refer to HES
			Circinate or group of exudates within the macula	
			Retinal thickening 01DD of the centre of the fovea (if stereo availa-ble).	
			Any microaneurysm or haemorrhage 01DD of the centre of the fovea with a best VA of 06/12 (if no stereo)	
Photo-coagulation	P	Photocoagula-tion	Only assigned if laser scars are identified (focal/grid to macula or peripheral scatter)	
Unclassifiable	U	Ungradable	E.g. If media opacity, poor photographs	Refer to HES

Central serous chorioretinopathy

The aetiology of central serous chorioretinopathy (*syn* central serous retinopathy, CSR) is unknown, but choroidal hyperpermeability appears to play a central role, leading to a variable combination of sub-RPE and SRF accumulation.

Risk factors

It typically affects adult men (20–50y) and is reportedly associated with type A personalities, psychosocial stress, pregnancy (usually third trimester), and Cushing's disease (5% prevalence). Numerous drugs (notably corticosteroids) are associated; it is vital to enquire about all medications, including tablets, creams and lotions, inhalers, plus any natural remedies.

Clinical features

- Unilateral sudden ↓VA, positive scotoma (usually central), metamorphopsia, increased hypermetropia.
- Shallow detachment of the sensory retina at the posterior pole, deeper small yellow-grey elevations RPE detachments (PEDs); multifocal or diffuse pigmentary changes suggest chronicity; occasionally, fluid tracks inferiorly from the posterior pole to cause a bullous non-rhegmatogenous detachment of the inferior peripheral retina.

Investigations

- In patients with chronic or recurrent disease, liaise with GP to rule out systemic causes (e.g. 24h urine collection for cortisol in cases of suspected Cushing's disease).
- *FFA* (see Fig. 13.3): one or more points of progressive leakage and pooling, classically in a smoke-stack or ink-blot pattern.
- *ICG*: when performed, shows choroidal hyperpermeability in late phase, with area of hyperfluorescence more widespread than the leakage point on FFA and commonly bilateral changes.
- *OCT*: shows neurosensory retinal detachment and accompanying small PEDs. The overlying retinal architecture typically appears intact, although cystoid degeneration may be present in severe, chronic cases. On EDI-OCT, the choroid is often markedly thickened, with dilatation of large choroidal vessels (now considered a disease hallmark by many).

Treatment

- *Conservative*: central serous chorioretinopathy has a high rate of spontaneous remission. Conservative management includes lifestyle counselling and the avoidance of glucocorticoid medication.
- *Indications for other intervention*: persistence >6mo, multiple recurrences, occupational needs, contralateral persistent visual impairment from central serous chorioretinopathy.
- *Argon laser treatment*: mild burns to the leakage site (usually <10 burns, 50–200 microns, 0.1s, power adjusted to produce very gentle blanching only).
- *PDT*: half-dose PDT may be beneficial for those with severe disease not amenable to argon laser (e.g. subfoveal).

Prognosis

In 80%, spontaneous recovery to near normal VA (≥6/12) within 1–6mo. Subtle metamorphopsia may persist. Chronic (5%) or recurrent episodes (in up to 45%) may be associated with more significant visual loss. A small risk (<2%/y) of CNV is reported. Pregnancy associated central serous chorioretinopathy usually resolves 1–2mo post-delivery.

Differential diagnosis

In all patients, it is important to examine the optic disc thoroughly for pits. Other differentials include: CNV, PCV, inflammatory disease causing serous detachments (VKH, posterior scleritis, sympathetic ophthalmia, uveal effusion syndrome), autoimmune disease (SLE, PAN), vascular disease (malignant hypertension, toxaemia of pregnancy, disseminated intravascular coagulation (DIC)), choroidal tumours (including lymphoma).

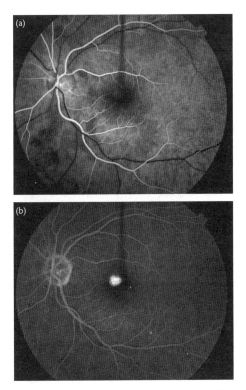

Fig. 13.3 FFA of central serous chorioretinopathy. (a) Early phase. (b) Late phase: ink blot pattern.

Cystoid macular oedema

This important macular disorder is a common pathological response to a wide variety of ocular insults, most commonly after cataract surgery (see ➲ Post-operative cystoid macular oedema, p. 339), or in association with retinal vascular or inflammatory disease (see Box 13.3). Knowledge of underlying mechanisms is essential to a rational therapeutic approach.

Mechanisms

- Increased vascular permeability:
  - Release of hyperpermeability factors (e.g. VEGF, prostaglandins)
  - Loss of vascular structure (e.g. loss of endothelial cells/pericytes in diabetic retinopathy).
  - Congenital vascular abnormalities (e.g. Coats' disease).
- Increased blood flow (e.g. post-operative states).
- Dysfunction of the RPE barrier/pump (e.g. inherited retinal dystrophies).
- Tractional stress (e.g. vitreomacular traction, ERM).
- Drug reactions.
- Fluid migration from abnormalities of the optic nerve head (e.g. optic disc pit).

Clinical features

- Asymptomatic, ↓VA (may be severe), metamorphopsia, scotomas.
- Loss of foveal contour, retinal thickening, cystoid spaces; central yellow spot, small intraretinal haemorrhages, and telangiectasia (occasional).
- Associated features depend on the underlying cause.
- *Complications*: lamellar hole (irreversible ↓VA).

Investigations

- *FFA*: typically dye leakage from the parafovea into the cystoid spaces (petalloid pattern) and from the optic disc. In certain conditions, CMO may develop in the absence of retinal capillary leakage on FFA (e.g. certain drug reactions and inherited dystrophies).
- *OCT*: detection rate is equal to FFA and can measure degree of retinal thickening and specific pathology, e.g. vitreomacular traction. OCT may also be useful in differentiating CMO from macular retinoschisis (e.g. XLRS).

Treatment

Although there may be some variation, according to the underlying cause and severity, a step-wise approach is recommended. Most experts would proceed directly to local or systemic therapy, unless the CMO is related to a recent insult (such as surgery or laser). Review the diagnosis if atypical or slow to respond. One approach is as follows:

1. *Topical (if CMO related to a recent insult)*: steroid (e.g. dexamethasone 0.1% 4×/d) + NSAID (e.g. ketorolac 0.3% 3×/d).

Review in 4–6wk; if persisting, then:

2. Periocular steroid (e.g. orbital floor/sub-Tenon's; methylprednisolone/ triamcinolone), and continue topical Rx.

Review in 4–6wk; if persisting, then:

3. *Consider*: repeating periocular or giving intravitreal steroid (e.g. triam-cinolone 2mg); vitrectomy; systemic steroids (e.g. prednisolone 40mg 1×/d, titrating over 3wk; or IVMP 500mg single dose; uveitic CMO may require higher doses); topical or oral carbonic anhydrase inhibitors (e.g. dorzolamide, acetazolamide; limited evidence).

Prognosis

Varies according to underlying pathology. Most patients with CMO arising after cataract surgery will attain VA ≥6/9 within 3–12mo of their operation.

Box 13.3 Causes of CMO

- Inflammatory disorders:
  - Post-operative (cataract/corneal/vitreoretinal surgery).
  - Post-laser (peripheral iridotomy, PRP).
  - Post-cryotherapy.
  - Uveitis.
- Retinal vascular disease:
  - RVO.
  - Diabetic retinopathy.
  - Hypertensive retinopathy.
  - Radiation retinopathy.
  - OIS.
  - Retinal vascular telangiectasia (e.g. MacTel).
- Choroidal vascular disease:
  - CNV.
- Drug reactions:
  - Nicotinic acid.
  - Topical adrenaline.
  - Prostaglandin analogues (e.g. latanoprost).
  - Chemotherapeutic agents (e.g. paclitaxel).
  - Glitazones.
- Inherited retinal dystrophies:
  - RP.
  - Autosomal dominantly inherited CMO.
- Disorders of vitreoretinal interface:
  - Vitreomacular traction syndrome.
  - ERM.
- Optic nerve head abnormalities:
  - Optic disc pit.
  - Optic disc coloboma.
- Tumours of the choroid/retina.
- Idiopathic.

Degenerative myopia

Myopia is common and is regarded as physiological if <–6D. Of those with high myopia (>–6D), there is a subset in whom the axial length may never stabilize (progressive or pathological myopia) and who are at risk of degenerative changes. Myopia has emerged as a major health issue in east Asia (affecting 80–90% in school-leavers) and because of the sight-threatening pathologies associated with high myopia (affecting 10–20% of those completing 2° schooling).[21] Excessive near work appears to be a risk factor, while increased time outdoors appears protective. Genetic risk factors may also play a role in high myopia, with the *CTNND2* gene on Chr 5p15 recently identified in genome-wide association studies.[22]

Clinical features

- Increasing myopia, ↓VA, metamorphopsia, photopsia (occasional).
- *Fundus*: pale, tessellated with areas of chorioretinal atrophy both centrally and peripherally; breaks in Bruch's membrane ('lacquer cracks') may permit CNV formation, spontaneous macular haemorrhage, and subsequent elevated pigmented scar (Förster–Fuchs' spot); posterior staphyloma; lattice degeneration.
- *Disc*: tilted, atrophy temporal to the disc ('temporal crescent'), peripapillary choroidal cavitation (appears clinically as a well-circumscribed yellow-orange thickening, commonly seen at the inferior border of the myopic conus).
- Vitreous syneresis; PVD (at younger age).
- *Other associations*: long axial length, deep AC, zonular dehiscence, PDS, and glaucoma (see Table 13.8).
- *Complications*: CNV (myopia is commonest cause of CNV in young patients), macular hole, peripheral retinal tears, RRD, macular retinoschisis. Macular hole retinal detachments may sometimes occur in eyes with posterior staphyloma.

Investigations

- *Posterior staphyloma*: US for confirmation and monitoring of axial length. A 'dome-shaped' macula variant may be seen on OCT in a minority.
- *Myopic CNV*: the appearance of myopic CNV on OCT differs from that seen in wet AMD, being smaller in size and associated with considerably less intraretinal or subretinal fluid. Sub-RPE fluid is typically negligible. As a result, assessment of CNV leakage using FFA is more frequently required, both for initial diagnosis and to guide retreatment.
- *Macular retinoschisis*: OCT is useful for differentiating macular retinoschisis from macular hole retinal detachment.

Table 13.8 Associations of myopia

| Stickler syndrome |
| Marfan's syndrome |
| Ehlers–Danlos |
| Down's syndrome |
| Gyrate atrophy |
| Congenital rubella |
| Albinism |

Treatment

- *Prevent progression*: trials of increased time spent outdoors are currently underway. Other interventions remain controversial (e.g. orthokeratology, atropine eye drops, scleral reinforcement procedures).
- *CNV*: preliminary results for use of anti-VEGF therapies (see ➲ Anti-vascular endothelial growth factor therapy, pp. 528–30) are supportive for 1° therapy of myopic CNV.[23] Alternative treatments are PDT (see ➲ Photodynamic therapy, p. 532) for subfoveal CNV, and argon laser photocoagulation for extrafoveal CNV (although use of the latter is limited due to the significant creep of the resultant atrophic zone that often occurs over time).

Prognosis

- High myopia is the commonest cause of CNV in young patients, accounting for >60% of CNV in those under 50y of age.
- Risk factors for CNV development are lacquer cracks (29% develop CNV) and patchy atrophy (20% develop CNV).
- Although the natural history of myopic CNV is highly variable, the long-term visual outcome is generally poor, in large part due to late atrophy. At 5y following onset of myopic CNV (untreated), about 90% of patients have a VA ≤6/60.[24] It is hoped that this will be improved by the advent of anti-VEGF therapies, although their long-term efficacy and safety are not yet known.

21. Morgan IG et al. Myopia. Lancet 2012;**379**:1739–48.

22. Li YJ et al. Genome-wide association studies reveal genetic variants in CTNND2 for high myopia in Singapore Chinese. Ophthalmology 2011;**118**:368–75.

23. Tufail A et al. Ranibizumab for the treatment of choroidal neovascularisation secondary to pathological myopia: interim analysis of the REPAIR study. Eye 2013;**27**:709–15.

24. Yoshida T et al. Myopic choroidal neovascularization: a 10-year follow-up. Ophthalmology 2003;**110**:1297–305.

Angioid streaks

Angioid streaks are breaks in an abnormally thickened and calcified Bruch's membrane that may be associated with a number of endocrine, metabolic, and connective tissue abnormalities, but, in about half, no underlying cause is found (see Table 13.9 for causes).

Pseudoxanthoma elasticum (PXE)

PXE is by far the most common systemic association of angioid streaks. PXE is an AR connective tissue disorder, causing calcification and degeneration of elastic fibres in the skin, eye, and CVS. In patients with angioid streaks, the skin of the neck, antecubital fossae, and axillae should be examined for the 'plucked chicken'/'cobblestone-like' appearance seen in PXE (skin is usually first organ system affected and leads to diagnosis in most cases).

Clinical features

- Asymptomatic; ↓VA, metamorphopsia.
- *Angioid streaks*: narrow irregular streaks radiating from a peripapillary ring; the colour of the streaks varies from red to dark brown, depending on background pigmentation (less visible in younger patients).
- *Associated features*: peripapillary chorioretinal atrophy; local/diffuse RPE mottling ('peau d'orange'; commonest in PXE); disc drusen.
- *Complications*: CNV, choroidal rupture (after minor trauma), subfoveal haemorrhage.

Investigations

- *FFA*: if CNV suspected; angioid streaks show hyperfluorescence due to window defect.

Treatment

- *Conservative*: advise to avoid contact sports/risk of trauma.
- *All CNV*: preliminary results suggest intravitreal anti-VEGF therapies may be beneficial and are now commonly used as first-line agents.
- *Extrafoveal/juxtafoveal CNV*: argon laser photocoagulation of PDT is also an option but often fail to prevent subfoveal progression.
- *Subfoveal CNV*: results suggest that PDT may be of benefit in the short term, but benefit is lost with a progressive decline in vision by 2y.

Table 13.9 Causes of angioid streaks

Pseudoxanthoma elasticum (PXE)
Ehlers–Danlos syndrome
Paget's disease
Acromegaly
Haemaglobinopathies
Hereditary spherocytosis
Abetalipoproteinaemia
Idiopathic (50%)

Choroidal folds

These are corrugations in the choroid and Bruch's membrane that are seen as a series of light and dark lines. They are usually horizontal and lie over the posterior pole, although they can be vertical, oblique, or jigsaw-like. They are distinguished from retinal striae by being deeper and broader. Although they may in themselves cause visual dysfunction, their main significance is to prompt thorough investigation for an underlying disease (see Table 13.10 for causes).

Investigations

- FFA shows alternating lines of hyperfluorescence (peaks) and hypofluorescence (troughs). At peaks, the RPE is stretched and thinned, allowing increased fluorescent signal from the underlying choroid, while, at troughs, the fluorescent signal is blocked by 'bunching up' of the RPE.
- On OCT, choroidal folds appear as undulations of the RPE, without evidence of separation from Bruch's membrane. OCT also allows easy differentiation between choroidal folds and retinal striae (e.g. as occurs in some eyes with ERM).
- Orbital US may allow detection of retrobulbar masses or other orbital pathology.
- CT/MRI scanning of the orbits and head may be useful for excluding orbital or intracranial pathology. The latter may be of particular value in patients with acquired 'idiopathic' hypermetropia, as raised intracranial pressure may sometimes cause choroidal folds in the absence of papilloedema.

Table 13.10 Causes of choroidal folds

- Idiopathic ('congenital')
  - Asymptomatic, bilateral folds in healthy, often hypermetropic, subjects
- Orbital
  - TED
  - Retrobulbar mass
  - Idiopathic orbital inflammatory disease
- Ocular
  - Hypotony
  - Posterior scleritis
  - Choroidal lesions (e.g. disciform scars or tumours)
  - Uveitis
- Intracranial
  - Raised intracranial pressure (ICP) (choroidal folds may sometimes occur in the absence of papilloedema)

Retinal vein occlusion (1)

RVOs are common, can occur at almost any age, and range in presentation from the asymptomatic to the painful blind eye. They are divided into branch (BRVO) or central retinal vein occlusions (CRVO) (equating to occlusion anterior or posterior to the cribriform plate), and 'ischaemic' or 'non-ischaemic' types. Most occur in those over 65y, but up to 15% may affect patients under 45y. BRVO are three times more common than CRVO.

CRVO

Although the division of non-ischaemic vs ischaemic CRVO is an arbitrary cut-off, based on FFA findings, it is a useful predictor of visual outcome and risk of neovascularization. The clinical picture also differs (see Table 13.11).

Clinical features

Non-ischaemic

- ↓VA (mild to moderate), painless, metamorphopsia.
- Dilated, tortuous retinal veins, with retinal haemorrhages in all four quadrants; occasional CWS; mild optic disc oedema.
- *Complications*: CMO.

Ischaemic

- ↓VA (severe); painless (unless NVG has developed).
- As for non-ischaemic, but RAPD, deeper and more extensive haemorrhages, widespread CWS; rarely vitreous haemorrhage, ERD.
- *Chronic*: venous sheathing, resorption of haemorrhages, macular pigment disturbance, collateral vessels (especially at disc).
- *Complications*: CMO, neovascularization (neovascularization of the iris (NVI) > NVD > NVE), neovascular ('90d') glaucoma (NVG). **NB** Vessels that occur in NVD are typically smaller calibre than collaterals, branch into a net-like vascular network, and leak on FFA.

Investigations

- *For all patients*: BP, FBC, ESR, U+E, Glu, lipids, protein electrophoresis, TFT, and ECG. Further investigation is directed by clinical indication and may include CRP, serum ACE, anticardiolipin, lupus anticoagulant, autoantibodies (RF, ANA, anti-DNA, ANCA), fasting homocysteine, CXR, and thrombophilia screen (e.g. proteins C and S, antithrombin, factor V).
- In the rare patient with simultaneous bilateral CRVOs, the possibility of an underlying hyperviscosity syndrome should be specifically excluded. Similarly, if gentle digital pressure on the globe produces retinal arterial pulsations (or they occur spontaneously), an underlying OIS should be excluded (see ➲ Ocular ischaemic syndrome, p. 562).

- *FFA*:
  - *All*: normal arm to eye time, slow AV phase acutely.
  - *Non-ischaemic*: vein wall staining, microaneurysms, dilated optic disc capillaries.
  - *Ischaemic*: as for non-ischaemic, but capillary closure (5–10DD is borderline; >10 is significantly ischaemic), hypofluorescence (blockage due to extensive haemorrhage), leakage (CMO, neovascularization),
- *OCT*: typically demonstrates substantial retinal thickening, with inner and outer retinal cysts and SRF at the fovea; allows diagnosis and monitoring of macular oedema.

Table 13.11 Associations of CRVO

Atherosclerotic	Hypertension
	Hypercholesterolaemia (including 2° to hypothyroidism)
	Diabetes
	Smoking
	Obesity
Haematological	Protein S, protein C, or antithrombin deficiency
	Activated protein C resistance
	Factor V Leiden
	Myeloma
	Waldenström's macroglobulinaemia
	Antiphospholipid syndrome
Inflammatory	Behçet's disease
	PAN
	Sarcoidosis
	Granulomatosis with polyangiitis (GPA)
	SLE
	Goodpasture syndrome
Pharmacological	Oral contraceptive pill (usually in context of prothrombotic state)
Ophthalmic	Glaucoma (open- or closed-angle)
	Trauma
	Optic disc drusen
	Orbital pathology

Treatment (See Table 13.12)
- *Underlying medical conditions*: liaise with a physician for investigation and treatment. NB In young adults with CRVO, a mortality of 12% due to vascular disease has been reported. The benefit of aspirin in RVO remains equivocal.
- *↓IOP*: if elevated (in either eye).
- *Macular oedema*: consider treatment with biodegradable dexamethasone intravitreal implant 0.7mg (Ozurdex®, Allergan), anti-VEGF therapies (ranibizumab, bevacizumab, aflibercept), or intravitreal triamcinolone acetonide 2–4mg.
- *NVA and/or NVI*: perform PRP ± anti-VEGF ± IOP control.

Prognosis[25]
- *Non-ischaemic recovery to normal VA*: is <10%.
- *Non-ischaemic progression to ischaemic*: 15% by 4mo, 34% by 3y.
- *Ischaemic progression to rubeosis*: 37% by 4mo. Highest risk if VA <6/60 or ≥30 disc areas of non-perfusion on FFA.
- *Risk of CRVO in contralateral eye*: 7% by 2y.

Table 13.12 Summary of Royal College of Ophthalmologists interim guidelines for management of CRVO 2010*

Non-ischaemic	If VA ≤6/12 + OCT ≥250 microns, consider Ozurdex® or ranibizumab. No Rx recommended if VA <6/96 or brisk RAPD (instead, manage as ischaemic CRVO). Retreat with Ozurdex® at 4–6mth intervals. For ranibizumab, consider monthly injections for first 6–12mo, and then prn. Can be discharged if stable by 24mo
Ischaemic with no neovasvularization	Examination (including gonioscopy) monthly for first 6mo, then every 3mo for 1y; can be discharged if stable by 24mo
Ischaemic with neovascularization (angle or iris)	PRP (1,500–2,000 × 500 microns × 0.05–0.1); consider combined use of bevacizumab; follow-up 6-weekly; repeat treatment if NVI/NVA persists
NVG with visual potential	↓IOP with topical agents or cycloablation (see ➲ Neovascular glaucoma, p. 370)
NVG in blind eye	Keep comfortable with topical agents (see ➲ Neovascular glaucoma, p. 370)

* Royal College of Ophthalmologists. *Interim guidelines for management of retinal vein occlusion.* (2010). Available at: ℗ http://www.rcophth.ac.uk/clinicalguidelines

25. The Central Vein Occlusion Study Group. Natural history and clinical management of central retinal vein occlusion. *Arch Ophthalmol* 1997;**115**:486–91.

Retinal vein occlusion (2)

BRVO

Clinical features
- Most commonly superotemporal, unilateral in 90%.
- May be asymptomatic; ↓VA, metamorphopsia, VF defect (usually altitudinal).
- *Acute*: retinal haemorrhages (dot, blot, flame), CWS, oedema in the distribution of a dilated, tortuous vein; superotemporal arcade most commonly affected; usually arise from an arteriovenous crossing.
- *Chronic*: venous sheathing, exudates, pigment disturbance, collateral vessels.
- *Complications*: CMO, neovascularization (NVE > NVD > NVI), recurrent vitreous haemorrhage.

Investigations
- Hypertension is the commonest association with BRVO (up to 75% of patients). BRVO may be investigated similarly to CRVO (see ➲ CRVO, p. 552).
- *FFA*: if uncertain diagnosis or where VA <6/12 at 3mo (>5DD is significantly ischaemic).
- *OCT*: useful for documenting macular oedema, which characteristically respects the horizontal raphe.

Treatment (See Table 13.13)
- *Macular oedema*: options include: macular grid laser (after FFA to determine perifoveal capillary perfusion), biodegradable dexamethasone intravitreal implant 0.7mg (Ozurdex®, Allergan), or anti-VEGF therapies (ranibizumab, bevacizumab, aflibercept), if VA ≤6/12.
- *Neovascularization*: sectoral PRP.

Prognosis[26]
- *Recovery of VA*: estimates vary widely, but around 50% appear to improve by ≥2 lines.
- *Risk of retinal neovascularization*: 20%, usually within the first 6–12mo.
- *Risk of NVD or NVI*: low.
- *Risk of BRVO in contralateral eye*: around 5% at baseline, increasing to 10% of fellow eye involvement over time.

Hemiretinal vein occlusion (HRVO)

HRVO has a similar appearance to BRVO, but the entire superior or inferior hemisphere is involved. HRVO has previously been classified as: (1) *hemi-central retinal vein occlusion*, in which the central retinal vein forms posterior to the lamina cribrosa from a dual trunk, with occlusion affecting a single trunk (thus a variant of CRVO), or (2) *hemispheric retinal vein occlusion*, in which a major branch of the central retinal vein is occluded at or near the optic disc (thus a variant of BRVO). However, use of this classification is limited by difficulty in identifying the site of occlusion in many cases of HRVO. Ischaemic hemispheric vein occlusions have an intermediate risk of rubeosis (compared with ischaemic BRVO and CRVO), but a greater risk of NVD than either ischaemic BRVO or CRVO. In the SCORE Study, HRVO was treated as BRVO and demonstrated a similar response to treatment.[27]

Table 13.13 Summary of Royal College of Ophthalmologists interim guidelines for management of BRVO 2010[*]

Macular oedema with no or minimal **macular** ischaemia	*Within 3mo of onset*: consider Ozurdex® or ranibizumab
	After 3mo of onset: consider macular grid laser (20–100 × 100–200 microns × 'gentle') or pharmacotherapy with Ozurdex® (licensed) or ranibizumab. Retreat with Ozurdex® at 4–6mo intervals. For ranibizumab, consider monthly injections for first 6mo and then prn. Retreatment with macular grid laser should be considered at 4-monthly intervals. If stable, can usually be discharged by 24mo
Macular oedema with marked **macular** ischaemia	No immediate treatment is recommended. Monitor for development of neovascularization
Ischaemic BRVO with no neovascularization	Review at 3mo, then every 3–4mo; if stable, can usually be discharged by 24mo
Ischaemic BRVO with NVD or NVE	Sectoral PRP (400–500 × 500 microns × 0.05–0.1) ± bevacizumab. Follow-up as described previously

[*] Royal College of Ophthalmologists. *Interim guidelines for management of retinal vein occlusion.* (2010). Available at: ✍ http://www.rcophth.ac.uk/clinicalguidelines

26. Rogers SL *et al.* Natural history of branch retinal vein occlusion: an evidence-based systematic review. *Ophthalmology* 2010;**117**:1094–101.

27. Scott IU *et al.* Baseline characteristics and response to treatment of participants with hemiretinal compared with branch retinal or central retinal vein occlusion in the Standard Care vs COrticosteroid for REtinal Vein Occlusion (SCORE) Study. SCORE Study Report 14. *Arch Ophthalmol* 2012;**130**:1517–24.

Retinal artery occlusion (1)

Retinal artery occlusion is an ocular emergency, in which rapidly instigated treatment *may* prevent irreversible loss of vision. Central retinal artery occlusion (CRAO) has an estimated incidence 0.85/100,000/y, with men twice as often affected as women and with a mean age of 60y. CRAO causes almost complete hypoxia of the inner retina. Experimental evidence shows that this causes lethal damage to the primate retina after 100min. Acute coagulative necrosis is followed by complete loss of the nerve fibre layer, ganglion cell layer, and inner plexiform layer.

Central retinal artery occlusion (CRAO)

Clinical features

- Sudden painless unilateral ↓VA (usually CF or worse).
- White swollen retina with a cherry-red spot at the macula; arteriolar attenuation + cattle-trucking; RAPD; visible emboli in up to 25%.
- A cilioretinal artery (present in 30%) may protect part of the papillomacular bundle, allowing relatively good vision.
- *Complications*: neovascularization (NVI in 18%; NVD in 2%); rubeotic glaucoma; optic atrophy; ocular ischaemic syndrome (OIS) (if ophthalmic artery occlusion).

Investigations

In the acute setting, the diagnosis is not usually in doubt, so the urgent priority is to rule out underlying disease (such as GCA) that may threaten the contralateral eye. When presentation is delayed, the clinical picture is less specific, with the fundus often appearing featureless. On OCT, however, inner retinal atrophy with outer retinal preservation may be clearly seen.

Identify cause

- Most importantly, consider GCA (if age >50y, then ESR, CRP, FBC, temporal artery biopsy; see ➲ Anterior ischaemic optic neuropathy, p. 666); more common causes are atherosclerosis (check for ↑BP, diabetes, hypercholesterolaemia, and smoking) and particularly carotid artery disease (may have carotid bruit).
- Further investigation is directed by clinical indication and may include PTT, APTT, thrombophilia screen (e.g. proteins C and S, antithrombin, factor V), antiphospholipid screen, vasculitis autoantibodies (ANA, ANCA, DNA, RF), syphilis serology (VDRL, TPHA), blood cultures, ECG, echocardiography, carotid Doppler scans (see Table 13.14). Where possible, 'fast-track' referral to a specialist stroke clinic is advisable.

NB On carotid Doppler scans, the presence or absence of a plaque is more important than whether significant stenosis is present (in terms of aetiology).

Treatment

- *Treat affected eye* (if within 24h of presentation):
  - ↓IOP with 500mg IV acetazolamide, ocular massage ± AC paracentesis (all common practice but no proven benefit); selective ophthalmic artery catheterization with thrombolysis is performed in some centres.

- *Protect other eye*: e.g. treat underlying GCA with systemic steroids immediately (see ➔ Anterior ischaemic optic neuropathy, p. 666).

Prognosis
- *Visual outcome*: 94% are CF or worse at presentation; about 1/3 show some improvement (with or without treatment).
- *Neovascularization*: NVI occurs in up to 18%; however; disc neovascularization is uncommon.

Table 13.14 Associations of CRAO

Atherosclerotic	Hypertension (60%)
	Diabetes (25%)
	Hypercholesterolaemia
	Smoking
Embolic sources	Carotid artery disease
	Aortic disease (including dissection)
	Cardiac valve vegetations (e.g. infective endocarditis)
	Cardiac or other tumours (e.g. atrial myxoma)
	Arrhythmias
	Cardiac septal defects
	Post-intervention (e.g. angiography/-plasty)
	Amniotic fluid
Haematological	Antiphospholipid syndrome
	Leukaemia or lymphoma
	Hyperhomocysteinaemia
Inflammatory	GCA
	PAN
	Granulomatosis with polyangiitis (GPA)
	SLE
	Kawasaki disease
	Susac's disease (retino-cochleo-cerebral vasculopathy)
Infective	Toxoplasmosis
	Mucormycosis
	Syphilis
	Lyme disease
Pharmacological	Oral contraceptive pill
	Cocaine
Ophthalmic	Trauma
	Optic nerve drusen
	Migraine

Retinal artery occlusion (2)

Branch retinal arteriolar occlusion (BRAO)

Most BRAO are due to emboli that are often visible clinically. The commonest emboli are:

- *Cholesterol (Hollenhorst plaque)*: small, yellow, refractile.
- *Fibrinoplatelet*: elongated, white, dull.
- *Calcific*: white, non-refractile, proximal to disc.
- Antiphospholipid syndrome is associated with multiple BRAO.

Clinical features

- Sudden painless unilateral altitudinal field defect.
- White swollen retina along a branch retinal arteriole; branch arteriolar attenuation + cattle-trucking; visible emboli common in over 60%.
- *Complications*: neovascularization may occur but is rare.

Investigations and treatment

- *OCT*: diagnosis is usually made clinically, but OCT may prove useful in selected cases, showing increased reflectivity and thickening of the inner retina (with blockage of signal from the underlying structures). In chronic cases, thinning and atrophy of the inner retina is seen.
- Identify underlying cause (as for CRAO). **NB** GCA is extremely rare as a cause of BRAO and does not need investigation in the absence of other supporting evidence.
- There is no proven treatment for BRAO.

Cilioretinal artery occlusion

Present in up to 30% of the population, this branch from the posterior ciliary circulation perfuses the posterior pole. Three distinct patterns of occlusion occur:

- *Isolated*: usually in the young, associated with systemic vasculitis, relatively good prognosis.
- *Combined with CRVO*: usually in the young, possibly a form of papillophlebitis, relatively good prognosis (as for non-ischaemic CRVO).
- *Combined with AION*: usually in the elderly, associated with GCA, very poor prognosis (GCA has a selective tendency to involve the posterior ciliary artery).

Ophthalmic artery occlusion

Ophthalmic artery occlusion may present with a similar picture to CRAO; however, profound choroidal ischaemia also occurs, with retinochoroidal whitening (no cherry-red spot) and complete loss of vision (usually NPL).

Combined retinal artery and vein occlusion

CRAO may sometimes be seen in association with CRVO (i.e. superficial retinal whitening plus cherry-red spot, in combination with signs of venous obstruction). May occur in CRVO where complete occlusion leads to 2° compromise of blood entry into the eye. On FFA, widespread retinal non-perfusion may be seen, with minimal macular leakage despite the clinical appearance. Prognosis is poor, and a careful search for underlying systemic disease is vital, e.g. antiphospholipid syndrome.

Purtscher's retinopathy

Uncommon disorder characterized by bilateral areas of polygonal retinal whitening (between retinal arteriole and venules) ± CWS, accompanied by minimal, if any, retinal haemorrhage and typically restricted to the posterior pole. Originally described in 1910 in patients with severe head trauma, but also seen following compressive chest injuries and in non-traumatic cases ('Purtscher-like' retinopathy). Non-traumatic aetiologies include acute pancreatitis, fat embolism syndrome following long bone fractures, and following childbirth. Suggested mechanism include fat embolism, leading to arterial occlusion, or angiospasm.

Acute retinal signs clear within months without treatment, leaving RPE changes, retinal vessel attenuation or sheathing and, commonly, optic disc pallor. Treatment with high-dose steroids has been advocated, but evidence for efficacy is limited.

Ocular ischaemic syndrome

OIS (*syn* venous stasis retinopathy) is an uncommon condition where ocular hypoperfusion occurs as a result of severe carotid artery obstruction.

The great majority of cases occur as a result of atherosclerosis of the carotid artery (common carotid or internal carotid); thus patients in their 60s and 70s, with other cardiovascular risk factors, are most commonly affected. >90% stenosis of the ipsilateral carotid system is typically present; severe bilateral occlusion may sometimes occur. Rarely, OIS may occur due to trauma, dissecting aneurysms, or vascular inflammatory disease.

Clinical features

- >90% of patients report subacute ↓VA in affected eye (occasionally more abrupt, with cherry-red spot on fundal exam). A history of amaurosis fugax is elicited in about 10%. Transient visual loss, with slow recovery, may occur following sudden exposure to bright light ('light-induced amaurosis fugax'). ~40% of patients report periorbital pain, typically described as a dull ache, on the affected side ('ocular angina').
- Prominent collateral vessels are occasionally seen on the forehead, connecting the external carotid artery on one side to that on the other.
- *Anterior segment findings*: anterior ischaemia leads to atrophic changes in the iris, with a poorly reactive pupil, AC flare, and occasionally mild AC cellular activity and KPs; NVI is seen in ~2/3 at presentation, although IOP may remain low due to ciliary body hypoperfusion.
- *Posterior segment findings*: narrowing of retinal arterioles; retinal veins are dilated but not tortuous (in contrast to CRVO); retinal haemorrhages and microaneurysms, commonly in mid-periphery; CWS; NVD/NVE. **NB** Spontaneous retinal arterial pulsations may be seen, especially with light digital pressure on the lid (in contrast to CRVO).

Investigations

- *FFA*: delayed and/or patchy choroidal filling; prolonged AV transit time; retinal vascular staining (due to chronic hypoxic damage to endothelial cells); macular leakage/oedema with optic disc hyperfluorescence; capillary non-perfusion, especially peripherally.
- *Carotid imaging*: duplex ultrasonography, CT or MR angiography.

Treatment

- *Carotid endarterectomy or stenting*: may stabilize or improve VA.
- *NVD/NVE/NVI*: full PRP.
- *NVG*: standard medical/surgical treatment (See ➲ Neovascular glaucoma, p. 370).

Takayasu's arteritis ('pulseless' disease)

This rare idiopathic large-vessel vasculitis affects the aorta and its 1° branches, causing narrowing/occlusion. Most commonly seen in women in their 20s/30s. Carotid involvement may lead to ocular hypoperfusion and OIS, while renal arterial involvement may lead to systemic hypertension and occasionally hypertensive retinopathy.

Hypertensive retinopathy

Systemic hypertension is one of the commonest diseases of the Western world where it may affect up to 60% of those aged over 60y.

- *Risk factors*: include age, gender (men > women), ethnic origin (African-Caribbean > white people), and society (industrialized > agricultural).
- Exercise is protective.

The majority of hypertension is chronic and of unknown cause ('essential'). It causes sclerosis and narrowing of the arterioles seen both in the retinal and, more severely, in the choroidal circulation. In about 1% of cases, hypertension is acute and severe (accelerated or 'malignant' hypertension). This causes fibrinoid necrosis of arterioles and accelerated end-organ damage.

- This medical emergency requires urgent assessment, treatment, and identification of an underlying cause. Untreated, accelerated hypertension carries a 90% mortality at 1y.

Chronic hypertension

There is no absolutely 'safe' BP and therefore no absolute definition of hypertension. However, intervention is currently recommended for BP >140mmHg systolic or >90mmHg diastolic on two occasions (see Table 13.15).

Clinical features

- *Systemic*: usually asymptomatic. May have evidence of end-organ damage (cardiovascular, cerebrovascular, peripheral vascular, renal disease).
- *Ophthalmic*: retinal arteriolar narrowing, sclerosis ('copper/silver wiring') and compression of venules ('nipping'), CWS, microaneurysms, retinal haemorrhages (commonly flame-shaped).
- *Complications*: macroaneurysms, non-arteritic AION, C/BRVO, C/BRAO, ocular motor nerve palsies. Uncontrolled BP may also adversely affect diabetic retinopathy progression.

Investigation and treatment

- Alert the 1° care physician who will monitor, assess vascular risk, and treat, as required (see Table 13.15 and Table 13.16).
- The target is <140/90 for most patients, <130/80 for those with diabetes, and <125/75 for diabetics with proteinuria.

Accelerated hypertension

Severe ↑BP (e.g. >220mmHg systolic or >120mmHg diastolic), with papilloedema or fundal haemorrhages and exudates.

Clinical features

- Systemic:
  - Headache.
  - Accelerated end-organ damage (e.g. myocardial infarct, cardiac failure, stroke, encephalopathy, renal failure).
- Ophthalmic:
  - Scotoma, diplopia, photopsia, ↓VA.
  - *Retinopathy*: focal arteriolar narrowing, CWS, flame haemorrhages.
  - *Choroidopathy*: infarcts, which may be focal (Elschnig's spots) or linear along choroidal arteries (Siegrist's streaks), serous retinal detachments.
  - *Optic neuropathy*: disc swelling ± macular star.

Investigation and treatment

Refer to medical team for admission and cautious lowering of BP; too rapid a reduction may be deleterious (e.g. stroke).

Table 13.15 Common antihypertensives

Group	Example	Contraindication	Side effects
Thiazide diuretic	Bendroflumethiazide	Renal/hepatic failure, persistent $\downarrow$K+, $\downarrow$Na+	$\downarrow$K+, $\downarrow$Na+, postural hypotension, impotence
β-blocker	Atenolol	Asthma; caution in cardiac failure	Bronchospasm, cardiac failure, lethargy, impotence
ACE inhibitor	Lisinopril	Renal artery stenosis, aortic stenosis	Cough, $\uparrow$K+, renal failure, angio-oedema
AIIR antagonist	Losartan	Caution in renal artery stenosis, aortic stenosis	Mild hypotension, $\uparrow$K+
Ca²⁺ channel antagonist	Nifedipine	Cardiogenic shock, within 1mth of MI	Dependent oedema, flushing, fatigue
α-blocker	Doxazosin	Aortic stenosis	Dependent oedema, fatigue, postural hypotension

Table 13.16 Treatment of hypertension (after Joint British Societies guidelines)*†

Systolic (mmHg)	Diastolic (mmHg)	Management
≥220	≥120	Admit and treat immediately
180–219	110–119	Treat if sustained over 1–2wk
160–179	100–109	*If high risk:* treat if sustained over 3–4wk *If low risk:* modify lifestyle, but treat if sustained over 4–12wk
140–159	90–99	*If high risk:* treat if sustained at up to 12wk *If low risk:* modify lifestyle; recheck monthly, and treat if cardiovascular risk is ≥20% in 10y

High risk = end-organ damage (e.g. renal impairment, left ventricular hypertrophy), cardiovascular complications, or diabetes.

* JBS 2: Joint British Societies' guidelines on prevention of cardiovascular disease in clinical practice. *Heart* 2005;**91**(Suppl V):v1–52.

† *BNF* 2013.

Haematological disease

Haemoglobinopathies

Normal adult Hb (HbA) comprises two α- and two β-globin chains associated with a haem ring. In sickle haemoglobinopathies, there is a mutant Hb, such as HbS (β-chain residue 6 Glu $\rightarrow$ Val), which behaves abnormally in response to hypoxia or acidosis. This causes 'sickling' and haemolysis of red blood cells. Many other mutant Hb have been described, in particular, HbC.

In thalassaemias, the problem is one of inadequate production of one or more of the α- or β-chains. Although systemic disease is most severe in sickle cell disease (HbSS), ocular disease is most severe in HbSC and HbS–Thal disease.

Sickle haemoglobinopathies are seen in Africans and their descendants; thalassaemias are mainly seen in Africans and Mediterranean countries.

Clinical features

- *Proliferative retinopathy* (see Table 13.17).
- *Non-proliferative retinopathy*: arteriosclerosis, vascular tortuosity; occasional CWS and microaneurysms; peripheral retinal non-perfusion; equatorial 'salmon patches' (preretinal/superficial intraretinal haemorrhages), and 'black sunbursts' (occur when retinal haemorrhage tracks into the subretinal space, leading to reactive RPE hyperplasia); macular ischaemia and atrophy ('macular depression sign').
- *Other*: periorbital swelling from orbital bone infarction/haematoma; 'comma-shaped' conjunctival capillaries; sectoral iris atrophy; angioid streaks.

Table 13.17 Goldberg staging of proliferative retinopathy

Stage 1	Peripheral arteriolar occlusions
Stage 2	AV anastomoses
Stage 3	Neovascular proliferation ('sea-fans')
Stage 4	Vitreous haemorrhage
Stage 5	Retinal detachment

Investigation

- Hb electrophoresis, FBC. **NB** Some patients with HbSC or HbS–Thal may be unaware of their disease.

Treatment

- No treatment required for small peripheral lesions, as high probability of spontaneous regression following autoinfarction.
- Consider scatter laser photocoagulation in patients with severe visual loss from the disease in the fellow eye or in cases of rapid growth of large elevated sea-fans with spontaneous haemorrhage (controversial, as most sea-fans spontaneously regress). Anti-VEGF therapy may have a role, although evidence to date is limited.
- Consider vitreoretinal surgery for persistent vitreous haemorrhage (e.g. >6mo) and TRD, although the results are generally disappointing and specialist perioperative care is required.

- Hyphaema in patients with sickle haemoglobinopathies is potentially sight-threatening, as even modest IOP increases can lead to retinal arterial occlusion; AC paracentesis may be required, and acetazolamide should be avoided, as it may promote sickling.

Anaemia and thrombocytopenia

Anaemia is a decrease in the number of circulating red blood cells or a decrease in the Hb content of each cell. Thrombocytopenia is a decrease in the number of platelets. Retinopathy is usually an incidental finding, although findings increase with severity of anaemia and with coexisting thrombocytopenia.

Clinical features

- *Retinopathy*: usually asymptomatic; retinal haemorrhages, CWS, venous tortuosity. Roth's spots are sometimes seen (retinal haemorrhages with white centres composed of coagulated fibrin).
- *Other*: subconjunctival haemorrhages, optic neuropathy (if ↓B12).

Leukaemia

Complications may be due to direct infiltration or 2° anaemia and hyperviscosity. Retinopathy is more common in acute leukaemia.

Clinical features

- *Retinopathy*: usually asymptomatic; haemorrhages, CWS, venous tortuosity, capillary non-perfusion, neovascularization (rare).
- *Other*: spontaneous haemorrhage (subconjunctival or hyphaema), infiltration (iris → anterior uveitis ± hypopyon; orbit → proptosis; optic nerve → optic neuropathy ± disc swelling; choroid → 'leopard spot' changes in overlying RPE).

Hyperviscosity

Hyperviscosity arises from abnormally high levels of blood constituents:
- Blood cells (e.g. 1° or 2° polycythaemia, leukaemias).
- Plasma proteins (e.g. multiple myeloma, Waldenström's macroglobulinaemia).

Clinical features

- *Retinopathy*: usually asymptomatic; retinal haemorrhages (may be peripheral), venous dilatation and tortuosity, CWS (may mimic appearance of RVO; however, retinal blood flow remains normal). Serous retinal detachments may sometimes occur.
- *Other*: disc swelling in polycythaemia and multiple myeloma, conjunctival/corneal crystals, iris/ciliary body cysts in multiple myeloma.

Coagulopathies

Coagulopathies are conditions in which there is increased bleeding diathesis (hypocoagulopathy) or an increased risk of thrombosis (hypercoagulopathy) and are commonly associated with RVO. Less commonly, DIC, idiopathic and thrombotic thrombocytopenic purpura (ITP/TTP), and toxaemia of pregnancy may result in choriocapillaris occlusion, with subsequent serous retinal detachment (commonly accompanied by subconjunctival, retinal, choroidal, or vitreous haemorrhages due to coexisting anaemia/thrombocytopenia).

Retinal telangiectasias

Retinal telangiectasias describe abnormalities of the retinal vasculature, usually with irregular dilation of the capillary bed and segmental dilation of neighbouring venules and arterioles (see Table 13.18). Most commonly, they are acquired 2° to another retinal disorder (e.g. BRVO), but 1° forms also exist (see Table 13.18).

Coats' disease and Leber's miliary aneurysms

Coats' disease, an uncommon condition first described in 1908, is the most severe of the telangiectasias. It affects mainly men (♂:♀ 3:1) and the young, although up to 1/3 may be asymptomatic until their 30s. Although often considered a unilateral disease, about 10% of cases are bilateral. In 1912, Leber described a localized, less severe form, which he termed 'miliary aneurysms'.

Clinical features

- May be asymptomatic; ↓VA, strabismus, leucocoria.
- Telangiectatic vessels, 'light bulb' aneurysms, capillary dropout, exudation (may be massive), scarring.
- *Complications*: ERD, neovascularization, vitreous haemorrhage, rubeosis, glaucoma, cataract.

Investigations

- FFA: highlights abnormal vessels, leakage, and areas of capillary dropout.

Treatment

- *Main aim is to control exudation*: consider laser photocoagulation (or cryotherapy) of leaking vessels; treat directly, rather than scatter approach (if exudate prevents adequate laser, consider anti-VEGF therapy and then laser once cleared).
- Scleral buckling with drainage of SRF may be performed for significant exudative detachment but carries a guarded prognosis.

MacTel type 1

MacTel type 1 (*syn* idiopathic juxtafoveal retinal telangiectasia type 1), first described by Gass in 1968, is a developmental or congenital, usually unilateral, retinal vascular anomaly, which may represent a mild variant of Coats' syndrome and Leber's miliary aneurysms.

Clinical features

- Visible aneurysmal dilation of retinal vasculature, mainly confined to an irregular or oval zone in the temporal macula, with surrounding CMO and yellowish exudates (in patients with diabetes, this may be mistaken for DMO).
- Presence of microaneurysms may help distinguish from MacTel type 2 where they are not a phenotypic feature (MacTel type 2 is also usually bilateral).
- The characteristic loss of central macular pigment seen in MacTel type 2 is also not present in MacTel type 1.

Treatment

- Direct laser photocoagulation of aneurysms has been reported to decrease vascular exudation and may improve VA.
- Use of intravitreal triamcinolone and anti-VEGF monotherapy has proven disappointing, albeit in small case series.

Table 13.18 Causes of retinal telangiectasias

1°	Congenital
	• Coats' disease
	• Leber's miliary aneurysms
	• MacTel type 1
	Acquired
	• MacTel type 2
2°	• BRVO
	• Diabetic retinopathy
	• Ocular inflammatory disease
	• Eales' disease
	• ROP
	• Sickle retinopathy
	• Radiation retinopathy

MacTel type 2

MacTel type 2 (*syn* idiopathic juxtafoveal retinal telangiectasia type 2), first described by Gass in 1977, is an acquired bilateral form of macular telangiectasia found in middle-aged and older patients. Beginning in 2005, the 'MacTel Project', an international consortium of investigators, has initiated major research activity on MacTel type 2.

Clinical features

- ↓VA, paracentral scotomas, metamorphopsia (despite mild ↓VA, vision-related quality of life is markedly reduced).
- Bilateral; occasionally asymmetric; tends to begin temporal to the foveal centre but subsequently involves entire parafoveolar area.
- Initially, reduced retinal transparency ('greying'), followed by dilatation of retinal capillaries and crystalline deposits at the vitreoretinal interface.
- Blunted, dilated venules develop adjacent to ectatic capillaries and dive down ('right-angled'); RPE hyperplasia and intraretinal pigment migration occurs along these vessels; subretinal neovascularization may develop.

Investigations

- *FAF*: characteristic loss of hypofluorescent foveal centre, seen normally with blue-light FAF, due to loss of central macular pigment.
- *FFA*: characteristic telangiectatic capillaries temporal to the fovea; early characteristic retinal leakage limited to the central macula and often more pronounced temporally. Signs of 2° CNV, if present.
- *OCT*: characteristic hyporeflective retinal cavities, with normal or subnormal retinal thickness despite angiographic leakage; disruption of photoreceptor IS-OS junction; hyperreflective intra- or subretinal lesions (pigment migration or neovascularization) in late stages; lamellar/full-thickness macular holes occasionally occur.

Treatment

- No generally accepted therapies for MacTel type 2 not associated with neovascularization.
- In patients with subretinal neovascularization, anti-VEGF therapies are commonly used, although evidence for efficacy is limited.

Other retinal vascular anomalies

Macroaneurysm

Focal dilatation of retinal arteriole, usually 100–250 microns in size, within first three orders of arterial tree. Typically occurs in hypertensive women >50.

Clinical features

- ↓VA (if macular exudate or vitreous haemorrhage); often asymptomatic.
- Saccular or fusiform dilatation of arteriole, often near AV crossing; haemorrhage (sub-/intra-/preretinal and vitreal). **NB** Consider the diagnosis in any presentation of 'hourglass' haemorrhage, i.e. simultaneous preretinal and subretinal haemorrhage; exudation ± circinate exudates.

Investigations

- FFA: immediate complete filling (partial filling suggests thrombosis) with late leakage.

Treatment

- High rate of spontaneous resolution, particularly of haemorrhagic lesions.
- Consider photocoagulation if symptomatic due to exudation at the macula (avoid laser in the presence of extensive retinal haemorrhage). Treat around the macroaneurysm with a single confluent laser barrier. If leakage persists, repeat procedure with direct laser of the lesion (although care is required if distal portion of the arteriole supplies the macula, as direct laser may lead to occlusion).
- Vitrectomy may be required for non-clearing vitreous haemorrhage.

Valsalva retinopathy

In Valsalva retinopathy, sudden increases in intrathoracic pressure (e.g. forced exhalation against a closed airway) result in premacular retinal haemorrhage due to increased pressure in the retinal venous system. On OCT, retinal haemorrhages may be seen to occur in sub-ILM, subhyaloid (preretinal), or a combination of both. Occasionally, breakthrough vitreous haemorrhage may occur.

Treatment options include: observation with spontaneous resolution, YAG posterior hyaloidotomy, or surgical removal of blood via vitrectomy in long-standing cases. For YAG laser, a Goldmann lens is used, and the laser is aimed at the inferior edge of the haemorrhage, away from the fovea and retinal vessels. Low energy is used initially and then increased in small steps until drainage of the haemorrhage occurs.

Terson's syndrome

Originally described as bilateral intraocular haemorrhage (intraretinal ± preretinal ± vitreous) with papilloedema in patients with subarachnoid haemorrhage. However, similar picture may occur with acute increases in intracranial pressure from other causes (retinal haemorrhage occurs due to increases in cavernous sinus pressure with retinal venous stasis).

Lipaemia retinalis

Lipaemia retinalis is a rare condition that occurs in patients with 1° or 2° hyperlipidaemia. Markedly elevated levels of triglycerides impart a creamy white-coloured appearance to retinal blood vessels (due to circulating chylomicrons).

Radiation retinopathy

Irradiation of the globe, orbit, sinuses, or nasopharynx may lead to retinal damage, predominantly through retinal vascular endothelial cell loss and resulting ischaemic retinopathy. Radiation retinopathy usually develops after a delay of 6mo–3y, which is thought to be the turnover time for retinal endothelial cells. Radiation-induced optic neuropathy occurs less frequently, with uncertain pathogenesis, but often results in blindness.

Risk factors

Risk of retinopathy increases with radiation dose and dose rate.

- 90% of brachytherapy patients receiving a macular dose of ≥7,500rad developed maculopathy.
- Over 50% of patients receiving orbital/nasopharyngeal irradiation may develop retinopathy.
- Retinopathy is unlikely after doses of ≤2,500rad, given in fractions of ≤200rad.

Presence of concomitant vascular disease (e.g. diabetes) and the use of radiation sensitizers (e.g. chemotherapy) also increase risk.

Clinical features

- *Ischaemic retinopathy*: initially microaneurysms; then intraretinal haemorrhages, capillary dilatation/non-perfusion, CWS, telangiectasia; exudation and hard exudates, often with macular oedema; large areas of capillary non-perfusion may result in neovascularization, with subsequent vitreous haemorrhage, TRD, and NVG. Retinochoroidal anastomoses (akin to RAP lesions) may occasionally develop. Acute severe responses to high-dose radiation may also sometimes occur.
- *Optic neuropathy*: acute disc hyperaemia, oedema, peripapillary haemorrhage, and CWS, commonly accompanied by retinopathy; subsequent severe optic atrophy; posterior optic neuropathy may sometimes occur after external beam irradiation of posterior optic nerve chiasm.

Treatment

- No widely accepted treatment protocol exists. Treatment to date is based on the similarities between radiation and diabetic retinopathy.
- *Macular oedema*: options include focal laser photocoagulation as per ETDRS, intravitreal triamcinolone, and anti-VEGF therapies. In patients undergoing plaque radiotherapy for uveal melanoma, prophylactic periocular injection of triamcinolone may be of benefit.
- *Retinal non-perfusion and neovascularization*: scatter laser photocoagulation may decrease macular oedema, neovascularization, and vitreous haemorrhages; prophylactic obliteration of ischaemic areas may be of benefit, even in the absence of neovascularization. Anti-VEGF therapies may also have a role in treatment of both neovascularization and its 2° complications.
- *Optic neuropathy*: guarded prognosis.

Retinitis pigmentosa (1)

RP is the commonest of the inherited retinal disorders, affecting about 1 in 3–4,000 of the population. RP is a group of conditions characterized by progressive dysfunction, cell loss, and atrophy of retinal tissue. Photoreceptors are affected initially (rods in the first instance, with cone involvement in the later stages), with subsequent atrophy of other retinal layers, although the nerve fibre layer is preserved till late in the disease process—which is exploited in retinal implant technology.

The relative frequency of the different modes of inheritance differs widely in different series, but ~50% of patients have no family history of RP. AD RP is often of later onset and less severe, whereas XL and AR disease is associated with an earlier onset and is more severe. Mutations in over 50 genes have been identified in RP to date (see Table 13.19).

The vast majority of RP is isolated (i.e. with no systemic features), with <25% having associated systemic disease (usually AR). A number of specific syndromes are also described (see Table 13.20).

Clinical features

- Nyctalopia, tunnel vision, ↓VA (later in the disease process).
- Mid-peripheral 'bone spicule' retinal pigmentation, waxy pallor of the optic disc, arteriolar attenuation.
- *Ocular associations*: cataract (esp. posterior subcapsular); myopia (especially in XL RP); POAG; optic disc drusen, keratoconus.
- *Complications*: CMO.

Investigations

- *ERG*: scotopic affected to a greater extent than photopic; can be used to monitor disease.
- *EOG* is abnormal—in keeping with generalized photoreceptor–RPE dysfunction.
- *VF*: recording progressive constriction of VF with kinetic testing is a reliable measure of change over time.

Variants

RP variants include unusual distributions (sectoral or pericentral RP) and characteristic patterns such as retinitis punctata albescens (scattered white dots predating more typical RP changes).

Differential diagnosis

A number of acquired and genetic conditions may cause a pigmentary retinopathy difficult to distinguish from advanced RP. These include: retinal inflammatory diseases (e.g. rubella, syphilis, infectious retinitis), auto-immune and paraneoplastic retinopathies, drug toxicity (e.g. chloroquine), pigmented paravenous chorioretinal atrophy, enhanced S-cone syndrome, traumatic retinopathy, and long-standing retinal detachment. Many cases previously attributed to 'unilateral' RP occurred as a result of DUSN.

Treatment

- Supportive measures, including genetic and psychological/emotional counselling, visual impairment registration, low vision aids, and provision of support from social services where needed.
- *Macular oedema*: carbonic anhydrase inhibitors; consider topical dorzolamide initially, proceeding to oral acetazolamide if no improvement (monitor renal function).
- *Cataract surgery*: reduce operating light levels; slowly taper post-operative topical steroids.
- *Disease progression*: role of nutritional supplements controversial; supplementation with vitamin A palmitate is no longer recommended; DHA (1200mg/d), and lutein (12mg/d), may be worth considering, although the current evidence base is limited.
- *Future therapies*: gene and stem cell therapies are promising with phase I/II clinical trials underway for various forms of LCA, Usher's and Stargardt's; the Argus II epiretinal prosthesis system has recently been licensed in Europe for use in advanced RP.

Retinitis pigmentosa (2)

LCA

LCA is a group of disorders, due to mutations in at least 18 genes, characterized by congenital blindness, nystagmus, often hypermetropia, and extinguished ERG responses. Pupillary light reflexes are absent or diminished. Systemic associations are uncommon. Most patients show normal fundus appearance or only subtle RPE changes/vessel attenuation in the early stages—although characteristic retinal phenotypes are seen with certain genes, including *RPE65*, *RDH12*, and *CRB1*-associated LCA. Also associated with oculodigital syndrome and keratoconus.

Bietti's crystalline dystrophy

Bietti's crystalline dystrophy is a rare AR chorioretinal dystrophy, characterized by multiple small intraretinal crystalline deposits. It is particularly common in East Asia, especially in Japan and China. Mutations are found in the *CYP4V2* gene, which are believed to result in disordered lipid metabolism. Patients either present following routine optician retinal evaluation or due to increasing night blindness and peripheral VF constriction.

Degenerative changes begin in the RPE and choriocapillaris, leading to the typical 'moth-eaten' appearance on FFA. Perilimbal subepithelial corneal deposits may also be seen. With extension of atrophy, there is gradual diminution of ERG responses, progressive VF constriction, and ↓VA. Patients often progress to legal blindness by the fifth or sixth decade.

Table 13.19 Genes involved in RP (selected)

AD RP*	Rhodopsin (e.g. Pro23His, Pro347Leu)
	RP1
	PRPF31
	PRPH2 (formerly called peripherin-RDS)
	NRL
AR RP†	*USH2A* (associated with AR RP and Usher syndrome type 2)
	PDE6B
	PDE6A
	CNGA1
	MERTK
	RLBP1
	TULP1 (AR, RP, and LCA)
	RPE65 (LCA)
	CRB1 (LCA)
	RDH12 (LCA)
	CEP290(LCA)
XL RP	*RPGR*
	RP2
Digenic RP	Mutation in *PRPH2* and *ROM1*

* Mutations in >20 genes have now been identified, accounting for ~60–70% of patients with AD RP, with mutations in the rhodopsin gene (*RHO*) being the commonest cause.

† Mutations in >30 genes have been identified to date in AR RP, believed to account for ~40–50% of patients with AR RP; with the commonest gene being *USH2A* (10–15% of AR RP), with more severe mutations in *USH2A* also causing Usher syndrome type 2.

Table 13.20 Associations of RP (selected)

Isolated	Sporadic
	Familial (AD, AR, XL)
Systemic	Usher syndrome
	Bardet–Biedl syndrome
	Laurence–Moon syndrome
	Kearns–Sayre syndrome
	Mucopolysaccharidoses I–III
	Abetalipoproteinaemia
	Refsum disease

Congenital stationary night blindness

A group of disorders that share the feature of early non-progressive nyctalopia. Additional ocular manifestations are variable but can include reduced VA, refractive error (commonly myopia but occasionally hyperopia), nystagmus, and strabismus. CSNB may be divided into those with a normal fundus, including myopic fundi (with AD, AR, and XL subtypes) and those with fundus abnormalities (Oguchi's disease and fundus albipunctatus).

CSNB with normal fundi

There are a number of different subclassifications, in large part based on characteristic ERG findings. In AD CSNB, the molecular defect is at the level of the rod phototransduction cascade; in AR and XL CSNB, the defect is in the transmission of the visual signal from photoreceptors to bipolar cells.

Classification

- XL and AR CSNB may be further subdivided into complete (cCSNB) and incomplete (iCSNB) forms, based on their ERG.
- Mutations in the genes *NYX*, *GRM6*, and *TRPM1* are associated with cCSNB, resulting in defects in the ON pathway. iCSNB is associated with mutations in genes involved in glutamate signalling between photoreceptors and bipolar cells (*CACNA1F*, *CABP4*, and *CACNA2D4*). Mutations in the genes encoding three components of the rod-specific phototransduction cascade have all been reported in association with AD CSNB (*RHO, GNAT1*, and *PDE6B*).

Investigations

- *cCSNB*: no detectable rod-specific ERG and a profoundly electronegative bright flash response (reduced b-wave to a-wave ratio—inner retinal dysfunction). Cone ERGs show subtle abnormalities now known to reflect ON-bipolar cell dysfunction.
- *iCSNB*: detectable rod-specific ERG and a profoundly negative bright flash response. Cone ERGs are much more abnormal than in complete CSNB, reflecting involvement of both ON- and OFF-bipolar pathways.
- ERG evidence of inner retinal rod system dysfunction may also occur in AD CSNB but in association with normal cone ERGs. In other cases of AD CSNB, ERG rod responses are attenuated with normal cone responses, but the standard bright flash response does not have a negative waveform.

Differential diagnosis

In patients with nyctalopia, other conditions to consider should include: vitamin A deficiency (may have grey-white fundus spots), RP (may have peripheral pigmentation), choroideraemia (may have choroidal atrophy), or autoimmune/paraneoplastic retinopathies.

CSNB with abnormal fundi

Oguchi's disease

This is a distinct form of AR CSNB, first described in Japan, with an abnormal fundus appearance—the fundus has a golden yellow metallic sheen but appears normal following prolonged dark adaptation (Mizuo phenomenon). On OCT, the parafoveal photoreceptor IS-OS junction only becomes visible after this dark adaptation. Two genes have been implicated, both of which are involved with rod phototransduction: *SAG* (encoding arrestin) and *GRK1* (encoding rhodopsin kinase).

Fundus albipunctatus

A rare AR CSNB due to mutations in three genes to date (*RDH5, RLBP1,* and *RPE65*) encoding components of the visual cycle; with *RDH5* encoding 11-cis retinol dehydrogenase being the most common cause. Numerous tiny radially distributed white dots/flecks cover most of the fundus and are usually absent at the macula; may represent accumulation of retinoids. Patients either present with night blindness or because the abnormal retinal appearance is noted on routine fundoscopy.

Inherited disorders of cone function

Inherited disorders of cone function may be non-progressive (typically with early infant/childhood onset) or progressive (typically with later onset). The former are termed cone dysfunction syndromes, including achromatopsia and blue cone monochromatism; the latter are termed progressive cone dystrophies.

Achromatopsia (rod monochromatism)

One in 30,000, AR disorder characterized by lack of cone function of all three subtypes. Complete or incomplete forms—with residual colour vision and slightly better VA (6/24–6/36) in the incomplete form.

Clinical features

- Patients have poor VA (6/36–6/60) and colour vision from birth, with pendular nystagmus and marked photophobia.
- Fundus appearance is usually normal or with mild RPE changes.

Investigations

- *ERG*: non-recordable cone responses, with normal rod responses (NB ERG essential to differentiate from LCA).
- *OCT*: a range of appearances, from normal to a hyporeflective, optically empty cavity, may be seen in the outer retina of the fovea; foveal hypoplasia may also be present.

Blue cone monochromatism

XL disorder, 1 in 100,000, characterized by absent L- and M-cone function, with normal S-cone and rod function.

Clinical features and investigations

- Similar presentation to achromatopsia but can be distinguished using S-cone-specific ERGs and psychophysical testing to identify relatively preserved tritan function. Family history may also be useful, as blue cone monochromatism is XL recessive (XR).

Progressive cone dystrophies

Heterogeneous group of disorders involving only the cones (cone dystrophy) or additional loss of rod function (cone–rod dystrophies); there is considerable overlap, with the majority of cone dystrophies having rod involvement at a later stage. Primarily non-syndromic, although cone–rod dystrophies may be associated with spinocerebellar ataxia, Bardet–Biedl, or Alstrom syndrome. Mutations in >30 genes have been identified to date, with AD, AR, and XL inheritance described.

Clinical features
- Typically present in the 2nd and 3rd decades of life with progressive symptoms, including ↓VA, colour vision loss, and mild photophobia.
- Rod involvement may lead to nyctalopia and peripheral field defects
- Fundus findings are variable, ranging from mild RPE changes and Bull's eye maculopathy to findings in keeping with advanced RP.

Investigations
- *ERG*: generalized retinal dysfunction affecting the cone system to a greater extent than the rod system, with early marked macular involvement. In early cone dystrophies, rod responses will be normal.

Macular dystrophies (1)

Macular dystrophies are characterized by bilateral symmetrical changes, often relatively confined to the posterior pole; although there may be electrophysiological, psychophysical, or histopathological evidence of more widespread retinal involvement. AD, AR, and XL inheritance has been described, with considerable variability, even within these categories.

Stargardt's disease and fundus flavimaculatus

Commonest macular dystrophy; represent two clinical presentations of the same disease. AR due to mutations in the ATP-binding cassette: *ABCA4* (*ABCA4* mutations also cause cone and cone–rod dystrophies). A rare Stargardt-like dominant disease associated with mutations in the gene *ELOVL4* has been described.. Histologically, in Stargardt's disease, there is diffuse accumulation of lipofuscin and A2E throughout the RPE; the clinical appearance may vary, depending on the sensitivity of the RPE to accumulation of these toxic bis-retinoids.

Clinical features

- *Stargardt's disease*: rapid ↓VA (6/18–6/60), usually in childhood, although can also present in early adulthood, initially with minimal fundus signs (but may have abnormal autofluorescence and pattern ERG); then changes, including pigmentary disturbance, 'beaten-bronze' atrophy, and yellowish white flecks.
- *Fundus flavimaculatus*: flecks of various shapes, including pisciform, at the posterior pole, usually occurring in adulthood, with relative preservation of vision, i.e. no macular atrophy.

Investigations

- *ERG*: three ERG groups have been identified: group 1 = isolated macular dysfunction; group 2 = macular and generalized cone dysfunction; group 3 = macular and both generalized cone and rod dysfunction; with a better prognosis associated with isolated macular disease. EOG abnormal in all groups.
- *FFA*: classically 'dark choroid', due to blockage of choroidal fluorescence by the RPE harbouring the aforementioned abnormal deposit.
- *FAF*: shows areas of RPE atrophy (including bull's eye maculopathy) and flecks, with peripapillary sparing (**NB** The latter is observed, even in very late *ABCA4*-associated retinal disease).
- *OCT*: demonstrates RPE atrophy and outer retinal loss.
- *Molecular testing*: becoming more sensitive and widely available.

Treatment

- Clinical trials of stem cell-derived RPE replacement are currently underway for patients with advanced RPE and photoreceptor loss. Gene therapy is also in trial for patients with better preserved retinal architecture.

Best's disease

Second most common macular dystrophy; onset usually in childhood, but highly variable expression. It is AD, associated with mutations in the *BEST1* gene (formerly *VMD2*). *BEST1* mutations are associated with several other phenotypes, including multifocal Best's disease and AR bestrophinopathy.

Clinical features
- Usually asymptomatic in early stages.
- The visual prognosis is surprisingly good, with most patients retaining reading vision beyond the 5th decade.
- Carriers who have minimal macular abnormality or a normal fundus appearance (but abnormal EOG) in early adult life usually retain good VA long term.
- Most easily recognized by yolk-like lesion at posterior pole; may later be replaced by non-specific scarring, atrophy, or CNV (see Table 13.21).

Investigations
- *EOG*: reduced Arden ratio.
- *ERG*: normal.
- *OCT*: classic lesions appear as homogenous hyperreflective material in the subretinal space; over time, some of this material is replaced by clear fluid which appears hyporeflective. In some patients, a hyperreflective 'pillar' in the sub-RPE space may elevate the retina like a circus tent. **NB** Therefore, SRF does not necessarily signify CNV, rather the failure of transport across the RPE that characterizes this disorder. FFA is required to determine the presence of a CNV.

Table 13.21 Staging of Best's disease

1	Pre-vitelliform	EOG findings only
2	Vitelliform	Yolk-like macular lesion
3	Pseudohypopyon	Partial absorption leaving level
4	Vitelliruptive	'Scrambled' appearance
5	End-stage	Scarring or atrophy

Adult vitelliform macular dystrophy (AVMD)
AVMD is often confused with Best's disease, although, as the name suggests, it usually has a later onset, lacks the typical course through different stages of macular disease seen in classical Best's disease, and the EOG is often normal. The typical clinical appearance is of bilateral, round or oval, yellow, symmetrical subretinal lesions, typically one-third to one-half optic DD in size. Mutations in the *PRPH2* gene have been identified in ~20% of patients with AVMD.

Adult exudative polymorphous dystrophy
Rare condition characterized by bilateral, multifocal vitelliform-like deposits with serous retinal detachments. May be distinguished from multifocal Best's dystrophy by the lack of mutations in *BEST1* and a normal EOG; it may represent an inflammatory/immune-mediated disorder.

Macular dystrophies (2)

Pattern dystrophy

This refers to a group of inherited conditions characterized by changes at the level of the RPE and encompassing a broad spectrum of clinical appearances. Inheritance is usually AD, with mutations identified in *PRPH2* (formerly peripherin-RDS) in some patients, encoding the outer segment structural protein peripherin; with further genes to be identified. Mutations in *PRPH2* are also associated with central areolar choroidal dystrophy and RP.

Clinical features
- Originally subtyped according to patterns of RPE changes:
  (1) butterfly-shaped dystrophy, (2) reticular dystrophy (net-like pattern), and (3) fundus pulverulentus (granular, mottled pigmentation).

Pattern ERG and EOG are usually abnormal, with variable full-field ERG ranging from normal to generalized cone and rod system dysfunction, suggesting widespread RPE–photoreceptor dysfunction.

The prognosis is generally good, although slowly progressive loss of central vision can occur. There is a low risk of CNV development.

Maternally inherited diabetes and deafness (MIDD)

MIDD is a subtype of diabetes associated with mutations in mitochondrial DNA. Patients commonly have normal or low body mass index (BMI), sensorineural deafness, and diabetes. An extensive macular and peripapillary pattern dystrophy may also be seen—often associated with a relatively good prognosis. Audiological testing and a fasting blood glucose may be warranted, because many patients report no hearing or metabolic abnormalities.

Autosomal dominant drusen

AD condition with a range of clinical appearances. Different patterns were originally described separately as Doyne's honeycomb dystrophy and malattia leventinese. However, these are now known to be a single disorder caused by a single point mutation (*R345W*) in the fibulin-3 gene. Marked inter- and intrafamilial variation, in terms of retinal appearance, severity, progression, and non-penetrance, have been identified.

Clinical features
- Usually asymptomatic (identified at routine optometrist review) or mild symptoms (except in advanced disease).
- Yellow-white drusen at the posterior pole; a radial distribution may infrequently be present. **NB** Drusen abutting the optic disc are characteristic—either seen clinically or on autofluorescence.
- Central atrophy may occur in late stage. CNV infrequently develops.

Sorsby's macular dystrophy

Rare AD disease characterized by early drusen-like deposition, arising from mutations in the *TIMP3* gene, a regulator of MMP activity. Altered TIMP3-mediated extracellular matrix turnover is thought to lead to thickening of Bruch's membrane and the widespread accumulation of abnormal material beneath the RPE that is seen histologically.

Clinical features
- Onset of night blindness in the 3rd decade and loss of central vision from macular atrophy or CNV, usually by the 5th decade.

North Carolina macular dystrophy

AD disease, initially described in North Carolina but now identified world-wide. The causative gene has not yet been identified, but links to a locus on Chr 6q (MCDR1). It is believed to be a developmental disorder, with lesions present at birth. Three North Carolina macular dystrophy-like phenotypes, mapping to different genetic loci than MCDR1, have been described, suggesting further genetic heterogeneity in the MCDR1 phenotype—MCDR3, North Carolina-like macular dystrophy and progressive sensorineural hearing loss (MCDR4), and North Carolina-like macular dystrophy and digital anomalies (Sorsby syndrome).

Clinical features
- Characterized by a variable macular phenotype and a non-progressive natural history. Bilaterally symmetrical fundus appearances, ranging from a few small (<50 microns), yellow, drusen-like lesions in the central macula (grade 1) to larger confluent lesions (grade 2) and macular colobomatous lesions (grade 3).
- Occasionally MCDR1 is complicated by CNV formation.
- EOG and ERG are normal, indicating that there is no generalized retinal dysfunction—unlike most other macular dystrophies where there is evidence of more widespread involvement.

Progressive bifocal chorioretinal atrophy

This rare AD disease has only been described in the UK to date, and, like North Carolina macular dystrophy, links to Chr 6q. This developmental disorder is characterized by infantile-onset nystagmus, myopia, poor vision, and slow progression. A large atrophic macular lesion and nasal subretinal deposits are present soon after birth. An atrophic area, nasal to the optic nerve head, appears in the 2nd decade of life and enlarges progressively. Marked photopsia in early/middle age and retinal detachment extending from the posterior pole are recognized complications. Unlike North Carolina macular dystrophy, the ERG and EOG are markedly abnormal.

Spotted cystic dystrophy

A recently described dystrophy, characterized by flat, pigmented spots with or without surrounding hypopigmentation, limited to the macula, with cysts in multiple retinal layers on OCT. Neovascularization may occur and may be treated with anti-VEGF therapies.

Membranoproliferative glomerulonephritis type II

Patients with membranoproliferative glomerulonephritis type II ('dense deposit' disease) commonly develop subretinal deposits with the appearance of drusen. These drusen-like deposits vary in size and tend to extend temporally from the macula, sometimes in association with RPE changes. VA is preserved, unless CNV occurs. In young adults with these findings, urinalysis may be of benefit in screening for this disease.

Chorioretinal dystrophies

These are inherited potentially blinding conditions, in which there is progressive chorioretinal atrophy; often initially involving the RPE, choriocapillaris and photoreceptors, and, in later stages, the larger choroidal vessels.

Gyrate atrophy

This rare AR condition arises from mutations in the *OAT* gene. This encodes for ornithine aminotransferase, which, with cofactor B6, catalyses the conversion of ornithine to glutamic-γ-semialdehyde, and thence to proline.

Two clinical subtypes are seen, according to whether treatment with B6 (pyridoxine) lowers plasma ornithine levels. Disease is usually symptomatic from late childhood. It is more common in Finland.

Clinical features
- Nyctalopia, peripheral field loss, later ↓VA.
- *RPE/choroidal atrophy*: well-defined, often circular patches, initially mid-peripheral and superficial (choriocapillaris); atrophic areas subsequently coalesce and enlarge towards the posterior pole, with a characteristic scalloped appearance at the leading edge, with deeper choroidal atrophy.
- ERM and CMO possible.
- *Other*: moderate to high myopia and cataract (posterior subcapsular).

Investigations
- Early reduction in ERG (rod responses affected before cone responses); less marked changes in B6-responsive group.
- *Plasma ornithine*: 10–15× normal level; also elevated in urine and CSF.
- *OCT*: demonstrates multiple intraretinal cystoid spaces, linear hyperreflective deposits in the ganglion cell layer, and outer retinal tubulations.

Treatment
Three different approaches to treatment have been used:
- A minority of patients are responsive to pyridoxine (B6) supplements and show reduced plasma ornithine levels and improvement in the ERG. Vitamin B6 should be used initially in all patients and continued in those who show a positive response.
- In non-responders, adhering to an arginine-restricted diet may reduce plasma ornithine levels.
- Proline supplementation has been reported to slow the progress of retinal degeneration in some patients.

Although the present treatment regimes are promising, more long-term studies are needed to assess whether such treatment will prevent retinal deterioration.

Choroideraemia

XR condition, causing significant visual impairment from childhood in ♂. ♀ carriers are usually asymptomatic but are readily recognized by widespread fine RPE atrophy and granular pigment deposition in the mid-peripheral retina.

Clinical features

- Nyctalopia, concentric VF loss, later ↓VA (variable, but often middle age).
- *RPE/choroidal atrophy*: initially mid-peripheral, patchy, and superficial (choriocapillaris); later central, diffuse, and deeper choroidal atrophy to expose the sclera.
- **NB** Relative sparing of retinal vessels and optic disc is characteristic.
- *Other*: cataract (posterior subcapsular), early vitreous degeneration.

Investigations

- Reduction in ERG (rod responses affected before cone responses). Useful vision may be retained until late in disease; supportive treatment and genetic counselling may be offered. Prenatal testing is possible.

Treatment

- There is no established treatment, but clinical trials of gene therapy are underway.

Differential diagnosis

A number of other retinal disorders may mimic the widespread retinal and choroidal atrophy seen in patients with choroideraemia. These include: severe XL RP, Bietti's crystalline dystrophy, thioridazine toxicity, and rarely advanced stages of Stargardt's disease and *PRPH2* retinopathy.

Central areolar choroidal dystrophy

In central areolar choroidal dystrophy, there is slowly progressive loss of central vision, with central, symmetric, sharply outlined geographic atrophy; the reddish orange colour of the large choroidal vessels also becomes yellow-white (previously termed 'choroidal sclerosis'). Mutations in *PRPH2* and *GUCY2D* have been found associated with this phenotype.

Albinism

Abnormalities in the synthesis of melanin result in pigment deficiency of the eye alone (ocular albinism) or of the eye, skin, and hair (oculocutaneous albinism). Although there is wide phenotypic variation, the VA is generally reduced due to foveal hypoplasia. These patients also have increased decussation of the temporal fibres at the chiasm (can be demonstrated using VEP, by predominance of response to monocular stimulation).

Ocular albinism

Classic ocular albinism (Nettleship–Falls albinism) represents 10% of all albinism. It is XL, the *OA1* gene being implicated in melanosome function.

♀ carriers may show mild, patchy features of the disease, including a 'mud-splattered' fundus.

Clinical features
- ↓VA, photophobia.
- Nystagmus, strabismus, ametropia, iris hypopigmentation/transillumination, foveal hypoplasia, fundus hypopigmentation.

Investigations
- *OCT*: at the fovea, the photoreceptor (outer) nuclear layer may be seen to bulge upwards, with the absence of an overlying central foveal depression. The normally absent inner retinal layers may also be seen to persist across the fovea.

Treatment
- The main priority is to correct ametropia (often with tinted lenses for photophobia) and prevent amblyopia.
- Consider surgery for strabismus and some cases of nystagmus.

Oculocutaneous albinism

Oculocutaneous albinism is AR and accounts for the majority of albinism. It arises from abnormalities in several components of melanogenesis, including: type I = tyrosinase (Chr 11q), type II = p product (Chr 15q, probably a transporter), and type III = tyrosinase-related protein 1 (Chr 9p). There is significant overlap of phenotype associated with the various genes identified to date. After the age of 5y, tyrosinase activity can be assessed using the hair bulb incubation test.

Clinical features
- *Ophthalmic*: as for ocular albinism.
- *Systemic*: there is variable hypopigmentation of skin and hair (blond).
- *Hermansky–Pudlak syndrome*: mild oculocutaneous albinism, with low platelets (easy bruising), pulmonary/renal/intestinal abnormalities in some cases, with increased incidence in people of Puerto Rican ancestry.
- *Chediak–Higashi syndrome*: mild oculocutaneous albinism, with leucocyte abnormalities resulting in recurrent pyogenic infections.

Treatment
- As for ocular albinism.

Toxic retinopathies (1)

A wide variety of prescribed and non-prescribed drugs results in retinal toxicity by a variety of mechanisms (see Table 13.23). Be alert to the possibility of toxicity when there is unusual pigmentary disturbance or crystal deposition. Coordinate with the prescribing physician before any drug withdrawal. If any pre-existing retinopathy is evident before starting treatment, then baseline imaging will be useful for monitoring (see Tables 13.22 to 13.24).

Chloroquine and hydroxychloroquine

These are aminoquinolones used as antimalarials and immunomodulators (e.g. in RA and SLE). Excretion from the body occurs very slowly (chloroquine has been detected in the body 5y after last known ingestion), with drugs becoming concentrated in melanin-containing structures of the eye (e.g. RPE), leading to RPE and retinal degeneration. Doses of >3.5mg/kg/d for chloroquine and >6.5mg/kg/d for hydroxychloroquine may result in retinopathy; risk increases with increasing dose, increasing duration, and reduced renal function. Toxicity occurs more commonly with chloroquine, and this drug is less commonly used.

Clinical features
- Asymptomatic, paracentral scotomas, ↓VA, decreased colour vision.
- Altered foveal reflex ± irregular central macular pigmentation →
  depigmentation of surrounding zone ('bull's eye maculopathy') →
  end-stage disease has appearance similar to end-stage RP (generalized atrophy, peripheral pigmentation, arteriolar attenuation, optic atrophy).
- *OCT*: subtle loss of the ellipsoid zone is seen in early toxicity, progressing to parafoveal thinning of the outer nuclear layer in moderate toxicity, and widespread RPE atrophy and retinal thinning in severe cases.
- *FAF*: commonly shows a ring of increased autofluorescence initially, with parafoveal hypoautofluorescence in severe cases.
- *FFA*: loss of RPE results in window defects; minimal loss of underlying choriocapillaris.
- *Associated features*: deposited in cornea, leading to enhanced Hudson–Stahli line, vortex keratopathy, CL intolerance.

Prevention and screening

Table 13.22 Summary of Royal College of Ophthalmologists recommendations for hydroxychloroquine, 2009

Recommendations for good practice in rheumatology and dermatology clinics

- Maximum dosage of hydroxychloroquine should not exceed 6.5mg/kg lean body weight (typically 200–400mg daily)
- Establish renal and liver function at baseline assessment
- Enquire about any visual impairment, and record reading performance

Examination by ophthalmologist

- Enquiry about any disturbance of central vision; measure VA and reading acuity
- Central VF, using an Amsler chart (preferably red on black) or automated perimetry (e.g. Humphrey 10-2 protocol)
- Slit-lamp examination of cornea and retina
- Other imaging may include fundus photography, FAF, OCT, and mfERG

Thioridazine and chlorpromazine

These are phenothiazines used in treatment of schizophrenia. Toxicity is more related to daily, rather than cumulative, dosages. Doses of thioridazine >1g/d for just a few weeks may result in retinopathy (see Table 13.23). Since 2005, Melleril® has been discontinued worldwide due to concerns about cardiotoxicity; however, it is still available in generic forms. Retinal toxicity from chlorpromazine is rare, except where massive doses are given (e.g. 2,400mg/d for 12mo; normal dose is 40–75mg/d).

Clinical features
- Commonly asymptomatic (especially chlorpromazine), scotomas (paracentral or ring), ↓VA, nyctalopia, reddish or brownish visual discoloration.
- *Thioridazine*: nummular areas of RPE loss from posterior pole to mid-periphery; associated loss of choriocapillaris on FFA; in late stages, widespread areas of depigmentation alternating with pigment plaques, vascular attenuation, and optic atrophy (may resemble choroideraemia).
- *Chlorpromazine*: corneal endothelial deposits and anterior lens granules commonly seen; pigmentary changes typically less severe than thioridazine.

Table 13.23 Mechanisms of toxic retinopathy

- Degeneration of RPE ± neurosensory retina ± choriocapillaris
  - Chloroquine/hydroxychloroquine
  - Phenothiazines (thioridazine, chlorpromazine)
  - Desferrioxamine
  - Clofazimine
  - Dideoxyinosine (DDI)
  - Quinine
- Retinal vasculopathy
  - Interferon retinopathy
  - Aminoglycoside antibiotics
  - Talc retinopathy
- CMO
  - Nicotinic acid
  - Topical adrenaline
  - Prostaglandin analogues (e.g. latanoprost)
  - Chemotherapeutic agents (e.g. paclitaxel)
  - Glitazones
- Crystalline retinopathy
  - Talc retinopathy
  - Tamoxifen
  - Canthaxanthin
  - Nitrofurantoin
  - Methoxyflurane
- Retinal folds
  - Topiramate and other sulfamated drugs

Toxic retinopathies (2)

Desferrioxamine

This chelating agent (*syn* deferoxamine) is given IV or SC to treat overload of iron (e.g. after multiple transfusions in chronic anaemias such as thalassaemia) and aluminium (e.g. dialysis patients). There appears to be no 'safe' dose, and retinopathy may occur within weeks of administration. An orally active agent deferasirox has recently become available that may also lead to retinopathy. A wide range of RPE changes may occur, which may be central and/or peripheral.

Interferon alfa retinopathy

Interferon alfa is used in treatment of chronic hepatitis C, cutaneous melanoma, Kaposi's sarcoma, renal cell carcinoma, and in chemotherapy protocols for leukaemia and lymphoma. Treatment may result in a microangiopathy, consisting of CWS and retinal haemorrhages and occurring particularly in diabetic and hypertensive patients. Visual loss may occur from retinal artery/venous occlusion or AION.

Aminoglycoside antibiotics

Aminoglycosides may result in retinal toxicity, particularly after inadvertent intraocular injection of large doses or when given as intravitreal injections for bacterial endophthalmitis. Gentamicin is the most toxic of the family. Large doses may result in acute macular necrosis, with FFA showing severe vascular non-perfusion. In later stages, rubeosis iridis and NVG may occur.

Talc retinopathy

IV drug abusers often inject aqueous suspensions of oral medications such as methylphenidate or methadone (they crush the tablets before adding water and heating the mixture). These medications contain talc as inert filler material. In talc retinopathy, these particles appear as small, white, glistening crystals in the end-arterioles of the posterior pole. Once a large number of arterioles are occluded, ischaemic retinopathy develops. In severe cases, neovascularization and vitreous haemorrhage may develop.

Nicotinic acid

This drug (*syn* niacin) is used to reduce serum lipid and cholesterol levels, often in combination with statins. At doses >1.5g/d, it may lead to CMO in a minority of patients. CMO occurs in the absence of vascular leakage on FFA, leading to speculation that the drug has a direct toxic effect on Müller cells, with resulting intracellular oedema.

Tamoxifen

This oestrogen antagonist is used in the treatment of breast cancer. Retinopathy most commonly occurs after 1y of therapy when a cumulative dose of >100g has been taken. Current prescribing practice (<40mg/d) very rarely leads to retinopathy, although a recent increase in cases has been seen, as patients with aggressive glioblastoma are treated with higher doses (100–200mg/d). Retinal toxicity consists of ↓VA, with white intraretinal crystalline deposits, CMO, and punctate RPE changes.

Canthaxanthine

Canthaxanthine is a naturally occurring carotenoid, used as a food-colouring agent, for skin pigmentation in the treatment of vitiligo, and as an OTC oral tanning agent. High doses may result in a characteristic ring-shaped deposition of yellow-orange crystals in the superficial retina. Patients are usually asymptomatic, and, with discontinuation of the drug, deposits slowly clear.

Topiramate

Topiramate is used in the treatment of epilepsy and in migraine prophylaxis, trigeminal neuralgia, bipolar disorder, and depression. Topiramate may cause a syndrome of transient acute myopia and AC shallowing, thought to occur as a result of ciliary body swelling, choroidal effusion, or both. Retinal folds are often seen in the macula in younger patients. AACG may occur, particularly in patients on selective serotonin reuptake inhibitors. A similar syndrome may occur with other sulfamated drugs.

'Poppers' retinopathy

'Poppers' is slang for the alkyl nitrite class of liquid chemicals, commonly used as recreational drugs. Amyl nitrate was originally supplied in small glass capsules that 'pop' open—hence the name. Repeated inhalation may result in prolonged bilateral vision loss, with foveal yellow spots on biomicroscopy and disruption of foveal cone outer segments on OCT.

Table 13.24 Causes of crystalline retinopathy

- Retinal vascular disease
  - Type 2, idiopathic macular telangiectasia
- Drugs
  - Tamoxifen
  - Canthaxanthine
  - Methoxyflurane
  - Talc retinopathy
  - Nitrofurantoin
- Inherited dystrophies/degenerations
  - Bietti's crystalline dystrophy
  - Kjellin syndrome
  - Sjögren–Larsson syndrome
  - Oxalosis
  - Cystinosis
- Other
  - West African crystalline maculopathy

Miscellaneous disorders

Flecked retina syndromes with systemic associations

In 1965, Krill and Klien introduced the term 'flecked retina syndrome' to describe retinal diseases with yellow or white deep retinal 'flecks' and without vascular or optic nerve abnormalities. Originally, this group consisted of four diseases—fundus albipunctatus, fundus flavimaculatus, familial drusen, and fleck retina of Kandori—but others were subsequently added.

This vague term has fallen out of favour now; however, retinal specialists should be aware of rare flecked retina syndromes with systemic associations. These include: neuro-ophthalmologic syndromes such as Kjellin's syndrome and Sjögren–Larsson syndrome, metabolic disorders such as Alport's syndrome, cystinosis, and oxalosis, and nutritional disorders such as vitamin A deficiency.

Solar maculopathy

Solar maculopathy is a form of photochemical retinal injury caused by prolonged, unprotected gaze at the sun. The retina is particularly at risk during solar eclipse observation, as pupillary dilatation can occur and increase retinal irradiance. It may also occur with drug abuse, psychosis, and in certain religious rituals. Retinal cell damage result from the photochemical generation of highly reactive oxygen radicals. A similar mechanism may result in welding arc maculopathy and in damage from operating microscopes or endoilluminators.

Clinical features
- ↓VA, central scotomas, erythopsia (objects appear red).
- VA usually returns to normal or near normal over the course of months.
- Small yellow-white foveolar lesions may be seen.

Investigations
- *OCT*: characteristic finding of small well-defined defect in photoreceptor IS-OS junction at fovea (sometimes termed 'microhole' or 'outer retinal hole').

Differential diagnosis
Similar findings may sometimes be seen as sequelae of blunt ocular trauma or whiplash injuries. Vitreomacular traction may occasionally produce this appearance, as rarely may closure of a full-thickness macular hole.

Orbit

Relevant pages
➲ Orbital and preseptal cellulitis 790

Anatomy and physiology

The bony orbit forms a pyramid, comprising a medial wall lying anteroposteriorly, a lateral wall at 45°, a roof, and a floor. It has a volume of about 30mL and contains most of the globe and associated structures: EOM (see ➲ p. 734), optic nerve (see ➲ Anatomy and physiology (1), p. 652), cranial nerves (see ➲ Anatomy and physiology (2), p. 654), vascular supply, and lacrimal system (see ➲ Anatomy and physiology, p. 168).

Being effectively a rigid box, the only room for expansion is forward. Most orbital pathology therefore presents initially with proptosis, followed by disruption of eye movements. The orbital septum, a connective tissue sheath representing the anatomic boundary between the lids and the orbit, acts as a barrier to the spread of infection (see Table 14.1, Table 14.2, Table 14.3, and Fig. 14.1).

Table 14.1 Orbital bones

Wall	Bones	Rim	Bones
Roof	Frontal	Superior	Frontal
	Sphenoid (lesser wing)		
Lateral	Sphenoid (greater wing)	Lateral	Zygomatic
	Zygomatic		Frontal
Floor	Zygomatic	Inferior	Zygomatic
	Maxilla		Maxilla
	Palatine		
Medial	Maxilla	Medial	Maxilla
	Lacrimal		Lacrimal
	Ethmoid		
	Sphenoid		

Table 14.2 Anatomic relations of the orbit walls

Wall	Relation
Roof	Anterior cranial fossa
	Frontal sinus
Lateral	Temporalis fossa
	Middle cranial fossa
Floor	Maxillary antrum
Medial	Ethmoid air cells
	Sphenoid sinus

Table 14.3 Orbital apertures

Aperture	Location	Contents
Optic canal	Apex (lesser wing sphenoid)	Optic n., sympathetic fibres Ophthalmic artery
Superior orbital fissure	Apex (greater/ lesser wings sphenoid)	III, IV, Va, VIn, sympathetic fibres Orbital veins
Inferior orbital fissure	Apex	Zygomatic and infraorbital n. (Vb) Orbital veins
Zygomaticofacial	Lateral wall	Zygomaticofacial n. (Vb) and vessels
Zygomaticotemporal	Lateral wall	Zygomaticotemporal n. (Vb) and vessels
Ethmoidal foramen	Medial wall (frontal/ ethmoidal bones)	Ethmoidal arteries (anterior, posterior)
Nasolacrimal canal	Medial wall (maxilla/lacrimal)	Nasolacrimal duct

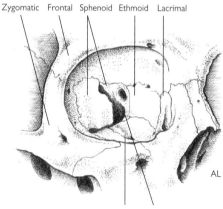

Fig. 14.1 The bones of the orbit.

Orbital and preseptal cellulitis

Orbital cellulitis is an ophthalmic and medical emergency that may cause loss of vision and even death. Assessment, imaging, and treatment should be under the combined care of an ophthalmologist and ENT specialist (and paediatrician in children). Part of the ophthalmologist's role is to assist in differentiating orbital cellulitis from the much more limited preseptal cellulitis.

In younger children, in whom the orbital septum is not fully developed, there is a high risk of progression and so should be treated similarly to orbital cellulitis. For orbital and preseptal cellulitis in children, see ➲ Orbital and preseptal cellulitis, p. 790 and Table 14.4.

Orbital cellulitis

Infective organisms include *Streptococcus pneumoniae*, *Staphylococcus aureus*, *Streptococcus pyogenes*, and *Haemophilus influenzae* (commoner in children, but reducing since Hib vaccination).

Risk factors
- *Sinus disease*: ethmoidal sinusitis (common), maxillary sinusitis.
  - *Infection of other adjacent structures*: preseptal or facial infection, dacryocystitis, dental abscess.
- *Trauma*: septal perforation, retained FB.
- *Surgical*: orbital, lacrimal, and vitreoretinal surgery.
- *Endogenous spread*: in immunocompromised patients.

Clinical features
- Fever, malaise, and periocular pain.
- Inflamed lids (swollen, red, tender, warm) ± chemosis, proptosis, painful restricted eye movements, diplopia, lagophthalmos, optic nerve dysfunction (↓VA, ↓colour vision, RAPD).
- *Complications*: exposure keratopathy, ↑IOP, CRAO, CRVO, inflammation of optic nerve.
- *Systemic*: orbital or periorbital abscess, cavernous sinus thrombosis, meningitis, cerebral abscess.

Investigation
- Temperature.
- FBC, blood culture (but yield is low; range 0–7% in recent studies[1]).
- *CT (orbit, sinuses, brain)*: orbital abscess, diffuse orbital infiltrate, proptosis ± sinus opacity.

Treatment
- Admit for IV antibiotics (e.g. either cefuroxime 750mg–1.5g 3×/d or ceftriaxone 1–2g 2×/d with metronidazole 500mg 3×/d if history of chronic sinus disease).
- Mark extent of skin inflammation to monitor status.
- Regular review of orbital and visual functions.
- ENT to assess for sinus drainage (required in up to 90% of adults).
- If any deterioration, repeat CT to exclude abscess formation.

Preseptal cellulitis

Preseptal cellulitis is not truly an orbital disease. It is much commoner than orbital cellulitis, from which it must be differentiated. It is commoner in children, with 80% cases are under 10y of age. The main causative organisms are staphylococci and streptococci spp. It is generally a much less severe disease, at least in adults and older children.

Risk factors

- Infection of adjacent structures (dacryocystitis, hordeolum) or systemic (e.g. upper respiratory tract infection, URTI).
- *Trauma*: laceration.

Clinical features

- Fever, malaise; painful, swollen lid/periorbital.
- Inflamed lids but no proptosis, normal eye movements, white conjunctiva, normal optic nerve function.

Investigation

- Investigation is not usually necessary, unles sthere is concern over possible orbital or sinus involvement.

Treatment

- Daily review until resolution (admit young/unwell children; see ➔ Orbital and preseptal cellulitis, p. 790).
- Treat with oral antibiotics (e.g. flucloxacillin 500mg 4×/d for 1wk).

Table 14.4 Orbital vs preseptal cellulitis

	Orbital	Preseptal
Proptosis	Present	Absent
Ocular motility	Painful + restricted	Normal
VA	↓ (in severe cases)	Normal
Colour vision	↓ (in severe cases)	Normal
RAPD	Present (in severe cases)	Absent (i.e. normal)

1. McKinley SH *et al.* Microbiology of pediatric orbital cellulitis. *Am J Ophthalmol* 2007;**144**:497–501.

Mucormycosis (phycomycosis)

This is a rare, very aggressive life-threatening fungal infection caused by *Mucor* spp. or *Rhizopus*. It is a disease of the immunosuppressed, most commonly seen in patients who are also acidotic such as in diabetic ketoacidosis or renal failure. However, it also occurs in the elderly, malignancy, HIV/AIDS, and therapeutic immunosuppression (e.g. organ transplant recipients). It represents fungal septic necrosis and infarction of tissues of nasopharynx and orbit.

Clinical features
- Black crusty material in nasopharynx, acute evolving cranial nerve palsies (III, IV, V, VI, IIn) ± obvious orbital inflammation.

Investigation
- *Biopsy*: fungal stains show non-septate branching hyphae.
- FBC, U+E, Glu.

Treatment
- Admit, and coordinate care with microbiologist/infectious disease specialist, ENT specialist ± physician.
- Correct underlying disease (e.g. diabetic ketoacidosis) where possible; without this, the prognosis is extremely poor.
- IV antifungals (as guided by microbiology, e.g. high-dose amphotericin).
- Some advocate hyperbaric oxygen therapy.
- Early and aggressive surgical debridement by ENT specialist ± orbital exenteration (for severe/unresponsive disease).

Thyroid eye disease: general

TED (also known as thyroid-associated ophthalmopathy, Graves's ophthalmopathy, dysthyroid eye disease) is an organ-specific autoimmune disease that may be both sight-threatening and disfiguring. Acute progressive TED is an ophthalmic emergency, as it may threaten the optic nerve and cornea (see Box 14.1).

While most patients with TED have clinical and/or biochemical evidence of hyperthyroidism or hypothyroidism, some are euthyroid—at least at the time of presentation. Thyroid dysfunction may precede, be coincident with, or follow TED. Incidence is about 10/100,000/y. About 30–50% of patients with Graves's disease develop TED, with the majority having mild features. In a small percentage (3–5%) of patients, the orbital inflammation may be very severe and lead to loss of vision and even blindness, if not treated promptly.

Risk factors

- ♀ sex (♀:♂ 6:1).
- HLA-DR3, HLA-B8, and the genes for CTLA4 and the thyroid-stimulating hormone (TSH) receptor.
- Smoking.
- Personal or family history of autoimmune thyroid disease.

Autoimmune thyroid disease

TED is most commonly associated with Graves's disease (90%) but may occur in 3% of Hashimoto's thyroiditis.

Graves's disease

The commonest cause of hyperthyroidism. Anti-TSH receptor antibodies cause overproduction of thyroxine (T4) and/or T3. Classic features include hyperthyroidism, goitre, TED, thyroid acropathy (finger clubbing), and pretibial myxoedema.

Autoimmune thyroiditis (e.g. Hashimoto's thyroiditis)

May have a transient hyperthyroid stage, before later hypothyroidism. Lymphocytic infiltration and fibrosis result in a firm, lobulated goitre.

Pathogenesis of TED

The cause is unclear. It is probable that the target antigen is shared between orbital tissues (extraocular muscles and adipose tissue) and the thyroid gland, with the binding and activation of antigens on orbital fibroblasts by autoantibodies (e.g. those to TSH receptor and insulin grown factor (IGF)-1 receptor) resulting in activation of inflammatory cascades, T-cell recruitment, cytokine production, and subsequent myofibroblast–adipocyte proliferation, adipogenesis, and glycosaminoglycan synthesis.

Box 14.1 Emergencies in TED

Acute progressive optic neuropathy

Optic neuropathy in TED may arise due to compression of the nerve by involved tissues (mainly muscles) or by proptosis-induced stretch.

- *Assess*: optic nerve function (VA, colour, VF, pupillary reactions).
- *Treatment*:
  - *Systemic immunosuppression*: this may be oral corticosteroids (e.g. 1mg/kg 1×/d PO prednisolone) or 'pulsed' (e.g. 500mg–1g IVMP 1×/d for the first 3d). Response rates for PO steroid ~50%, and IV steroid ~80%. Monitor response over 1–2wk.
  - Repeat doses of IVMP may be given. The total dose should not exceed 8g in one course of therapy to avoid small risk (0.8%) of acute liver damage.[2]
  - If this fails, then urgent surgical decompression is required. This varies in extent but must decompress the orbital apex where compression is often maximal.

Exposure keratopathy

Exposure keratopathy in TED may arise due to proptosis and lid retraction.

- *Assess*: corneal integrity, tear film, lid closure, proptosis.
- *Treatment*: lubricants, taping/Frost suture/tarsorrhaphy, acute immunosuppression (e.g. systemic corticosteroids) ± orbital decompression.

Clinical features

Ophthalmic

- *Symptoms*: ocular irritation, ache (worse in mornings), red eyes, pain on eye movement, cosmetic changes, diplopia, visual loss.
- *Signs*: proptosis (exophthalmos), lid retraction (upper > lower), lid lag (on downgaze), lagophthalmos, conjunctival and caruncular injection and/or chemosis, orbital fat prolapse, keratopathy (exposure/superior limbic/KCS), restrictive myopathy, optic neuropathy.

Systemic

- Systemic signs depend on the thyroid status (over-/underactivity) and underlying disease (goitre in Graves's or Hashimoto's; pretibial myxoedema, thyroid acropachy in Graves's) (see Table 14.5).
- There is an increased frequency of other autoimmune diseases, e.g. MG, pernicious anaemia, vitiligo, diabetes mellitus, Addison's disease, etc.

2. Bartalena L *et al.* Consensus Statement of the European Group on Graves' Orbitopathy (EUGOGO) on management of Graves' orbitopathy. *Thyroid* 2008;**18**:333–46.

Table 14.5 Common systemic features of thyroid dysfunction

	Hyperthyroidism	Hypothyroidism
Symptoms	Weight loss	Weight gain
	Heat intolerance	Cold intolerance
	Restlessness	Fatigue
	Diarrhoea	Constipation
	Poor libido	Poor libido
	Amenorrhoea	Menorrhagia
	Poor concentration	Poor memory
	Irritability	Depression
Signs	Warm peripheries	Dry coarse skin
	Hair loss	Dry thin hair
	Tachycardia	Bradycardia
	Atrial fibrillation (AF)	Pericardial/pleural effusions
	Proximal myopathy	Muscle cramps
	Tremor	Slow relaxing reflexes
	Osteoporosis	Deafness

Thyroid eye disease: assessment

The diagnosis and management of TED depends on accurate clinical assessment. Grading systems aim to formalize this process but generally are not a substitute for careful clinical documentation of disease status (severity and activity). Similarly, while investigations may support a diagnosis of TED, they are not diagnostic in their own right.

Rundle's curve

The natural history of TED can be described in terms of an active phase of increasing severity, a regression phase of declining severity, and an inactive plateau phase (Rundle's curve). While specific to each patient, these time courses can be plotted graphically and broadly categorized according to mild, moderate, marked, or severe disease (Rundle a to d).

Type 1 and type 2 TED

Some classify TED into type 1 (predominant orbital fat expansion) and type 2 (predominant EOM expansion and restrictive myopathy), with the latter being found in an older age group.

Assessment of disease severity

Grading systems that attempt to document severity include the NOSPECS classification (see Table 14.6). This is now little used by ophthalmologists who generally wish to document disease activity/inflammation in greater detail. It is still widely used by GPs and endocrinologists.

The European Group on Graves' Ophthalmopathy (EUGOGO)[3] classifies TED severity as: sight-threatening—dysthyroid optic neuropathy and/or corneal breakdown; moderate to severe—no sight-threatening TED but sufficient impact on quality of life to justify immunosuppression (if active) or surgery (if inactive); mild—features of TED have only a minor impact on daily life, insufficient to justify immunosuppression or surgery. Other TED severity classifications include VISA, advocated by the International Thyroid Eye Disease Society (ITEDS).

Table 14.6 NOSPECS disease severity score

0	N	No signs or symptoms
1	O	Only signs, no symptoms
2	S	Soft tissue involvement
3	P	Proptosis
4	E	EOM involvement
5	C	Corneal involvement
6	S	Sight loss (↓VA)

On Werner's modified NOSPECS, categories II–VI can be further graded as o, a, b, or c (e.g. degree of visual loss for category VI).

Werner SC. Modification of the classification of the eye changes of Graves' disease. *J Clin Endocrinol Metab* 1977;**44**:203–4.

Assessment of disease activity

The most widely used score of clinical activity is the *Mourits* system (see Table 14.7).

Table 14.7 Mourits *et al.* clinical activity score (CAS)[*]

Pain	Painful, oppressive feeling on or behind globe	+1
	Pain on eye movement	+1
Redness	Eyelid redness	+1
	Conjunctival redness	+1
Swelling	Swelling of lids	+1
	Chemosis	+1
	Swelling of caruncle	+1
	Increasing proptosis (≥2mm in 1–3mo)	+1
Impaired function	Decreasing eye movement (≥5° in 1–3mo)	+1
	Decreasing vision (≥1 line pinhole VA on Snellen chart in 1–3mo)	+1
Total		/10

[*] Mourits MP *et al.* Clinical criteria for the assessment of disease activity in Graves' ophthalmopathy. *Br J Ophthalmol* 1989;**73**:639–44.

Investigations

- *TFTs* (see Table 14.8): usually TSH and free T4, but check free T3 (the active metabolite) if strong clinical suspicion.
- *Thyroid autoantibodies*: anti-TSH receptor, anti-thyroid peroxidase, and anti-thyroglobulin antibodies (see Table 14.9).
- *Orbital imaging*: CT orbits gives better bony resolution and is preferred for planning decompression; MRI (T2-weighted and STIR) gives better soft tissue resolution. Classically, the bellies of the muscles show enlargement and inflammation, but the tendons are spared.
- *Orthoptic review*: may include field of binocular single vision, field of uniocular fixation, Hess/Lees chart, VF.

Table 14.8 Biochemical investigations in TED

TFT	Hyperthyroid	Hypothyroid
TSH	↓	↑
Free T4	↑	↓

In subclinical hyper- or hypothyroidism, free T4 will be normal, but the TSH will still be ↓ or ↑, respectively.

Table 14.9 Immunological investigations in TED

Autoantibody	Association	
Anti-TSH receptor	>95% Graves's disease 40–95% TED	
Anti-thyroid peroxidase	80% Graves's disease	90% Hashimoto's thyroiditis
Anti-thyroglobulin	25% Graves's disease	55% Hashimoto's thyroiditis

3. Bartalena L *et al.* Consensus Statement of the European Group on Graves' Orbitopathy (EUGOGO) on management of Graves' orbitopathy. *Thyroid* 2008;**18**:333–46.

Thyroid eye disease: management

Treatment of eye disease

General

- Multidisciplinary input from endocrinologist and orthoptist. Meticulous control of thyroid function is associated with reduced TED severity.
- *Supportive*: counselling, ocular lubricants, tinted glasses, nocturnal eyelid taping, bed-head elevation, prisms for diplopia, support groups (e.g. British Thyroid Foundation, ℜ http://www.btf-thyroid.org).
- *Smoking cessation*: smokers have more severe TED, are less likely to respond to treatment, and may have worse outcomes.

Medical

- Consider immunosuppression in active disease (CAS ≥3; see Table 14.7). Early aggressive treatment in the active phase can prevent much of the morbidity associated with TED.
- Treatment is usually with systemic corticosteroids, but ciclosporin, methotrexate, azathioprine, and newer agents, such as etanercept (anti-TNF) and rituximab (anti-CD20), have also been used.
- Radiotherapy (e.g. 20Gy in ten daily doses of 2Gy) may be used, with response rates ~60%, although alone it is not advised for sight-threatening optic neuropathy and is contraindicated in those with severe hypertension or diabetes mellitus.

Surgical

- *For acute disease*: acute progressive optic neuropathy or corneal exposure may require emergency orbital decompression.
- *For burnt-out disease*: surgery (usually staged) may improve function and cosmesis. Decompression, motility, or lid surgery is performed, as required and in that order. Decompression can be 1-, 2-, or 3-wall and by a variety of approaches (e.g. endoscopic, swinging lower lid flap, etc.) to hide scars.

Prognosis

- A self-limiting disease that usually resolves within 1–5y.
- Once stable, dramatic improvements in ocular motility and appearance can be achieved with a staged surgical approach.
- Good long-term vision, however, depends on successfully guarding against sight-threatening complications in the acute phase (see Box 14.2).

Box 14.2 Poor prognostic factors in TED

- Older age of onset.
- ♂.
- Smoker.
- Diabetes.
- ↓VA.
- Rapid progression at onset.
- Longer duration of active disease.

Treatment of hyperthyroidism

Carbimazole and propylthiouracil

Carbimazole or propylthiouracil are thionamide drugs used to block the production of thyroid hormones. The initial dose (15–40mg for carbimazole; 200–400mg for propylthiouracil) is continued until the patient is euthyroid and then gradually reduced, while maintaining normal free T4 levels. Therapy is generally required for 12–18mo.

An alternative regimen is blocking–replacement where higher doses of carbimazole are given simultaneously with thyroxine replacement.

Patients should be warned of the risk of agranulocytosis and to seek medical review (including an FBC) if they develop infections, particularly sore throat.

Radioactive iodine

- A single oral dose (typically 400 or 600MBq) of radioactive sodium iodide (^{131}I) is given. The patient must avoid close contact with others, particularly children, for a period afterwards. Subsequent hypothyroidism is common, should be avoided, and requires thyroxine replacement.
- Some studies have shown that ~15% will develop new eye disease or experience TED progression within 6mo after [131]I. This risk is reduced by a short course (~3mo) of 'prophylactic' oral steroids.

Surgical thyroidectomy

This may be total or subtotal. It may be preceded by radioactive iodine to shrink the goitre.

In pregnancy and breastfeeding

- Carbimazole and propylthiouracil cross the placenta and can cause fetal hypothyroidism. Consequently, the lowest dose possible should be used and the blocking–replacement regimen avoided.
- Radioactive iodine is contraindicated in pregnancy.

Treatment of hypothyroidism

Levothyroxine

- Thyroxine replacement is started at a dose of 25–100 micrograms (50 micrograms if >50y of age; 25 micrograms if cardiac disease or elderly) and cautiously increased at intervals of 4wk to a maintenance dose of 100–200 micrograms.
- Treatment is monitored against TFT (aim to normalize, but not suppress, TSH) and clinical status.
- Rapid increases or excessive doses may result in angina, arrhythmias, and features of hyperthyroidism.

Selenium and mild TED

A large randomized, double-blind, placebo-controlled trial of 159 patients with mild TED found that, at 6 and 12mo, those who took the antioxidant selenium (100 micrograms bd) for 6mo had comparatively better quality of life, less ophthalmic involvement, and reduced TED progression, with no adverse effects.[4]

4. Marcocci C *et al.* Selenium and the course of mild Graves' orbitopathy. *N Engl J Med* 2011;364:1920–31.

Other orbital inflammations (1)

A number of inflammatory diseases may affect the orbit. These may be purely orbital or related to systemic disease (e.g. TED). The purely orbital diseases may be diffuse (e.g. idiopathic orbital inflammatory disease) or focal (e.g. myositis).

The classification of orbital inflammations is continuing to evolve as our understanding of immunogenetic and clinical features of orbital diseases improves (see Table 14.10).

Table 14.10 Inflammatory diseases affecting the orbit (selected)

Isolated	Diffuse	Idiopathic orbital inflammatory disease
		IgG4-related orbitopathy
	Focal	Myositis
		Dacryoadenitis
		Tolosa–Hunt syndrome
Systemic		TED
		Granulomatosis with polyangiitis (GPA; formerly Wegener's granulomatosis)
		Sarcoidosis

Idiopathic orbital inflammatory disease

An uncommon chronic inflammatory process of unknown aetiology. The pattern of inflammation may be predominantly anterior orbit (more common) or diffuse. It may simulate a neoplastic mass (hence the former term pseudotumour), but histology shows a pure inflammatory response with no cellular atypia. It is a diagnosis of exclusion (see Box 14.3) and may represent a number of poorly understood entities. It may occur at almost any age and is usually unilateral.

Clinical features
• Acute pain, redness, lid swelling, diplopia.
• Conjunctival injection, chemosis, lid oedema, proptosis, restrictive myopathy, orbital mass.

Investigation
• *Orbital imaging*: B-scan (low-medium reflectivity, acoustic homogeneity); MRI (hypointense, cf. muscle on T1; hyperintense, cf. muscle on T2; moderate enhancement with gadolinium).
• *Biopsy*: required to confirm diagnosis.

Treatment
• *Immunosuppression*: usually systemic corticosteroids, although cytotoxics (e.g. cyclophosphamide) and radiotherapy are sometimes used.

Box 14.3 Differential diagnosis of idiopathic orbital inflammatory disease
- Orbital cellulitis.
- TED.
- GPA (Wegener's granulomatosis).
- Haemorrhage within a vascular lesion.
- Rhabdomyosarcoma.
- Metastatic neuroblastoma.
- Leukaemic infiltration.

Myositis

Idiopathic inflammatory process, usually restricted to one or more EOM, most commonly the superior or lateral rectus. It may occur at almost any age. It is usually unilateral.

Clinical features

Acute pain (especially on movement in the direction of the involved muscle), injection over muscle ± mild proptosis. Repeated episodes may lead to EOM fibrosis and subsequent squint.

Investigations

- *Orbital imaging*: may be diagnosed on CT scan, although MRI gives better soft tissue resolution; classically, the whole of the muscle and tendon insertion shows enlargement and inflammation (cf. TED).

Treatment

- *Immunosuppression*: normally very sensitive to systemic corticosteroids.
- Radiotherapy if recurrent/chronic or poor response to steroids.
- Biopsy if treatment response poor/persistent symptoms.

Other orbital inflammations (2)

Dacryoadenitis

- Lacrimal gland inflammation may be isolated or occur as part of diffuse idiopathic orbital inflammatory disease.
- Presents with an acutely painful swollen lacrimal gland that is tender to palpation, has reduced tear production, and results in an S-shaped deformity to the lid and upper lid ptosis.
- It must be differentiated from infection (e.g. mumps, EBV, CMV), sarcoidosis, Sjögren's syndrome, tumours of the lacrimal gland, and ruptured dermoid cyst.
- Isolated dacryoadenitis responds well to oral NSAIDs (flurbiprofen 100mg 3×/d) or oral corticosteroids.
- Complete resolution may take up to 3 mo.
- Orbital imaging and biopsy is indicated if inflammation persists.

Tolosa–Hunt syndrome

- A rare idiopathic condition; there is focal inflammation of the superior orbital fissure ± orbital apex ± cavernous sinus.
- Presents with orbital pain, multiple cranial nerve palsies, periocular sensory disturbance (Va and Vb), and sometimes proptosis.
- It must be differentiated from other causes of the superior orbital fissure syndrome: carotid–cavernous fistula, cavernous sinus thrombosis, GPA, pituitary apoplexy, sarcoidosis, mucormycosis, and other infections.
- It is very sensitive to steroids.

Granulomatosis with polyangiitis (GPA; formerly Wegener's granulomatosis)

This is an uncommon, severe necrotizing granulomatous vasculitis that may have ophthalmic involvement in up to 50% of cases and orbital involvement in up to 22%. It is commonest in ♂ (♂:♀ 2:1) and in middle age.

Clinical features
Ophthalmic

- *Orbital disease*: pain, proptosis, restrictive myopathy, disc swelling, and ↓VA.
- *Other ocular disease*: epi-/scleritis, PUK, uveitis, and vasculitis.

Systemic

- Pneumonitis, glomerulonephritis, sinusitis, and nasopharyngeal ulceration.

Investigation
- *ANCA*: most cases are c-ANCA positive.
- *CT scan*: obliteration of orbital fat planes by a plaque-like infiltrative mass. Erosion and destruction of sinus and nasal bones.

Treatment
Treatment (coordinated by rheumatologist/physician) is usually combined corticosteroids, cyclophosphamide, or rituximab.

IgG4-related orbitopathy

An immune-mediated systemic syndrome with orbital infiltration of IgG4-expressing plasma cells and subsequent fibrosis and sclerosis.[5] It may affect any ocular adnexal structure. Multi-organ involvement (pancreas, liver, salivary glands, retroperitoneum) may coexist. There may be a history of asthma/allergic rhinitis/drug allergy.

Clinical features

- Proptosis, lid swelling, ocular movement restriction.

Investigation

- *CT/MRI*: solid homogeneous mass, indistinguishable from muscle.
- *Biopsy*: IgG4+ lymphoplasmacytic infiltrate, follicular hyperplasia, eosinophils, sclerosis, and fibrosis.

Treatment

- Excellent response to corticosteroids.
- Radiotherapy and immunomodulatory treatments (e.g. rituximab have also been used).

Adult orbital xanthogranulomatous diseases

Four rare overlapping, poorly understood entities.[6] Yellow-orange, elevated xanthomatous eyelid and/or orbital masses may extend into the orbital fat, EOM, and/or the lacrimal gland(s). May be associated with lymphoproliferative disorders.

Clinical features

In terms of frequency: NBX > ECD > AAPOX > AOX.

- *Adult-onset xanthogranuloma (AOX)*: solitary lesion, no systemic findings, ♂ = ♀, usually self-limiting.
- *Adult-onset asthma and periocular xanthogranuloma (AAPOX)*: xanthomatous eyelid/orbit masses, ♂:♀ 2:1, asthma develops months to years afterwards, associated with lymphoproliferative disorders.
- *Necrobiotic xanthogranuloma (NBX)*: subcutaneous skin lesions may ulcerate and fibrose, ♂ = ♀, associated with paraproteinaemia.
- *Erdheim–Chester disease (ECD)*: lymphohistiocytic orbital infiltration, may also affect heart, lungs, bone, retroperitoneum, ♂:♀ 2:1, often fatal.

Investigation

- *Biopsy*: characteristic histopathology with foamy histiocytes, Touton giant cells, varying degrees of fibrosis/necrosis.

Treatment

- Optimal treatment unclear—surgical debulking/orbital radiotherapy/intralesional or systemic steroids/ciclosporin/biologic agents.

5. Plaza JA et al. Orbital inflammation with IgG4-positive plasma cells: manifestation of IgG4 systemic disease. Arch Ophthalmol 2011;**129**:421–8.

6. Guo J et al. Adult orbital xanthogranulomatous disease: review of the literature. Arch Pathol Lab Med 2009;**133**:1994–7.

Cystic lesions

Dacryops (lacrimal ductal cyst)

These cysts of the lacrimal duct tissue are relatively common and may arise from any lacrimal tissue (including the accessory lacrimal glands of Krause and Wolfring). They represent obstruction and subsequent expansion of lacrimal gland ductules and are filled with serous fluid.

Clinical features
- Painless, smooth-walled, bluish grey, transilluminable areas in the superolateral fornix. They may be bilateral.

Treatment
- Aspiration, if required.

Dermoid cyst

Dermoids are a type of choristoma (congenital tumours of tissues abnormal to that location). They probably represent surface ectoderm trapped at lines of embryonic closure and suture lines. They are most commonly located on the superotemporal orbital rim (69%) in the vicinity of the temporal–zygomatic suture line but may extend deceptively far posteriorly. They are less commonly found superonasally (30%).[7] They comprise stratified squamous epithelium (with epidermal structures such as hair follicles and sebaceous glands) surrounding a cavity that may contain keratin and hair. Accidental traumatic rupture may lead to episodes of inflammation and skin discharge.

Clinical features
Superficial dermoids
- Present in infancy.
- Slowly growing, firm, smooth, round, non-tender mass.

Deep dermoids
- Present from childhood onwards.
- Gradual proptosis, motility disturbance, ↓VA.
- Can present with recurrent orbital inflammation.
- May extend beyond the orbit into the frontal sinus, temporal fossa, or cranium.

Investigation
- *Orbital imaging*: CT shows well-circumscribed lesion with heterogeneous centre; B-scan US shows well-defined lesion with high internal reflectivity.

Treatment
- They should be excised completely without rupture of the capsule to avoid severe inflammation and recurrence.
- Intracranial spread of deep dermoid cysts requires coordination with neurosurgeons.

Mucocele

A mucocele is a slowly expanding collection of secretions due to blockage of the sinus opening. This may be due to a congenital narrowing or arise 2° to infection, inflammation, tumour, or trauma. Over time, erosion of the sinus walls permits the mucocele to encroach into the orbit. Orbit-involving mucoceles usually arise from frontal, ethmoidal, or occasionally the maxillary sinus.

Clinical features
- Headache, gradual non-axial proptosis or horizontal displacement, fluctuant tender mass in medial or superomedial orbit.

Investigation
- *Orbital imaging*: CT shows opacification of frontal or ethmoidal sinus (+ loss of ethmoidal septae), with a bony defect allowing intraorbital protrusion; B-scan US shows a well-defined lesion with low internal reflectivity.

Treatment
- Referral to ENT specialist to excise the mucocele, restore sinus drainage, or obliterate the sinus cavity (in recurrent cases).

Cephalocele

These are rare developmental malformations resulting in herniation into the orbit of brain (encephalocele), meninges (meningocele), or both (meningoencephalocele). They may be anterior (fronto-ethmoidal bony defects) or posterior (sphenoid dysplasia). They usually present as congenital lesions but, if in the deep orbit, may present later in life. Encephaloceles may be associated with other craniofacial or ocular abnormalities, particularly involving midline structures; posterior encephaloceles may be associated with neurofibromatosis-1 and morning glory syndrome.

Clinical features
- *Pulsatile proptosis*, which may increase with Valsalva manoeuvre but without a bruit (cf. AV fistulae).
- *Anterior lesions*: the encephalocele may be visible, transilluminable, and proptosis is usually anterotemporal.
- *Posterior lesions*: the encephalocele is not visible, and the proptosis is usually anteroinferior.

Investigation
- *Orbital imaging*: CT shows a defect in the orbital wall.

Treatment
- Excision/closure/ligation of the base, with patching of the bony defect from the orbital side.

7. Chawda SJ et al. Computed tomography of orbital dermoids: a 20-year review. *Clin Radiol* 1999;**54**:821–5.

Orbital tumours: lacrimal and neural

Lacrimal gland

Pleomorphic adenoma

The commonest lacrimal neoplasm. Accounts for up to 20% of all lacrimal fossa lesions. They are derived from epithelial and mesenchymal tissue, hence the term benign mixed cell tumour. They may arise from either lobe, most commonly the orbital.

They occur in middle age, with a slight ♂ bias (♂:♀ 1.5:1). Malignant transformation occurs in <3% in 10y and 10–20% in 20y.

Clinical features

Gradual painless proptosis (inferonasal), upper lid swelling, diplopia, palpable mass (orbital lobe tumours may not be palpable), globe indentation may cause choroidal folds ± hypermetropic shift.

Investigation

- *US*: round, lobulated lesion, typically medium/high reflectivity.
- *CT/MRI*: expansion of the lacrimal fossa, indentation of the globe, well-circumscribed slightly nodular tumour, calcification in 3%.

Treatment

- Surgical removal of whole tumour with intact pseudocapsule without prior biopsy (risk of seeding). This is usually by an anterior (palpebral lobe tumours) or lateral (orbital lobe tumours) orbitotomy.
- Patient needs to be warned regarding subsequent KCS.
- Prognosis is excellent with complete excision but needs prolonged follow-up for malignant transformation, even if complete clearance.

Lacrimal carcinomas

Commonest malignant tumour of the lacrimal gland is the adenoid cystic carcinoma, followed by the mucoepidermoid carcinoma and the pleomorphic adenocarcinoma. Occur at a similar age to adenomas but cause more rapid proptosis and ophthalmoparesis, and orbital pain or sensory disturbance from perineural spread is common.

- Imaging shows an irregular poorly defined lesion, with bony destruction and possibly calcification (20–30%).
- *Treatment*: seldom curative but consists of exenteration ± radiotherapy.
- Prognosis is very poor, with high mortality.

Neural

Optic nerve glioma

An uncommon slow-growing tumour of glial tissue that usually occurs in children and has a strong association to neurofibromatosis-1.

- Usually present with gradual ↓VA (although this often stabilizes), disc swelling or atrophy, and proptosis.
- Isolated optic nerve involvement occurs in 22%, but most involve the chiasm (72%), often with midbrain and hypothalamic involvement.
- Imaging shows fusiform enlargement of the optic nerve ± chiasmal mass.

- Observation is recommended for patients with isolated optic nerve involvement distant from the chiasm, good vision, and non-disfiguring proptosis.
- Progress is monitored with serial MRI scans.
- Surgical excision is indicated for reduced vision, pain, severe proptosis, or posterior spread threatening the chiasm.
- Chiasmal or midbrain involvement may be an indication for chemotherapy or radiotherapy
- Prognosis for life is good for optic nerve-restricted tumours but worsens with more posterior involvement.

Optic nerve sheath meningioma

A rare benign tumour of meningothelial cells of the meninges that usually occurs in middle age and has a slight ♀ bias (♀:♂ 1.5:1). There is an association with neurofibromatosis-2.

- Usually present with gradual ↓VA, disc swelling or atrophy, optic disc collateral vessels (30%), proptosis, and ophthalmoparesis.
- Imaging shows tubular enlargement of the nerve with 'tram-track' enhancement of the sheath ± calcification.
- Observation is recommended if VA is good.
- Surgical excision is indicated for blind eyes, severe proptosis, or threat to the chiasm
- Prognosis for life is good.

Neurofibroma

Neurofibromas are uncommon benign tumours of peripheral nerves.

- *Plexiform neurofibroma*: presents in childhood and is strongly associated with neurofibromatosis-1. Anterior involvement results in a 'bag-of-worms' mass, causing an S-shaped lid deformity. The tumour is poorly defined and not encapsulated. Surgical excision is difficult and may require repeated debulking.
- *Isolated neurofibroma*: presents in adulthood with gradual proptosis. The tumour is well circumscribed, and surgical excision is usually straightforward.

Schwannoma

Uncommon slow-growing tumours of peripheral or cranial nerves that are usually benign but may be malignant.

- Usually present in adulthood.
- There is an association with neurofibromatosis.
- It is usually located in the superior orbit and presents as a gradually enlarging non-tender mass (often cystic), with proptosis, ↓VA, and restricted motility.
- Treatment is with complete surgical excision, with good prognosis.

Orbital tumours: vascular

Cavernous haemangioma

The commonest benign orbital neoplasm of adults. It is a hamartoma composed of dilated large vascular spaces lined by endothelial cells. Does not usually present until young adulthood, most notably during pregnancy (accelerated growth). It is usually intraconal (80%).

Clinical features

- Proptosis (usually axial); later restricted motility, globe indentation (resulting in choroidal folds or hypermetropic shift), and ↓VA. Rarely, apical retrobulbar lesions may result in gaze-evoked amaurosis.

Investigation

- US: well-defined, round intraconal lesion with high internal reflectivity
- CT/MRI: well-circumscribed intraconal lesion with mild/moderate enhancement. There may be areas of thrombosis within.

Treatment

- Most may be observed, but symptomatic lesions should be excised.

Capillary haemangioma

This is a type of hamartoma (congenital tumour of tissues normal to that location). Very large tumours may be consumptive (Kasabach–Merritt syndrome: ↓plt, ↓Hb, ↓clotting factors) or cause high-output cardiac failure.

Superficial lesions ('strawberry naevus')—confined to dermis

- Bright red tumours that usually appear before 2mo of age, reach full size by 1y, and involute by around 6y.
- May be disfiguring and/or cause amblyopia by obscuring the visual axis or causing astigmatism. In these cases, treatment may be indicated.

Deep lesions—posterior to orbital septum

- May not be visible but cause variable (axial or non-axial) proptosis (worsens with Valsalva manoeuvre/crying).
- With time, partial involution occurs, but large tumours may be treated.

Treatment

- Topical/intralesional/systemic corticosteroids.
- Systemic propranolol.
- Surgical excision.

Lymphangioma

This is a rare hamartoma of lymph vessels that usually presents in childhood. They increase in size with head-down posture and the Valsalva manoeuvre.

Superficial lesions are visible as transilluminable cystic spaces of the lid or conjunctiva that may also contain blood. Deep lesions may cause gradual proptosis or present acutely with orbital pain and ↓VA due to haemorrhage ('chocolate cyst'). Most lesions are observed.

CT shows low-density, cyst-like mass, with associated enlargement of the orbit. If a sight-threatening bleed occurs, they may be drained, but surgery is difficult, as lesions are often large and friable.

Orbital tumours: lymphoproliferative

Orbital lymphoid diseases range from benign hyperplasia to malignant lymphomas, the latter being solid tumours that arise from malignant transformation of leucocytes, particularly B-lymphocytes (about 85%).

Lymphoproliferative tumours are now classified according to the WHO consensus classification system.[8]

Benign reactive lymphoid hyperplasia

An uncommon polyclonal proliferation of lymphoid tissue that usually occurs in the superolateral orbit, often involving the lacrimal gland. It may present with gradual proptosis, ptosis, and/or a palpable firm rubbery mass.

It usually responds to corticosteroids or radiotherapy, although some cases require cytotoxics or monoclonal antibody therapy (e.g. rituximab). Progression to lymphoma occurs in up to 25% by 5y.

Atypical lymphoid hyperplasia

This is intermediate between benign reactive hyperplasia and lymphoma and is characterized by a very homogeneous pattern with larger nuclei.

Malignant orbital lymphoma

An uncommon low-grade proliferation of B-cells (non-Hodgkin's type), usually arising in the elderly. The most common subtype is the marginal zone B-cell lymphoma of MALT, which accounts for 40–70% of all orbital lymphomas.

About half of orbital B-cell lymphomas are 1° tumours (arising solely within orbital structures).[9] Usually presents with gradual proptosis, ptosis, and/or a palpable firm rubbery mass. Usually unilateral, but bilateral involvement occurs in 25%; systemic involvement is present in up to 40% at diagnosis and in up to 60% within 5y.[9,10]

Treatment (radiotherapy, chemotherapy, monoclonal antibody) depends on grade and spread of tumour; a systemic work-up by haematologist/oncologist is necessary in all cases.

Langerhans cell histiocytosis

A rare proliferative disorder of childhood. It comprises a spectrum of disease from the unifocal, relatively benign, unifocal 'eosinophilic granuloma' to the disseminated Letterer–Siwe form.

In eosinophilic granuloma, orbital involvement is common and presents as rapid proptosis with a superotemporal swelling. Bilateral proptosis may occur in disseminated Langerhans cell histiocytosis.

Surgical excision is usually curative.

8. Swerdlow SH et al. *WHO classification of tumours of haemopoietic and lymphoid tissues* (4th edition). Lyon: IARC Press; 2008.

9. Coupland SE et al. Lymphoproliferative lesions of the ocular adnexa. Analysis of 112 cases. *Ophthalmology* 1998;**105**:1430–41.

10. Demirci H et al. Orbital lymphoproliferative tumors analysis of clinical features and systemic involvement in 160 cases. *Ophthalmology* 2008; **115**:1626–31.

Orbital tumours: other

Rhabdomyosarcoma

This is the commonest 1° orbital malignancy in children. It usually arises in the first decade and has a slight ♂ bias (♂:♀ 1.6:1). 87% present before the age of 15y.

It arises from pluripotent mesenchymal tissue. Histologically, it may be differentiated into embryonal (commonest), alveolar, and pleomorphic types. It is usually intraconal (50%) or within the superior orbit (25%).

Clinical features

- Acute/subacute proptosis, ptosis, and orbital inflammation; it may therefore mimic inflammatory conditions such as orbital cellulitis.

Investigation

- B-scan US: irregular but well-defined edges, low/medium reflectivity. Colour Doppler shows very high internal flow.
- CT/MRI: irregular, but well-defined, mass ± bony erosion.

Treatment

- A biopsy (to confirm diagnosis) and systemic work-up (to establish spread) are necessary in all cases.
- Surgical excision is possible for well-circumscribed localized tumours.
- Combined radiotherapy and chemotherapy is given for more extensive tumours.

Fibrous histiocytoma

Uncommon but is the commonest adult mesenchymal orbital tumour. May affect middle-aged adults or children who have had orbital radiotherapy. It may be benign or malignant, is usually located superonasally, and may infiltrate locally.

It presents with gradual proptosis, pain, ↓VA, and restricted motility. Treatment is by complete surgical excision. Recurrences are common, but metastases rare.

Metastases

Orbital metastases (see Table 14.11) are uncommon. In about half of all cases, they precede the diagnosis of the underlying tumour.

Usually present aggressively, with fairly rapid proptosis, restricted motility, cranial nerve involvement, and orbital inflammation. Scirrhous tumours (e.g. some breast and gastric tumours) may cause enophthalmos.

Table 14.11 1° tumours metastasizing to the orbit

Adults	Children
Breast	Neuroblastoma
Lung	Nephroblastoma
Prostate	Ewing sarcoma
Gastrointestinal	

Vascular lesions

Orbital varices

Uncommon congenital venous enlargements that may present from childhood onwards. They are usually unilateral and located in the medial orbit.

Clinical features
- Intermittent proptosis and/or visible varix (worse with increased venous pressure, i.e. Valsalva manoeuvre, coughing, or in head-down position).
- Occasional thrombosis or haemorrhage.

Investigation
- CT/MRI shows multiple ill-defined, irregular masses. There may be expansion of the orbital walls and the presence of phleboliths.

Treatment
- Surgery difficult, but indicated if painful, disfiguring, or sight-threatening. Radiological endovascular injection of sclerosant/coil may be possible.

AV fistula

These are abnormal anastamoses between the arterial and venous circulation. The carotid–cavernous fistula is a high-flow system arising from direct communication between the intracavernous internal carotid artery and the cavernous sinus. The dural shunt (also known as indirect carotid–cavernous fistula) is a low-flow system arising from dural arteries (branches of the internal and external carotid arteries) communicating with the cavernous sinus.

AV fistulae may be congenital (e.g. Wyburn–Mason syndrome), 2° to trauma (particularly in young adults), or occur spontaneously (usually due to hypertension in older people).

Clinical features
Carotid–cavernous fistula (direct)
- ↓VA, diplopia, audible bruit.
- Pulsatile proptosis with a bruit, orbital oedema, injected chemotic conjunctiva, ↑IOP, variable ophthalmoparesis (usually III and VI), retinal vein engorgement, RAPD, disc swelling, anterior segment ischaemia.

Dural shunt (indirect carotid–cavernous fistula)
- May be asymptomatic; pain, cosmesis.
- Chemosis, episcleral venous engorgement/arterialization, ↑IOP.

Investigation
- *Orbital imaging*: B-scan/Doppler US, CT, MRI show a dilated superior ophthalmic vein and mild thickening of the EOM.

Treatment
- High-flow carotid–cavernous fistula may cause visual loss in up to 50% cases and require closure by catheter embolization, with success rate >85%.
- Low-flow dural shunts spontaneously thrombose in up to 40%. Intervention is reserved for cases with glaucoma, ↓VA, diplopia, or severe pain.

Disorders of the anophthalmic socket

Indications for eye removal

- Malignant tumours (e.g. retinoblastoma, choroidal melanoma).
- Painful or cosmetically unacceptable (e.g. phthisical) blind eye.
- Severe ocular trauma.
- Untreatable intraocular infection (e.g. severe endophthalmitis).
- Prevention or treatment of sympathetic ophthalmitis.

Enucleation: eye removal, leaving EOM intact.
Evisceration: eye content removal, leaving sclera and EOM.
Exenteration: removal of eye and parts of the orbit (lids, orbital tissue, bone).
Placement of an orbital implant (acrylic or hydroxyapatite) is almost always performed in conjunction with enucleation/evisceration. The principal of implant placement is to choose the largest possible for that patient's socket.

Post-enucleation socket syndrome (PESS)

A combination of features that result from the deficient, shrunken volume of orbital tissues surrounding an enucleated/eviscerated socket.

Clinical features
- Loss of orbital volume.
- Superior sulcus deformity (hollowing above the upper eyelid).
- Upper lid ptosis.
- Lower lid laxity.

Treatment
Inadequate volume
- Prosthetist to modify or replace the existing prosthesis.
- Exchange orbital implant for one of a larger volume.
- Subperiosteal orbital floor implant.
- Orbital injection of filler material (i.e. hyaluronic acid-based).
- Dermis fat graft (autogenous dermis and subdermal fat, e.g. from abdomen, left inguinal region, or buttocks).

Abnormal lid position
- Lateral or medial tarsal strip.
- Levator resection.

The discharging socket and socket infection

A small amount of discharge is a common problem that needs to be differentiated from socket infection or giant papillary conjunctivitis. Discharge is usually due to socket dryness, the very presence of a prosthesis, and the resulting abrasion of the socket conjunctiva. Hallmarks of implant infection are recurrent discharge resistant to multiple drops, implant discomfort (to touch), and recurrent pyogenic granuloma.

Treatment

- Ensure regular cleaning and polishing of the prosthesis (e.g. annual).
- Advise patient not to remove prosthesis too frequently.
- Ensure no exposed sutures or implant exposure.
- Short course of topical lubricants, antibiotics, and steroids.
- True deep socket infection responds poorly to topical/PO/IV antibiotics and requires implant removal.

Implant exposure, migration, or extrusion

Problems may range from conjunctival thinning to implant exposure or eventual extrusion. Predisposing factors include inadequate surgical closure (wound closure under tension, inadequate or poor wound closure technique), infection, mechanical or inflammatory irritation, previous radiotherapy, abnormally small socket (e.g. previous microphthalmos).

Treatment

- Revision or resuturing does not work—requires orbital implant exchange.
- Dermis fat graft if orbital implant exchange fails.

Poor prosthesis mobility

This is more common for horizontal, rather than vertical, gaze (as the fornices are shorter), but less common after evisceration than enucleation. May be related to poor prosthesis movement, rather than that of the implant. Pegged implants exist but have higher complication rates.

Treatment

- Prosthetist to review the fitting of the prosthesis.
- Increased size of orbital implant.

Shortening of the fornices

Recurring socket infection and/or scarring 2° to trauma can result in fornix shortening (lower > upper). This may be associated with lower lid retraction, difficulty fitting the prosthesis, or the prosthesis recurrently falling out.

Treatment

- Fornix deepening sutures—generally do not work.
- Amniotic membrane graft.
- Hard palate/ear cartilage/donor sclera graft.

Intraocular tumours

Iris tumours

Uveal melanoma

Uveal melanoma is the commonest primary malignant intraocular tumour of Caucasian adults, with a lifetime incidence of about 0.05%. Risk factors include race (light >> dark pigmentation), age (old > young), UV light exposure (possible risk factor), and underlying disorders such as ocular melanocytosis and dysplastic naevus syndrome. It is slightly more common in men than women. Tumours arise from neuroectodermal melanocytes of the choroid, ciliary body, or iris.

Iris melanoma

Compared with the other uveal melanomas, iris tumours are less common (8% of all uveal tumours), present younger (age 40–50y), and have a better prognosis. They are more common in ♀. Histologically, they usually comprise spindle cells alone or spindle cells with benign naevus cells (see Table 15.1).

Clinical features
- Usually asymptomatic; patient may note a spot or diffuse colour change.
- *Iris nodule*: most commonly light to dark brown, well-circumscribed, usually inferior iris; may be associated with hyphaema, ↑IOP (tumour or pigment cell blockage of trabecular meshwork), cataract; transpupillary or transcleral illumination may help demarcate posterior extension.

Risk factors for malignancy (See Box 15.1)
- Size (>3mm diameter, >1mm thickness), rapid growth, prominent intrinsic vascularity, pigment dispersion, ↑IOP, pupillary peaking, ectropion uveae, iris splinting (uneven dilation).

Investigations
- *Anterior segment US*: assess ciliary body involvement.
- *Biopsy*: consider fine-needle aspiration (FNA) (simple, safe, but scanty sample with no architecture) or incisional biopsy (corneal/limbal wound, risk of hyphaema).

Treatment
Specialist advice should be sought. Options include:
- *Observation*: in small asymptomatic tumours with no convincing growth, intervention may not be necessary.
- *Excision*: consider iridectomy/iridocyclectomy ± cosmetic contact lens (artificial pupil).
- *Radiotherapy*: proton beam radiotherapy.
- *Enucleation*: rarely indicated (non-resectable, extensive aqueous seeding, or painful blind eye).

Prognosis
- Most patients do well and rarely (1–2%) develop metastatic disease.
- Poor prognostic features include large size, ciliary body, or extrascleral extension, and diffuse or annular growth pattern.

Table 15.1 Differential diagnosis of iris mass

Pigmented	Iris melanoma
	Naevus
	ICE syndrome
	Adenoma
	Ciliary body tumours
Non-pigmented	Iris melanoma
	Iris cyst
	Iris granulomas
	IOFB
	Juvenile xanthogranuloma
	Leiomyoma
	Ciliary body tumours
	Iris metastasis

Iris naevus

These common lesions do not require regular ophthalmic observation, unless there are suspicious features. Patients will usually detect any worrying change in a lesion themselves.

Clinical features

- Usually asymptomatic; patient may note a spot on the iris.
- Small (<3mm diameter, <0.5mm thick) defined pigmented stromal lesion; pupillary peaking, iris splinting (uneven dilation), or ectropion uveae occasionally occur in naevi but may be suspicious features.

Iris metastases

These are typically amelanotic solid tumours that may cause complications such as 2° open-angle glaucoma (clogging or infiltration of trabecular meshwork with tumour cells), hyphaema, and pseudohypopyon (see Box 15.1).

In most cases, patients are already known to have a malignancy elsewhere, the commonest sites being 1° breast or bronchogenic carcinoma. However, in some patients, the iris lesion is the presenting feature and requires extensive work-up with an oncologist.[1]

Box 15.1 Suspicious features in an iris naevus

- Size (>3mm diameter, >1mm thickness).
- Rapid growth.
- Prominent intrinsic vascularity.
- Pigment dispersion.
- ↑IOP.
- Spontaneous hyphaema.
- Satellite lesions.

---

1. IG Rennie. Don't it make my blue eyes brown: heterochromia and other abnormalities of the iris. *Eye* 2012;**26**:29–50.

Ciliary body tumours

Ciliary body melanoma

These account for about 12% of all uveal melanomas. They most commonly present at about 50–60y. In contrast to iris melanomas, they usually contain the more anaplastic epithelioid melanoma cells and carry a worse prognosis. Cytogenetic analysis of tumour cells can allow stratification of the prognostic risk.

Clinical features
- Usually asymptomatic; occasionally visual symptoms.
- Ciliary body mass (may only be visible with full dilation; see Table 15.2); dilated episcleral sentinel vessels; anterior extension onto the iris or globe; lens subluxation or 2° cataract; anterior uveitis.

Investigation
- *US* (ocular/anterior segment): size, extension, composition.
- *Biopsy*: consider FNA.

Treatment
Specialist advice should be sought. Options include:
- *Excision*: may be possible for smaller lesions.
- *Radiotherapy*: brachytherapy or proton beam.
- *Enucleation*: for larger lesions or significant extension.

Medulloepithelioma

This is a rare slow-growing tumour derived from immature epithelial cells of the embryonic optic cup. It usually arises from the non-pigmented ciliary epithelium, but iris and retinal sites are occasionally seen. They may be benign (1/3) or malignant (2/3), and teratoid (e.g. containing cartilage, brain, bone) or non-teratoid.

Overall, invasion is common, but metastasis is rare. Age of onset ranges from congenital to adult but is usually under the age of 10; both sexes are equally affected.

Clinical features
- Red eye, ↓VA, iris colour change/mass.
- Injection, ciliary body mass (amelanotic, often cystic; see Table 15.2).
- *Complications*: NVG, lens coloboma/subluxation/cataract.

Investigation and treatment
Diagnosis may be assisted by US. Iridocyclectomy may be curative for small, well-defined benign tumours; for most others, enucleation is still required.

Table 15.2 Differential diagnosis of ciliary body mass

Pigmented	Ciliary body melanoma
	Metastases
	Ciliary body adenoma
Non-pigmented	Ciliary body melanoma
	Ciliary body cyst
	Uveal effusion syndrome
	Medulloepithelioma
	Leiomyoma
	Metastases

Choroidal melanoma

Choroidal melanomas account for 80% of all uveal melanoma. They usually present at about 50–60y of age.

They are classified according to size: small (<10mm diameter), medium (10–15mm diameter), and large (>15mm diameter). Histologically, they may comprise spindle cells (types A and B), epithelioid cells, or a mixture (commonest type). Necrosis may prevent cell typing in 5%.

Clinical features

- Often asymptomatic; ↓VA, field loss, 'ball of light' slowly moving across vision.
- *Elevated sub-RPE mass*: commonly brown but may be amelanotic; commonly associated with orange pigment (lipofuscin) and ERD; some (20%) may rupture through Bruch's membrane and RPE to form a subretinal 'mushroom'; occasional vitreous haemorrhage, ↑IOP, cataract, uveitis. **NB** The key diagnostic dilemma is to distinguish a malignant melanoma from a benign naevus (see ⟳ Choroidal naevus, p. 632). Suspicious features are listed in Box 15.2 (see Table 15.3 for differential diagnosis.).

> **Box 15.2 Suspicious features suggestive of choroidal melanoma**
> - Symptomatic.
> - Juxtapapillary.
> - SRF/retinal detachment.
> - Lipofuscin on the surface.
> - Large size (e.g. >2mm thickness).
> - Significant growth.

Investigations

- *US*: solid, acoustically hollow, low internal reflectivity, with choroidal excavation.
- *CT and MRI*: may detect extraglobar extension but cannot reliably differentiate between types of tumour.
- *Biopsy*: incisional biopsy or FNA may be performed in selected cases.
- *Systemic assessment*: FBC, LFT, liver/abdominal US (or CT, MRI).

At the time of presentation, most (98%) do not have detectable metastatic disease.

Treatment

Specialist advice should be sought. Options include:
- *Observation*: for small asymptomatic lesions without suspicious features. Collaborative Ocular Melanoma Study (COMS) showed growth in only 31% of small melanomas by 5y.
- *Radiotherapy*: plaques (3mm larger in diameter than the lesion; deliver about 80–100Gy to the tumour apex) or proton beam irradiation (usually 50–70Gy in 4–5 fractions). Plaque radiotherapy has fewer local

side effects than proton beam and was shown to be as effective as enucleation for medium-sized melanomas (COMS). Side effects include dry eyes, radiation retinopathy, cataracts, and NVG.

- *Local resection:* may be suitable for smaller anterior tumours. Unlike enucleation, it preserves vision and cosmesis and avoids long-term complications of irradiation. However, surgery is difficult, with significant risk of complications (vitreous haemorrhage, retinal detachment, cataract), and requires hypotensive anaesthesia, rendering it unsuitable for patients with cardiovascular comorbidities.
- *Enucleation:* usually performed for large tumours (>15mm diameter, 10mm thick), optic nerve involvement, or painful blind eyes. No benefit demonstrated for pre-enucleation radiotherapy.
- *Orbital exenteration:* occasionally performed for extrascleral and orbital extension or recurrence after enucleation.
- *Transpupillary thermotherapy:* has previously been used as 1° treatment, but this has been largely abandoned due to high rates of local recurrence. However, it still has a role as an adjunct to other therapeutic modalities.

Prognosis

Poor prognostic features include large size, extrascleral extension, greater age of the patient, epithelioid cell type, high mitotic count, and certain genetic mutations in the tumour cells. The most important genetic predictors of mortality are Chr 3 loss (monosomy 3) and partial duplication of Chr 8q. Microarray analysis can further stratify the metastatic risk of an individual choroidal melanoma, based on the pattern of expression of multiple genes.

Table 15.3 Differential diagnosis of choroidal mass

Pigmented	Choroidal melanoma
	Naevus
	CHRPE
	Melanocytoma
	Metastasis (rare)
	Bilateral diffuse uveal melanocytic proliferation (BDUMP) syndrome
Non-pigmented	Choroidal melanoma
	Choroidal granuloma
	Posterior scleritis
	Retinal detachment
	Choroidal detachment
	Choroidal neovascular membrane
	Haematoma (subretinal/sub-RPE/suprachoroidal)
	Choroidal osteoma
	Choroidal haemangioma
	Metastasis

Choroidal naevus

Uveal naevi are benign melanocytic tumours. They may occur in up to 10% of adult Caucasians, making them the commonest of all intraocular tumours. Rarely, they may become malignant (1 in 5,000).

Their main significance lies in the need to differentiate them from a malignant melanoma. Choroidal naevi are usually incidental findings.

Clinical features

- Usually asymptomatic (89% of cases).
- Rarely ↓VA from serous retinal detachment (50%), photoreceptor atrophy (42%), or CNV (8%).
- Small (<5mm diameter, <1mm thick), homogeneous grey-brown; may have drusen; absence of lipofuscin or SRF (cf. choroidal melanoma).

Differentiating a naevus from a malignant melanoma

With time, a malignant melanoma may declare itself by continued, often rapid, growth. However, it may be possible to identify probable melanomas at the time of presentation due to the presence of suspicious characteristics. Features suggestive of malignancy include:

- Thickness (>2mm).
- Fluid (subretinal).
- Symptoms.
- Orange pigment.
- Margin touching disc.

In the absence of any of the first five features, a small melanocytic lesion is very unlikely to be a choroidal melanoma (only 3% show significant growth at 5y). The presence of one feature increases the risk to 38%, and of two or more to >50%. The following mnemonic has been suggested: TFSOM—'To Find Small Ocular Melanomas'.[2] Documented growth would also suggest malignancy.

Investigation and treatment

If no suspicious features are present, these lesions do not require regular ophthalmic review. The naevus should be photographed and the patient provided with a copy to permit their own optometrist to monitor the lesion (e.g. annually) as part of their routine optometric review.

Melanocytoma

These comprise a distinctive cell type—the polyhedral naevus cell. They are heavily pigmented benign tumours, usually involving the optic disc, which may cause axonal compression and consequent VF defects. Occasionally, the choroid, ciliary body, or iris can be involved, but these are often asymptomatic. Rarely, malignant transformation may occur.

---

2. Shields CL et al. Clinical features of small choroidal melanoma. Curr Opin Ophthalmol 2002;**13**:135.

Choroidal haemangiomas

Choroidal haemangiomas are benign vascular hamartomas. Although congenital, they are usually asymptomatic until adulthood when secondary degenerative changes of the overlying RPE and retina, or the development of SRF, may cause visual loss. Two clinical patterns are seen: circumscribed and diffuse.

Histologically, they comprise mainly cavernous vascular channels (with normal endothelial cells and supporting fibrous septa) but with some capillary-like vessels (especially in the diffuse form).

Circumscribed choroidal haemangioma

This form is isolated, may be asymptomatic, and has no systemic associations. It is usually static but may grow in pregnancy.

Clinical features

- Poorly demarcated, elevated, orange-red choroidal mass; usually 3–7mm diameter, 1–3mm thick; located around the posterior pole (within 2DD of disc or foveola).
- *Complications*: fibrous change of RPE, cystic change, or serous detachment of the retina.

Investigations

- *US*: very high internal reflectivity.
- *FFA*: early hyperfluorescence of intralesional choroidal vessels, followed by hyperfluorescence of the whole lesion.
- *ICG*: early cyanescence of intralesional choroidal vessels, followed by intense cyanescence of the whole lesion and subsequent central fading.

Treatment

- Specialist advice should be sought. Options include observation, PDT, transpupillary thermotherapy, or irradiation (usually proton beam).

Diffuse choroidal haemangioma

This form is usually associated with other ocular and systemic abnormalities, forming part of the Sturge–Weber syndrome (see Table 15.4).

Clinical features

- Deep red (cf. normal other eye), thickened choroid, particularly at the posterior pole; may have tortuous retinal vessels, fibrous change of RPE, cystic change, or serous detachment of the retina and disc cupping.
- *Complications*: subretinal fibrosis, cystic change or serous detachment of the retina, glaucoma.

Investigations

- *US*: diffuse choroidal thickening with high internal reflectivity.
- *MRI brain*: if CNS haemangioma suspected as part of Sturge–Weber syndrome.

Treatment

- Specialist advice should be sought.
- Options include PDT, transpupillary thermotherapy, or irradiation.
- Liaise with neurologist, if cerebral involvement.

Table 15.4 Features of Sturge–Weber syndrome

Ocular	Extraocular
Episcleral haemangioma	Naevus flammeus of the face
Ciliary body/iris haemangioma	CNS haemangioma
Choroidal haemangioma (diffuse)	
Glaucoma	

Other choroidal tumours

Choroidal osteoma

This is a rare benign tumour of the choroid. Originally thought to be a choristoma, it is now felt to be an acquired neoplasm in which mature bone replaces choroid, with damage to overlying RPE and retina.

Typically, it is seen in young adult women ($\female$:$\male$ 9:1); it may be bilateral in 20%.[3]

Clinical features

- Gradual ↓VA (<6/60 in 58% of cases by 10y), metamorphopsia.
- Yellow, well-defined geographic lesion, usually abutting or surrounding the optic disc; superficial abnormalities include prominent inner choroidal vessels and irregular RPE changes.
- *Complications*: CNV (47% by 10y, 56% by 20y).

Investigations and treatment

- US: highly reflective with acoustic shadow.
- CT: bone-like signal from posterior globe.
- FFA: early mottled hyperfluorescence and late diffuse hyperfluorescence.
- Although treatment of the tumour itself is not indicated, CNV may be treated conventionally.

Choroidal metastases

These are the commonest intraocular malignant neoplasms. Usually, the patients are already known to have a primary tumour, but, in about 25%, the first clinical manifestation may be an ocular problem.

Although the choroid is the commonest site (see Box 15.3), metastases may occur in the iris, ciliary body (rare), retina, vitreous (cutaneous melanoma), and optic nerve may be involved. Bilateral involvement is seen in about 30%.

Clinical features

- ↓VA, metamorphopsia; may be asymptomatic.
- Yellow-white (breast, bronchus, bowel), ill-defined lesion; usually fairly flat but may have associated ERD.
- *Colour variation*: consider cutaneous malignant melanoma if lesion is black, renal cell carcinoma or follicular thyroid carcinoma if red-orange, and carcinoid if golden orange.

Investigations

Ocular

- US: high internal reflectivity.
- FFA: no/few large vessels within the tumour, early hypofluorescence, and late diffuse hyperfluorescence. ICG may show tumours not detected on FFA.
- FNA: consider FNA if diagnostic uncertainty and no extraocular tissue available for biopsy.

Systemic

This should be coordinated with a general physician or oncologist and would include a complete examination (including breasts, prostate, lymph nodes, skin) and selected investigations (e.g. CXR, mammography).

Treatment

This will depend on the lesion, the visual status of the eye, and the general health of the patient; options include observation, chemotherapy, radiotherapy (plaque, proton beam), or occasionally enucleation.

Box 15.3 Commonest 1° tumours metastasizing to the eye

- Bronchus.
- Breast.
- Bowel.
- Kidney.
- Thyroid.
- Testis.
- Skin.

3. Aylward GW *et al.* A long-term follow-up of choroidal osteoma. *Arch Ophthalmol* 1998:**116**;1337–41.

Retinoblastoma (1)

This is the commonest primary malignant intraocular tumour of childhood. The tumour arises from primitive retinoblasts of the developing retina, with loss of function of the *Rb* tumour suppressor gene (Chr 13q14).

Lifetime incidence is 1 in 15–20,000, and there is no gender or racial predilection. The median age at presentation is under 12mo in heritable cases, and closer to 24mo in sporadic cases. Presentation after the age of 6y is extremely rare.

Genetics

Understanding the genetics of retinoblastoma is critical in planning management. Two separate mutational events M1 and M2, which result in loss or inactivation of both *Rb* gene copies, are required to initiate the tumour (Knudson's 'two-hit' hypothesis). Recent evidence suggests the occurrence of subsequent mutations (M3–Mn) that determine the progression of tumour. The two hits can occur in one of two situations:

- In the genetic (also referred to as the germline or heritable) form, every cell in the body is missing one copy of the *Rb* gene, the mutation occurring at the zygote stage. Every photoreceptor cell can potentially give rise to a tumour.
- In the somatic (non-heritable) form, a single developing retinal cell loses one copy of the *Rb* gene during retinal development (the first hit); the rest of the body cells are normal. The second hit is a random event and gives rise to a tumour.

Therefore, genetic cases often have multiple tumours in one or both eyes (unilateral multifocal or bilateral), while somatic cases are always unilateral and unifocal.

Inherited vs sporadic retinoblastoma

Retinoblastoma may be inherited or occur sporadically.

- Over 90% cases are sporadic (with no FH). In most of these cases, the mutation is somatic and gives rise to isolated unilateral disease.
- A third of the sporadic cases arise from new germline mutations that are heritable (can be passed on to their offspring) but not inherited from the parents.
- 40% of all cases are bilateral (and necessarily germline), and 60% are unilateral (which could be somatic or germline).
- Of the unilateral cases, 15% are germline and carry the same risks as bilateral germline cases. Germline mutations are highly penetrant.
- Over 90% of children carrying the *Rb* gene defect will develop retinoblastoma.

Histology

Characteristic histological features include abnormal patterns of retinoblasts such as the Flexner–Wintersteiner rosettes, Homer Wright rosettes, and fleurettes.

Clinical features
- Leucocoria (see Table 18.18) (60%), strabismus (20%), ↓VA, acute red eye, orbital inflammation, excess watering.
- White, round retinal mass, with one of the following growth patterns: endophytic (growth towards vitreous with vitreous seeds), exophytic (growth towards RPE/choroid with subretinal seeds), mixed or diffuse infiltrating (generalized retinal thickening) ± visible calcification.
- Visible calcification on ophthalmoscopy or detectable on ultrasonography.

Complications (in order of frequency)
- Optic nerve (± CNS) invasion.
- *Anterior segment involvement*: glaucoma ± buphthalmos/corneal oedema, iris invasion manifesting as heterochromia, phthisis bulbi ± pseudohypopyon, rubeosis ± hyphaema.
- *Extraocular spread*, e.g. orbital inflammation.
- *Systemic metastasis*: to bone marrow, liver, and lungs.

Investigations
- *US*: intralesional calcification with high internal reflectivity and acoustic shadow (best detected with low gain setting).
- *CT/MRI*: apart from ultrasonography, routine imaging is not indicated. CT is best avoided, as any dose of radiation magnifies the risk of developing 2° malignancies in germline cases. MRI may be useful if there is suspicion of extraocular (particularly intracranial) spread, if the child presents with signs of ↑ICP (to look for pineal blastoma–trilateral retinoblastoma), or if the diagnosis is in doubt.
- *Mutation testing*: is an essential investigation and can be performed on peripheral blood and tumour tissue, if available (from the enucleated eye). The information gained often helps distinguish between germline and somatic cases, which has major implications for determining the risk to the fellow eye, unaffected relatives, and future siblings and offspring.

Staging
The international classification of intraocular retinoblastoma has five groups A–E of increasing severity and guides initial management. There is a separate staging system for extraocular disease.

Treatment principles
- Retinoblastoma is a unique cancer by virtue of its confinement within the scleral envelope and has >95% cure rate with appropriate treatment.
- The diagnosis is clinical, and it is important to avoid any intraocular procedure (e.g. diagnostic biopsy), as it may lead to extraocular spread, which could result in death.
- A combination of treatment modalities, e.g. chemotherapy with laser/cryotherapy/plaque brachytherapy, helps minimize adverse effects.
- Close monitoring with examination under anaesthesia (EUA) at decreasing frequency as the child grows older is important for early detection of recurrent or new tumours, with awake exams for older children.
- During active treatment, chemotherapy is given over 4–6 cycles at 3-weekly intervals, with EUAs before each cycle to monitor response and apply local treatment (laser or cryo).
- Local treatment may be continued at further EUAs until all tumours are inactive.

Retinoblastoma (2)

Treatment

This requires significant multidisciplinary input and should be coordinated by a specialized centre. Options include:

Laser treatment

- *Using green laser (532nm) for photocoagulation or large spot infrared (810nm) laser for transpupillary thermotherapy*: suitable for smaller tumours or larger tumours after they have been shrunken to a treatable size with chemotherapy (chemoreduction).
- Laser treatment is not effective for vitreous seeds.

Cryotherapy

- Suitable for larger peripheral tumours or localized vitreous disease close to the retina.

Radiotherapy

- *External beam radiotherapy (teletherapy)*: once the mainstay of treatment, this is now reserved for diffuse disease in the only remaining eye or recurrent disease not responsive to all other forms of treatment. *Disadvantages*: large dose of diffuse radiation causing ↑risk of inducing 2° malignancies (major risk in germline cases), soft tissue/bony atrophy, cataracts, and dry eyes.
- *Plaque brachytherapy*: involves suturing a radioactive plaque on to the sclera for a specified period of a few hours to 3–4d, which delivers a high dose of radiation to a very localized area, with no risk of 2° tumours. It is highly effective against localized vitreous disease and for elevated tumours where laser is ineffective.

Chemotherapy

- The main role of chemotherapy is to shrink the tumour(s) to a size where laser treatment can be effective (chemoreduction). It is also very effective against vitreous and subretinal disease, and invaluable for extraocular involvement and metastases.
- Common regimens include carboplatin, etoposide, and vincristine. Significant short- and long-term side effects of chemotherapy (e.g. hearing loss with carboplatin and nephrotoxicity). Usually given over 4–6 sessions at 3-weekly intervals.

Enucleation

- The oldest and most effective treatment, enucleation is curative for intraocular retinoblastoma and is the treatment of choice for advanced uniocular disease or the worse eye of bilateral cases.
- The eye is removed with a long segment of optic nerve and sent for histology and tumour DNA studies to identify the mutations; comparison with peripheral blood can then differentiate germline vs somatic cases.
- An orbital implant of 18–22mm diameter (porous polyethylene (Medpor®), hydroxyapatite, or bioceramic) is inserted at the same time to restore lost volume; later, a cosmetic prosthetic shell (matched to the other eye) is fitted.

Intra-arterial chemotherapy
- A relatively new interventional radiology technique of delivering chemotherapeutic drugs directly into the ophthalmic artery after transfemoral artery catheterization. Useful in recurrent and resistant disease. Melphalan and topotecan are commonly used agents.

Intravitreal chemotherapy
- The newest technique of delivering melphalan into the vitreous cavity via pars plana injection to treat resistant vitreous disease in selected cases. This is still undergoing evaluation in some centres and not widely used due to risk of disseminating disease.

Supportive treatment
- *Prosthesis fitting for enucleated eyes*: is an important part of rehabilitation, usually 6wk after surgery.
- *Psychological support for children and families*: to deal with loss of eye, vision, and a chronic illness.
- *Protective eye wear*: for the better/remaining eye during contact sport.
- *Long-term oncological surveillance, especially for germline cases*: this is best undertaken by the oncologists.
- *Counselling*: genetic counselling (including risk to siblings and offspring) and advice regarding the risk of 2° malignancies (including advice about risk factors, such as smoking, and how to look out for early warning signs). Parents should be counselled soon after diagnosis, and the patients usually when they reach adolescence.
- *Cataract surgery*: if needed, should be delayed for at least 1–2y after active treatment.

Screening for retinoblastoma
Screening close relatives of retinoblastoma patients is invaluable in early detection and treatment, saving eyes and lives. If the mutation for the index case is known, mutation testing (see ⮕ Retinoblastoma (1), p. 638) can be offered to relatives to determine if they are at risk of suffering/passing on the disease.

Screening is offered if: (1) mutation positive or (2) if the mutation is not known for the index case and risk cannot be excluded. Screening is not needed if the relative tests negative for the mutation. This approach helps avoid unnecessary screening and saves resources.

Prognosis
- Most untreated tumours proceed to local invasion and metastasis, causing death within 2y. Occasionally, however, the tumour may spontaneously stop growing to form a retinoma or necrose to cause phthisis bulbi.
- Most small/medium tumours without vitreous seeding can be successfully treated while preserving useful vision. Overall, there is a 95% survival rate (in the developed world). *Poor prognostic factors include*: size of tumour, optic nerve involvement, extraocular spread, and older age of child.
- Patients with germinal mutations are at increased risk of pineoblastoma (trilateral retinoblastoma), ectopic intracranial retinoblastoma, and osteogenic or soft tissue sarcomas. This risk is increased with radiation exposure.

Retinal vascular tumours (1)

Capillary haemangioma

This is an uncommon benign hamartoma of the retinal (or optic disc) vasculature, consisting of capillary-like vessels. It may present at any age but is most commonly diagnosed in young adults. Isolated capillary haemangiomas are usually not related to systemic disease, but most multiple/bilateral tumours are seen in the context of von Hippel–Lindau syndrome (VHL) (see Table 15.5).

Histologically, there are endothelial cells, pericytes, and stromal cells. The VHL mutation may be restricted to the stromal cells, suggesting that, despite their innocent appearance, they are the underlying neoplastic cell.

Clinical features

- ↓VA; asymptomatic (may be diagnosed on family screening).
- Red nodular lesion, with tortuosity and dilatation (often irregular) of feeding artery and draining vein ± exudation, ERD, rubeosis/NVG, ERM, TRD, vitreous haemorrhage.
- Optic disc haemangiomas are less well defined and do not have obvious feeder vessels.

Investigation

- *FFA*: rapid sequential filling of artery, haemangioma, and vein, with extensive late leakage; leakage into vitreous may make late images hazy.

Treatment

- *Systemic disease*: if VHL is suspected, multidisciplinary care with physician and clinical geneticist is required.
- *Ocular disease*:
  - *Photocoagulation*: for small (<3mm diameter) tumours; requires confluent white burns covering the entire tumour ± feeder vessel; multiple treatment sessions are usually required.
  - *Cryotherapy*: for peripheral or larger tumours; usually double freeze-thaw technique; multiple treatment sessions are usually required.
  - *Radiotherapy*.
  - *Excision*.

Cavernous haemangioma

This is an uncommon benign hamartoma of the retinal (or optic disc) vasculature, consisting of large-calibre, thin-walled vessels. It is usually isolated, but familial bilateral cases do occur.

Clinical features

- Usually asymptomatic; occasional ↓VA or floaters.
- Cluster of intraretinal blood-filled saccules (a plasma level may separate out due to the slow flow); otherwise, normal retinal vasculature; ± vitreous haemorrhage.

Investigation and treatment

- *FFA*: slow-filling, remain hyperfluorescent, no leakage.
- Treatment is not usually necessary.

Table 15.5 Features of VHL syndrome

Ocular	Extraocular
Retinal capillary haemangioma	Haemangioblastoma of cerebellum, spinal cord, or brainstem
	Renal cell carcinoma
	Phaeochromocytoma
	Islet cell carcinoma
	Epididymal cysts/adenomas
	Visceral cysts

Racemose haemangioma

These are rare retinal AVMs and are therefore not true tumours. Although congenital, they progress with age and are usually detected in early adulthood. These may be isolated or associated with ipsilateral AVMs of the CNS (Wyburn–Mason syndrome; see Table 15.6).

Clinical features

- Usually asymptomatic; occasional ↓VA.
- Enlarged tortuous vascular abnormality, with direct connection between arterial and venous circulations, with similar colour throughout.

Investigation and treatment

- This is usually a clinical diagnosis.
- There is no effective treatment for retinal AVMs, although intracranial AVMs have been successfully treated by surgery, radiotherapy, and embolization.

Table 15.6 Features of Wyburn–Mason syndrome

Ocular	Extraocular
Retinal AVM	Cerebral/brainstem AVM
Orbital/periorbital AVM	

Retinal vascular tumours (2)

Vasoproliferative tumours

These are uncommon sporadic retinal lesions which can occur in isolation (primary lesions, 74%) or in association with another ocular condition (secondary lesions, 26%) (see Box 15.4). Primary lesions are usually solitary (87%), whereas secondary lesions are often multiple and bilateral. They can present at any age but usually within the third and fourth decade.[4]

Clinical features

- Usually ↓VA due to epiretinal fibrosis (31%), CMO (18%), or subretinal exudation.
- Globular or dome-shaped lesion in the peripheral retina (often inferior temporal), with telangiectatic vessels over the surface and retinal 'feeder' vessels.
- Sub- and intraretinal exudation (80%) which can lead to ERD (50%).

Investigation and treatment

- This is usually a clinical diagnosis.
- Symptomatic lesions can be treated with PDT, plaque brachytherapy, or occasionally triple freeze-thaw transconjunctival cryotherapy.

Box 15.4 Conditions associated with 2° vasoproliferative tumours

- Intermediate uveitis.
- RP.
- Toxoplasmosis.
- Toxocariasis.
- Retinal detachment surgery.
- Sickle cell disease.
- Retinochoroidal coloboma.
- Coats' disease.
- ROP.
- Waardenburg syndrome.

---

4. Rennie IG. Retinal vasoproliferative tumours. *Eye* 2010;24:468–71.

Other retinal tumours

Astrocytoma

This is a rare benign tumour of the neurosensory retina, composed of astrocytes. There is debate as to whether it is acquired or is actually a hamartoma.

Typically, it presents in childhood/adolescence; both sexes are equally affected. Isolated astrocytomas are usually not associated with systemic disease, but most multiple/bilateral tumours are seen in the context of tuberous sclerosis (see Table 15.7). An association with neurofibromatosis (type 1) is also suggested.

Clinical features

- ↓VA but often asymptomatic.
- Superficial white, well-defined lesion (translucent to calcified 'mulberry' type; flat or nodular) ± ERD.

Investigation and treatment

- Further evaluation is not usually required, other than ruling out possible syndromic associations.

Table 15.7 Features of tuberous sclerosis

Ocular	Extraocular
Retinal astrocytoma	Adenoma sebaceum
	Ash leaf spots
	Shagreen patches
	Subungual fibromas
	Cerebral astrocytomas (with epilepsy and ↓IQ)
	Visceral hamartomas (e.g. renal angiomyolipoma, cardiac rhabdomyoma)
	Visceral cysts
	Pulmonary lymphangioleiomyomatosis

Retinal pigment epithelium tumours

CHRPE

This is a common benign congenital proliferation of the RPE, occurring in about 1% of the population (typical form). The typical form is unilateral and either solitary or, more commonly, grouped ('bear tracks'). They are unrelated to systemic disease. The atypical form is bilateral and multifocal and is associated both with familial adenomatous polyposis (see Table 15.8) and its variants.

Histologically, the RPE cells are of increased height with increased numbers of melanin granules.

Clinical features

Typical CHRPE

- *Solitary*: black, well-defined, flat, round lesion, often with depigmented 'lacunae' within it, deep to the neurosensory retina; usually 2–5mm. May show slow progressive enlargement. Rarely give rise to elevated solid neoplasms of the RPE.[5]
- *Grouped*: similar smaller lesions, grouped to form 'bear tracks'; usually <2mm.

Atypical CHRPE

- Bilateral, multiple, widely separated, black oval lesions with irregular depigmentation; usually <2mm.

Investigation and treatment

Typical CHRPE does not require investigation. Atypical CHRPE should prompt an investigation of family history and consideration of referral to a gastroenterologist. If familial adenomatous polyposis is diagnosed (by a gastroenterologist), prophylactic colectomy is recommended. In untreated familial adenomatous polyposis, the development of colonic carcinoma is almost universal.

Combined hamartoma of the RPE and retina

This is a rare benign hamartoma of the RPE, retinal astrocytes, and retinal vasculature. It is usually not related to systemic disease but may be associated with neurofibromatosis type 2 (NF-2) and rarely type 1 (NF-1).

Clinical features

- ↓VA, floaters, leucocoria.
- Elevated lesion, with whitish sheen superficially (ERM and intraretinal gliosis), tortuous vessels, and variable deeper pigmentation; usually juxtapapillary but may be peripheral; usually 4–6mm in diameter.

Investigation and treatment

- Assess for the possibility of underlying neurofibromatosis (see Table 15.9 and Table 15.10).

Table 15.8 Features of familial adenomatous polyposis

Ocular	Extraocular
Atypical CHRPE	Colonic polyps and carcinoma
	Gardner's variant: bone cysts, hamartomas, soft tissue tumours .
	Turcot's variant: CNS neuroepithelial tumours

Table 15.9 Features of NF-1[*]

Ocular	Extraocular
Optic glioma	Café-au-lait spots (≥6; each >0.5cm pre-puberty or >1.5cm post-puberty)
Lisch nodules (≥2)	
Lid neurofibroma	Axillary/inguinal freckling
Choroidal naevi	Neurofibromas (≥1 plexiform type or ≥2 any type)
Retinal astrocytoma	Characteristic bony lesion (sphenoid dysplasia, which may → pulsatile proptosis; long bone cortex thinning/dysplasia)
	First-degree relative with NF-1

[*] Diagnosis requires two or more of the features in bold.

Table 15.10 Features of NF-2

Ocular	Extraocular
Early-onset posterior subcapsular or cortical cataracts	Acoustic neuroma
	Meningioma
Combined hamartoma of the RPE and retina	Glioma
	Schwannoma
	First-degree relative with NF-2

Definite NF-2:

- Bilateral acoustic neuroma, OR
- First-degree relative with NF-2 AND either unilateral acoustic neuroma (at <30y) or two of the other diagnostic features.

Probable NF-2:

- Unilateral acoustic neuroma (at <30y) AND one of the other diagnostic features, OR
- Multiple meningiomas AND one of the other diagnostic features.

5. Shields JA et al. Adenocarcinoma arising from congenital hypertrophy of retinal pigment epithelium. Arch Ophthalmol 2001;**119**:597–602.

Lymphoma (1)

Although this is an uncommon tumour of the eye, ocular lymphoma is increasing in incidence.

- It is both sight-threatening and life-threatening and is easily missed, as it may masquerade as a number of other conditions such as uveitis.
- Risk factors include immunosuppression (e.g. therapeutic, AIDS, etc.).

Classification

In ocular disease, lymphoma may be divided according to clinical pattern (vitreoretinal, choroidal, ciliary, or iridal) and whether they are primary or secondary to either CNS lymphoma or systemic disease. They are then subtyped histomorphologically, according to the WHO Lymphoma Classification.

Hodgkin's lymphoma

Hodgkin's lymphoma is characterized by the Reed–Sternberg cell (thought to be an abnormal B-cell) and accounts for 20% of lymphomas (about 1,500 new cases/y in the UK).

Non-Hodgkin's lymphoma

This comprises all other lymphomas (80%; about 9,700 new cases/y in the UK). It is usually subclassified, according to cell type. Most non-Hodgkin's lymphomas are B-cell lymphomas, but some are T-cell lymphomas.

- *B-cell non-Hodgkin's lymphoma*: the commonest types of B-cell lymphoma are diffuse large B-cell lymphoma and follicular lymphoma; other types include Burkitt's lymphoma, MALToma (extranodal marginal zone B-cell lymphoma), nodal marginal zone B-cell lymphoma, mantle cell lymphoma, mediastinal large B-cell lymphoma, small lymphocytic lymphoma, and Waldenström's macroglobulinaemia.
- *T-cell non-Hodgkin's lymphoma*: T-cell lymphomas include cutaneous lymphoma (mycosis fungoides; Sézáry syndrome), peripheral T-cell lymphoma, anaplastic large cell lymphoma, and lymphoblastic lymphoma.

Primary vitreoretinal lymphoma (PVRL)

PVRL (also known as primary intraocular lymphoma, primary CNS lymphoma with ocular involvement) is the commonest type of intraocular lymphoma.[6]

Histology

This is usually an intermediate/high-grade non-Hodgkin's lymphoma of diffuse large B-cell type.

Disease distribution and presentation

- *Disease distribution*: bilateral ophthalmic disease occurs in 90%; coexistent intracranial disease occurs in up to 85% of patients with primary intraocular disease; conversely, up to 20% who present with primary CNS lymphoma develop concurrent ocular disease.
- *Disease presentation*: the ocular disease is the presenting feature in 50–65% (and can precede CNS disease by months or years), whereas, in 35–50%, it is found concurrent with or after presentation of CNS disease.

Risk factors

- May occur in both immunocompetent and immunocompromised individuals.
- In patients on immunosuppressive drugs, risk is related to degree and duration of immunosuppression.

- In patients with HIV, it is normally associated with CD4+ counts of <30/mm³; EBV is strongly associated with ocular CNS lymphoma in AIDS patients.

Clinical features

- Typically, PVRL presents with a 'vitreoretinal' pattern of disease, sometimes being described as a uveitis 'masquerade' syndrome.

Ophthalmic features

- *Typical*: 'vitritis' (cellular infiltrate), yellowish sub-RPE plaques with overlying pigment clumping ('leopard spotting'), usually bilateral; may be misdiagnosed as a refractory 'uveitis' (although corticosteroid treatment may initially be successful).
- *Atypical*: ERD; retinitis, which may mimic diseases seen with CMV, ARN, sarcoidosis, TB, and syphilis; NVG.

CNS features

- *Typical*: progressive focal symptoms indicative of a space-occupying lesion ± seizures, mental state change.
- *Atypical presentations*: meningeal (may present with headache, isolated cranial neuropathy, spinal nerve root problems); progressive dementia; intravascular malignant lymphomatosis (multiple stroke-like episodes); neurolymphotasis (CNS lymphoma with peripheral nerve infiltration); relapsing-remitting form.

Investigation

- *Ophthalmic*: full diagnostic vitrectomy is recommended as the 1° investigation over fine-needle vitreous aspiration (25G needle), as the cellular yield is much greater and more likely to be diagnostic.[7] Incisional biopsy may also be considered if chorioretinal involvement. The vitreous specimen requires expert handling with immediate fixing in theatre, where possible (ensuring maximum cellular viability), and centrifugation. Levels of interleukin 10 are generally elevated. In one study of 159 patients (51 with intraocular lymphoma), elevated interleukin 10 was a useful predictor of intraocular lymphoma; an interleukin 10:interleukin 6 ratio of >1.0 indicates likely lymphoma.[8] Clonal bcl-2/IgH translocations may be detected by PCR in up to two-thirds of cases.
- *Systemic*: assessment and treatment should be coordinated by an oncologist and would usually include MRI brain ± LP (for ocular-CNS type) and abdomen–pelvis imaging (for systemic involvement).

Treatment

Treatment options include radiotherapy (external beam or plaque) and chemotherapy (intravitreal, e.g. methotrexate or systemic). CNS involvement may require aggressive treatment with combined intrathecal and IV chemotherapy and radiotherapy.

6. Mudhar HS et al. Diagnostic cellular yield is superior with full pars plana vitrectomy compared with core vitreous biopsy. *Eye (Lond)* 2013;**27**:50–5.

7. Cassoux N et al. IL-10 measurement in aqueous humor for screening patients with suspicion of primary intraocular lymphoma. *Invest Ophthalmol Vis Sci* 2007;**48**:3253–9.

8. Chan CC et al. Primary vitreoretinal lymphoma: a report from an International Primary Central Nervous System Lymphoma Collaborative Group symposium. *Oncologist* 2011;**16**:1589–99.

Lymphoma (2)

Primary uveal lymphoma

Primary uveal lymphoma may arise in the choroid, ciliary body, or iris. They are all rare; uveal lymphoma is much more likely to be due to systemic disseminated disease. Primary uveal lymphomas are usually of low grade, extranodal, marginal zone B-cell type.

Secondary uveal lymphoma

Secondary intraocular involvement may occur with systemic lymphoma. Uveal lymphoma is much less common than PVRL; it may be associated with involvement of other orbital structures.

Histology

The most common systemic lymphoma types to involve the eye is diffuse large B-cell lymphoma, multiple myeloma, and Waldenström's macroglobulinaemia.

Clinical features

- *Typical*: more diffuse yellowish choroidal thickening (may be multifocal), with minimal if any vitritis.
- *Atypical*: may mimic melanoma (or other choroidal tumours), posterior scleritis, uni-/multifocal choroiditis.

Investigation

- *Ophthalmic:* in most cases, tissue diagnosis of lymphoma has already been made from non-ocular tissue, although ocular fluid/tissue may be obtained, as described for primary intraocular disease. Orbital imaging (US/MRI) may be helpful in assessing extent of disease.
- *Systemic:* assessment and treatment should be coordinated by an oncologist. It is likely to include extensive imaging (e.g. abdomen–pelvis), with a view to assessing extent of disease and identifying suitable tissue for biopsy. MRI brain and LP (suspected CNS involvement).

Treatment

- Treatment options include radiotherapy and chemotherapy, as directed by histological grade of lymphoma and extent of systemic and intraocular disease.

Neuro-ophthalmology

Anatomy and physiology (1)

Within the retina, photoreceptors transduce photons into electrical impulses, which are relayed via bipolar cells to the retinal ganglion cell.

The ganglion cells can be divided into two populations: parvocellular system for fine VA and colour, and the magnocellular system for motion detection and coarser form vision. This division is preserved both in the lateral geniculate nucleus (LGN) and the visual cortex.

Optic nerve

The optic nerve is about 50mm long, carries 1.2 million axons, and runs from the optic disc to the chiasm. It may be divided into:

- *Intraocular part (1mm long)*: unmyelinated axons pass through the channels of the lamina cribrosa to become myelinated, so doubling in diameter (1.5mm prelaminar to 3.0mm retrolaminar).
- *Intraorbital part (25mm long)*: this portion has a full meningeal sheath of tough outer dura (continuous with sclera anteriorly and periosteum of sphenoid posteriorly), arachnoid, subarachnoid space, and inner pia mater. It has about 8mm of 'slack' permitting free ocular motility.
- *Intracanalicular part (5–9mm long)*: the nerve enters the optic foramen to travel through the optic canal within the lesser wing of the sphenoid.
- *Intracranial part (12–16mm long; 4.5mm diameter)*: the nerve runs up, posteriorly and medially, to form the chiasm. Neighbouring structures include the frontal lobes superiorly, the internal carotid artery (ICA) laterally, and the ophthalmic artery inferolaterally.

Blood supply

The ophthalmic artery originates from the ICA. It lies inferolaterally to the intracranial optic nerve, inferiorly to the intracanalicular part, and perforates the intraorbital part 8–12mm behind the globe to become the central retinal artery. The intracranial, intracanalicular, and intraorbital portions of the optic nerve are supplied by the pial plexus fed by branches of the ophthalmic artery and, most posteriorly, by the superior hypophyseal artery. The intraocular part (the optic nerve head) is supplied by the circle of Zinn–Haller, an anastomosis fed mainly by the short posterior ciliary arteries.

Optic chiasm

The optic chiasm (8mm long, 12mm wide) represents the joining of both optic nerves, the hemidecussation of the nasal fibres, and the emergence of the optic tracts. The chiasm usually lies directly above the pituitary gland (80%) but may be relatively anterior (prefixed) or posterior (post-fixed). The pituitary itself lies within the sella turcica of the sphenoid, roofed by the diaphragma sellae, a sheet of dura between anterior and posterior clinoids. Neighbouring structures include the cavernous sinus and ICA inferolaterally and the third ventricle lying posteriorly.

Within the chiasm, fibres from superonasal retina are found to decussate relatively posteriorly, while inferonasal fibres decussate more anteriorly; some of these inferonasal fibres appear to loop so far forward as to join the contralateral optic nerve to form Wilbrand's knee. Macular fibres decussate in the central and posterior chiasm.

Optic tract and LGN

The optic tract runs from the chiasm to the LGN, during which axons from corresponding locations of each retina start to become associated. Within the tract, parvocellular fibres run centrally with magnocellular fibres on the outside. The LGN is organized into six layers: contralateral fibres synapse with 1 (magnocellular), and 4 and 6 (parvocellular); ipsilateral fibres with 2 (magnocellular), and 3 and 5 (parvocellular). There may be other modifying pathways (akin to K cells in primates) located between these layers. Axons from the superior retina synapse medially, inferior retina laterally. Macular fibres synapse in the central and posterior LGN. Blood supply is from branches of the middle cerebral artery and thalamogeniculate branches of the posterior cerebral artery.

Optic radiation

Axons of the optic radiation project from the LGN to the visual cortex.

Fibres from the superior retina project posteriorly through the parietal lobe. Fibres from the inferior retina project through the temporal lobe but deviate laterally round the inferior horn of the lateral ventricle to form Meyer's loop. Macular fibres generally lie between these two courses.

The blood supply is from the internal carotid, middle, and posterior cerebral arteries.

Visual cortex

The 1° visual cortex (V1, Brodmann area 17, striate cortex) is located on the medial surfaces of both occipital lobes on either side of the calcarine sulcus.

V1 is organized into six layers; optic radiations synapse mainly with layer IV; layers II and III project to 2° visual cortex; layer IV to superior colliculus; and layer VI back to LGN.

Superior retina is represented superiorly, inferior retina inferiorly, macula most posteriorly, and extreme temporal periphery (temporal crescent) anteriorly. Blood supply is mainly from the posterior cerebral artery but with middle cerebral artery contributions at the anterior and lateral margins.

The visual cortex cells are arranged into basic processing units representing discrete areas of the VF. These hypercolumns comprise right and left ocular dominance columns, and orientation columns. The orientation columns are divided into blobs (colour) and interblobs (orientation). Cell types range in complexity. Least discriminatory are the circularly symmetrical cells that respond to small central stimulus, regardless of orientation and movement. Simple cells require a centrally located single contrast stimulus that must be correctly orientated and moving in the correct direction. Complex cells are similar but do not require the stimulus to be centrally located. Hypercomplex cells require that the stimulus is also of a particular length.

Further processing occurs in the visual association areas, which may also integrate information from nuclei involved with head and eye movement. Subspecialization occurs in V3 (depth perception, dynamic form), V4 (colour), and V5 (motion, maintenance of fixation).

Anatomy and physiology (2)

Ocular motor nerves (See Fig. 16.1)

Third nerve (oculomotor nerve)

The III nucleus lies in the midbrain, anterior to the periaqueductal grey matter, at the level of the superior colliculus. It consists of a single central nucleus, innervating both LPS muscles, and separate subnuclei for each superior rectus (SR; contralateral innervation), medial rectus (MR), inferior rectus (IR), and inferior oblique (IO) (all ipsilateral innervation).

The IIIn fasciculus travels anteriorly through the medial longitudinal fasciculus (MLF), the red nucleus, and the cerebral peduncle. On leaving the midbrain, it emerges within the interpeduncular fossa and passes anteriorly beneath the posterior cerebral artery, above the superior cerebellar artery and lateral to the posterior communicating artery. It travels within the lateral wall of the cavernous sinus, dividing into superior and inferior branches that enter the orbit via the superior orbital fissure and annulus of Zinn. The superior branch innervates LPS and SR, whereas the inferior branch innervates MR, IR, IO, and the pupillary sphincter.

Parasympathetic fibres from the Edinger–Westphal nucleus travel in the IO branch as far as the ciliary ganglion and then in the short ciliary nerves to the globe where they innervate the ciliary muscle and pupillary sphincter.

Fourth nerve (trochlear nerve)

The IV nucleus lies just below the III nucleus in the lower midbrain at the level of inferior colliculus.

The fasciculus decussates within the anterior medullary velum and exits the midbrain posteriorly. It then curves round the midbrain, passes anteriorly between the posterior cerebral and superior cerebellar arteries, travels within the lateral wall of the cavernous sinus (inferolateral to III, superior to Va). It then enters the orbit through the SO fissure (but superior to the annulus of Zinn) and terminates in the SO.

Sixth nerve (abducens nerve)

The VI nucleus lies in the lower pons, anterior to the fourth ventricle, at the level of the facial colliculus. Although most axons innervate the ipsilateral lateral rectus (LR), about 40% of axons project via the MLF to the contralateral MR subnucleus.

The fasciculus travels anteriorly through the medial lemniscus and corticospinal tract, just medial to the trigeminal nuclear complex and vestibular nuclei. After emerging at the pontomedullary junction, it ascends in the subarachnoid space between the pons and the clivus, before turning anterior over the petrous apex of the temporal bone and under the petroclinoid ligament to enter the cavernous sinus. Here it runs within the sinus itself, just lateral to the ICA and inferomedial to III, IV, and Va, which run in the sinus wall. It then enters the orbit via the superior orbital fissure and annulus of Zinn to terminate in LR.

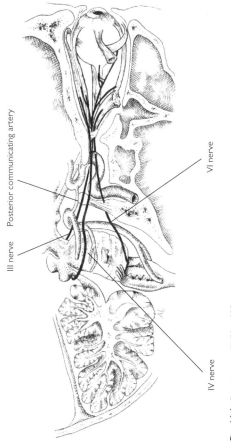

Posterior communicating artery

III nerve

IV nerve

VI nerve

Fig. 16.1 Cranial nerves III, IV, and VI.

Anatomy and physiology (3)

Seventh nerve (facial nerve)

The facial nerve nuclei are located in the lower pons below the level of the fourth ventricle. There are three nuclei: (1) the main motor nucleus; (2) the parasympathetic superior salivatory and lacrimal nuclei (nucleus salivatorius superior); and (3) the sensory nucleus (nucleus of tractus solitarius). Fibres from the latter two nuclei form the nervus intermedius.

The main motor nucleus is bilaterally innervated by the cerebral cortex, and the neurones pass around the VI nerve nuclei before emerging anteriorly from the brainstem with the nervus intermedius, at the lower border of the pons. Passing above the VIII nerve, they pass over the cerebellopontine angle into the internal auditory canal. They transverse the petrous temporal bone and exit behind the stylomastoid process through the stylomastoid foramen. They terminate in the temporal, zygomatic, buccal, mandibular, and cervical branches.

- *Motor functions:* muscles of facial expression and movement; superficial platysma muscles of the neck and the stapedius ear muscles.
- *Sensory and secretory functions (nerve intermedius and geniculate ganglion):* lacrimal gland (via the greater superficial petrosal nerve) and salivary glands (via the chorda tympani, mediating taste for the anterior two-thirds of the tongue).

Autonomic supply

Sympathetic

The first-order neurones originate in the posterior hypothalamus, descend through the brainstem to synapse in the spinal cord at the ciliospinal centre of Budge (C8–T2).

The second-order neurones emerge anteriorly in the ventral root (close to the lung apex) and then ascend in the sympathetic chain to synapse at the superior cervical ganglion.

The third-order neurones ascend along the ICA to the cavernous sinus, and then via the nasociliary branch of Va into the orbit, and subsequently the long ciliary nerves to terminate in the dilator pupillae.

Parasympathetic

The light and near reflexes are both mediated by the parasympathetic supply from the Edinger–Westphal nucleus. The afferent arm for the light reflex is by: (1) retinal ganglion cells that synapse in the ipsilateral pretectal nucleus and then (2) interneurones that innervate bilateral Edinger–Westphal nuclei. The inputs for the near reflex are less well defined but probably include cortical influences (frontal and occipital lobes) mediated by a midbrain centre (anterior to the pretectal nucleus).

The efferent arm for both reflexes comprise: (1) preganglionic neurones from the Edinger–Westphal nucleus, which travel in III, then inferior division of III, then nerve to IO before synapsing at the ciliary ganglion, and (2) post-ganglionic neurones, which run via the short ciliary nerves to terminate in the constrictor pupillae and ciliary muscle.

CSF

CSF is produced by the choroid plexus in the lateral ventricles and the third ventricle. It flows from the lateral ventricles via the foramen of Munro to the third ventricle, and then via the aqueduct of Sylvius to the fourth ventricle. From there, it leaves, either via the lateral foramina of Luschka or the medial foramen of Magendie, to bathe the spinal cord and cerebral hemispheres in the subarachnoid space. It is then absorbed into the cerebral venous system by the arachnoid granulations.

The subarachnoid space is continuous with the optic nerve sheath.

Optic neuropathy: assessment

The optic nerve is vulnerable to injury from numerous local and systemic diseases. Clinical features include ↓VA, relative/complete afferent pupillary defect, ↓light sensitivity, ↓colour vision, VF defects, and optic disc abnormalities such as swelling (early) and pallor (late) (see Table 16.1).

Table 16.1 An approach to assessing optic nerve disease

PC	Blurring, 'washout' of colours, 'blind spots'; may be asymptomatic; check duration, speed of onset/recovery, precipitants, associations (diplopia, proptosis, red eye)
HPC	Recent trauma or surgery
POH	Previous/current eye disease; refractive error
PMH	Vascular risk factors and disease; neurological disease (e.g. MS); connective tissue disease (e.g. SLE, RA); granulomatous disease (e.g. sarcoid, TB)
SR	Detailed review of all systems; particularly any headache or abnormalities of sensation/motor system/speech/balance/hearing
SH	Driver; profession; diet, tobacco consumption, alcohol intake, toxin exposure(e.g. lead, tin, or carbon monoxide)
FH	Family members with visual problems
Dx	Previous/current toxic drugs (e.g. anti-TB)
Ax	Allergies or relevant drug contraindications
VA	Best corrected/pinhole/near
Retinoscopy	Rule out refractive error
Visual function	Check for RAPD, colour vision, red desaturation, VF (confrontation VF and formal perimetry)
Orbit	Proptosis, palpable mass, globe displacement, pulsation/bruit
AS	Features suggestive of glaucoma, uveitis, carotid–cavernous fistula
Tonometry	IOP
Optic disc	Size, cup, colour, oedema, congenital abnormalities, flat/elevated/tilted, crowding, peripapillary oedema or haemorrhages, retinociliary collateral vessels, SVP
Macula	Abnormalities which may cause central scotoma
Fundus	Abnormalities (e.g. retinoschisis) that may cause peripheral field loss; posterior uveitis or vasculitis
Vessels	Arteriosclerosis, hypertensive changes, occlusions and emboli
CNS/PNS	Cranial nerves (incl. ocular motility), sensory, motor, cerebellar function, speech, mental state
CVS	Pulse, heart sounds, carotid bruits
Systemic review	Including respiratory, GI, GU, ENT systems

Diagnosis is more difficult in early symmetric disease where there may be no objective signs. EDTs may be helpful in such cases. Also typical 'optic neuropathy' features may be seen in other diseases (e.g. central scotoma, ↓colour vision, or 2° optic atrophy in retinal disorders). The challenge is thus first to recognize the optic neuropathy and then elucidate the cause (see Table 16.1 and Table 16.2).

Unexplained optic neuropathy requires urgent investigation (see ➜ Atypical optic neuritis, p. 665) to elucidate the cause and rule out serious disease such as compression 2° to a tumour.

Table 16.2 Clinical features of optic nerve vs macular disease

	Optic neuropathy	Macular disease
Hx		
Main complaint	Grey/darkness	Distortion
Scotoma	Negative	Positive
Associated symptoms	May have retrobulbar pain, e.g. on eye movement	May have micropsia, hyperopic shift
Examination		
VA	Variable ↓	↓↓
Colour vision*	↓ or ↓↓	Normal or mild ↓
RAPD	+ to ++++	– or (–/+)
Testing		
Perimetry	Central, centrocaecal, arcuate, or altitudinal defects	Central scotoma
Amsler chart	Scotoma	Metamorphopsia
VEP latency	↑	Normal or mild ↑

* Classically, optic neuropathies preferentially affect the red-green axis and macular disease the blue-yellow axis, but there are many exceptions to this (e.g. glaucoma preferentially affects the blue-yellow axis).

Typical optic neuritis

Inflammation of the optic nerve may be divided into papillitis (where the disc is swollen), retrobulbar neuritis (where the disc is spared), and neuro-retinitis (with retinal involvement, 'macular star').

The most common cause of optic neuritis is demyelination, although a number of important differential diagnoses must be considered.

Acute demyelinating optic neuritis

Incidence within the general population is 1–3/100,000/y but occurs in up to 70% of patients with known MS and is often the presenting symptom of MS. The majority are ♀ (♀:♂ 3:1) and are usually aged 20–50. The disease is usually unilateral, although bilateral involvement may be seen in children.

Clinical features

- Rapid ↓VA over hours/days (rarely become NPL); recovery starts within 2wk and may continue for a few months; ↓contrast sensitivity, ↓colour vision, field loss (variable pattern), retrobulbar pain (present in 90%; often worse on eye movement, may be very severe, usually precedes ↓VA), photopsia.
- RAPD (may be absent if pre-existing contralateral disease), disc swelling (only 1/3 of cases); disc should not be pale in the acute stages of a first episode; may have few haemorrhages, retinal exudates, and mild vitritis.

Investigations

- If episode is entirely typical (see Box 16.1), the diagnosis may be made on clinical grounds alone.
- If episode is atypical, investigate to rule out a progressive optic neuropathy (see ➲ Atypical optic neuritis, p. 665).

Box 16.1 Features of typical optic neuritis (Optic Neuritis Treatment Trial, ONTT)[*]

- Age 20–50.
- Unilateral.
- Worsens over hours/days.
- Recovery starts within 2wk.
- Retrobulbar pain (may be worse on eye movement).
- ↓colour vision.
- RAPD.

[*] Beck RW *et al.* A randomized, controlled trial of corticosteroids in the treatment of acute optic neuritis. The Optic Neuritis Study Group. *N Engl J Med* 1992;**326**:581–8.

Treatment

This remains controversial. IVMP may hasten visual recovery but does not affect final VA (ONTT).[1] There is no conclusive evidence that corticosteroids (IV or PO) are beneficial in terms of recovery to normal VA, VF, or contrast sensitivity.[2] On this basis, it may be offered to those with poor vision in the other eye or with severe pain.

Prognosis

- *Visual recovery*: all patients will have some improvement, with >90% attaining 6/9 in the affected eye. However, even if RAPD resolves and VA recovers to >6/6, abnormalities of colour perception, contrast sensitivity, stereopsis, or field may persist. About a third have a further episode (either eye) within 5y. On MRI, poor visual prognosis is associated with length of optic nerve involvement and intracanalicular segment involvement.
- *Probability of developing MS*: risk factors are ♀ sex, multiple white matter lesions on MRI, and CSF oligoclonal bands.
- 15y probability of MS increases from 25%, if normal MRI at baseline, to 72%, if >1 white matter lesion.[3]

1. Beck RW et al. A randomized, controlled trial of corticosteroids in the treatment of acute optic neuritis. The Optic Neuritis Study Group. *N Engl J Med* 1992;**326**:581–8.

2. Vedula SS et al. Corticosteroids for treating optic neuritis. *Cochrane Database Syst Rev* 2007;**1**:CD001430.

3. Optic Neuritis Study Group. Visual function 15 years after optic neuritis: a final followup report from the Optic Neuritis Treatment Trial. *Ophthalmology* 2008;**115**:1079–82.e5.

Multiple sclerosis

MS is a T-cell-mediated autoimmune neurodegenerative disorder where there is inflammation in the CNS myelin, followed by hardening (sclerosis) of the affected areas. It is more common in people with northern European ancestry. The UK incidence within the general population is between 3–7/100,000/y (see Table 16.3).

Clinical features (ophthalmic)

- Optic neuritis.
- Internuclear ophthalmoplegia.
- Isolated VF defects (lesions affecting any part of the afferent visual system).
- Uveitis (periphlebitis and intermediate uveitis are the most common).
- Nystagmus.

Diagnosis

- Based on clinical history and examination consistent with demyelination, supported by investigations (MRI/CSF analysis) where typical white matter lesions are seen on MRI that are disseminated in time (≥2 episodes) and disseminated in space (≥2 separate locations) and alternate diagnoses are excluded.[4]

Classification

Table 16.3 MS subtypes (adapted from NICE CG8)[*]

Relapsing/remitting MS (RRMS)	80% of people at onset	Symptomatic neurological event that lasts ≥24h, followed by complete or almost complete resolution, with periods of remission in between
2° progressive MS	50% of RRMS develop 2° progressive MS during the first 10y	Gradually more symptomatic attacks, with fewer remission periods
1° progressive MS	10–15% of people at onset	Symptoms occur without remission within 1y

NB The subtypes are further defined within the revised 2010 McDonald Criteria (Polman CH et al. Diagnostic criteria for multiple sclerosis: 2010 revisions to the McDonald criteria. *Ann Neurol* 2011;**69**:292–302).

[*] National Institute for Clinical Excellence. *Multiple sclerosis—management of multiple sclerosis in primary and secondary care. NICE clinical guideline No. 8.* (2003). London: National Institute for Clinical Excellence. Available at: ⅁ http://www.nice.org.uk

Treatment

Under the care of a physician with expertise in MS, acute attacks can be treated with high-dose IVMP. Immunomodulatory drugs are the mainstay of preventative treatment. They aim to ↓attacks, ↑remission, and ↓disability.

First-line therapies

- Glatiramer acetate (SC) ↓risk of developing clinically definite MS (45% vs placebo) and ↓time to development of definite MS (>1y vs placebo) (PreCISe).[5]
- Interferon beta (IM or SC) and glatiramer ↓risk of relapse by one-third at 2y in RRMS (CHAMPS;[6] ETOMS).[7]

Second-line therapies

- Mitoxantrone (IV infusion) is moderately effective in ↓relapses (adverse effects include cardiac events).
- Natalizumab (IV infusion) should be considered in rapidly evolving aggressive RRMS (adverse events include progressive multifocal leukoencephalopathy).

Oral therapies

- Fingolimod is licensed for RRMS (adverse effects include cardiac events).
- Teriflunomide, laquinimod, and dimethyl fumarate (BG-12) are under evaluation.

Diet

- Polyunsaturated fatty acids and antioxidants currently lack evidence for disease modification.[8]
- *Vitamin D*: well-documented link between MS and vitamin D; however, only recent small studies are showing a reduction in MRI lesion load with vitamin D supplementation. Further RCTs are required.

Prognosis

MS is a very variable condition where individuals can have a unique combination of symptoms and neurological deficits. White matter lesion load and activity do not correlate well with relapse rate or disability score. Life expectancy is normal or near normal.

4. Polman CH et al. Diagnostic criteria for multiple sclerosis: 2010 revisions to the McDonald criteria. Ann Neurol 2011;69:292–302.

5. Comi G et al. Effect of glatiramer acetate on conversion to clinically definite multiple sclerosis in patients with clinically isolated syndrome (PreCISe study): a randomised, double-blind, placebo-controlled trial. Lancet 2009;374:1503–11.

6. Galetta SL. The controlled high risk Avonex multiple sclerosis trial (CHAMPS Study). J Neuroophthalmol 2001;21:292–5.

7. Comi G et al. Hommes and the early treatment of MS study group. Effect of early interferon treatment on conversion to definite multiple sclerosis; a randomised study. Lancet 2001;357:1576–82.

8. Farinotti M et al. Dietary interventions for multiple sclerosis. Cochrane Database Syst Rev 2007;1:CD004192.

Neuromyelitis optica (NMO) spectrum disorder

Formally known as Devic's disease, this is an idiopathic antibody-mediated inflammatory disease of the CNS. There is a predilection for the optic nerves and spinal cord; the brain is relatively spared. 15% have a discrete episode (monophasic) of unilateral or bilateral optic neuritis, accompanied by transverse myelitis and no further events. 85% have a relapsing form. There is a ♀ preponderance and mean age of onset is late 30y. Typically, the optic neuritis is profound but, at onset, can be indistinguishable from MS-related optic neuritis.

Diagnosis

NMO should be considered if there is:

- Simultaneous bilateral optic neuritis or sequential recurrent optic neuritis in the presence of a normal contrasted MRI head.
- A single attack or recurrence of longitudinally extensive transverse myelitis (contiguous ≥3 segment spinal cord MRI lesion).

Investigations

- MRI head and spine (cervical and thoracic) with contrast.
- CSF analysis shows pleocytosis (>50 WBC).
- Serum NMO-IgG (target antigen is the aquaporin-4 water channel).
- Consider serum glial fibrillary acidic protein (if available).

Treatment

- *Acute*: treatment is with high-dose IVMP (e.g. 1g 1×/d for 3–5d) and long oral taper. Consider plasmapheresis if severe manifestations or if non-responsive to steroids.
- *Longer term*: steroid-sparing immunosuppressive agents are used (e.g. azathioprine ↓relapse rate by around 70%). The role of biologics which target B-cells (e.g. rituximab) or complement (e.g. eculizumab) is under investigation. **NB** NMO does not respond to the immunomodulatory treatments that are used in MS.

Prognosis[9]

Untreated, prognosis is poor. High cervical spine lesions can cause neurogenic respiratory failure.

Monophasic NMO

- 20% will have permanent visual loss (VA 6/60 in at least one eye).
- 30% will have permanent paralysis in one or both legs.
- 5y survival is 90%.

Relapsing NMO

- 55% relapse within 1y and 90% within 5y.
- 50% will have permanent visual loss (VA 6/60 in at least one eye) or paralysis within 5y.
- 5y survival is around 70%.

9. Wingerchuk DM *et al.* The clinical course of neuromyelitis optica (Devic's syndrome). *Neurology* 1999; **53**:1107–14.

Atypical optic neuritis

If an acute optic neuropathy does not fulfil the criteria for typical optical neuritis (see Box 16.1; see ➋ Typical optic neuritis, p. 660), then it must be investigated further to exclude a compressive lesion or other serious pathology (see Table 16.4).

Investigations may include: MRI (gadolinium-enhanced), CXR, FBC, ESR, CRP, U+E, Glu, LFT, ACE, ANA, ANCA, syphilis serology, genetic testing for LHON, LP (CSF analysis for microscopy, protein, Glu, oligoclonal bands, and cytology).

Table 16.4 Differential diagnosis of acute/subacute optic neuropathy

Optic neuritis (typical)	Age 20–50, unilateral, ↓VA over hours/days, recovery starts within 2wk, retrobulbar pain (see Box 16.1)
Compressive	Progressive ↓VA, disc pallor ± pain, involvement of other local structures
Sphenoid sinus disease	Persistent severe pain, pyrexia, history of sinusitis; consider fungal disease in the immunosuppressed, in diabetic ketoacidosis, or in the elderly. NB Can present silently in non-pyrexial individuals
Sarcoidosis	Progressive ↓VA ± uveitis, symptoms or signs of sarcoidosis, very steroid-sensitive
Vasculitis (e.g. SLE)	Progressive ↓VA ± uveitis, symptoms or signs of vasculitis
Syphilis	Progressive ↓VA, disc swelling, ± uveitis; leucocytosis in CSF; symptoms or signs of syphilis; may be HIV +ve
AION	Sudden painless ↓VA, altitudinal field loss, swollen disc (may be segmental), usually older age group; features of arteritic or non-arteritic disease
Toxic or nutritional	Slowly progressive symmetrical ↓VA with central scotomas; relevant nutritional, therapeutic, or toxic history
LHON	Severe sequential ↓VA over weeks/months, telangiectatic vessels around disc (acutely); usually young adult ♂; FH
Post-viral demyelination	Often bilateral ↓VA few weeks post-viral or post-vaccination, usually in children/young adults; ± acute disseminated encephalomyelitis

Anterior ischaemic optic neuropathy

This is a significant cause of acute visual loss in the elderly population, affecting up to 10/100,000/y of those over 50y. In 5–10%, the aetiology is arteritic, in which the majority of these are caused by GCA, and, in 90–95%, the aetiology is non-arteritic (see Table 16.5). The vascular supply to the anterior optic nerve is from the short posterior ciliary artery and the choroidal circulation.

Table 16.5 Arteritic and non-arteritic AION

	Arteritic AION	Non-arteritic AION
Incidence/y	1/100,000	10/100,000
Cause/ possible associations	**Major:** GCA	**Major:** Hypertension Diabetes Disc morphology 'disc at risk'
	Minor: Churg–Strauss PAN GPA RA Relapsing polychondritis Other connective tissue disorders (e.g. SLE)	**Minor:** Smoking Hyperlipidaemia Acute hypotension Anaemia Obstructive sleep apnoea Optic disc drusen Cataract surgery Non-ocular surgery (e.g. cardiac, spinal) Drugs (e.g. amiodarone, erectile dysfunction drugs) Radiation-induced optic neuropathy
Age (mean)	70y	60y
VA + VF	Sudden ↓ Usually <6/60	Sudden ↓ Usually >6/60 Often altitudinal field loss
Associated symptoms	Scalp tenderness, jaw claudication, headache	Usually none
Disc	Swollen Commonly pale	Swollen (often sectoral) Commonly hyperaemic Predisposed (small + crowded)
ESR	↑↑ (mean = 70mmHg)	Normal
CRP	↑↑	Normal
Plt	↑	Normal
Risk to fellow eye	10% (if treated) to ≤95% (untreated)	
Prognosis	Up to 15% improve	40% improve (by ≥2 Snellen lines)

Arteritic AION and giant cell arteritis

GCA

GCA or temporal arteritis is an ophthalmic emergency, requiring immediate assessment and appropriate institution of systemic steroid treatment. Mean onset is 70y; it is rare before 50y. It commonly occurs in Caucasians and is three times more likely to occur in ♀. In arteritic AION, short posterior ciliary artery vasculitis leads to ischaemic necrosis of the optic nerve head (Box 16.2).

> **Box 16.2 Traditional criteria for the diagnosis of GCA***
> * Age ≥50y at disease onset.
> * New onset of localized headache.
> * Temporal artery tenderness or decreased pulse.
> * ESR ≥50mm/h by the Westerngren method.
> * Arterial biopsy with necrotizing arteritis with a predominance of mononuclear cell infiltrates or granulomatous process with multinuclear giant cells.
>
> **NB** The presence of three or more of five of these criteria was associated with 93.5% sensitivity and 91.2% specificity.
>
> * Hunder GG et al. The American College of Rheumatology 1990 criteria for the classification of giant cell arteritis. Arthritis Rheum 1990;**33**:1122–8.

Clinical features
* Sudden ↓VA (<6/60 in 76%); new-onset headache, scalp tenderness, jaw claudication, weight loss, night sweats, myalgia (association with polymyalgia rheumatica); may have a warning episode of transient ↓VA (short obscurations or longer amaurosis fugax-like episodes).
* RAPD, swollen disc (typically pale; rarely segmental), ± peripapillary haemorrhages and CWS, abnormal temporal arteries (thickened, tender, non-pulsatile).
* *Associations*: CRAO, BRAO, cilioretinal artery occlusion; III, IV, VIn palsy.

Investigations
* *Immediate ESR, CRP, FBC*: ↑ESR, ↑CRP, and ↑Plt are all supportive of GCA. Interpret ESR in context (see Table 16.5).
* *Prompt temporal artery biopsy (TAB)* (see Box 16.4): recommend biopsy length ≥2cm, no <1cm (to avoid likelihood of skip lesions). Aim for within 1wk, although positive results may be obtained up to 2–6wk after treatment is commenced.
* *Additional tests include*: U+E, LFT, CXR, and urinalysis.[10]

Consider:
* *Duplex ultrasonography*: hypoechoic 'halo' due to vessel wall oedema in affected temporal arteries (positive for over 2wk post-steroid initiation) + arterial stenosis/occlusion. At present, US is user-dependent and requires high level of expertise, but ongoing studies are assessing its utility to replace TAB.

- *High-resolution MR imaging (with IV contrast)* of the superficial cranial and extracranial arteries demonstrates increased vessel wall thickness and oedema, with increased mural enhancement post-contrast and luminal stenosis.
- *Fluoro-deoxyglucose PET*: may have a role in assessing disease activity and extent in GCA, assessing activity of polymyalgia rheumatica and large vessel vasculitis.

Long-term

In suspected large-vessel GCA, investigations should include:[11]

- 2-yearly CXR for aneurysm detection.

Treatment

- Immediate systemic corticosteroid treatment (e.g. 1g IVMP 1×/d for 1–3d), followed by PO prednisolone 1–2mg/kg 1×/d).
- Low-dose aspirin (if no contraindications).
- Careful explanation of the side effects of steroids is mandatory (see ➲ Systemic corticosteroids: general, p. 994), and note recommendations re gastric and bone protection. Once disease is controlled, steroids may be titrated, according to symptoms and inflammatory markers (CRP responds more quickly than ESR).

When the TAB is negative

If there is a typical clinical and laboratory picture of GCA, with a positive response to high-dose steroid therapy in the presence of a negative TAB, patients should be managed as having GCA. However, if the clinical history and inflammatory markers are atypical in presence of the negative TAB, then alternate diagnoses (see Box 16.3) and an appropriate referral to a specialist team should be considered. Steroids can be rapidly tapered (within 2wk).[11]

Prognosis

The risk of second eye involvement ranges from 10% (if treated) to 95% (untreated). Other complications of GCA include: TIA, stroke, myocardial infarcts, neuropathies, mesenteric artery occlusion, thoracic artery aneurysms, and death.

> **Box 16.3 Differential diagnosis of GCA**
>
> Granulomatosis with polyangitis
> Polyarteritis Nodosa
> Systemic Lupus Erythematosus
> Rheumatoid Arthritis
> Takayasu Arteritis

10. Dasgupta B *et al.* BSR and BHPR guidelines for the management of giant cell arteritis. *Rheumatology (Oxford)* 2010;**49**:1594–7.

11. Hunder GG *et al.* The American College of Rheumatology 1990 criteria for the classification of giant cell arteritis. *Arthritis Rheum* 1990;**33**:1122–8.

Temporal artery biopsy

See Table 16.6 and Box 16.4.

Indication

Superficial TAB remains the gold standard for diagnosis of GCA (see ➲ Arteritic AION and giant cell arteritis, p. 668).

Table 16.6 Investigations in GCA

	Sensitivity	Specificity
Histological TAB	80–90% (unilateral biopsy, Bx) 95–97% (bilateral Bx)	≤100%
Haematological		
*Bx-proven GCA vs normal controls (Hayreh)**		
↑ESR	92%	94%
↑CRP	100%	97%
↑ESR + ↑CRP		
Bx-positive vs negative patients with clinical suspicion of GCA (Foroozan)†		
↑ESR + ↑Plt	51%	91%
Imaging		
Duplex US		
Characteristic 'halo rings' = oedematous wall swellings (Karassa)‡		
US compared with Bx-proven GCA	69%	82%
US compared with the ACR§ criteria	55%	94%
High-resolution MRI (Bley)¶		
MRI compared with the ACR§ criteria	80.6%	97%

* Hayreh SS et al. Giant cell arteritis: validity and reliability of various diagnostic criteria. Am J Ophthalmol 1997;**123**:285–96.

† Foroozan R et al. Thrombocytosis in patients with biopsy-proven giant cell arteritis. Ophthalmology 2002;**109**:1267–71.

‡ Karassa FB et al. Meta-analysis: test performance of ultrasonography for giant-cell arteritis. Ann Intern Med 2005;**142**:359–69.

§ American College of Rheumatology.

¶ Bley TA et al. Diagnostic value of high-resolution MR imaging in giant cell arteritis. Am J Neuroradiol 2007;**28**:1722–7.

Consent

Discuss what the procedure involves, its rationale, and possible complications, including:

- Visible scarring (particularly if incision is pretrichial and not parallel to Langer's lines).
- Haematoma.
- Wound infection.
- Scalp or skin necrosis.
- Facial nerve injury, with variable recovery (particularly if pretrichial incision).
- Biopsy does not include temporal artery (up to 1.25% of specimens in one report were vein or peripheral nerve).
- Cerebral infarction (rare; possibly related to collateral blood flow to the brain from the superficial temporal artery).

Box 16.4 An approach to superficial TAB

Preoperative

- Choose side (side of visual loss and/or where artery is abnormal).
- Ensure that the artery is mapped, either by palpation and/or with US Doppler. The skin overlying the artery should be marked.
- Adequate hair removal is recommended for good surgical exposure.

Procedure

- Skin should be cleaned with cleaning preparation.
- Skin should be infiltrated with local anaesthetic using a fine-bore needle (e.g. 27G). Some surgeons include adrenaline; others exclude it. In our experience, if the artery is adequately marked, using adrenaline helps with local haemostasis and visualization of tissues.
- Skin incision should be of adequate length and parallel to Langer's lines.
- Blunt dissection to artery, ensuring not to totally breach the superficial temporalis facia (as the artery lies superficially within this facia).
- 4-0 silk or Vicryl® should be tied twice around the distal and proximal end of the artery. The suture should either be passed with the needle mounted backwards or the suture without needle doubled and passed under with the help of an artery clip and then cut to make two ties. The second tie should be passed over the first (towards the open lumen) so that biopsy length is maximized. Any other tributaries local to the specimen should be tied off
- Care should be taken not to crush the specimen by repeatedly regrasping the biopsy.
- The subcutaneous tissue is closed with 5-0 interrupted Vicryl® and the skin closed with a running 6-0 Vicryl® subcuticular suture.

Post-operative care

- Compression bandage for 24h.
- Some advocate antibiotic ointment to the wound site for 3–4d.

Non-arteritic AION

Non-arteritic AION comprises 90–95% of AION. Although the exact mechanism is unclear, there is perfusion insufficiency in the short posterior ciliary arteries, which leads to infarction of the retrolaminar portion of the disc.

Identified vascular risk factors should be modified to try to prevent further ophthalmic and systemic complications.

Risk factors

These are multiple and include: diabetes, atherosclerosis, disc morphology ('disc at risk'—crowded disc with a small cup), hypertension, hyperlipidaemia, hypotension, haemoconcentration, haemodilution, and hypercoagulable states.

Clinical features

- ↓VA (usually sudden but can be progressive; VA >6/60 in 61%; >6/12 in 18%); commonly occur overnight; occasional pain.
- RAPD, field loss (45% inferior altitudinal; 15% superior altitudinal), swollen disc (typically hyperaemic ± segmental, telangiectasia)
- *Associations*: 'disc at risk' in fellow eye.

Investigations

- *First:* rule out GCA (for assessment, see ➲ Arteritic AION and giant cell arteritis, p. 668).
- *If non-arteritic, then*: BP, Glu, lipids, FBC. If patient <50y, then consider also vasculitis screen.

Treatment

- No proven benefit for any treatment (including steroids, optic nerve sheath defenestration, hyperbaric oxygen, dopamine, and aspirin); however, low-dose aspirin (e.g. 75mg/d) is commonly prescribed.
- Refer to physician for vascular assessment and treatment.

Prognosis

The natural history of non-arteritic AION can be determined from the control group of the Ischemic Optic Neuropathy Decompression Trial[12] which reported that at 6mo 43% experienced improvement of three or more lines of acuity, compared with 12% who lost three or more lines of acuity.

The risk of second eye involvement is about 14.7% over 5y. Poor baseline VA and diabetes were risk factors for second eye involvement.[13]

There is an increased risk of non-arteritic ischaemic optic neuropathy in the fellow eye after cataract surgery.[14]

12. The Ischemic Optic Neuropathy Decompression Trial Research Group. Optic nerve decompression surgery for nonarteritic ischemic optic neuropathy (NAION) is not effective and may be harmful. *JAMA* 1995;**273**:625–32.

13. Newman NJ *et al.* The fellow eye in NAION: report from the ischemic optic neuropathy decompression trial follow-up study. *Am J Ophthalmol* 2002;**134**:317–28.

14. Lam BL *et al.* Risk of non-arteritic anterior ischaemic optic neuropathy (NAION) after cataract extraction in the fellow eye of patients with prior unilateral NAION. *Br J Ophthalmol* 2007;**91**:585–7.

Posterior ischaemic optic neuropathy (PION)

PION is a rare condition; it describes abrupt ischaemia of the more posterior (retrolaminar) optic nerve. The blood supply to the retrobulbar portion of the optic nerve is from the plial plexus arising from the ophthalmic artery.

Causes

- *Perioperative/shock*: blood loss, hypotension, anaemia (see Table 16.7).
- *Arteritic*: GCA; rarely other vasculitides.

Clinical features

- Sudden visual loss with an RAPD (if unilateral) but normal appearing optic disc; bilateral involvement is common.
- Occasionally disc swelling which develops subsequent to the visual loss.
- Associations include anaemia and acute hypotension. Occasionally seen dialysis patients.

Investigations

- *First*: rule out GCA (for assessment, see ➲ Arteritic AION and giant cell arteritis, p. 668).
- *If non-arteritic, then*: BP, Glu, lipids, FBC. If patient <50y, then consider also vasculitis screen.
- Low threshold for MRI head and orbits with contrast to exclude compressive and infiltration.

Perioperative visual loss

A very rare, but devastating, complication following non-ocular surgery. Presumed mechanism is ischaemic optic neuropathy, with AION more commonly reported following cardiac procedures and PION reported following prolonged spinal surgery in the prone position. The exact aetiology is not known.

NB Perioperative CRAO has been reported 2° to compression of the periorbita during prolonged prone position surgeries.

Clinical features

- Most have bilateral simultaneous involvement, usually associated with very poor visual function.

Treatment

- Prompt fluid replacement and transfusion of blood products is appropriate; however, there is no evidence that it reverses the insult.
- This complication warrants senior review and careful medical documentation; such cases may have medicolegal sequelae.[15]

Ischaemic optic neuropathy 2° to hypotension

This usually presents in chronic renal failure or patients undergoing dialysis. Presumed mechanism is acute hypotension in the setting of a compromised vascular system (such as arteriosclerosis), with most patients being chronically anaemic. Both AION and PION can be seen. This should be treated with prompt normalization of hypotension, fluid replacement, and transfusion of blood products, as appropriate.

Table 16.7 Identifying PION

	Arteritic AION	Non-arteritic AION	PION
Cause/possible associations	Major: GCA	Major: Hypertension Diabetes Disc morphology 'disc at risk'	Major: *Perioperative/shock:* Blood loss/anaemia Acute hypotension Cardiac or spinal surgery *Arteritic:* GCA
	Minor: Other vasculitides/ connective tissue disorders	Minor: Smoking Hyperlipidaemia Acute hypotension Anaemia Obstructive sleep apnoea Optic disc drusen Surgery, drugs, radiation	Minor: Hypertension Diabetes Smoking Hyperlipidaemia
Disc appearance	Swollen; often pale	Swollen; often segmental; usually hyperaemic	Normal
ESR	↑↑ (mean = 70mmHg)	Normal	Normal (unless arteritic)
CRP	↑↑	Normal	Normal (unless arteritic)
Plt	↑	Normal	Normal (unless arteritic)
MRI head/ orbits (contrast)	Enhancement of optic nerve	No enhancement of optic nerve	No enhancement of optic nerve

15. American Society of Anesthesiologists Task Force on Perioperative Blindness. Practice advisory for perioperative visual loss associated with spine surgery: a report by the American Society of Anesthesiologists Task Force on Perioperative Blindness. *Anesthesiology* 2006;104:1319–28.

Other optic neuropathies/atrophies

There are many causes of optic atrophy (see Table 16.8). Careful history, examination, and specific investigations may help to identify the cause.

LHON

This rare condition is maternally inherited, arising from point mutations in mitochondrial DNA. It may present at almost any age but typically in young adult ♂ (♂:♀ 3:1). FH is present in around 50%. The mutations identified are at nucleotide positions 11778 (the commonest comprising 95%), 3460, and 14484, all of which affect complex I of the respiratory chain. LHON has some similarities to nutritional and toxic neuropathies, and indeed the presentation of LHON may be precipitated by a toxic insult.

Clinical features
- Sudden painless sequential ↓VA (usually affects second eye within 2mo; typically 6/60 HM).
- Large dense centrocaecal scotoma, ↓colour vision; disc may show peripapillary telangiectasia and peripapillary nerve fibre layer swelling (early) and temporal pallor (late). **NB** Pupillary reactions are usually normal.

Investigations and treatment
Mitochondrial DNA analysis for LHON mutations (peripheral blood); consider also screening for differential diagnosis, including toxins/deficiencies. There is no effective treatment. The majority has a poor visual prognosis, although some spontaneous recovery is seen with the uncommon 14484 mutation.

Nutritional and toxic optic neuropathies

These uncommon acquired optic neuropathies all behave in a similar manner, probably due to a common disruption of mitochondrial oxidative phosphorylation.

Tobacco–alcohol amblyopia may represent a combination of toxin (cyanide in tobacco smoke) and nutritional deficiency (low B12 associated with alcohol excess). Numerous other agents have been identified (see Table 16.8).

Clinical features
- Subacute painless bilateral ↓VA (typically 6/9–6/60).
- Small central/centrocaecal scotomas, ↓colour vision; ± swelling of disc/ peripapillary nerve fibre layer (early) and temporal pallor (late).

Investigations and treatment
- A detailed history may reveal the cause.
- *Consider*: B1, B2, B12, folic acid levels (peripheral blood), and heavy metal screening (including 24h urine).
- Treat deficiency with oral supplementation, other than B12 (IM and must be given with folate). In alcoholics, consider prophylactic vitamin supplementation.
- Identify and prevent route of toxin exposure (may affect others, e.g. family members).

Table 16.8 Causes of optic atrophy

Inherited		Kjer syndrome
		Behr syndrome
		Wolfram syndrome
		LHON
Compression	Extrinsic tumour	Pituitary
		Craniopharyngioma
		Meningioma
		Metastasis
	Intrinsic tumour	Optic nerve glioma
		Optic nerve sheath meningioma
	Other	Aneurysm
		Mucocele
Vascular		CRAO
		AION or PION
Inflammatory		Acute demyelinating optic neuritis
		Sarcoidosis
		Vasculitis (e.g. SLE, PAN)
Infection		Bacterial (e.g. TB, syphilis)
		Rickettsial (e.g. Lyme disease)
		Viral (e.g. measles, mumps, varicella)
		Fungal (e.g. *Aspergillus*)
Nutritional		B1 (thiamine) deficiency
		B2 (riboflavin) deficiency
		B6 deficiency
		B12 deficiency
		Folate deficiency
Toxic		Amiodarone
		Ethambutol
		Methanol
		Carbon monoxide
		Cyanide
		Isoniazid
		Lead
		Triethyl tin
Other		Trauma
		Disc oedema (e.g. papilloedema)
		Retinal disease (e.g. RP)

Inherited optic atrophy

AD

Kjer syndrome is the commonest isolated optic atrophy and is due to a mutation in 3q. Bilateral symmetrical ↓VA (usually 6/9–6/36) occurs insidiously in mid/late childhood.

AR

- *Isolated*: this is rare, severe, and presents early (age <4y).
- *Behr syndrome*: optic atrophy ± nystagmus, ataxia, spasticity, ↓IQ.
- *Wolfram syndrome (DIDMOAD)*: diabetes insipidus, diabetes mellitus, optic atrophy, deafness.

Papilloedema

Papilloedema describes optic disc swelling (usually bilateral) arising from raised ICP; the term should not be used to describe other causes of disc oedema (see Table 16.9 and Table 16.10). Raised ICP is transmitted from the subarachnoid space via the optic nerve sheath to cause axoplasmic hold-up and consequent disc oedema. The urgent priority is to rule out an intracranial mass (e.g. tumour, abscess, haemorrhage).

Clinical features

- Visual obscurations (transient ↓VA, few seconds' duration, up to 30×/d, uni-/bilateral, may be precipitated by posture/straining, etc.); diplopia; field defects (usually enlarged blind spot); sustained ↓VA is a serious sign of irreversible damage—it may occur early in aggressive disease or late in chronic papilloedema.
- ↑ICP leads to headache (often worse lying down/straining), nausea, vomiting, pulsatile tinnitus.
- *Disc swelling*: usually bilateral; however, swelling may not occur in an already abnormal disc/nerve sheath (e.g. congenital anomaly, optic atrophy, high myopia).

Staging of papilloedema

- *Early*: hyperaemic, blurred + elevated margin, subtle peripapillary nerve fibre layer oedema, dilated disc capillaries, distended retinal veins, absent SVP. Paton's lines are circumferential retinochoroidal folds that can be sometimes seen around the disc.
- *Acute*: as for 'early' + peripapillary haemorrhages, CWS, increased nerve fibre layer oedema (may obscure retinal vessels), macular changes with SRF.
- *Chronic*: ↓hyperaemia, ↓CWS/haemorrhages, variable swelling, usually still elevated; ± drusen-like deposits and optociliary collateral vessels at the disc (in which case sometimes called vintage papilloedema); RPE atrophy.
- *Atrophic/late*: pale atrophic disc, ↓swelling, attenuated arterioles.

Investigation

Urgent neuroimaging (preferably MRI with gadolinium enhancement): may reveal 1° pathology, hydrocephalus, or empty sella. Consider:

- *MRV or CTV*: to check patency of the cerebral venous sinuses.
- *LP*: check opening pressure (normal <20cmH$_2$O or <25cmH$_2$O in the obese), Glu, protein, protein electrophoresis, microscopy, culture.
- *FFA (if diagnostic uncertainty)*: late leakage from dilated disc capillaries.

Treatment

- Intervention depends on the underlying cause and severity. It may range from weight loss to extensive neurosurgery.
- Shared care with another speciality (neurosurgery, neurology, oncology, medicine) is often necessary.
- Regular ophthalmic assessment of acuity, colour vision, pupils, VF, and disc status is invaluable to preserving vision.

Table 16.9 Causes of raised ICP

Mass effect	Tumour
	Haemorrhage
	Trauma (haematoma/oedema)
Increased CSF production	Choroid plexus tumour
Reduced CSF drainage	Stenosis of foramen/aqueduct (congenital or 2° to tumour, cyst, infection, etc.)
	Damage to arachnoid granulations (meningitis, subarachnoid haemorrhage)
	Idiopathic intracranial hypertension (IIH)
Other	Malignant hypertension
	2° causes of intracranial hypertension (see Table 16.10)

Table 16.10 Conditions associated with intracranial hypertension

Drugs	Tetracycline and derivatives
	Corticosteroid withdrawal
	Oral contraceptive pill
	Vitamin A derivatives
	Nalidixic acid
	Nitrofurantoin
	Lithium
	Growth hormone
	Indometacin
	Rofecoxib (now withdrawn)
	Cimetidine
Systemic disorders	Hypoparathyroidism
	Adrenal adenomas
	Renal failure
	Addison's disease
	Obstructive sleep apnoea syndrome
	COPD
Habitus	Obesity
Haematological	Anaemia
	Cerebral venous sinus thrombosis (CVST)

Idiopathic intracranial hypertension

IIH (also known as pseudotumour cerebri and benign intracranial hypertension) is the commonest cause of papilloedema. It is a diagnosis of exclusion, made in the presence of normal neuroimaging (MRI/MRV) and CSF analysis, but with an elevated CSF opening pressure (see Table 16.11). The prevalence is about 0.9/100,000 in the general population but increases to 19/100,000 in obese young women. IIH does rarely occur in pre-pubertal children, but typically the phenotype is different (non-obese and equal sex ratio) and may therefore represent a different underlying process.

Risk factors

It typically affects obese young women, but there is a wide age range of presentation. The strongest risk factors are obesity and recent weight gain.

Clinical features

- Visual obscurations (transient ↓VA, few seconds' duration, uni-/bilateral, up to 30×/d, may be precipitated by posture/straining, etc.); diplopia; field defects (usually enlarged blind spot); sustained ↓VA may be early in aggressive disease (usually an indication for shunting).
- Headache (in 94%; often worse lying down/straining), retrobulbar pain, pulsatile tinnitus.
- Disc swelling (usually bilateral).
- Occasional unilateral or bilateral sixth nerve palsy or rarely CSF rhinorrhoea.

Investigations

- *MRI with gadolinium enhancement and MRV or CTV*: aim to rule out all other causes of ↑ICP.
- *LP* (only proceed to LP if MRI/CT shows no intracranial mass) measured in the lateral decubitus position: check opening pressure, Glu, protein, protein electrophoresis, microscopy, culture. Normal opening pressure in adults is usually <20cmH$_2$O or <25cmH$_2$O in the obese; in children, lower levels are normal.
- *VF*: to assess size of physiological blind spot and detect any other VF defect.
- *OCT*: may be useful in monitoring of extent of papilloedema and macular involvement.

Table 16.11 Diagnostic criteria for IIH*

Symptoms and signs of raised intracranial hypertension
Raised ICP, as measured on LP in the lateral decubitus position
CSF composition is normal
Neuroimaging with no evidence of hydrocephalus, mass, structural or vascular lesion
No other cause of intracranial hypertension found (see Table 16.9)

* Friedman DI et al. Diagnostic criteria for idiopathic intracranial hypertension. *Neurology* 2002;**59**:1492–5.

Treatment

Current management may include:

- *Weight loss.*
- *Medical*: acetazolamide (up to 500mg 4×/d) or consider furosemide.
- *Surgical*: optic nerve sheath fenestration.
- *Neurosurgical*: CSF diversions using a lumboperitoneal, ventriculoperitoneal, or ventriculoatrial shunting.

Titrate treatment against symptoms and risk of visual loss (monitor VA, colour vision, pupils, fields, discs).

- *If pregnant*: acetazolamide appears to be safe after 20wk gestation; weight loss is not advised. Opinion from neuro-ophthalmologist should be sought regarding delivery advice.

Prognosis

- In the majority, this is good. In the UK, a British Ophthalmic Surveillance Unit study found the incidence of blindness was 1–2%.
- IIH can recur at any time after the original episode has resolved.

Cerebral venous sinus thrombosis (CVST)

An important differential of IIH is CVST. CVST can present in the same way as IIH, but its treatment and prognosis are dramatically different. *Causes*: include prothrombotic tendencies; drugs such as hormone replacement therapy (HRT) and the oral contraceptive pill; factor V Leiden mutations, protein S and C, and antithrombin III deficiencies; pregnancy (with Caesarean section and increasing maternal age being risk factors); and regional infective causes.

ICP may be very high and require urgent CSF shunting. Treatment is with anticoagulation therapies (currently heparin or low molecular weight heparin, followed by warfarin).

Pseudopapilloedema

A number of disc anomalies may resemble papilloedema (see Table 16.12).

Clinical features

- Usually seen on a routine examination in an asymptomatic patient, whereas papilloedema is often accompanied with clinical symptoms and signs.
- *SVP*: the central retinal vein can be seen to pulsate in about 80% of normal patients.

Differential diagnosis

- *Disc drusen*: may cause most diagnostic confusion, as they may not be clinically obvious (buried) and may cause visual loss. Their prevalence is about 0.5% in Caucasians. They may be inherited (AD). They are usually bilateral and become more obvious throughout life. The disc has a lumpy appearance, absent cup, and the vessels emerge centrally and then show abnormal branching (trifurcation); optociliary shunt vessels may be present. VA is usually normal, but field defects occur in 75% (arcuate, blind spot enlargement, generalized constriction). They are associated with CNV. Their presence may be demonstrated by their autofluorescence, or on B-scan US or CT.
- *Hypermetropic* discs may appear crowded and elevated.
- *Myopic* discs are often elevated nasally and may show leakage on FFA. Tilted discs are usually elevated superotemporally.

Table 16.12 Causes of apparent disc swelling

True disc swelling	Papilloedema	↑ICP	Tumours, etc. (see Table 16.9)
	Local disc swelling	Inflammatory	Optic neuritis Uveitis Scleritis
		Granulomatous	TB Sarcoid
		Infiltrative	Leukaemia Lymphoma
		Vascular	AION CRVO Diabetic papillitis
		Trauma	Causing hypotony
		Tumours	Of optic nerve (meningioma, glioma) Of orbit
		Hereditary	LHON
		Iatrogenic	Ocular surgery causing hypotony
No true disc swelling	Pseudo-papilloedema	Structural	Disc drusen Tilted discs Hypermetropic discs Myopic discs Myelinated peripapillary nerve fibres

Congenital optic disc anomalies

Congenital optic disc anomalies range from common variations with minimal sequelae (e.g. tilted discs) to severe abnormalities associated with poor vision and CNS abnormalities (e.g. morning glory anomaly).

Tilted disc

In this common bilateral, but often asymmetric, condition, the optic nerves insert obliquely into the globe. It is often associated with myopia and oblique astigmatism.

The bitemporal field defects are unlike chiasmal lesions; they do not respect the vertical midline, are static, and, in some cases, may be resolved with refractive correction.

Clinical features
- Normal VA; may have superotemporal field defects.
- Disc usually orientated inferonasally with elevation of the superotemporal rim, thinning of the inferonasal RPE/choroid, and situs inversus of the retinal blood vessels.

Optic disc pit

This rare, usually unilateral, condition may cause significant visual problems. Its origin is unclear but it represents a herniation of neuroectodermal tissue into a depression within the optic nerve.

Clinical features
- Often asymptomatic; ↓VA if complications; field defects (commonly paracentral arcuate scotoma).
- Grey pit usually in the temporal part of the disc; disc itself is larger than in the unaffected eye.
- *Complications*: macular retinoschisis and subsequent serous retinal detachment may occur in up to 45%; this can be treated with vitrectomy and gas tamponade.

Optic nerve hypoplasia

This describes a reduced number of axons within the optic nerve. It is a significant cause of poor vision in childhood. It may be isolated or be associated with a range of CNS abnormalities (see Table 16.13).

Clinical features
- Variable VA (normal to NPL), field defects, colour vision, pupil reactions.
- Small grey disc surrounded by an inner yellow ring of chorioretinal atrophy and an outer pigment ring (double-ring sign).
- Other features may include aniridia, microphthalmos, strabismus, nystagmus.

Table 16.13 Associations of optic disc hypoplasia

Syndromic	De Morsier syndrome (septo-optic dysplasia)
Non-syndromic	Isolated midline CNS abnormalities
	Endocrine abnormalities

Sectorial optic disc hypoplasia

Typically, the nasal portion of the disc is affected, but superior 'topless' optic disc hypoplasia has been reported. In nasal optic disc hypolasia, there is bilateral or unilateral wedge-shaped temporal VF defects that expand from the blind spot which correspond to the abnormal nasal portion of the disc.

Optic disc coloboma

This rare condition arises from incomplete closure of the embryonic fissure (inferonasal), with variable involvement of the adjacent retina and choroid. It may be sporadic or AD and may be isolated, part of a syndrome, or occasionally associated with trans-sphenoidal encephalocele (see Table 16.14).

Clinical features
- ↓VA (according to severity of coloboma), superior field defect.
- Glistening white bowl-shaped excavation within the disc (inferior part predominantly affected) ± chorioretinal/ciliary body/iris colobomas.

Table 16.14 Associations of optic disc coloboma

Chromosomal	Patau syndrome (trisomy 13)
	Edward syndrome (trisomy 18)
	Cat-eye syndrome (trisomy 22)
Other syndromes	Aicardi syndrome
	CHARGE syndrome
	Walker–Warburg syndrome
	Goltz syndrome
	Goldenhar syndrome
	Meckel–Gruber syndrome

Morning glory anomaly

This very rare condition describes a usually unilateral excavation of the posterior globe that includes the optic disc and may even include the macula ('macula capture').

Clinical features
- Severe ↓VA.
- Enlarged pink disc located within the excavation and surrounded by an elevated and irregularly pigmented annular zone; vessels are abnormally straight, with arteries and veins being of similar appearance.
- *Complications*: serous retinal detachments may occur in 30%.
- *Associations*: include a syndrome of trans-sphenoidal encephalocele with hypertelorism, flat nasal bridge, midline cleft lip/palate, and often panhypopituitarism.

Megalopapilla

Megalopapilla describes an unusually large, but essentially normal, disc. They have a high C/D ratio that may be confused with glaucomatous change.

Chiasmal disorders

The chiasm permits the hemidecussation of visual information from the temporal fields so that information from the right VF of both eyes is processed in the left visual cortex and vice versa. It lies in an anatomically crowded region, so chiasmal syndromes may be accompanied by other neurological or endocrine abnormalities.

The commonest and best known disorder of the chiasm is a pituitary adenoma causing bitemporal hemianopia; however, a wide range of other lesions and clinical presentations may be seen (see Table 16.15 and Table 16.16).

Clinical features

- Often asymptomatic unless central ($\downarrow$VA) or advanced peripheral field loss.
- *Field loss*: classically bitemporal but often asymmetric and dependent on exact site of lesion (see Table 16.16).
- *Headache* (usually frontal): if acute and severe, consider apoplexy.
- *Hemifield slide*: can occur in cases with advanced field loss and a pre-exisiting phoria. The normal nasotemporal field overlap of the two eyes is absent, leading to loss of fusion. This can cause horizontal or vertical diplopia to be described in the absence of any extraocular muscle misalignment.
- *Post-fixation blindness*: can occur during close work where an object placed just beyond fixation (therefore in the temporal field) may disappear.

Associated features

Involvement of III, IV, Va, Vb, VI, and sympathetic nerve fibres: may result in abnormalities of pupils (including Horner's syndrome), ocular motility, and facial sensation. Rarely see-saw nystagmus may occur.

- $\uparrow$ICP: may cause nausea, vomiting, pulsatile tinnitus, and papilloedema; hydrocephalus (blockage of foramen of Munro from posterior chiasmal lesions) may cause abnormal gait, urinary incontinence, drowsiness, and Parinaud syndrome.
- *Functioning pituitary tumours*: may cause acromegaly or gigantism ($\uparrow$growth hormone; large hands/feet and coarsening of features or abnormal height), Cushing's syndrome ($\uparrow$adrenocorticotrophic hormone; moon face, truncal obesity, hypertension), hyperprolactinaemia (impotence and galactorrhoea).
- Pituitary destruction causes hypopituitarism, with loss of luteinizing hormone (LH)/follicle-stimulating hormone (FSH) ($\downarrow$libido, amenorrhoea; may present as 1° infertility), growth hormone (silent unless pubertal), TSH (hypothyroidism), and adrenocorticotrophic hormone (2° hypoadrenalism with collapse). Hypothalamic involvement may cause diabetes insipidus ($\downarrow$antidiuretic hormone; polydipsia, polyuria).

Table 16.15 Causes of chiasmal syndromes

Pituitary	Adenoma (functioning or non-functioning)
	Apoplexy
	Sheehan's syndrome (pregnancy-related pituitary infarction)
	Lymphocytic hypophysitis
Suprasellar	Meningioma
	Craniopharyngioma
Chiasm	Optic glioma
	Chiasmatic neuritis (chiasmitis)
Other	ICA aneurysm
	AVM (e.g. Wyburn–Mason syndrome)
	Cavernous haemangioma
	Germinoma
	Lymphoma
	Sarcoidosis
	Langerhans cell histiocytosis
	Metastasis
	Radionecrosis

Table 16.16 Localization by field defect

Superior bitemporal loss	Inferior lesion, e.g. pituitary adenoma
Inferior bitemporal loss	Superior lesion, e.g. craniopharyngioma
Junctional (central scotoma with superotemporal field loss in contralateral eye)	Anterior chiasmal lesion to side of central scotoma, e.g. sphenoid meningioma
Bitemporal central hemianopic scotomas	Posterior chiasmal lesion, e.g. hydrocephalus
Nasal loss	Lateral lesion, e.g. ectasia of the ICA

Investigations

- Accurate field testing and interpretation are vital.
- Urgent neuroimaging: MRI (gadolinium-enhanced) is preferred, although CT is better at detecting bony involvement.
- Prolactin levels.
- Consider endocrinological assessment and LP for CSF analysis.

Treatment

The ophthalmologist's role is first to diagnose, second to refer for appropriate treatment (e.g. to endocrinology, neurosurgery, or often to a multispeciality pituitary team), and third to monitor the patient's vision long-term (VA, colour vision, pupils, VF). Late loss of vision may represent tumour recurrence or may be as a result of treatment (radiotherapy) (see Table 16.17).

Table 16.17 Treatment options for chiasmal lesions

Pituitary adenoma	Medical (cabergoline or bromocriptine if prolactin-secreting; octreotide if growth hormone-secreting)
	Surgical resection (e.g. trans-sphenoidal route)
	Radiotherapy
Pituitary apoplexy	Hormone replacement (including high-dose corticosteroids)
	Trans-sphenoidal decompression
Meningioma	Surgical resection ± radiotherapy
Craniopharyngioma	Surgical resection ± radiotherapy
Optic glioma	Depends on whether it is benign or malignant (conservative vs surgery vs radiotherapy)
Lymphocytic hypophysitis	Medical (steroids)

Retrochiasmal disorders

Most retrochiasmal disorders are associated with significant additional neurological morbidity, and hence such patients tend to have already been assessed by physicians prior to seeing an ophthalmologist. However, lesions that are otherwise clinically silent (e.g. some occipital pathology) may present first to the ophthalmologist.

The patient will usually be vague as to the problem with their vision, and even a dense hemianopia may be missed, unless VFs are routinely assessed (e.g. by confrontational testing).

Clinical features

Optic tracts

- Incongruous homonymous hemianopia, optic atrophy, contralateral RAPD, larger pupil on the side of the hemianopia (Behr pupil), pupillary hemiakinesia (Wernicke's pupil).

LGN

- Incongruous homonymous hemianopia, normal pupils; often associated with thalamic and corticospinal signs (mild hemiparesis).

Optic radiations

- *Parietal lesions*: inferior incongruous homonymous defect, usually sparing fixation (macula fibres pass between parietal and temporal lobes); may be associated with damage to the posterior limb of the internal capsule (contralateral hemiparesis + hemianaesthesia), injury to the pursuit pathways (fails to pursue to the side of the lesion; cannot follow an optokinetic (OKN) drum rotated to the side of the lesion), and Gerstmann syndrome (dominant parietal lobe only).
- *Temporal lesions*: superior incongruous homonymous defect ('pie in sky'), usually sparing central vision; may be associated with memory loss, hallucinations (olfactory, gustatory, auditory), and receptive dysphasia.
- *Calcarine cortex (occipital) lesions*: congruous homonymous defect; variants include sparing of the temporal crescent (represented anteriorly), sparing of the macula (represented posteriorly), or a congruous homonymous macular lesion (selective injury to the occipital tip); may be associated with visual hallucinations (usually in the hemianopic field) and denial of blindness (Anton syndrome).

Investigations

- *Urgent neuroimaging*: MRI (gadolinium-enhanced) is preferable, although CT may be adequate for many lesions and may be advantageous in the presence of extensive haemorrhage.
- Further investigations will be directed by the nature of the lesion found.

Treatment

After diagnosis, the main role of the ophthalmologist is to refer for appropriate treatment of the underlying cause (e.g. to stroke unit, neurosurgery, oncology). A 2° role is in coordinating visual rehabilitation/support (may include visual impairment registration).

Primary headache disorders

Migraine is a very common recurrent headache disorder that may be severely disabling. Its prevalence is estimated at up to 20% for men and 40% for women. About 25% cases present before the age of 10y, and 90% before the age of 40y. Overall, it is commoner in women but, under 12y of age, is slightly more common in boys. A first-degree relative confers a relative risk of 3.8 for classic migraine and 1.9 for common migraine.

The mechanism is uncertain; migraineurs appear to have an inherited susceptibility to environmental factors that trigger norA and serotonin release. These cause constriction of cortical vessels (spreading neuronal depression → aura) and dilation of extracranial vasculature (perivascular pain receptors → headache).

Clinical features

Migraine without aura

(See Box 16.5.)

- *Prodrome*: mood/autonomic system disturbance (e.g. fatigue, hunger, irritability).
- *Headache*: unilateral (may generalize), throbbing, moderate to severe intensity, worsens over 1–2h, usually subsides over 4–8h but may last 1–3d; may be associated with nausea, photophobia, and sensitivity to noise ('phonophobia').
- *Termination and postdrome phase*: recovery stages marked by fatigue.

Box 16.5 Diagnostic criteria for migraine without aura (International Headache Society, IHS)*

At least five attacks fulfilling the following criteria:
1. Headache attacks lasting 4–72h (untreated or unsuccessfully treated).
2. Headache has at least two of the following:
    i. Unilateral location.
    ii. Pulsating quality.
    iii. Moderate or severe pain intensity.
    iv. Aggravated by, or causing avoidance of, routine physical activity (e.g. walking or climbing stairs).
3. During headache, at least one of the following:
    i. Nausea and/or vomiting.
    ii. Photophobia and phonophobia.
4. No other cause found.

* Headache Classification Subcommittee of the International Headache Society. The International Classification of Headache Disorders (2nd edition). *Cephalalgia* 2004;24:9–160.

Migraine with aura (See Box 16.6)

This is characterized by an aura that usually precedes the headache phase but may coincide with or follow it. The aura is most often visual but may be somatosensory, motor, or speech.

- *Visual (99% of migraineurs)*: typically starts paracentrally and expands temporally; the advancing edge forms a positive scotoma (flickering/

shimmering/zigzag/multicoloured lights), whereas the trailing edge is negatively scotomatous; other visual phenomena include foggy vision, 'heat waves', tunnel vision, and complete loss of vision.

- *Somatosensory (40%)*: hemisensory paraesthesiae/anaesthesia.
- *Motor (18%)*: hemiparesis.
- *Speech (20%)*: dysphasia.

Box 16.6 Diagnostic criteria for migraine with aura (IHS)[*]

At least two attacks fulfilling the criteria of clinical symptoms of either typical aura with migraine; typical aura with non-migraine; typical aura without headache; familial hemiplegic migraine; sporadic hemiplegic migraine; or a basilar type migraine. With no other cause found.

[*] Headache Classification Subcommittee of the International Headache Society. The International Classification of Headache Disorders (2nd edition). *Cephalalgia* 2004;**24**:9–160.

Retinal migraine (See Box 16.7)

Repeated attacks of monocular visual disturbance, such as scintillations, scotomas, or blindness, associated with migraine headache.

Box 16.7 Diagnostic criteria of retinal migraine (IHS)[*]

- At least two attacks of a fully reversible monocular positive and/or negative visual phenomena (e.g. scintillations, scotomas, or blindness), confirmed by examination during an attack or from the patient history.
- The headache must fulfil the criteria 1–4 in Box 16.5, and migraine without aura begins during the visual symptoms or follows them within 60min.
- A normal ophthalmology exam between attacks and not attributed to another disorder.

[*] Headache Classification Subcommittee of the International Headache Society. The International Classification of Headache Disorders (2nd edition). *Cephalalgia* 2004;**24**:9–160.

Investigation

Migraine (with or without aura) may be diagnosed on the basis of a typical history in the presence of a normal neurological examination. Atypical features in the history (e.g. age >55y, occipitobasal headache) or persistent neurological deficits require further assessment by a neurologist (may include neuroimaging, carotid Doppler scan, ECG, echocardiography, vasculitis screen).

Treatment

- *Prophylactic*: avoid trigger factors (e.g. foods containing tyramine (cheese and red wine), monosodium glutamate, or nitrates (salami and smoked meats). Pickled or fermented food, alcoholic or caffeinated beverages.
- *Therapeutic*: relax in a dark quiet room; aspirin, NSAIDs, or combination analgesics; consider 5HT1 agonist (e.g. sumatriptan 50mg PO or 10mg nasally stat) for more severe attacks.
- Medical treatment is considered if >2 disabling attacks/mth (e.g. propranolol, amitriptyline, sodium valproate).

Supranuclear eye movement disorders (1)

Eye movements serve to either bring an object of interest on to the fovea (saccades, quick phase of nystagmus) or maintain it there (vestibular, OKN, pursuit, vergences) (see Fig. 16.2).

Movement of the globe requires sufficient contraction of the EOM to first overcome orbital viscosity and then to sustain the new position against the elastic restoring force. The ocular motor neurones (originating from III, IV, VI nuclei) achieve this by pulse-step innervation whereby they generate first a phasic and then a tonic stimulus. For example, in saccades, a high-frequency signal from excitatory burst neurones excites the ocular motor nucleus directly (resulting in a 'pulse'), but also indirectly via neural integrators (which mathematically integrate the signal to give a 'step'). Pause cells act as dampers to prevent unwanted saccadic activity. Supranuclear pathways control this activity. Horizontal conjugate gaze requires the VI nucleus to simultaneously drive ipsilateral LR, to drive contralateral MR (via the MLF to contralateral III nucleus), and to inhibit the contralateral LR (via inhibitory burst cells to contralateral VI nucleus). Saccades originate in the contralateral frontal eye field (FEF).

Pursuit eye movements originate in the ipsilateral parieto-occipito-temporal junction. Vestibular input (e.g. for vestibulo-ocular reflex, VOR) is from the contralateral vestibular nucleus complex. Convergence input is directly to both III nuclei, avoiding the MLF. Control of vertical eye movements are more complex, as the system is effectively a torsional one that has been subverted to permit vertical movements.

Disorders of horizontal gaze

Horizontal gaze palsy

Lesions of the paramedian pontine reticular formation (PPRF) or VI nucleus result in failure to move the eyes beyond the midline to the side of the lesion (**NB** may not be complete); the VOR is preserved in a PPRF lesion but lost in a VI nucleus lesion.

Internuclear ophthalmoplegia

Lesions of the MLF (connecting the III and contralateral VI nerve nuclei) result in failure of ipsilateral adduction and overshoot of the contralateral eye ('ataxic nystagmus'), which are best demonstrated on saccadic movements; may be associated with upbeat and torsional nystagmus, loss of vertical smooth pursuit, abnormal VOR, and skew deviation. Convergence is preserved in unilateral lesions.

One and a half syndrome

Lesions of the MLF and the PPRF (or VI nucleus) on the same side result in an ipsilateral gaze palsy and an ipsilateral internuclear ophthalmoplegia. There is loss of horizontal movements other than abduction of the contralateral eye.

Tonic gaze deviation

Destructive lesions of the FEF (e.g. acute strokes) cause loss of gaze initiation to the contralateral side, with the result that the eyes deviate to the side of the lesion. Irritative lesions (e.g. trauma, tumour) cause transient deviations to the contralateral side.

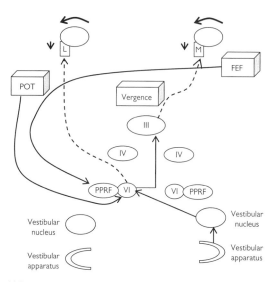

Fig. 16.2 Supranuclear inputs for horizontal eye movements.

Connections are shown for eye movements to the left (including saccades from FEF, smooth pursuit from POT, and VOR from vestibular nucleus). For convergence movements, the III nuclei are innervated directly to drive both MR. For further explanation, see text. PPRF, paramedian pontine reticular formation; L, lateral rectus; M, medial rectus.

Locked-in syndrome

Large lesions of the ventral pons may destroy bilateral PPRF and the corticospinal pathways, resulting in loss of all voluntary motor activity, except lid movements and vertical eye movements (cf. coma where all voluntary movements are lost).

Selective loss of pursuits

Lesions of the parieto-occipito-temporal junction cause failure of pursuit to the side of the lesion. This can also be demonstrated by inability to follow an OKN drum rotated to the side of the lesion. It is often associated with a contralateral homonymous field defect (usually superior).

Selective loss of saccades

Selective saccadic loss may occur in congenital or acquired ocular motor apraxia. In the congenital form, the child learns after a few months to compensate by 'head thrusts' (± blinks) beyond the target; these become less noticeable with age. In the acquired form, head thrusts are not a major feature; it may occur in bilateral frontoparietal injuries or diffuse cerebral disease.

Supranuclear eye movement disorders (2)

See Table 16.18 for location of ocular premotor and motor neurones.

Vertical gaze palsies

Parinaud dorsal midbrain syndrome

Lesions of the posterior commissure and pretectal area result in supranuclear upgaze palsy (saccades affected first, then pursuits, and finally VOR),
light-near dissociation, lid retraction, and convergence retraction nystagmus.

Causes include hydrocephalus, tumour, trauma, AVM, CVA,
demyelination.

Progressive supranuclear palsy (PSP; Steele–Richardson–Olszewski syndrome)

PSP is a rare progressive neurodegenerative disease caused by abnormal
accumulation of tau proteins (microtubule-binding proteins) proteins. Age
of onset is >40y.

- *Clinical features include*: vertical supranuclear palsy, with slowing of
  vertical saccades (ultimately involves horizontal eye movements). Lid
  apraxia is a very early sign and may lead to corneal exposure from
  failure of lid closure. Other useful signs include frequent or continuous
  square wave jerks, abnormal vertical OKN and reduced blink rate.
  There is prominent postural instability, usually within the first year, and
  early cognitive impairment.

There is no effective treatment at present.

Other supranuclear gaze palsies

Selective upgaze palsy may occur in Wilson's disease. Selective downgaze
palsy with athetosis and ataxia occurs in Niemann–Pick disease type C.

Tonic gaze deviation

Raised ICP or thalamic haemorrhage may cause forced downgaze ('sunset
sign'), although it may occur as a transient phenomenon in healthy neonates.

Selective loss of saccades

In Huntington's disease, there is selective loss of saccades (vertical more so
than horizontal), which may be compensated for by head thrusts and blinks.

Skew deviation

This is a vertical deviation that is usually concomitant and associated with
torsion. Dysfunctions of the vertical VOR pathways are usually caused by
lesions of the pons or lateral medulla (e.g. CVA, demyelination). Incomitant
skews may be confused with IVn (or IIIn) palsies.

Table 16.18 Location of ocular premotor and motor neurones

Pause cell	Nucleus raphe interpositus
Horizontal burst cell	PPRF
Horizontal inhibitory burst cell	Nucleus paragigantocellularis dorsalis
Horizontal integrator	Medial vestibular nucleus Nucleus prepositus hypoglossi
Horizontal ocular motor nucleus	VIn nucleus
Vertical burst cell	Rostral interstitial nucleus of MLF
Vertical inhibitory burst cell	Rostral interstitial nucleus of MLF (probable)
Vertical integrator	Interstitial nucleus of Cajal
Vertical ocular motor nuclei	III nucleus, IV nucleus

Third nerve disorders

A third nerve palsy may be the first sign of an aneurysm of the posterior communicating artery. Unfortunately, it may also be the last sign before the aneurysm ruptures, causing subarachnoid haemorrhage and often death.

- *Diagnosis may be difficult*: a partial palsy may be caused by a number of other conditions. Classical teaching associates painful, pupil-involving, progressive lesions with compressive disease (e.g. an expanding aneurysm). However, the differentiation of a compressive from an ischaemic third nerve palsy may not be possible on clinical grounds alone (see Box 16.8).

Anatomy

See ➲ Anatomy and physiology (2), p. 654.

Classification

Accurate localization greatly assists diagnosis. Identify whether it is:
- Complete vs partial (including aberrant regeneration).
- Pupil-sparing vs pupil-involving.
- Nuclear, fascicular, or peripheral (nerve palsy).
- Isolated vs complex (other neurological defects).

Clinical features

- Variable presentation, according to extent of loss of third nerve function. May include: pain, diplopia (due to horizontal and/or vertical ophthalmoplegia), ptosis, and pupil dilation.

What is the character of the pain/headache?

- A severe headache ('worst pain in my life', 'like someone kicked me in the back of the head') in this context should be assumed to be due to subarachnoid haemorrhage until proven otherwise; pain is classically associated with compressive lesions but may also occur in ischaemia.

Is it complete or partial?

- *Complete*: diplopia (horizontal and often vertical); complete ptosis, eye abducted, and usually depressed.
- *Partial*: any of the above features from near-complete involvement to isolated ptosis or single muscle paresis (rare).
- *Aberrant regeneration* is usually associated with long-standing compressive lesions. In lid-gaze dyskinesia, there is lid elevation on adduction ('inverse Duane's') or on depression ('pseudo von Graefe'). In pupil-gaze dyskinesia, there is pupil constriction on adduction or depression. Pure eye movement dyskinesias may also occur (e.g. elevation when trying to adduct).

Is it pupil-involving or pupil-sparing?

- *Pupil-involving*: mydriasis (no light or near response), difficulty focusing.

Is it nuclear, fascicular, or peripheral (nerve palsy)?

- Certain patterns of IIIn disorder are localizing (see Table 16.19).

Is it isolated or complex?

- Check for involvement of all other cranial nerves, including IIn (especially fields, discs), VIn (abduction), IVn (intorsion), cerebellum, and PNS. Other neurological signs may be local (e.g. compressive lesion) or disseminated (e.g. demyelination).

Investigation

- *Pupil-involving or partial IIIn palsies* (often compressive): emergency neuroimaging (MRI with MRA or high-resolution CTA). If normal, consider further investigation such as LP (CSF for oligoclonal bands, Glu, protein, xanthochromia, MC&S, cytology).
- *Pupil-sparing complete IIIn palsies* (usually ischaemic): assess vascular risk factors (atherosclerosis or arteritis; BP, Glu, lipids, ESR, CRP, FBC), and monitor closely for first week (e.g. every 2d) to ensure no developing pupil involvement. Likelihood of ischaemic cause increased if age >40y, known vasculopath, acute onset, non-progressive, and no other neurological abnormality. If no recovery at 3mo, then investigate further (including MRI). Monitor in conjunction with orthoptists (including Hess/Lees charts and fields of BSV).

Treatment

This is dependent on the underlying cause. Posterior communicating artery aneurysms require immediate transfer to neurosurgical unit for open (clips) or endovascular (coils, balloons) treatment. Other pathologies may require referral to neurology, neurosurgery, oncology, or medicine. Diplopia may be relieved by intrinsic ptosis or occlusion (patch or CL).

Surgery is dictated by any residual function and may comprise staged lid and muscle procedures. While this may improve cosmesis, its effect on the field of BSV is less predictable; it may even worsen diplopia.

Prognosis

Untreated posterior communicating artery aneurysms rupture in two-thirds of cases, of which half are fatal. Treatment reduces mortality rate to <5%.

After surgery, compressive IIIn palsies usually recover (at least partially) over 6mo. Ischaemic IIIn palsies usually spontaneously recover over 4mo.

Box 16.8 Causes of IIIn palsy

- Aneurysms (usually of the posterior communicating artery).
- Microvascular ischaemia.
- Tumour (e.g. parasellar).
- Trauma.
- Demyelination.
- Vasculitis.
- Congenital.

Table 16.19 Nuclear and fascicular IIIn syndromes

Nuclear	
Definitely nuclear	Unilateral palsy with contralateral SR paresis and bilateral partial ptosis
	Bilateral palsy without ptosis

Fascicular	
Red nucleus (paramedian midbrain)	Ipsilateral IIIn palsy
	Contralateral intention tremor + ataxia ± contralateral anaesthesia (Benedikt syndrome)
Cerebral peduncle (anterior midbrain)	Ipsilateral IIIn palsy
	Contralateral hemiparesis (Weber syndrome)

Fourth nerve disorders

SO weakness 2° to IVn palsy is a common cause of vertical strabismus. A third of cases are congenital but may not present until adulthood. Acquired cases are commonly traumatic or due to microvascular infarction (see Box 16.9). Bilateral IVn palsy is most commonly due to head injury.

Anatomy

See ➲ Anatomy and physiology (2), p. 654.

Clinical features

- Diplopia (vertical and torsional; worse on downgaze), head tilt (to opposite side), aesthenopia.
- Ipsilateral hypertropia/phoria worse on downgaze or on ipsilateral head tilt; compensatory head tilt to opposite side; limited depression in adduction; extorsion (examine fundus: normal foveal position is level with lower third of disc; measure angle with double Maddox rod); may have V pattern.
- See Parks–Bielschowsky 3-step test (see ➲ Ocular motility examination, p. 28).

Is it congenital or acquired?

A large vertical prism fusion range and high concomitance suggest that the paresis is either congenital or, if acquired, a long-standing lesion.

Is it unilateral or bilateral?

SO palsy may be bilateral (particularly after head injury) but may be asymmetric. Typically, there is a reversing hypertropia, with L/R on right gaze and R/L on left gaze, a prominent V pattern, and significant excyclotorsion (>10°) (see Box 16.10).

Is it isolated or complex?

Check for involvement of all other cranial nerves, including IIn (especially fields, discs), IIIn, Vn, and VIn, pupils (Horner's, RAPD), cerebellum, and PNS. Other neurological signs may be local (e.g. orbital apex lesion) or disseminated (e.g. demyelination).

Investigation

A history of abnormal head posture (check old photographs) or recent trauma may identify the cause. Assess vascular risk factors (atherosclerosis or arteritis; BP, Glu, lipids, ESR, CRP, FBC). Likelihood of ischaemic cause increased if age >40y, known vasculopath, acute onset, non-progressive, and no other neurological abnormality.

If aetiology unclear or no recovery at 3mo, then investigate further (including MRI). Monitor in conjunction with orthoptists (including Hess/Lees charts and fields of BSV) (see Table 16.20).

Treatment

Manage underlying cause (see Box 16.9) with appropriate team. Symptomatic management includes orthoptic intervention with a vertical prism (or occlusion) and may satisfactorily control diplopia.

Surgical options include ipsilateral IO weakening (myectomy or recession), contralateral IR recession, SO tuck, and the Fells modified Harada–Ito procedure. SO tuck carries a significant risk of inducing an iatrogenic Brown syndrome.

Box 16.9 Causes of IVn palsy

- Congenital.
- Trauma.
- Presumed microvascular ischaemia.
- Idiopathic.
- Iatrogenic (following ENT, neuro- or ophthalmic surgery).
- Tumour (e.g. pinealoma, tentorial meningioma).
- Demyelination.
- Vasculitis.
- Meningitis.
- Cavernous sinus lesions.
- Tolosa–Hunt syndrome.
- HZO.

Box 16.10 Features suggestive of bilateral IVn palsy

- Chin-down head posture (without much tilt).
- Reversing hyperdeviation.
- Excyclotorsion >10°.
- Prominent V pattern.
- Bilateral failure of adduction in depression.

Table 16.20 Nuclear and fascicular IVn syndromes

Sympathetic pathways	Ipsilateral Horner's syndrome Contralateral SO palsy
MLF	Ipsilateral internuclear ophthalmoplegia Contralateral SO palsy
Superior cerebellar peduncle	Ipsilateral ataxia, intention tremor Contralateral SO palsy

Sixth nerve disorders

Sixth nerve palsy is the commonest cause of neurogenic strabismus (see Box 16.11). Although VIn palsy results in an easily recognized abduction deficit, other pathologies may give a similar picture, notably Duane syndrome, medial wall orbital fracture, and TED (see Box 16.12).

Anatomy

See ➔ Anatomy and physiology (2), p. 654.

Clinical features

- Diplopia (horizontal; worse for distance and on looking to the side of the lesion), head turn (to same side).
- Esophoria/tropia (worse for distance and on ipsilateral gaze); ipsilateral abduction deficit (ranges from saccadic slowing only to complete loss of all movement beyond the midline).

Isolated or complex?

Check for involvement of all other cranial nerves, including IIn (especially fields, discs), IIIn, IVn, Vn, and VIIn, pupils (Horner's), cerebellum, and PNS. Other neurological signs may be local (e.g. the now very rare Gradenigo syndrome), disseminated (e.g. demyelination), or reflect ↑ICP (if the VIn palsy is a false localizing sign). (See Table 16.21.)

Investigation

Assess vascular risk factors (atherosclerosis or arteritis; BP, Glu, lipids, ESR, CRP, FBC). Likelihood of ischaemic cause increased if age >40y, known vasculopath, acute onset, non-progressive, and no other neurological abnormality.

If aetiology unclear or no recovery at 3mo, then investigate further (including MRI). Monitor in conjunction with orthoptists (including prism cover test, Hess charts, and fields of BSV).

Treatment

- Orthoptic intervention with a base-out prism (or occlusion) may satisfactorily control diplopia. Botulinum toxin injection into ipsilateral MR has both a therapeutic and diagnostic role. It may restore BSV and, if only temporary, may be repeated. In any event, it reveals any residual VIn function that might be augmented by an LR resection/MR recession.
- If there is no residual function, then vertical muscle transposition would be required.
- If there is residual LR function, transposition surgery will cause exotropia and should be avoided.

Box 16.11 Causes of VIn palsy

- Idiopathic.
- Microvascular ischaemia.
- Tumour (e.g. clivus, cerebellopontine angle, pituitary, nasopharyngeal).
- ↑ICP.
- Trauma (basal skull fracture).
- Demyelination.
- Vasculitis.
- Meningitis.
- Cavernous sinus thrombosis.
- Carotid–cavernous fistula.
- Congenital.

Box 16.12 Differential diagnosis of abduction deficit

- Duane syndrome.
- Convergence spasm.
- TED.
- Myasthenia.
- Myositis.
- Medial wall fracture.
- Distance esotropia of high myopia.

Table 16.21 Nuclear and fascicular VIn syndromes

Nuclear	
PPRF (dorsal pons)	Ipsilateral gaze palsy
PPRF + MLF (dorsomedial pons)	Ipsilateral gaze palsy Ipsilateral INO *(one and a half syndrome)*
AICA territory (dorsolateral pons)	Ipsilateral gaze palsy Ipsilateral VIIn palsy Ipsilateral Vn palsy Contralateral hemianaesthesia *(Foville syndrome)*
Fascicular	
Corticospinal tract (ventral pons)	Ipsilateral VIn palsy
Facial colliculus (dorsal pons)	Contralateral hemiparesis *(Raymond syndrome)* Ipsilateral VIn palsy; ipsilateral VIIn palsy *(Millard–Gubler syndrome)*

AICA, anterior inferior cerebellar artery.

Seventh nerve disorders

The seventh or facial nerve has a number of important motor, sensory, and secretory functions. Of these, it is the facial nerve's ability to close the eyelids (i.e. innervation of orbicularis oculi) that make it so important to the ophthalmologist.

Facial nerve palsy should not be underestimated. Do not automatically assume that every facial nerve palsy is a 'Bell's palsy', and be alert to its capacity to cause blinding exposure keratopathy (see Box 16.13).

Anatomy

See ➲ Anatomy and physiology (3), p. 656.

Function

- *Motor*: muscles of facial expression and movement; superficial platysma muscles of the neck and the stapedius ear muscles.
- *Sensory and secretory functions* (nerve intermedius and geniculate ganglion): lacrimal gland (via the greater superficial petrosal nerve) and salivary glands (via the chorda tympani, mediating taste for the anterior two-thirds of the tongue).

Clinical features

- Weakness of one side of the face/facial asymmetry (if unilateral).
- Lagophthalmos, with or without lower lid ectropion.
- Corneal surface exposure.

NB Specifically assess corneal sensation, tear film, and signs of exposure keratopathy, lid closure, orbicularis strength, Bell's phenomenon.

Is it isolated or complex?

Check for involvement of all other cranial nerves, including Vn (cerebellopontine lesions), VIn (lesion in pons), and VIIn (cerebellopontine angle lesions). Check for alteration of taste, salivation, and lacrimation.

Is it an upper motor neurone or lower motor neurone lesion?

- In upper motor neurone lesions, the upper facial muscles still function (e.g. can still raise eyebrows) due to the bilateral innervation (see ➲ Anatomy and physiology (3), p. 656). In lower motor neurone lesions, both upper and lower facial muscles are involved.

Investigation

ENT or neurology referral to establish a cause for all new-onset facial nerve palsies. All recurrent facial nerve palsy should undergo neuroimaging to exclude inflammatory or neoplastic causes.

Treatment

- *Lubricants*: often requires intensive preservative-free artificial tears during the day and ointment at night.
- *Lid closure*: consider taping lid closed at night as a temporary measure, but have a low threshold for performing a temporary tarsorrhaphy; in chronic cases, insertion of gold weights to the upper lid can be helpful.

Box 16.13 Causes of VIIn palsy

- Bell's palsy (idiopathic).
- Ramsay–Hunt syndrome (varicella-zoster infection).
- Cerebellopontine angle lesions.
- Trauma.
- Otitis.
- Neurofibroma (neurofibromatosis type 2).
- Parotid gland mass.
- Congenital (e.g. Moebius' syndrome).
- Guillain–Barré syndrome.*
- Lyme disease.*
- Saroidoisis.*
- Meningitis.*

* Commonly present with bilateral VIIn weakness.

Bell's palsy (idiopathic facial paralysis)

Although the majority of facial nerve palsy (up to 70%) are idiopathic, this is a diagnosis of exclusion. It can affect any age group (peak 40y), with ♂ and ♀ equally affected. Associations include diabetes and pregnancy. Symptoms reach their peak at 48h; most start recovery at 3wk. A large RCT reported 65% of patients fully recovered at 3mo and 85% at 9mo with no intervention.[16]

Investigation

- Assess and investigate as for unexplained facial nerve palsy.

Treatment

Early treatment

- Within 72h after the onset of symptoms, Bell's palsy treated with oral prednisolone (25mg bd) has increased recovery rates from 64% to 83% at 3mo and from 82% to 94% at 9mo.[16]
- Anti-herpes simplex antivirals treatment alone confers no recovery benefit, compared to placebo.[17]
- Combination therapy of oral steroids plus aciclovir has been investigated, and no benefit was observed over steroids alone.[18,19,20]
- Treat corneal exposure with lubricants and lid closure, as needed (see ➲ Exposure keratopathy, p. 270).

Late treatment

- Surgical treatment can improve facial function and cosmesis to some degree. Options include facial nerve repair, nerve substitution, and muscle transposition.
- Crocodile tears (gustatory hyperlacrimation 2° to aberrant regeneration) have been successfully treated with transcutaneous injection of botulinum toxin to the lacrimal gland.

16. Sullivan FM et al. Early treatment with prednisolone or acyclovir in Bell's palsy. N Engl J Med 2007;357:1598–607. 17. Lockhart P et al. Antiviral treatment for Bell's palsy (idiopathic facial paralysis). Cochrane Database Syst Rev 2009;7:CD001869. 18. Sullivan FM et al. Early treatment with prednisolone or acyclovir in Bell's palsy. N Engl J Med 2007;357:1598–607. 19. Lockhart P et al. Antiviral treatment for Bell's palsy (idiopathic facial paralysis). Cochrane Database Syst Rev 2009;7:CD001869. 20. Quant EC et al. The benefits of steroids versus steroids plus antivirals for treatment of Bell's palsy: a meta-analysis. BMJ 2009;339:3354.

Anisocoria

Assessing unequal pupils begins with a detailed history, including when and who noticed the difference in the pupil size, whether there are associated ophthalmic or neurological symptoms, any previous ophthalmic history and systemic history (see also ➔ Anisocoria, p. 884).

Differential diagnosis of unequal pupils
- Physiological anisocoria.
- Iris pathology.
- Pharmacological.
- Sympathetic chain pathology (see ➔ Anisocoria: sympathetic chain, p. 710).
- Parasympathetic chain pathology (see ➔ Anisocoria: parasympathetic chain, p. 713).

Investigations
(See ➔ Pupils examination, p. 26).

Physiological anisocoria
This is a common cause of unequal pupils, affecting 15–20% of the normal population. As involutional ptosis (from LPS disinsertion) is also common, it is not infrequent to see the two conditions coexist, so mimicking a Horner's syndrome.

Clinical features
Classically, the patient is asymptomatic.
- Pupils have brisk response to light.
- Pupils have brisk response to accommodation.
- Pupils briskly redilate after testing with light and accommodation.
- Clinically isolated, with no associated ptosis or ocular motility problems.

Prognosis is good; reassure patient.

Iris pathology
Secondary to intraocular surgery or trauma.

Pharmacological anisocoria
This is due to local instillation/inoculation (inadvertent or intentional).

Clinical features
- Fixed large (parasympathetic agents) or fixed small pupils.
- Unreactive to light or accommodation.
- Clinically isolated, with no associated ptosis or ocular motility problems.

Investigation
- *Dilated pupils*: 1% pilocarpine, wait for 45min. Pharmacological anisocoria is confirmed when there is refusal to fully constrict.
- *Constricted pupils*: 1% tropicamide, wait for 45min. Pharmacological anisocoria is confirmed when there is refusal to fully dilate.

Sympathetic chain and parasympathetic chain pathology

For anisocoria arising from disorders of the sympathetic and parasympathetic chains, see ➲ Anisocoria: sympathetic chain, p. 710 and ➲ Anisocoria: parasympathetic chain, p. 713).

Anisocoria: sympathetic chain

Horner's syndrome

The ocular sympathetic supply may be damaged anywhere along its route. The extent of sympathetic dysfunction, associated neurological signs, and pharmacological tests help to identify the level of the injury.

Clinical features

- Pupil is miotic with normal light and near reaction.
- Anisocoria is most marked in dim conditions.
- Also ptosis, apparent enophthalmos (due to 1–2mm upper lid ptosis and 1mm elevation of lower lid), ↓IOP, conjunctival injection; facial anyhydrosis suggests lesion of the first- or second-order neurone; iris hypochromia suggests a congenital lesion (also in long-standing acquired lesions).

Is it isolated or complex?

Check for involvement of all other cranial nerves, including IIn (especially fields, discs), IIIn, IVn, Vn, and VIn, cerebellum, and PNS. Other neurological signs may be local (e.g. cavernous sinus pathology) or disseminated (e.g. demyelination).

Also check for history of pain (headache, neck pain, arm pain), trauma or surgery, and any other physical signs, e.g. scars and masses (lung apices, neck, thyroid).

Investigation

- **Confirm diagnosis:**
  - *With apraclonidine:* apraclonidine has weak α1-agonist activity, with little effect on the normal pupil. At 0 and 60min, measure pupil sizes when fixing on a distant target in identical ambient lighting conditions (bright and dim). Instil 1% or 0.5% apraclonidine to both eyes after first measurement. Positive for Horner's if pupil dilates (there may also be reversal of the ptosis).
  - *With cocaine:* cocaine blocks reuptake of norA at the dilator pupillae neuromuscular junction. At 0 and 60min, measure pupil sizes when fixing on a distant target in identical ambient lighting conditions (bright and dim). Instil 4% cocaine to both eyes after first measurement; repeat at 1min. Positive for Horner's if no/poor pupillary dilation.
- **Identify level:** 1% hydroxyamfetamine to both eyes. If first- or second-order neurone lesion, there will be normal dilation; if third-order neurone lesion, then there will be no/poor dilation. This test is seldom performed in clinical practice. Topical hydroxyamfetamine is expensive and may not be readily available. The test is not reliable if performed within 48h of cocaine test.
- **Identify cause:** further investigation is directed by the likely cause and level of lesion (see Table 16.22 and Table 16.23).
- **Identify if** *congenital or acquired:* old photographs may show changes to be long-standing (view with a 20D to see pupils); also look for additional clinical features (see ➲ Congenital Horner's syndrome, p. 711).

Treatment and prognosis
- This is dependent on the underlying cause and may involve urgent referral to other specialities. Any recovery of Horner's also depends on the underlying cause and treatment.
- In cases associated with cluster headaches (Raeder syndrome), recovery may occur within a few hours.
- Other causes (e.g. invasive tumours) may cause relentless, irreversible progression.

Congenital Horner's syndrome

Usually idiopathic but can be secondary to birth trauma (such as forceps delivery).

Clinical features
- Miosis, ptosis, and apparent enophthalmos, as for adult Horner's syndrome.
- Heterochromia: lighter iris pigmentation on ipsilateral side.
- Facial flushing ('harlequin' sign), particularly seen on cycloplegic refraction or crying, due to ipsilateral anhydrosis. Generally, the affected side is pale.

Caution
Acquired Horner's syndrome in childhood, should be investigated for neuroblastoma.

Table 16.22 Investigations of Horner's syndrome

Lesion type	Investigations may include
Central	MRI brain/spinal cord
Preganglionic	CXR
	CT thorax
	Carotid Doppler
	MRI/MRA head/neck
	LN biopsy
Post-ganglionic	Carotid Doppler
	MRI/MRA head/neck
	MRI orbits
	ENT assessment

Table 16.23 Causes of Horner's syndrome

Lesion type	Location	Cause
Central	Brainstem	CVA
		Tumour
		Demyelination
	Spinal cord	Tumour
		Syringomyelia
		Trauma
Preganglionic	Lung apex	Pancoast tumour
		Trauma
	Neck	Trauma
		Surgery
		Tumour (thyroid, cervical LN)
		CCA dissection
Post-ganglionic	ICA	ICA dissection
	Middle ear	Otitis media
		Herpes zoster
	Cavernous sinus	Thrombosis
		Tumour
	Orbit	Tolosa–Hunt
		Tumour
		Cluster headache

NB Many acquired and congenital cases are idiopathic.

CCA, common carotid artery; ICA, internal carotid artery; LN, lymph node.

Anisocoria: parasympathetic chain

Adie's tonic pupil

In Adie's pupil, the parasympathetic supply from the ciliary ganglion to the iris and ciliary muscle is abnormal. It is thought that this arises due to acute viral denervation and aberrant regeneration.

It is most commonly unilateral (80%), occurring in otherwise healthy young women.

Clinical features

- Classically, pupil is mydriatic, poor response to light, with vermiform movements seen at the slit-lamp, and exaggerated, but slow and sustained (tonic), response to near/light-near dissociation.
- *Variants*: early lesions may show no response to light or near; late lesions are usually miotic; segmental lesions are common; there may be additional absence of deep tendon reflexes (Holmes–Adie syndrome) or patchy hypohidrosis (Ross syndrome); with time, the pupil becomes miotic.

Investigations

- *Confirm diagnosis*: 0.125% pilocarpine to both eyes. At 0 and 30min, measure pupil size when fixing on a distant target in identical dim lighting conditions.
- In Adie's, the response is greater in the affected eye (denervation hypersensitivity of sphincter pupillae).

Treatment

- Reassure patient.
- Weak-strength pilocarpine (e.g. 0.1%, as often as required) may help treat mydriatic blurring and accommodative problems.
- Mydriasis may also be helped by a painted CL acting as an artificial pupil.
- Reading glasses may also help with the accommodative dysfunction.

Idiopathic intermittent unilateral mydriasis

One pupil transiently becomes large, lasting between 15min to hours. Patients complain of blurred vision, ocular pain, and photosensitivity. On examination, the large pupil is clinically isolated. More commonly occurs in women and is associated with migraine, with nearly 50% having history of migraines.

Aetiology is either parasympathetic insufficiency of the iris sphincter, or sympathetic hyperactivity of the iris dilator.[21]

---

21. Jacobson DM. Benign episodic unilateral mydriasis. Clinical characteristics. *Ophthalmology* 1995;**102**:1623–7.

Argyll Robertson pupils

Argyll Robertson pupils present in the tertiary stage of neurosyphilis are now uncommon due to the introduction of penicillin.

Clinical features

- Initially unilateral, then bilateral, irregular miosed pupils.
- React poorly to light.
- Light-near dissociation.
- Iris can be atrophic on slit-lamp examination.

Investigations

- *Non-treponemal serology*: VDRL tests disease activity; it may become negative in later disease syphilis. RPR is a simple test used in screening.
- *Treponemal serology*: fluorescent treponemal antibody absorption (FTA-ABS) and haemagglutination tests (TPHA) test previous or current infection. They do not distinguish from other treponematoses (e.g. yaws).

Treatment

Management of syphilitic eye disease should be in conjunction with a GU physician. Treatment requires high-dose penicillin, with an extended regimen for late latent and tertiary syphilis. Benzathine benzylpenicillin is now the preferred preparation for syphilis in the UK (unlicensed indication).[22] Spirochaete death may transiently worsen inflammation (Jarish–Herxheimer reaction).

22. *British National Formulary* (March 2013). London: BMJ Publishing Group.

Nystagmus (1)

Nystagmus, oscillations, and saccadic intrusions are a group of involuntary abnormalities of fixation.

- In nystagmus, there is an abnormal slow movement away from fixation that is then corrected by a fast movement (jerk nystagmus) or by another slow movement (pendular nystagmus).
- In oscillations and intrusions, there is an abnormal saccade away from fixation, followed by a corrective saccade, i.e. both movements are fast.
- The corrective saccade may be immediate (oscillation) or delayed (intrusion).

Classification

Analyse the movement disorder in a logical manner.

- *History*: early or late onset; presence of oscillopsia (see Table 16.24).
- *Abnormal movement away from fixation*: slow or fast.
- *Corrective movement*: slow or fast.
- *Direction*: horizontal, vertical, or rotatory.
- *Symmetry*: conjugate or disconjugate (see Table 16.27 and Table 16.28).
- *Effect on direction/amplitude of*: time, direction of gaze, fixation, head position.
- *VA*.
- *Associated involuntary movements*: palate, head, and neck.

Nystagmus with onset in infancy

This is not usually associated with oscillopsia; however, a minority of patients do get oscillopsia, especially when looking in the direction of greatest nystagmus.

Idiopathic infantile nystagmus (idiopathic congenital nystagmus)

- Conjugate horizontal (usually) jerk nystagmus, worsens with fixation but improves within 'null zone' and on convergence. The null zone is a direction of gaze in which the nystagmus is damped down.
- It has a very early onset (usually by 2mo of age) and may initially be pendular.
- It can occasionally be vertical or rotatory.
- There is usually only mild ↓VA; strabismus is common.
- It may be inherited (AD, AR, XL).

Nystagmus associated with retinal disease (sensory deprivation)

Erratic waveform ± roving eye movements; moderate/severe ↓VA due to ocular or anterior visual pathway disease.

- *Common retinal diseases associated include*: albinism, CSNB, cone–rod dystrophy, LCA.

Latent/manifest latent nystagmus

- Conjugate horizontal jerk nystagmus, with fast phase towards fixing eye, worsens with occlusion of non-fixing eye and with gaze towards fast phase but improves with gaze towards slow phase.
- It alternates if opposite eye takes up fixation; often associated with infantile esotropia.

Table 16.24 Early-onset nystagmus

Waveform	Effect of occlusion	Nystagmus type
Horizontal jerk	Already evident	Idiopathic congenital
	Becomes manifest	Manifest latent
Erratic ± roving	No effect	Sensory deprivation

Nystagmus (2)

Acquired nystagmus: conjugate (See Table 16.25)

Late-onset or acquired nystagmus is usually associated with oscillopsia and is often associated with other neurological abnormalities.

Gaze-evoked nystagmus

- Conjugate horizontal (usually) jerk nystagmus on eccentric gaze, with fast phase towards direction of gaze; it occurs at smaller angles than physiological end-point nystagmus, i.e. <45°.
- Asymmetric gaze-evoked nystagmus usually indicates failure of ipsilateral neural integrator/cerebellar dysfunction (see ➔ Supranuclear eye movement disorders (1), p. 696); symmetric gaze-evoked nystagmus may be due to CNS depression (fatigue, alcohol, anticonvulsants, barbiturates) (see Box 16.14) or structural pathology (e.g. brainstem, cerebellum).

Periodic alternating nystagmus

- Conjugate horizontal jerk nystagmus present in 1° position, with waxing–waning nystagmus lasting for 90s in each direction, with a 10s gap or 'null' period.
- Periodic alternating nystagmus is usually due to vestibulocerebellar disease (e.g. demyelination, Arnold–Chiari malformation). An alternating nystagmus without such regular periodicity may also be seen in severe ↓VA.

NB Periodic alternating nystagmus is easily missed if too brief an assessment of the pattern of nystagmus is made.

Peripheral vestibular nystagmus

- Conjugate horizontal jerk nystagmus, improves with fixation and with time since injury, worsens with gaze towards fast phase (Alexander's law) or change in head position.
- Nystagmus with fast phase away from the lesion is associated with destructive lesions of the vestibular system (e.g. labyrinthitis, vestibular neuritis), whereas nystagmus to the same side may be seen in irritative lesions (e.g. Ménière's disease). It may be associated with vertigo, deafness, or tinnitus.

Central vestibular/cerebellar/brainstem nystagmus

- Conjugate jerk (usually) nystagmus that may be horizontal, vertical, or torsional and that does not improve with fixation.
  - Horizontal central vestibular nystagmus is usually due to lesions of the vestibular nuclei, the cerebellum, or their connections.
  - Upbeat nystagmus in 1° position is usually due to cerebellar or lower brainstem pathology (e.g. demyelination, infarction, tumour, encephalitis, Wernicke's syndrome).
  - Downbeat nystagmus in 1° position is usually due to pathology of the craniocervical junction (e.g. Arnold–Chiari malformation, spinocerebellar degenerations, infarction, tumour, demyelination) or drug-induced (Box 16.14).

Box 16.14 Pharmacological agents that induce nystagmus

- Carbamazepine.
- Lithium carbonate.
- Phenytoin.
- Amiodarone.
- Morphine.
- Fomepizole.
- Ketamine abuse.
- Nutmeg.

Table 16.25 Late onset nystagmus—conjugate

Effect of gaze	Effect of time	Direction	Effect of fixation	Nystagmus type
Present in 1° position	Sustained	Horizontal	Improves	Peripheral vestibular
			Worsens/no effect	Central vestibular
		Vertical	N/A	Upbeat
				Downbeat
	Periodic	Horizontal	N/A	Periodic alternating
Only present in eccentric gaze	N/A	Usually horizontal	N/A	Gaze evoked

Table 16.26 Late-onset nystagmus—disconjugate

Extent	Waveform	Nystagmus type
Unilateral	Torsional	SO myokymia
	Horizontal in abducting eye	INO-associated
Bilateral	Pendular	Acquired pendular
	See-saw	See-saw

INO, internuclear ophthalmoplegia.

Nystagmus (3)

Acquired nystagmus: disconjugate (See Table 16.26)

Acquired pendular nystagmus
- Usually disconjugate with horizontal, vertical, and torsional components.
- It is associated with brainstem and cerebellar disease, including toluene abuse.
- It may be associated with involuntary repetitive movement of palate, pharynx, and face (oculopalatal myoclonus).

SO myokymia
- Unilateral high-frequency, low-amplitude torsional nystagmus.
- This movement is so small that it may only be detectable at the slit-lamp.
- May cause occasional diplopia.
- It is rarely associated with underlying disease, although it has been reported after SO palsy, and associated with MS and pontine tumours.

Internuclear ophthalmoplegia
- Nystagmus of the abducting (and occasionally adducting) eye.
- The mechanism is uncertain, possibly being due to gaze paresis or ataxia.

See-saw nystagmus
- Vertical and torsional components, with one eye elevating and intorting while the other depresses and extorts.
- It is usually a slow pendular waveform, although a jerk see-saw nystagmus may also be seen. In the congenital form, the torsional element is reversed, i.e. the elevating eye extorts.

Treatment
- Treatment is difficult and often disappointing.
- Treatment options depend on visual potential, presence of visual symptoms (oscillopsia), and the location of a null position.
- Drug treatment includes GABA-ergics (e.g. gabapentin), anticholinergics (e.g. hyoscine), and memantine (antiglutamatergic, antiserotonergic, and anticholinergic).
- Optical devices aim to stabilize (e.g. high plus spectacle lens with high minus CL) or optimize the null position (e.g. prisms to move null position towards the 1° position).
- Surgical procedures may generally stabilize (e.g. bilateral weakening procedures—usually only a transient benefit) or move the null position and reduce the corrective head posture (horizontal, vertical, or torsional Kestenbaum procedures).
- Retrobulbar botulinum toxin causes general dampening of ipsilateral nystagmus; however, it is associated with ptosis, diplopia, and vertigo (hence may not be suitable for ambulatory patients).

Saccadic oscillations and intrusions

In oscillations and intrusions, there is an abnormal saccade away from fixation, followed by a corrective saccade, i.e. both movements are fast. The corrective saccade may be immediate (oscillation) or delayed (intrusion).

Saccadic oscillations

Ocular flutter
- Bursts of moderate-amplitude horizontal saccades without intersaccadic interval.
- It is associated with cerebellar and brainstem disease.

Opsoclonus
- Bursts of large-amplitude multidirectional saccades without intersaccadic interval.
- It is associated with loss of pause cell activity that may be caused by viruses, myoclonic encephalopathy, paraneoplastic syndromes (neuroblastoma in children, small cell lung cancer in adults), and demyelination.

Saccadic intrusions

Small, infrequent square-wave jerks may be physiological. However, other intrusions are usually pathological, most commonly due to cerebellar disease.

Square-wave jerks and macrosquare-wave jerks
Horizontal 1–5° (square wave) or 10–40° (macro) excursions from fixation and back again.

Macrosaccadic oscillations
Series of hypermetric saccades attempting to narrow in on the target; 'ocular past-pointing'.

Coma-associated eye movements

Ocular bobbing
- Conjugate fast downward movements, with slow drift upward.
- Ocular bobbing may be caused by large lesions of the pons, metabolic encephalopathies, or hydrocephalus.

Ocular dipping
- Conjugate slow downward movements, with fast saccade upward.
- This and other variants of ocular bobbing are fairly non-specific.

Ping-pong gaze
- Conjugate horizontal movements, alternating side every few seconds.
- This is associated with bilateral cerebral hemispheric lesions.

Myasthenia gravis

MG is an uncommon autoimmune disease, characterized by weakness and fatiguability of skeletal muscle. Antibodies against post-synaptic acetylcholine (Ach) receptors cause loss of receptors and structural abnormalities of the neuromuscular junction.

Its prevalence is estimated as up to 1 in 10,000. It may occur at any age but has a bimodal distribution, with peaks at about 20y and 60y. In the younger group, it is more common in ♀, but, in the older group, it is more common in ♂.

It may be associated with thymic hyperplasia, and other autoimmune disease (e.g. Graves's disease in 4–10%).

Clinical features

MG is a great mimic. Consider it when confronted with ocular motility abnormalities that 'do not fit', particularly when these seem to be highly variable.

Ocular signs are the presenting feature in 70% and are present at some point in 90% of MG. Ocular MG becomes generalized in 80% of patients (usually within 2y).

Ocular

- Variable diplopia or ptosis (usually worsening towards evening/with exercise).
- Variable and fatiguable ptosis or ocular motility disturbance (any pattern); sustained eccentric gaze of ≥1min or repeated saccades demonstrate fatigue, e.g. attempted prolonged upward gaze demonstrates fatigue of LPS and elevators; Cogan's twitch (ask patient to look down for 20s and then at object in the 1° position: positive if lid 'overshoots'); spontaneous twitching is a sign of severe fatigue.

Systemic

- Fatiguable weakness of limbs, speech, chewing, swallowing, breathing; choking, fluids going up nose when swallowing.

NB MG is potentially fatal due to respiratory failure or choking. Take breathlessness or any choking episodes seriously.

Investigations

- *Ice-pack test*: measure ptosis; use ice pack or place ice, wrapped in a towel/glove, on the closed eyelid for 2min; remeasure ptosis; test significantly positive if ≥2mm.
- *Tensilon® (edrophonium) test*: ensure that IV atropine (0.5–1mg), resuscitation equipment, and trained staff are on hand. Cardiac monitoring essential. Give 2mg edrophonium IV (test dose); if no ill effects at 30s, give further 8mg edrophonium IV (slow injection). Compare pre- and post-test ptosis or motility disturbance (consider Hess chart). The objectivity of this test may be improved by having a second syringe of 0.9% saline and using an independent observer, who is unaware of which agent is being administered, to comment on the effects of each.

- *Serum antibodies*: anti-ACh receptor is present in >95% patients with generalized myasthenia, but only 50% of ocular myasthenia; anti-skeletal muscle is present in 85% of patients with thymoma; anti-thyroid antibodies and ANA may detect associated disease.
- *Single fibre electromyography (EMG)*: repetitive supramaximal stimuli demonstrate reduction in action potential amplitude; also jitter (the EMG equivalent of twitch).

Treatment

- Liaise with a neurologist to assess systemic involvement (may include a CT chest to assess the thymus gland) and to optimize care.
- *Anticholinesterases*: pyridostigmine—start 30–60mg PO 1–2×/d, gradually increasing, if required, to maximum of 450mg/d. GI disturbance may occur but can be treated by propantheline.
- *Immunosuppression*: if generalized disease, refer to a physician for further assessment and immunosuppression; this may include corticosteroids, azathioprine, IV immunoglobulin, plasmapheresis, and thymectomy.
- Thymectomy is associated with quicker remission of MG. Full benefit may not be seen until 1y post-surgery. Thymic hyperplasia is seen in about 70% of MG cases, and thymoma found in 10% of all MG patients. Thymoma is an absolute indication for thymectomy.

Prognosis

- Fatal cardiorespiratory failure may rarely occur, usually during the first year of disease. Death may also occur from choking episodes. At-risk patients should be nursed sitting upright and require a nasogastric tube.
- Prognosis is worse for those with thymoma and with a late onset of disease.
- Most patients are well controlled on treatment; some spontaneously remit.

Other disorders of the neuromuscular junction

See Table 16.27.

Congenital myasthenia syndromes

Heterogeneous group of disorders that can occur throughout childhood. They are usually caused by presynaptic, synaptic, or post-synaptic defects of the ACh receptor. Commonly have purely ocular disease.

Lambert–Eaton myasthenic syndrome (LEMS)

A disorder of the presynaptic calcium channels, causing impaired release of ACh. It is usually associated with malignancy (e.g. small cell lung cancer) but may be an isolated autoimmune disorder. The main ocular feature is decreased lacrimation, although ocular motility abnormalities and tonic pupils may occur. In contrast to MG, repeated or sustained testing may cause improvement in any abnormalities.

Toxins

Toxins may act presynaptically to either impair ACh release (botulism, tick paralysis) or increase its release (black widow spider, scorpion bite). Organophosphates (fertilizers, nerve gas) act within the cleft to inhibit acetylcholinesterase. Treatment includes supportive measures, antitoxin (if available), and, for the excitatory syndromes, atropine blockade.

Table 16.27 Neuromuscular junction disorders

Syndrome	Pathogenesis	Ocular features	Systemic features
Inhibitory syndromes			
MG	Antibodies to post-synaptic AChR	Fatiguable ptosis, abnormal motility	Fatigue of limbs, bulbar function, respiratory failure
LEMS	Paraneoplastic presynaptic ↓ACh release	↓Lacrimation, tonic pupils, abnormal motility	Proximal weakness Autonomic dysfunction
Botulism	Toxin presynaptic ↓ACh release	Ptosis, tonic pupils, abnormal motility	Weakness of bulbar function Autonomic dysfunction
Excitatory syndromes			
Organophosphate	Toxin inhibits acetylcholinesterase	Miosis	Respiratory failure Fasciculation Paralysis
Scorpion toxin	Toxin Presynaptic ↑ACh release	↓VA, abnormal motility	Respiratory failure Mental disturbance

AChR, acetylcholine receptor.

Myopathies

Inherited myopathies are rare, insidious, and easily missed in their early stages. Diplopia is uncommon, and patients may adopt exaggerated head movements. It is important to consider the diagnosis in all patients with bilateral ptosis, partly because a more cautious approach to lid surgery is necessary.

Acquired myopathies due to orbital inflammation or infiltration (e.g. TED and myositis; see ➲ Thyroid eye disease: general, p. 600) are much more common. Florid cases are easily recognized, but early cases may cause a non-specific restrictive pattern.

Chronic progressive external ophthalmoplegia (CPEO)

This is a rare group of conditions in which there is progressive failure of eye movement. Mutations of mitochondrial DNA lead to abnormalities of oxidative phosphorylation and consequent muscle and CNS injury.

Clinical features
- Bilateral ptosis, ↓smooth pursuits/saccades/reflex eye movements (downgaze usually affected last; diplopia uncommon); weakness of orbicularis oculi and facial muscles.

Variants
- *Kearns–Sayre syndrome*: CPEO, pigmentary retinopathy (granular pigmentation, PPA), and heart block; usually presents before 20y.
- *MELAS syndrome*: mitochondrial encephalopathy, lactic acidosis, stroke-like episodes; also CPEO, hemianopia, cortical blindness.

Investigations
- *ECG*: check for conduction abnormalities.
- Consider skeletal muscle biopsy (ragged red fibres with peripheral concentration of mitochondria); peripheral blood (mitochondrial DNA analysis; fasting sample for Glu, lactate, pyruvate, pH); MRI, EMG (to rule out other diagnoses).

Treatment
Management of CPEO may involve liaison with neurologists (who may perform the muscle Bx), clinical geneticists, and cardiologists. Symptomatic ptosis or diplopia may be relieved by cautious surgery (beware weak orbicularis oculi and poor Bell's phenomenon). Conduction abnormalities may require pacemaker insertion. Coenzyme Q10 has some benefit on the systemic features of Kearns–Sayre syndrome.

Oculopharyngeal dystrophy

This rare AD (occasionally sporadic) condition is associated with an expanded GCG repeat in the poly(A) binding protein 2 gene. It typically presents in the sixth decade and has been identified in a large French Canadian pedigree. It is a form of myotonia, i.e. there is a delay in muscle relaxation post-contraction. The condition progresses from dysphagia to bilateral ptosis to external ophthalmoplegia and orbicularis weakness.

Myotonic dystrophy

This uncommon AD dystrophy arises due to an expanded CTG repeat in the dystrophica myotonica protein kinase (*DMPK*) gene (Chr 19q). 'Anticipation' occurs whereby the triplet expansion increases in successive generations, leading to earlier and more severe disease. Prevalence is estimated at about 5/100,000, being highest among French Canadians. It is characterized by a failure of muscle relaxation after contraction.

Clinical features

- *Ocular*: bilateral ptosis, cataracts (polychromatic 'Christmas tree cataracts' or posterior subcapsular), orbicularis oculi weakness; rarely pigmentary retinopathy ('butterfly' pigmentation centrally, reticular at mid-periphery, and atrophic far periphery) and myotonia of EOM.
- *Systemic*: 'mournful' facies, dysphasia, dysphagia, muscle weakness with delayed relaxation ('myotonic grip'), testicular atrophy, frontal baldness, ↓IQ, cardiac myopathy, and conduction abnormalities (may lead to fatal cardiac failure).

Investigations

- *DNA analysis*: confirms diagnosis.
- *ECG*: should be performed annually for conduction abnormalities; these may occur in otherwise minimally affected individuals.

Treatment

- Multidisciplinary management may include neurology, cardiology, physiotherapy, occupational therapy, and speech therapy.
- Offer genetic counselling, annual influenza vaccination, and cataract surgery (when symptomatic).
- **NB** General anaesthesia may unmask subclinical respiratory failure, leading to problems of ventilatory weaning.

Blepharospasm and other dystonias

Blepharospasm is a relatively common condition, which, in its severe form, can be very disabling both in terms of vision and social function. It is more common in women ($♀:♂$ 2:1) and increases with age. It is a type of focal dystonia in which there is tonic spasm of the orbicularis oculi. It may be idiopathic (essential blepharospasm) or 2° to ocular or periocular disease. Blepharospasm may be associated with dystonias involving other facial muscles (see Table 16.28 for causes).

Essential blepharospasm

Clinical features

- Bilateral involuntary lid closure, ↑frequency of lid closure (normal is about 10–20×/min); may be precipitated by stress, fatigue, social interactions; may be relieved by relaxation or 'distraction', e.g. touching face or whistling; often marked fluctuations from day to day but generally worsens over years.
- Associated ocular disease may include underlying precipitants (particularly lid and ocular surface) and 2° anatomical changes of the lid (ptosis or entropion) or brow (brow ptosis or dermatochalasis).

Investigations

- Typical isolated blepharospasm does not usually require investigation.
- If atypical (e.g. associated weakness or any other neurological abnormality), liaise with a neurologist and consider imaging (e.g. MRI) and other tests (e.g. EMG).

Treatment

- *Botulinum toxin Type A*: this is usually given as multiple injections of the upper and lower lid; it has high rate of success in the short term (up to 98%) but generally only lasts for 3mo; complications include ptosis, epiphora, keratitis, dry eyes, and ocular motility disorders (diplopia).
- Treat any underlying ocular disease.
- Other treatment options include medical (e.g. benzodiazepines) and surgical (myectomy or chemomyectomy with doxorubicin).

Other dystonias of the face and neck

- *Meige syndrome*: blepharospasm with mid-facial spasm; regarded as a 'spill-over' of essential blepharospasm to involve the mid-facial musculature; may compromise speech and eating/drinking.
- *Torticollis*: tonic spasm of sternocleidomastoid causes sudden sustained movement of the head to one side.

Table 16.28 Causes of blepharospasm

Type	Cause
Essential	Idiopathic
2°	**Blepharitis**
	Trichiasis
	Dry eyes/KCS
	Other chronic lid disease
	Other chronic ocular surface disease
	Glaucoma
	Uveitis

Common causes are shown in bold.

Other involuntary facial movement disorders

- *Hemifacial spasm*: tonic-clonic spasm of facial musculature, which, unlike blepharospasm or Meige syndrome, is unilateral, may occur during sleep, and typically affects a younger age group. It suggests irritation of the root of VIIn by a compressive lesion (usually an abnormal vessel but needs imaging to rule out a posterior fossa tumour).
- *Facial myokymia*: fleeting movements of facial musculature that may be associated with caffeine, stress, MS, or rarely tumours of the brainstem.
- *Facial tic*: brief, repetitive stereotypic movements, which are suppressible (at least initially); may be associated with Gilles de la Tourette syndrome.

Lid 'apraxia'

Normal blinking requires both the inhibition of LPS and the activation of orbicularis oculi. In lid opening 'apraxia', there is total inhibition of LPS, with no activation of orbicularis oculi. This results in sustained lid closure, with difficulty in initiating lid opening.

It is associated with extrapyramidal diseases (e.g. Parkinson's disease, progressive supranuclear palsy (PSP), Huntington's disease, Wilson's disease).

Lid retraction and poor initiation of lid closure may also be seen in Parkinson's disease, PSP, and Parinaud syndrome.

Functional visual loss

Functional visual loss (syn non-organic visual loss, psychogenic visual impairment) is a diagnosis of exclusion. It can often coexist with genuine pathology.

Suspecting functional visual loss

Consider this diagnosis when the patient reports poor vision but some of the following features are present.

Visual function and history

- Visual functioning obviously does not correlate with history, e.g. reported blindness but able to easily navigate around the waiting room; however, be cautious, as some patients with low vision due to organic visual loss can navigate surprisingly well.
- Patient cannot perform tasks that he/she may consider to be visual but actually are not, e.g. signing name.
- Recent stressful event elicited in history, e.g. impending exams.

Normal examination

- No apparent pathology after detailed examination.
- Absence of RAPD in the context of profound reported asymmetrical visual loss. **NB** Bilateral symmetrical pathology may give slow ('sluggish') pupillary light responses but no RAPD.
- Retinoscopy and subjective refraction shows absence of uncorrected refractive error.
- OKN nystagmus is demonstrable using field stimulus which patient reports not to be able to discern.

Inconsistent abnormalities in the examination

- *Goldmann perimetry features*: 'spiralling' isopters regress towards fixation as test progresses; crossed isopters show that a dimmer or smaller target is surprisingly seen further in the periphery than a brighter or larger target; crowded isopters show that targets of greatly differing size or brightness are suddenly seen when they reach about the same eccentricity within the VF.
- *Ishihara plates*: patient may give inconsistent responses, e.g. recognize '12' but no other numbers, yet repeatably trace the plates correctly. (**NB** This can also be seen in associative visual agnosia.) It is important to exclude defective colour vision in the 'normal eye' in order to validate RAPD observations.

Diagnosing functional visual loss

Diagnose functional visual loss only when the patient has demonstrated normal vision. This requires an encouraging, empathic approach and a slick examination. Consider:

Tests of stereoacuity

- Normal stereoacuity implies normal VA.

The 'crossed cylinder technique'

- Fog good eye with +6D lens in trial frame, +0.25 before 'blind' eye.
- Rotate a crossed +3D cyl before a −3.0 cyl.
- See if patient can be encouraged to read with the 'blind' eye when the cylinders are superimposed to negate each other.

Tests of reading vision

In some cases, normal reading vision can be demonstrated, proving normal visual potential despite apparently impaired Snellen acuities.

Tests of colour vision

If the patient gives normal Ishihara plate responses, then their VA is at least 6/24. For those with congenital red-green colour blindness, the presence of a red filter should enable them to read the plates, provided they have an acuity of at least 6/24.

Causes

- *Conversion disorder*: visual loss may be a manifestation of psychological or social difficulties.
- *Malingering*: feigned visual loss for other (usually material) benefit.

Management

- Patients suspected of functional visual loss will often need encouragement, reassurance, and follow-up.
- If the diagnosis remains uncertain, use a term, such as visual loss of unknown cause, in the notes.
- Referral to an ophthalmologist familiar with unexplained visual loss (e.g. neuro-ophthalmologist or paediatric ophthalmologist) may avoid unnecessary investigations.

Investigations

Investigation is mandatory when there is diagnostic uncertainty. Consider:

- *EDTs*: normal VEP results support reasonable vision, but abnormal results can be found in the absence of genuine pathology; EDTs may identify early Stargardt's disease or cone dystrophy.
- *Neuroimaging*, e.g. contrast-enhanced MRI of visual pathway.
- Investigation as a chronic optic neuropathy of unknown cause, e.g. for Leber's mutations.
- In exceptional circumstances (when cortical injury is suspected), PET can reveal organic disease when other imaging techniques give normal results.

Treatment

- When functional visual loss is diagnosed, the patient should be counselled carefully. The physician faces the unusual situation of contesting the patient's symptoms. However, an adversarial scenario can be both disagreeable and entirely counterproductive. The patient can be reassured that they have healthy eyes and that the return of normal visual functioning is expected.
- With support, patience, and reassurance, the patient can be allowed to resolve their visual functioning.
- The underlying problem may be far beyond the scope of most ophthalmologists' expertise. In some cases, a clinical psychologist may be helpful.

Strabismus

Anatomy and physiology (1)

EOM

The orbit forms a pyramid, in which the lateral and medial walls are at 45° to each other and the central axis thus at 22.5° (approximated to 23°). The four rectus muscles originate from the annulus of Zinn (see Fig. 17.1, Fig. 17.2, and Table 17.1).

The SO (like the LPS) originates from the orbital apex outside the annulus; in contrast, the IO arises from the nasal orbital floor. The obliques lie inferior to their corresponding rectus muscle, i.e. SO lies inferior to SR and IO inferior to IR. The SO tendon and sheath uniquely pass through a cartilaginous rigid pulley attached to the superonasal orbital wall.

The spiral of Tillaux describes the way the recti insert increasingly posterior to the limbus (MR, IR, LR, then SR). Innervation is by IIIn for SR, MR, IR, IO, by IVn for SO, and by VIn for LR.

Each rectus muscle carries two anterior ciliary arteries, except the lateral which carries only one. These are important for anterior segment perfusion.

Tenon's capsule is a diffuse fascial layer between the conjunctiva and globe which envelops the EOM. Condensations of this layer are classically understood to form check ligaments (spanning radially from the globe to the lateral and medial orbital wall and between muscles), Lockwood's ligament (slung below and supporting the globe), and the intermuscular septum (concentrically surrounding the anterior globe between muscles). Our understanding of the function of these structures has been improved by high-resolution imaging. MRI shows EOM do not pass in a straight line from origin to insertion and that pulleys and associated passive and active sling structures control the muscle paths.[1]

Table 17.1 Anatomy of EOM

	Origin	Muscle length (mm)	Tendon length	Insertion (mm from limbus)*
MR	Annulus of Zinn	40	3.6mm	5.5
LR	Annulus of Zinn	40	8.4mm	6.9
SR	Annulus of Zinn	41	5.4mm	7.7
IR	Annulus of Zinn	40	5.0mm	6.5
SO	Sphenoid	32	From 10mm pre-trochlea	Posterior superotemporal
IO	Orbital floor	34	Minimal	Posterior temporal

* Distance to mid-point of insertion.

1. Demer JL. Pivotal role of orbital connective tissues in binocular alignment and strabismus. The Friedenwald Lecture. *Invest Ophthalmol Vis Sci* 2004;**45**:729–38.

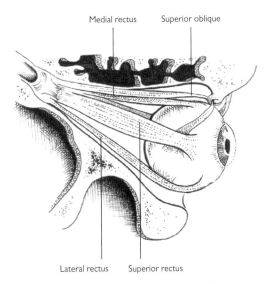

Fig. 17.1 Superior view of the right globe showing muscle insertions (LPS removed).

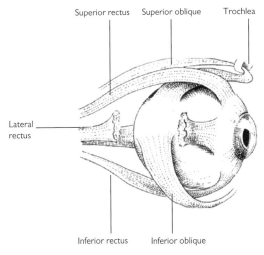

Fig. 17.2 Lateral view of the right globe showing muscle insertions (LR partly removed).

Anatomy and physiology (2)

Eye movements

Eye movements may be monocular (ductions) or binocular (versions and vergences).

Versions are conjugate eye movements, i.e. eyes move in the same direction, whereas vergences are disconjugate, i.e. eyes move in opposing directions. Eye movements may be described as rotations of the globe around horizontal (x), anteroposterior (y), and vertical (z) axes—the axes of Fick (see Fig. 17.3).

Ductions comprise abduction (outward), adduction (inward), supraduction (upward), infraduction (downward), intorsion (superior limbus moves inward), and extorsion (superior limbus moves outward).

Versions include dextroversion (right gaze), laevoversion (left gaze), supraversion (upgaze), infraversion (downgaze), dextrocycloversion (superior limbus moves right), and laevocycloversion (superior limbus moves left). Vergences are limited to convergence (inward) or divergence (outward) (see Fig. 17.4).

The EOM do not act in isolation. Thus, each agonist (e.g. LR) has an antagonist that acts in the opposite direction on the same eye (i.e. ipsilateral MR). Increased innervation of the agonist is accompanied by decreased innervation of its antagonist (Sherrington's law). Each agonist also has a yoke muscle that acts in the same direction on the other eye (i.e. contralateral MR in this example). During conjugate movement, yoke muscles receive equal and simultaneous innervation (Hering's law) (see Table 17.2).

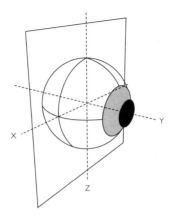

Fig. 17.3 The axes of Fick.

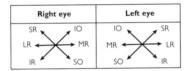

Fig. 17.4 The six cardinal positions of gaze (from observer's perspective).

Table 17.2 Actions of EOM

	In 1° position (subsidiary actions)	In abduction	In adduction
MR	Adduction	Adduction	Adduction
LR	Abduction	Abduction	Abduction
SR	Elevation (intorsion, adduction)	Elevation (isolated at 23° abduction)	Intorsion (isolated at 67° adduction)
IR	Depression (extorsion, adduction)	Depression (isolated at 23° abduction)	Extorsion (isolated at 67° adduction)
SO	Intorsion (depression, abduction)	Intorsion (isolated at 39° abduction)	Depression (isolated at 51° adduction)
IO	Extorsion (elevation, abduction)	Extorsion (isolated at 39° abduction)	Elevation (isolated at 51° adduction)

Amblyopia

Amblyopia is a developmental defect of central visual processing, leading to reduced visual form sense. In essence, during the first 6y of life, our capacity for high-level vision is vulnerable. Anything less than perfect, balanced foveal images from both eyes can lead to loss of vision in one/both eyes. With increasing age, this is harder to reverse and, by about 7–8y of age, is usually permanent. The aetiology of amblyopia is related to interocular competitive disadvantage, thus bilateral foveal image deprivation is less amblyogenic than uniocular.

Causes of amblyopia

No/reduced image

- *Stimulus-deprivation amblyopia*: constant monocular occlusion for >1wk/y of life is very likely to lead to amblyopia in those <6y.

Most congenital cataracts, especially unilateral, are highly amblyogenic. Outcome is closely linked to expedient removal; however, post-operative glaucoma risk diminishes exponentially with age at surgery. Most operate at about 6wks of age.

Image blurring from refractive error

Although usually a 1° phenomenon, consider 2° causes and the need to address these (e.g. eyelid chalazion or infantile haemangiomas when the corrective 'plus' axis of the corrective prescription points at the lesion).

- *Anisometropic amblyopia*: unequal refractive power of the eyes (usually referring to spherical equivalent). High risk if difference in refraction of >2.5D but may be significant with differences as low as 1D; increased risk if present >2y; this is a highly amblyogenic stimulus.
- *Ametropic amblyopia*: significant though symmetrical, refractive error >+5.00DS or –10.00DS likely to confer significant risk; bilateral amblyopia may occur, if uncorrected.
- *Astigmatic/meridional amblyopia*: significant risk if >0.75D cylinder; risk is increased if different axis and/or magnitude between the two eyes.

Abnormal binocular interaction

- *Strabismic amblyopia*: significant risk if one eye preferred for fixation; if freely alternating, then low risk; more common in esotropia than exotropia.

Clinical features

- Reduced VA in the absence of an organic cause and despite correction of refractive error if present.
- Exaggeration of the crowding phenomenon (scores better with single optotypes).
- Tolerance of a neutral density filter. Classically, in amblyopia, VA is reduced less by the addition of neutral density filters than in other causes of ↓VA. This phenomenon is better demonstrated in strabismic amblyopia than anisometropic amblyopia.
- Failure to respond, following compliance with treatment, should prompt reconsideration of the diagnosis.

Treatment

The critical period during which visual development may be influenced is up to 8y. At younger ages, there is more rapid response to treatment of amblyopia, but increased risk of inducing occlusion (or 'reversal') amblyopia in the covered eye.

The general approach is spectacle adaptation first and then either patching or atropine penalization.

Spectacle adaptation is the period of visual improvement which will occur from refractive correction alone and plateaus before 3mo of compliant glasses wear.

Occlusion

Adjust for age, acuity, and social factors. Practice is very variable, but, in general, longer episodes (time/d) and longer treatment (weeks of patching) have been used for older patients and those with worse VA. There is some evidence that there is little excess benefit in patching for >4h/d, and this is used as an upper limit in some centres.

Penalization

Atropinization is gaining an increased role. It may reduce the VA in the better eye to about 6/18 so is maximally effective if the amblyopic eye has VA >6/18. It is most effective when there is a hypermetropic refractive error in the atropine-treated eye.

Binocular single vision

In essence, BSV is the ability to view the world with two eyes, form two separate images (one from each eye), and yet fuse these centrally to create a single percept. The development of BSV depends on correct alignment and similar image clarity of both eyes from the neonatal period. Thus, a prerequisite for high-quality BSV is *normal retinal correspondence*, in which an image stimulates anatomically corresponding points on each retina with subsequent stimulation of functionally corresponding points in the occipital cortex producing a single perception. The points in space that project to these corresponding retinal points lie on an imaginary plane known as the *horopter*. Panum's fusional area is the narrow region around the horopter in which, despite disparity, points will be seen as single.

Levels of BSV

Characteristics of binocularity in order of increasing quality are:
1. *Simultaneous perception*: perception of a single image due to simultaneous formation of an image on each retina.
2. *Fusion*: stimulation of corresponding points in each retina allows central fusion of image.
3. *Stereopsis*: disparity in fused images gives a perception of depth.

Fusion has sensory and motor components. Whereas sensory fusion generates a single image from corresponding points, motor fusion adjusts eye position to maintain sensory fusion. Fusional reserves indicate the level beyond which these mechanisms break down (usually seen as diplopia) (see Table 17.3).

Table 17.3 Normal fusional reserves (approximate values)

Horizontal	Near	Convergent	32Δ	BO
		Divergent	16Δ	BI
	Distance	Convergent	16Δ	BO
		Divergent	8Δ	BI
Vertical			4Δ	BU and BD

Abnormalities of BSV

Confusion and diplopia

These are abnormalities of simultaneous perception.
• *Confusion* is the stimulation of corresponding points by dissimilar images, i.e. two images appear to be on top of each other.
• *Diplopia* is the stimulation of non-corresponding points by the same image, i.e. double vision.

Adaptive mechanisms

Adaptive mechanisms include suppression, abnormal retinal correspondence, and abnormal head posture.

- *Suppression*: a cortical mechanism to extinguish one of the images causing confusion (central suppression at the fovea) or diplopia (peripheral suppression). Monocular foveal suppression leads to amblyopia, if not treated; alternating suppression (between the two eyes) does not. The size and density of the suppression scotoma are variable. Density can be measured with a Sbiza filter bar by successively using denser filters in front of the better eye until fixation switch occurs.
- *Abnormal retinal correspondence (ARC)*: a cortical mechanism to remap anatomically non-corresponding points of each retina to stimulate functionally corresponding points in the occipital cortex to produce a single perception. It permits a degree of BSV despite a manifest deviation.
- *Abnormal head posture*: a behavioural mechanism that brings the field of single vision to a more central location.

Microtropia

The advantages of adaptive mechanisms are seen in a microtropia. This is a small manifest deviation, usually with a degree of BSV created by a combination of ARC, eccentric fixation, and a central suppression scotoma.

There is usually no movement on cover test (microtropia with identity), unless the eccentric fixation is not absolute (microtropia without identity).

Strabismus: assessment

Although the patient's (or parents') primary concern is likely to be the 'squint', it is imperative to step back and consider the whole child, their visual development, and their ophthalmic status. Assessment requires taking a history (visual/birth/developmental), appropriate measurement of vision, refraction and ophthalmic examination, and consideration of any amblyogenic risk. A 'squint' may be the first presentation of serious ocular pathology (e.g. retinoblastoma, cataract), and thus careful ophthalmic examination (including dilated fundoscopy) is essential.

Your general 'ophthalmic' approach to examining the child (see ➋ Ophthalmic assessment in a child (1), p. 768) must be adapted to include orthoptic examination and refraction. Turn the examination into a game wherever possible. Efficient examination helps reduce patient (and examiner) fatigue. Where there is concern about possible systemic abnormalities, refer the child to a paediatrician (see Table 17.4 and Table 17.5).

The individual tests are discussed as part of clinical methods (see ➋ Ocular motility examination, p. 28).

History

Table 17.4 An approach to assessing strabismus—history

Visual symptoms	Duration, variability and direction of squint, precipitants, fatiguability, associations (VA/development, diplopia, abnormal head position)
POH	Previous/current eye disease; refractive error
PMH	Obstetric/perinatal history; developmental history
SR	Any other systemic (especially CNS) abnormalities, in particular tumours or trauma
SH	Family support (for children)
FH	FH of strabismus/other visual problems
Dx	Drugs
Ax	Allergies

Examination

Table 17.5 An approach to assessing strabismus—examination

Observation	Whole patient (e.g. dysmorphic features, use of limbs, gait), face (e.g. asymmetry), abnormal head posture, globes (e.g. proptosis), lids (e.g. ptosis)
VA	Use age-appropriate test (see Table 1.1)
	Where quantitative not possible, grade ability to fix and follow (i.e. is it central, steady, and maintained?)
Visual function	Check for RAPD
Corneal reflexes	Check for normal position and symmetry
Cover test	Near/distance/far distance
Deviation	Measure with prism cover test or estimate with Krimsky or Hirschberg test; may be measured with synoptophore
Fusional reserves	Measure prism (horizontal and vertical) tolerated before diplopia/blurring
Motility	Ductions/versions (9 positions of gaze)
	Convergence
	Saccades
	VOR ('doll's eye movements' or 'manual spinning')
Accommodation	
Fixation	Fixation behaviour, normal vs eccentric, visuscope
Binocularity	Check for simultaneous perception with Worth 4-dot test or Bagolini glasses
Suppression	Detect with Worth 4-dot test, 4Δ base-out prism test, or Bagolini glasses
Correspondence	Detect anomalous retinal correspondence with Worth 4-dot, Bagolini glasses, or after-image test
Stereopsis	Measure level with Titmus, TNO, Lang or Frisby tests, or synoptophore
Refraction	Cycloplegic refraction (for children)
Ophthalmic	This should include dilated fundoscopy. Identify any cause of ↓VA or associated abnormalities
Systemic review	Notably cranial nerves, sensory/motor/cerebellar function, speech, mental state

Strabismus: outline

Is there a deviation?

Abnormalities of the face, globe, or retina may simulate an esodeviation. Angle kappa (the difference between the pupillary axis and the optical axis) is usually slightly positive. A negative angle occurs due to abnormal nasal positioning of the fovea (high myopia, traction, etc.). This simulates an esodeviation (see Table 17.6).

Esodeviations: the 'in-turning' eye

Esophoria vs esotropia

Phorias are latent deviations that are controlled by fusion. In certain circumstances (specific visual tasks, fatigue, illness, etc.), fusion can no longer be maintained and decompensation occurs. Tropias are manifest deviations. Some individuals may be phoric in one situation (e.g. for distance) and tropic in another (e.g. for near) (see Table 17.7).

Exodeviations: the 'out-turning' eye

Exophoria vs exotropia

Exophorias are latent deviations that are generally asymptomatic. However, when fusion can no longer be maintained, they decompensate with symptoms of asthenopia, blurred vision, photalgia (closing one eye in bright light), or diplopia.

Exotropias are manifest deviations that may be variable or constant. Fusion often allows control at one viewing distance, with a manifest deviation at a different viewing distance (i.e. simulated distance exotropia) (see Table 17.8).

Table 17.6 Causes of pseudosquint

	Pseudoesotropia	Pseudoexotropia
Specific	Epicanthic folds	Wide IPD
	Narrow IPD	Positive angle kappa
	Negative angle kappa	
General	Face—asymmetry	
	Globe—proptosis/enophthalmos	
	Pupils—miosis/mydriasis/heterochromia	

Table 17.7 Esotropia

Primary			
Accommodative	Varies with accommodation	Normal AC:A ratio Resolves with hypermetropic correction	*Fully accommodative esotropia*
		Normal AC:A ratio Improves with hypermetropic correction	*Partially accommodative esotropia*
		High AC:A ratio	*Convergence excess esotropia*
Non-accommodative	Constant	Starting <6mo	*Infantile esotropia*
		Starting >6mo	*Basic esotropia*
	Varies with fixation distance despite relief of accommodation	Near fixation only	*Near esotropia (non-accommodative convergence excess)*
		Distance fixation only	*Distance esotropia (divergence insufficiency)*
	Varies with time	Cyclical	*Cyclic esotropia*
Secondary		Organic ↓VA (e.g. media opacities)	*2° esotropia(sensory)*
Post-exo		Previous surgery for exotropia	*Consecutive esotropia*

Table 17.8 Exotropia

Primary	Constant	Starting <6mo	*Infantile exotropia*
		Starting >6mo	*Basic exotropia*
	Variable	Worse for near	*Near exotropia*
		Worse for distance High AC:A ratio	*Simulated distance exotropia*
		Worse for distance Normal AC:A ratio	*True distance exotropia*
Secondary		Organic ↓VA (e.g. media opacities)	*2° exotropia*
Post-eso		Develops with time in absence of fusion	*Consecutive exotropia*

Concomitant strabismus: esotropia (1)

Esotropia is a manifest inward deviation of the visual axes. It is the most common form of childhood strabismus in the UK. It may be primary, secondary (most commonly due to poor vision), or consecutive (after surgery for an exodeviation). Primary esotropias are classified as accommodative or non-accommodative.

As with all strabismus, the assessment should include refraction, full ophthalmic examination, and addressing of amblyopic risk. It is essential to detect/rule out underlying pathology (e.g. intraocular tumour or cataract) at the outset.

Accommodative esotropia

Accommodation and convergence are neurologically linked. The AC:A ratio is a measure of accommodative convergence per unit of accommodation and varies between individuals. Young, uncorrected hypermetropes accommodate to see clearly but may develop esotropia through convergent drive, particularly at near if they have a high AC:A ratio.

Accommodative esotropia usually presents between 1 and 5y of age. It may be refractive or non-refractive. If there is a refractive element, spectacles improve alignment. The non-refractive group often have an abnormally high AC:A ratio. There may, however, be overlap between these groups.

Refractive: fully accommodative esotropia

Esotropia fully corrected for distance and near by hypermetropic (usually +2 to +7D) correction; normal AC:A ratio; normal BSV if corrected; often intermittent initially (e.g. with fatigue, illness).

Treatment

Full hypermetropic correction; allow time for spectacle adaptation (the period over which vision improves in an amblyopic eye after onset of refractive correction, usually about 12wk); treat any associated amblyopia.

Refractive: partially accommodative esotropia

Esotropia only partially corrected by full hypermetropic correction; BSV absent or limited with ARC; ± bilateral IO overaction.

Treatment

Full hypermetropic correction; treat amblyopia; consider surgery if potential for BSV or for cosmesis (if cosmetically unacceptable despite glasses).

Non-refractive: convergence excess esotropia

Esotropia for near due to high AC:A ratio; ortho-/esophoric for distance; ↓BSV for near, normal BSV for distance; usually hypermetropic.

Treatment

Treat any associated hypermetropia or amblyopia; consider orthoptic exercises, executive bifocal glasses, surgery (bilateral MR recession and/or posterior fixation sutures), or miotics.

Non-accommodative esotropia

The commonest esotropia is the non-accommodative 'infantile esotropia' (*syn* congenital esotropia). Other non-accommodative esotropias usually present later, i.e. after 6mo of age.

Infantile esotropia

Esotropia presenting before 6mo, large angle (>30Δ), alternating fixation (so low risk of amblyopia), poor BSV potential, The following features often indicate congenital or infantile failure of binocularity development (but are not exclusively seen in infantile esotropia):

- *DVD (dissociated vertical deviation)*: an incomitant tendency for an occluded eye to elevate and extort which resolves on uncovering.
- *LN (latent nystagmus)*: a horizontal, conjugate jerk nystagmus apparent upon occluding one eye, with fast phase *away* from covered eye (ACE) (see → Nystagmus (1), p. 716).
- *IOOA (inferior oblique overaction)*: a hyperdeviation in adduction, greatest in the field of the IO.

Treatment

- Treat any associated amblyopia (e.g. occlusion of better eye, if not freely alternating); correct hypermetropia if >2D; surgery aims for ocular alignment by 18mo (with better potential BSV) and usually comprises symmetrical MR recessions (± LR resection).
- 1° or 2° surgery for significant IOOA may be required or surgical treatment of DVD (usually after horizontal correction).

Other non-accommodative esotropias

- *Basic esotropia*: constant esotropia for near and distance; treat surgically.
- *Near esotropia (non-accommodative convergence excess)*: esotropia for near, ortho/esophoria for distance but with normal AC:A ratio. *Treatment*, if any, is surgical (MR > LR).
- *Distance esotropia (divergence insufficiency)*: esophoria (or small esotropia) for near, larger esotropia for distance; associated with poor fusional divergence. **NB** Exclude bilateral VIn palsies. Treat with orthoptic exercises initially.
- *Cyclic esotropia—rare, periodic (e.g. alternate days)* : may proceed to constant esotropia.
- *Nystagmus blockage syndrome and Cianca syndrome*: have considerable overlap and are used to describe large angle infantile onset esotropia, nystagmus increasing on abduction, head turn towards the fixing eye.

Concomitant strabismus: esotropia (2)

2° esotropias

Esotropia may arise 2° to ↓VA, and thus full ocular examination is vital in all cases. Some esotropic syndromes may arise 2° to intracranial pathology.

- *Sensory deprivation*: 2° to unilateral/bilateral ↓VA.
- *Divergence paralysis*: 2° to tumour, trauma, or stroke. Unlike a bilateral VI palsy, the esodeviation remains constant or even decreases on lateral gaze.
- *Convergence spasm*: usually intermittent and associated with blurred vision (pseudomyopia due to associated accommodation) and pupillary miosis. If encouraged, ductions (in the absence of miosis) will be normal. In children, upper midbrain pathology must be excluded; however, this condition is often non-organic in origin. Attempt treatment with cycloplegia.

Pseudoesotropia

Various conditions may mimic an esotropia (see Table 17.6).

Concomitant strabismus: exotropia

Exotropia is a manifest outward deviation of the visual axes. It is the commonest form of childhood strabismus in South East Asia. It may be 1°, 2° (associated with poor vision), or consecutive (may follow an esotropia with time or after surgical correction). 1° exotropias may be constant or intermittent.

As with all strabismus, the assessment should include refraction, full ophthalmic examination, and addressing of amblyopic risk. It is essential to detect/rule out underlying pathology (e.g. intraocular tumour, cataract) at the outset.

Constant exotropia

Infantile (or congenital) exotropia

- Constant large angle exotropia, presenting at 2–6mo of age; often associated with ocular/CNS abnormalities; rarely exotropia is present at birth (congenital exotropia).
- *Treatment* is usually surgical (e.g. bilateral LR recessions ± MR resection).

Basic exotropia

- Constant exotropia for near and distance, presenting after 6mo of age.
- *Treatment* is usually surgical (e.g. unilateral LR recession + MR resection).

Intermittent exotropia

This is the commonest form of exotropia.

True distance exotropia

- Exotropia worse for distance, with normal AC:A ratio; rare.

Simulated distance exotropia

Exotropia worse for distance, as ↑AC:A ratio and/or fusional reserves fully or partially corrects for near; much more common than true distance exotropia. Tenacious proximal convergence (TPC) may mask a larger angle for near. TPC contamination of the near angle is removed/reduced by 1h of monocular occlusion ('patch test') or prism adaptation testing (PAT, in which base-in prisms are gradually increased on alternate cover testing to reveal a maximum angle). Similarly, the near exotropia may be increased by +3.0D lenses (or pharmacological cycloplegia) if patient is achieving near control by accommodative drive.

Treatment

- Myopic correction; treat amblyopia; orthoptic exercises; consider prisms, minus lenses, bifocals, botulinum toxin, or surgery for more severe cases.
- Surgery is generally performed before 5y of age.
- Unilateral LR recession and MR resection for simulated distance exotropia.
- Bilateral LR recession is traditionally reserved for true distance exotropia.

Near exotropia

Exotropia worse for near, often exophoric for distance; commoner in young adults who report aesthenopia or diplopia for reading; may be associated with myopia.

Treatment
- Full myopic correction.
- Orthoptic exercises if poor fusional reserves.
- Consider surgical treatment (e.g. bimedial MR resection).

Convergence insufficiency
- This is not an exotropia but is considered here as an important differential diagnosis.
- Near point of convergence greater than age normal; no manifest deviation but may be exophoric for near; commoner in teenagers who report aesthenopia.

Treatment
- Full myopic correction; convergence exercises (e.g. pencil push-ups); consider prisms, botulinum toxin, or surgery for more severe cases.

Secondary exotropia

Exotropia is the commonest strabismic outcome of ipsilateral ↓VA, although sensory esotropia may occur in young children (see ➲ Secondary esotropias, p. 748). Full ocular examination is vital in all cases.

Consecutive exotropia

With time, an esotropia, in which fusion has not been established, may become an exotropia. Surgical correction may also result in a consecutive exotropia.

Pseudoexotropia

Various conditions may mimic an exotropia (see Table 17.6).

Incomitant strabismus

In incomitant strabismus, the angle between the visual axes changes according to the direction of gaze. Incomitant strabismus is often grouped into neurogenic or mechanical types; however, the abnormality may occur in the brainstem, nerve, neuromuscular junction, muscle, or orbit.

In assessing incomitant strabismus, the aims are to identify the pattern and cause of the strabismus and address any actual or potential complications such as amblyopia, diplopia, or poor cosmesis (see Table 17.9).

Neurogenic strabismus

Underaction with reduced of saccadic velocity in the field of action of the paretic muscle (underaction may be more marked for versions than ductions); may develop full sequelae with time.

Investigations

• *Hess chart*: inner and outer fields are equally affected; full sequelae, if long-standing, comprise:
  • Underaction of palsied muscle.
  • Overaction of contralateral synergist (yoke muscle).
  • Underaction of contralateral antagonist.
• *Forced duction test*: full passive movement, unless chronic contracture of ipsilateral antagonist.
• *Further investigation and treatment*: according to cause (see ➔ Third nerve disorders, p. 700; ➔ Fourth nerve disorders, p. 702; ➔ Sixth nerve disorders, p. 704).

Mechanical strabismus

Limitation in direction away from restricted muscle (equal for ductions and versions); saccades of normal speed, but sudden early stop due to restriction; IOP increase in direction of limitation, often with globe retraction.

Investigations

• *Hess chart*: inner and outer fields are compressed in direction of limitation; outer affected more than inner; sequelae limited to overaction of contralateral synergist.
• *Forced duction test*: reduced passive movement in direction of limitation.
• *Further investigation and treatment*: according to cause (see ➔ Thyroid eye disease, pp. 600–4; ➔ Orbital fractures, pp. 112–14; ➔ Duane syndrome, p. 754; ➔ Congenital fibrosis of the EOM (CFEOM), p. 755).

Myasthenic strabismus

Variable and fatiguable ocular motility disturbance (any pattern), often associated with ptosis; sustained eccentric gaze of ≥1min or repeated saccades demonstrate fatigue; Cogan's lid twitch (ask patient to look down for 20s and then at object in the primary position; positive if lid 'overshoots'); may have systemic involvement (e.g. proximal muscle weakness, speech, breathing).

Investigations
- *Hess chart*: range from normal to highly variable/frustrating for operator.
- *Forced duction test*: full passive movement.
- *Ice-pack test*: measure ptosis; place ice, wrapped in a towel/glove, on the closed eyelid for 2min; remeasure ptosis; test significantly positive if ≥2mm improvement.
- *Further investigation (including Tensilon® test, serum antibodies, and EMG) and treatment* (see ➜ Myasthenia gravis, p. 722).

Myopathic strabismus

Gradual, symmetrical, non-fatiguable loss of movement associated with ptosis is seen in the inherited myopathies (e.g. CPEO group). Acquired myopathies (e.g. TED and myositis) may be regarded as causing a mechanical strabismus pattern.

Investigations
- *Hess chart*: symmetrical and proportional reduction in inner and outer fields.
- *Further investigation and treatment*: according to cause (see ➜ Myopathies, p. 726).

Table 17.9 Features of neurogenic and mechanical incomitant strabismus

	Neurogenic	Mechanical
Ductions/versions	Ductions > versions	Ductions ≈ versions
		May be painful
Saccades	Slow in paretic direction	Normal speed with sudden stop
Sequelae	Full sequelae with time	Sequelae limited to overaction of contralateral synergist
IOP change	IOP ± constant	IOP increases in the direction of limitation
Globe	No change	May retract on movement in direction of limitation
Hess	Inner and outer fields are proportional. The smaller field is of the affected eye (but sequelae reduce this effect with time)	Inner and outer fields are compressed in direction of limitation
Forced duction testing	Full passive movement (but antagonist contracture with time)	Reduced passive movement in direction of limitation

Restriction syndromes

Syndromic patterns of mechanical restriction are uncommon causes of strabismus. They are usually congenital, although later presentations may occur.

Duane syndrome

This is thought to arise due to aberrant co-innervation of LR and MR by IIIn, which may be associated with VI nucleus hypoplasia. It is usually sporadic but may be AD. The most common form (type I) preferentially affects girls (60%) and the left eye (60%). It is bilateral (usually asymmetric) in at least 20%.

Clinical features

- Retraction of globe (with reduction of palpebral aperture) on attempted adduction; ± up-/downshoots on attempted adduction; additional features according to type (see Table 17.10).
- *Systemic associations (30%)*: deafness, Goldenhar syndrome, Klippel–Feil syndrome, Wilderwank syndrome (Duane, Klippel–Feil, and deafness).

Classification

Types of Duane syndrome can be described according to the Huber classification (see Table 17.10), based on EMG findings, or the Brown classification, which was based on clinical features alone (see Table 17.11).

Table 17.10 Huber classification of Duane syndrome

Type	Frequency (%)	1° position	1° feature	Globe retraction
I	85	Eso or ortho	↓abduction	Mild
II	14	Exo or ortho	↓adduction	Severe
III	1	Eso or ortho	↓abduction and ↓adduction	Moderate

Table 17.11 Brown classification of Duane syndrome

Type	Key features
A	Limited abduction and adduction—adduction less limited than abduction
B	Limited abduction only
C	Limited abduction and adduction—adduction more limited than abduction

Treatment

Assess and treat for refractive error and potential amblyopia; reassure if managing well with minimal/mild compensatory head posture; most require no further intervention; consider prisms for comfort or to improve head position; consider surgery to improve BSV and improve head position.

Usual practice is uni-/bilateral MR recession for esotropic Duane and uni-/bilateral LR recession for exotropic Duane. Avoid LR resection, as it increases retraction more than improving abduction.

Brown syndrome

This is a mechanical restriction syndrome that Brown attributed to the SO tendon sheath. It appears to arise from structural or developmental abnormalities of the SO muscle/tendon or the trochlea, leading to limitation in the direction of its antagonist (IO) due to apparent failure of relaxation of the SO. In most cases, it is congenital (or at least infantile) and usually improves or resolves by 12y of age. Acquired cases may arise due to trauma, surgery (e.g. SO tuck, buckling, orbital), or inflammation (e.g. RA, sinusitis).

Clinical features

Limited elevation in adduction ± pain/click ('click' often occurs during resolution); limited sequelae (i.e. overaction of contralateral SR only); V pattern; may downshoot in adduction (swan dive); positive forced duction test.

Treatment

Reassure if managing well with minimal/mild compensatory head posture; it usually improves with age, and upgaze is less of an issue with increased patient vertical growth. Consider surgery if significant abnormal head posture or if strabismus in 1° position. The aim is to release the restriction, e.g. with SO tenotomy, until a repeated traction test demonstrates free rotation of the globe. Complications include SO palsy, and results are often disappointing. Acquired causes may be treated with periocular or oral corticosteroids.

Moebius syndrome (syn Möbius syndrome)

This rare sporadic congenital syndrome includes bilateral nuclear VI and VIIn palsies and often other neurological abnormalities. It is included here, as it may be associated with bilateral tight MR causing restriction, in addition to the horizontal gaze palsy.

Clinical features

- Bilateral failure of abduction; may be pure gaze palsy, or bilateral tight MR can lead to esotropia and positive forced duction test.
- *Systemic associations*: bilateral VII palsy (expressionless face), bilateral XII palsy (atrophic tongue), ↓IQ, digital abnormalities.

Congenital fibrosis of the EOM (CFEOM)

This rare congenital syndrome probably arises due to abnormal development of the oculomotor nuclei. Classic CFEOM (CFEOM1) is AD Chr 12q. There is bilateral restrictive ophthalmoplegia and ptosis, with an inability to elevate the globes above the midline. CFEOM2 is AR Chr 11q. There is bilateral ptosis, wide angle exotropia, and severe limitation of horizontal and vertical movements. In CFEOM3 Chr 16q, there are more variable motility defects.

Myopic strabismus fixus

This is a rare, well-recognized acquired syndrome seen in high myopes. The eye is often fixed in adduction with hypotropia. MRI shows deviated courses of the EOM, with globe prolapse between LR and SR. Surgery involves ipsilateral myopexy of LR and SR (after Yokoyama) ± MR recession.

Alphabet patterns

Horizontal deviations may vary in size according to vertical position. The deviation is measured at 30° upgaze, 1° position, and 30° downgaze, while fixing on a distance target. Significant incomitance is labelled according to the 'alphabet' patterns described in Table 17.12. The mechanism of alphabet strabismus varies from patient to patient. Postulated explanations include:

- Imbalance in tertiary abducting action of the obliques causes greatest effect in upgaze from inferior oblique overaction (IOOA) and downgaze from SO overaction.
- MR action causes greater adduction in depression, LR greater abduction in elevation.
- The adducting force from the vertical recti causes greatest adduction in their field of action.

V pattern

This is defined as a horizontal deviation, which is more divergent (or less convergent) in upgaze than in downgaze.

Clinical features

- *V-pattern esotropia*: usually arises from IOOA or SO palsy; it is also associated with antimongoloid palpebral fissures (perhaps altering the recti insertions). Patients may adopt a chin-down posture.
- *V-pattern exotropia*: usually arises from IOOA. Patients adopt a chin-up posture.

Treatment

Surgical treatment for significant V patterns may require IO weakening (if overacting), vertical translations of the horizontal recti (when operating on paired recti; upward for LR, downward for MR), and correction of the horizontal component (e.g. MR recession for esotropia; LR recession for exotropia). For both A and V patterns, the acronym *MALE* identifies the direction of vertical translation: *MR to Apex, LR to Ends*.

A pattern

This is defined as a horizontal deviation, which is less divergent (or more convergent) in upgaze than in downgaze.

Clinical features

- *A-pattern esotropia*: usually arises from SO overaction; it may also be associated with mongoloid palpebral fissures. Patients may adopt a chin-up posture.
- *A-pattern exotropia*: usually arises from SO overaction. Patients adopt a chin-down posture.

Treatment

Surgical treatment for significant A patterns may require SO weakening (if overacting) with a posterior disinsertion (division of posterior fibres, with preservation of the anterior torsion fibres), vertical translations of the horizontal recti (when operating on paired recti; upward for MR, downward for LR), and correction of the horizontal component (e.g. MR recession for esotropia; LR recession for exotropia).

Other patterns

Y pattern

Exotropia in upgaze only. It is usually due to IOOA, in which case it can be treated by IO weakening alone.

λ pattern

Exotropia in downgaze only. It may be treated by downward translation of both LR.

X pattern

Exotropia in upgaze and downgaze but straight in the 1° position. It usually arises in a long-standing exotropia with overaction of all four oblique muscles or is iatrogenic.

Table 17.12 Causes of alphabet patterns

		A pattern	V pattern
Esotropia	Obliques	SO+, IO–	IO+, SO–
	Horizontal recti	LR–	MR+
	Vertical recti	SR+, IR–	IR+, SR–
Exotropia	Obliques	SO+, IO–	IO+, SO–
	Horizontal recti	MR–	LR+
	Vertical recti	SR+, IR–	IR+, SR–

+, overaction, e.g. IO+ = inferior oblique overaction.

–, underaction, e.g. SO– = superior oblique underaction.

Strabismus surgery: general

Surgery should only be performed after full assessment and treatment of causative factors (e.g. refractive error) and consideration of non-surgical alternatives (e.g. orthoptic exercises, prisms, botulinum toxin).

The main role for surgery is where significant deviation remains despite appropriate refraction, where the deviation is stable over time, and where further improvement is not anticipated.

Surgical options involve weakening, strengthening, or transposing the EOM. These procedures adjust the effective pull of the muscle (by changing stretch and torque) and/or direction of action. The aim is to produce eyes that are straight in the 1° position and downgaze while keeping the largest possible field of BSV. It may be necessary to sacrifice BSV in lower priority gaze positions (e.g. upgaze) to achieve this (see Table 17.13).

General principles

- *Identify*: (1) direction of overaction; (2) any incomitance; and (3) any oblique muscle dysfunction.
- Weaken overacting muscle, and strengthen its antagonist.
- Balance these procedures to prevent induced incomitance.
- Treat pre-existing incomitance with an unbalanced procedure to have maximal effect in the area of greatest incomitance.
- Reduce oblique muscle overaction.

Adjustable sutures

Surgical results may be improved by the use of adjustable sutures. These can be used in conjunction with recessions, resections, and advancements. They are of particular value in redo operations, mechanical strabismus, and where there is a significant risk of post-operative diplopia.

Complications

Complications include suture granuloma, globe perforation (0.5%), slipped or lost muscle, anterior segment ischaemia, consecutive strabismus, post-operative diplopia, retinal detachment, and endophthalmitis.

Table 17.13 Overview of common strabismus operations

Operation	Muscles	Procedure
Weakening		
Recession	Recti or IO	Moves insertion closer to origin
Disinsertion	IO (SO)	Divide tendon (or part) at its insertion
Myotomy/myectomy	IO	Divide muscle (myotomy) or remove a portion of it (myectomy)
'Z' myotomy	Recti	Two alternate incisions of about 80% width; weakens muscle without changing insertion
Faden procedure	SR or MR (very rarely IR)	Post-equatorial fixation suture (non-absorbable); weakens action of muscle without affecting 1° position
Tenotomy	SO	Division of tendon (partial or total)
Strengthening		
Resection	Recti	Shortens/stretches muscle
Advancement	Recti/SO	Moves insertion anteriorly (often of previously recessed muscle)
Tuck	SO	Loop tendon
Transposition		
To improve abduction (particularly in complete VIn palsy)		
Toxin transposition	Toxin to MR, then SR and IR	Complete transposition of SR and IR to superior and inferior border of LR after toxin injection into MR.
Hummelsheim	SR and IR	Lateral half of SR and IR disinserted and attached to LR; MR may also be weakened
Jensen	LR, SR, and IR	Split LR, SR, and IR; suture neighbouring belly of LR + SR, and LR + IR together
To improve elevation		
Knapp	LR and MR	LR and MR disinserted and attached adjacent to SR insertion
To improve depression		
Inverse Knapp	LR and MR	LR and MR disinserted and attached adjacent to IR insertion
To improve intorsion		
Fells modification of Harado–Ito	SO	Disinsert anterior half of SO tendon; advance towards the superior margin of LR

Strabismus surgery: horizontal

The most common deviations (esotropia and exotropia) are horizontal and are therefore generally amenable to surgery on the horizontal recti (see Table 17.14). The most common procedure is a unilateral 'recess/resect', although the options range from single muscle procedures to bilateral (simultaneous or staged) surgery involving multiple muscles.

'Recess/resect'

An MR recession/LR resection will turn the visual angles away from each other, whereas an LR recession/MR resection will turn them towards each other. Estimation of the amount of surgical correction (in mm) required for the size of strabismus (in Δ) may be assisted by surgical tables. However, such tables are only a guide and should be modified by each surgeon, according to their own outcomes.

Table 17.14 Outline of horizontal muscle surgery

Recession	Local conjunctival peritomy
	Identify and expose muscle
	Free muscle from Tenon's layer
	Place two locking bites of an absorbable suture through the outer thirds of the muscle (e.g. 6-0 Vicryl®)
	Disinsert tendon, and measure recession
	Suture in new position, either directly to adjacent sclera or to the insertion (hang back technique)
	Close conjunctiva (e.g. 8-0 Vicryl®)
Resection	Local conjunctival peritomy
	Identify and expose muscle
	Free muscle from Tenon's layer
	Measure and place two locking bites of an absorbable suture (e.g. 6-0 Vicryl®), posterior to intended resection
	Resect desired length of muscle
	Suture remaining muscle to insertion
	Close conjunctiva (e.g. 8-0 Vicryl®)

Paediatric ophthalmology

Embryology (1)

The normal eye forms from an outpouching of the embryonic forebrain (neuroectoderm), with contributions from neural crest cells, surface ecto-derm, and, to a lesser extent, mesoderm. The interactions between these layers are complex, and failure may result in serious developmental abnor-malities (see ➔ Developmental abnormalities, pp. 810–14).

General

The developing embryo comprises three germinal layers: ectoderm, meso-derm, and endoderm (see Table 18.1). The ectoderm differentiates into outer surface ectoderm and inner neuroectoderm. The neuroectoderm continues to develop, forming first a ridge (neural crest), then a cylinder (neural tube), and finally vesicles within the cranial part of the tube, to form the fore-, mid-, and hindbrain (prosencephalon, mesencephalon, telenceph-alon). The neural crest cells also migrate to contribute widely to ocular and orbital structures.

The globe

The optic vesicle develops as a neuroectodermal protrusion of the pros-encephalon. It induces the overlying surface ectoderm to thicken into the lens placode. Then (*week 4*) both these structures invaginate to form a double-layered optic cup and lens vesicle, respectively. The cup is not com-plete but retains a deep inferior groove (optic fissure), in which mesodermal elements develop into the hyaloid and other vessels. Closure starts at the equator (*week 5*) and proceeds anteroposteriorly; failure of closure results in colobomas.

Anterior segment

Lens

The lens placode forms from surface ectoderm and invaginates to form the lens vesicle (*week 5*). At this point, it is a unicellular layer surrounded by a BM (the future capsule). This layer continues to divide throughout life. The posterior cells elongate and differentiate into primary lens fibres. The anterior cells migrate to the equator and elongate, forming the secondary lens fibres. These meet at the lens sutures.

Cornea

After separation of the lens vesicle, the surface ectoderm reforms as an epithelial bilayer with basement membrane. It is joined by three waves of migrating neural crest cells: the first (*week 6*) forms the corneal and trabecu-lar endothelium; the second (*week 7*) forms the stroma; the third (*also week 7*) forms the iridopupillary membrane. This process is strongly influenced by the interplay between the genes *PITX2* (4q25) and *FOXC1* (6p25).

Sclera

The sclera develops from a condensation of mesenchymal tissue situated at the anterior rim of the optic cup. This forms first at the limbus (*week 7*) and proceeds posteriorly to surround the optic nerve (*week 12*).

Iris, trabecular meshwork, and angle

The optic cup grows around the developing lens such that the cup rims meet the iridopupillary membrane. The optic cup rims give rise to the epithelial layers of the iris that are therefore continuous with the ciliary body and retina/RPE layers. The mesenchymal iridopupillary membrane develops into the iris stroma. The dilator and sphincter muscles are both neuroectodermal. The trabecular meshwork and Schlemm's canal arises from 'first wave' neural crest tissue located in the angle (*week 5*).

Ciliary body

The ciliary body forms as a kink in the optic cup rim (contributing an epithelial bilayer) and associated neural crest tissue (ciliary muscles and vasculature). The longitudinal musculature appears first (*month 3*); the circular musculature continues to develop after birth (*year 1 post-natal*).

Embryology (2)

Posterior segment

Retina

All retinal tissues develop from the optic cup (neuroectoderm). The inner layer of the cup divides into two zones: a superficial non-nucleated 'marginal zone' and a deeper nucleated 'primitive zone'. Mitosis and migration from the primitive zone leads to the formation of an inner neuroblastic layer (giving rise to Müller cells, ganglion cells, and amacrine cells) and an outer neuroblastic layer (giving rise to bipolar cells, horizontal cells, and primitive photoreceptor cells).

Familiar retinal organization starts with the formation of the ganglion cell layer and continues at the deeper levels with both cellular and acellular zones (nuclear and plexiform layers). This wave of retinal development starts at the posterior pole and proceeds anteriorly.

The photoreceptors arise from the outermost cells of the inner layer. Originally ciliated, these are replaced by distinctive outer segments. Cones develop first (*months 4–6*), rods later (*month 7–*). These photoreceptor cells project towards the outer layer of the cup. The outer layer (the RPE) thins to become one-cell thick and becomes pigmented, the first structure in the body to do so.

Retinal vasculature arises from the hyaloid circulation and spreads in an anterior wave, reaching the nasal periphery before the temporal periphery (*month 9*); it may therefore not be fully developed in premature infants.

Choroid

This vascular layer arises from: endothelial blood spaces around the optic cup; the extension of posterior ciliary arteries to join the primitive choroidal vasculature; and the consolidation of venous networks to form the four vortex veins.

Optic nerve

Vacuolization of cells within the optic stalk allows ganglion cell axons to grow through from the retina. The appearance of crossed and uncrossed fibres results in the formation of the chiasm (*months 2–4*). Myelination proceeds anteriorly from the LGN (*month 5*) to the lamina cribrosa (*month 1 post-natal*). The inner layer of the stalk gives rise to supportive glial cells; the outer layer contributes to the lamina cribrosa.

Vitreous

The 1° vitreous (*week 5*) forms in the retrolental space. It contains collagen fibrils, mesenchymal elements, and the hyaloid vasculature (which forms the tunica vasculosa lentis). Later (*week 6*), this is surrounded by the 2° vitreous and effectively forms Cloquet's canal.

The 2° vitreous is avascular, transparent, and is composed of very fine organized fibres. Failure of the vascular system to regress causes Mittendorf's dot, Bergmeister's papilla, persistent hyaloid artery, and persistent fetal vasculature (formerly known as persistent hyperplastic primary vitreous).

Traditionally, 'tertiary vitreous' was used to describe a relatively anterior condensation associated with the formation of lens zonules (which in fact arise from the ciliary body).

Nasolacrimal drainage system

This arises from a cord of surface ectoderm that is met by proliferating cords of cells, both from the lids above and from the nasal fossa below. Cannulation of the cord may be delayed distally, causing congenital obstruction. More commonly, there is simply an imperforate mucus membrane at the valve of Hasna that disappears within the first year.

Table 18.1 Summary of germinal layers

Ectoderm	Neuroectoderm	Iris epithelium
		Iris sphincter/dilator
		Ciliary body epithelium
		Neural retina
		RPE
		Optic nerve
	Neural crest	Corneal stroma
		Corneal endothelium
		Trabecular meshwork
		Ciliary musculature
		Sclera
		Choroidal stroma
	Surface ectoderm	Skin/lids
		Conjunctival epithelium
		Corneal epithelium
		Lacrimal gland
		Nasolacrimal duct
		Lens
Mesoderm		EOM
		Ocular vasculature

Genetics

Genetic disorders can be divided into single gene disorders, chromosome abnormalities (entire chromosomes or large parts of them are missing, duplicated, or otherwise altered), or multifactorial disorders (mutations in multiple genes coupled with environmental causes).

Single gene disorders may be autosomal, XL, or from abnormal mitochondrial DNA. Autosomal disorders obey the laws of segregation and independent assortment noted by Mendel, which results in predictable patterns of inheritance. More complex patterns arise from XL and mitochondrial disease. Most common conditions appear to be polygenic, with additional contributions from environmental factors.

Even for single gene disorders, the pattern of disease may be unpredictable. Such conditions may have incomplete *penetrance* (i.e. genotype present without the phenotype) or variable *expressivity* (i.e. wide range within the phenotype). In some conditions, *anticipation* may occur where succeeding generations develop earlier and more severe disease. This is due to 'triplet repeats', in which the number of repeats of a particular codon (e.g. CTG in the myotonic dystrophy gene) increases from generation to generation (see Table 18.2 and Table 18.3).

Inheritance patterns

Table 18.2 Inheritance patterns for single gene defect with 100% penetrance

AD	One parent carries the gene mutation and usually has the phenotype
	50% chance of inheriting the gene mutation and of developing the phenotype
AR	Both parents carry the gene mutation, but neither has the phenotype
	50% chance of inheriting one copy of gene mutation (i.e. carrier without the phenotype)
	25% chance of inheriting two copies of gene mutation and of developing the phenotype
XR	*If mother carries the gene with the mutation:*
	50% chance of inheriting the mutation and developing the phenotype for a son
	50% chance of inheriting the mutation and becoming a carrier for a daughter
	If father carries the mutation:
	100% chance of inheriting the mutation and becoming a carrier for a daughter
	0% chance of inheriting the gene for a son
Mitochondrial	The mother carries the gene with the mutation
	Variable probability of inheritance, dependent on proportion of abnormal mitochondria in the oocyte that becomes fertilized (heteroplasmy)

Table 18.3 Chromosomal locations of genes involved in selected ophthalmic disease (associated gene in parentheses)

1	Schnyder dystrophy (*UBIAD1*) Stargardt's disease/fundus flavimaculatus (*ABCA4*) LCA, RP (*RPE65*)
2	Oguchi disease 1 (*SAG*) Waardenburg syndrome (*PAX3*)
3	VHL (*VHL*) CSNB AD1 (*RHO*)
4	Anterior segment dysgenesis (*PITX2*)
5	Reis–Bucklers, Thiel–Behnke, granular, lattice I dystrophies (*TGFBI*)
6	Anterior segment dysgenesis (*FOXC1*)
7	Tritanopia (*OPN1SW*)
8	RP (*RP1*)
9	Tuberous sclerosis (*TSC1*) Oculocutaneous albinism type III (*TYRP1*)
10	Gyrate atrophy (*OAT*)
11	Best's macular dystrophy, AD vitreochoroidopathy (*BEST1*) Aniridia, Peter's anomaly (*PAX6*) Oculocutaneous albinism type I (*TYR*)
12	Meesman dystrophy (*KRT3*) CFEOM 1 (*KIF21A*)
13	Wilson's disease (*ATP7B*) Retinoblastoma (*RB1*)
14	
15	Marfan's syndrome (*FBN1*) Oculocutaneous albinism type II (*OCA2*)
16	Tuberous sclerosis (*TSC2*)
17	Neurofibromatosis-1 (*NF1*) Meesman (*KRT12*)
18	
19	Myotonic dystrophy (*DMPK*)
20	
21	Homocystinuria type 1 (*CBS*)
22	Neurofibromatosis-2 (*NF2*) Sorsby fundus dystrophy (*TIMP3*)
X	Ocular albinism type I (*GPR143*) XL RP (*RP2*) XL juvenile retinoschisis (*RS1*) Choroideraemia (*CHM*)

Ophthalmic assessment in a child (1)

The assessment of children requires a flexible approach, responsive to the child, parents, and extended family, to maximize the family's feeling of trust in their doctor. Without this trust, it is very difficult achieve diagnostic accuracy and institute appropriate treatment.

The awake child

Children often come to the clinic accompanied by a number of different people. Start by introducing yourself, and find out who everyone is—the person you assume to be mum may actually be an aunt while 'dad' may actually be the hospital interpreter.

The clinic is often a daunting place for a child, and it is important to make the process as pleasant as possible. Have simple indestructible toys available, and let them play with these while taking a history from them and the family. When examining the child, it is important not to be in a hurry. Start with the less daunting equipment and important clinical findings before trying the slit-lamp lest the child gets tired and disengage. A good system is to begin with the direct ophthalmoscope to look from a distance at red reflexes and pupils and then the retinoscope, if required, before using the indirect ophthalmoscope to examine the fundus. Most children will then be happy to be examined at the slit-lamp (standing, kneeling on the chair, or sitting on carer's knee), and, if this is not possible, consider a portable slit-lamp for the anterior segment.

IOP measurement is important, particularly in children using steroid drops. Rebound tonometry (eg. iCare) has dramatically reduced the need for IOP measurements under anaesthesia, and, where IOP is a critical finding, it should be measured early in the consultation. GAT may not be possible, although gentle attempts at each visit often desensitizes the child and will make it possible in the future.

Restraining the child to examine them, i.e. physically holding them still, is rarely indicated and should only be done after a detailed discussion with the parents and with their consent. The relationship between child and ophthalmologist may need to last for many years. This can be destroyed by one overzealous, frightening examination.

The anaesthetized child

An EUA may be indicated, if detailed examination is impossible with the child awake. It may be possible to perform this when the child is anaesthetized for a different procedure, so liaison with other specialists involved with the child is essential. The anaesthetist should have appropriate experience of paediatric anaesthesia. Inhalational anaesthesia progressively lowers IOP measurements with time (more than ketamine sedation).

The presence of the speculum may affect IOP and refraction. Tonometry (Tonopen, Perkins, or rebound devices) and retinoscopy should therefore be performed early in the examination before insertion of the speculum. Devices which only function with the barrel parallel to the floor may require the child's head to be turned 'ear to pillow'.

Examine the anterior segment with the portable slit-lamp, the operating microscope, and gonioscope. Examine the posterior segment with the direct and indirect ophthalmoscope. Consider A- and B-scan ultrasonography, corneal diameter measurements, keratometry (if planning cataract surgery), pachymetry, retinal photography (Retcam), fluorescein angiography, depending upon the clinical scenario.

Developmental milestones

It is often important that the paediatric ophthalmologist can evaluate in general terms whether a child has 'developmental delay'. If there is any suspicion that this is the case (see Table 18.4), refer to a paediatrician for further assessment.[1] Determining a child's developmental progress requires experience and expertise, and specialist help can avert unnecessary investigation (see Table 18.5).

Table 18.4 Warning signs of developmental delay

6wk	Unresponsive to visual or auditory stimuli
3mo	Unresponsive to social stimuli; lack of vocalization
6mo	Floppiness; poor head control; not reaching for objects
12mo	Not weight-bearing; not using gestures to communicate
18mo	Not walking; no words
2y	Not running; not joining two words
3y	Not climbing stairs; not communicating with words

Table 18.5 Visual milestones

6wk	Can fix and follow a light source, smiling responsively.
3mo	Can fix and follow a slow target, and converge
6mo	Reaches out accurately for toys
2y	Picture matching
3y	Letter matching of single letters (e.g. Sheridan Gardiner)
5y	Snellen/LogMAR chart by matching or naming

---

1. A useful review of the assessment of development in children is: Bellman M *et al*. Developmental assessment of children. *BMJ* 2013;**346**:e8687.

Ophthalmic assessment in a child (2)

See Table 18.6 for taking an ophthalmic history and Table 18.7 for taking an examination.

Table 18.6 Taking an ophthalmic history in a child

History	
Visual symptoms	History of poor visual behaviour for their age, strabismus, nystagmus, head nodding, red eye, epiphora, photophobia, asymmetry of pupils/corneas/ globes/red reflexes—sometimes first noted in photographs
POH	Previous/current eye disease; refractive error
PMH	Obstetric/perinatal history; developmental history; document which other health professionals are involved in their care
SR	Any other systemic (especially CNS, including hearing*) abnormalities
SH	Family support
FH	Family history of strabismus/other visual problems
Dx	Drugs
Ax	Allergies

* Up to 50% children with moderate/severe sensorineural deafness have an associated ophthalmic problem.

Table 18.7 An approach to an ophthalmic examination in a child

Examination	
VA	Select test according to age (see Table 1.1); where quantitative not possible, grade ability to fix and follow (i.e. is it central, steady, and maintained?)
Visual function	Check for RAPD, binocularity, stereopsis, suppression, and retinal correspondence (see ➲ Assessment of vision: clinical tests in children and tests of binocular status, p. 8)
Cover test	Near/distance/prism cover test
Motility	Ductions, versions, convergence, saccades, doll's eye movements
Accommodation	AC/A ratio
BSV	Level of BSV
Fixation	Fixation behaviour, visuscope
Refraction	Cycloplegic refraction
Orbit	Proptosis, inflammation, masses
Lids	Ptosis, skin crease, lid lag, additional skin folds, puncta
Conjunctiva	Inflammation, adhesions, subtarsal papillae
Cornea	Diameter, thickness, opacity, staining, 'brightness of reflex'
AC	Flare, cells, hypopyon, hyphaema, depth
Gonioscopy	(may require EUA) angle, dysgenesis
Iris	Coloboma, anisocoria, polycoria, corectopia, Lisch nodules, transillumination, peripheral iridectomy
Lens	Lens opacity, shape, position
Tonometry	Applanation (may require EUA) rebound or digital
Vitreous	Hyaloid remnants, inflammation, optically empty
Optic disc	Size, cup, congenital anomaly, oedema, pallor
Fundus	Macula, vessels, retina (e.g. tumours, inflammation, dystrophies, exudation)
Systemic review	For dysmorhpic features (including face, ears, teeth, hair), developmental progress or any other systemic abnormalities

The child who does not see

Worldwide, there are over 1.5 million children who are blind or severely visually impaired. Only 6.5% live in the more affluent regions of the world. Major causes include inherited abnormalities (e.g. cataracts, glaucoma, retinal dystrophies), intrauterine insults (e.g. infection), and acquired problems (e.g. ROP, trauma).

The ophthalmologist's primary aim—best possible vision for the child—must be seen in the context of the child's overall health, quality of life, and family support. Likewise, the ophthalmologist's contribution should be seen in the context of the multidisciplinary team, which may include paediatricians, optometrists, orthoptists, primary care physicians, specialist nurses, social workers, and teachers. The challenge to provide best possible care for the child (and family) will depend on the following factors.

Disability

Is the visual impairment the only problem, or are there associated disabilities? These may range from mild developmental delay (e.g. motor, speech, social) to profound neurological or systemic abnormalities. In some severe diseases, life expectancy may also be considerably reduced. Such children require the full benefit of the multidisciplinary team, usually coordinated by a paediatrician.

Treatment

What treatment might be possible now or in the future? Be realistic about what is and what is not currently possible. Ensure best visual potential with refraction, visual aids, and other supportive measures. Where more invasive treatment is indicated, ensure that the parents are fully aware of the risks, realistic outcome, and the extent of care that they will need to give in the perioperative period (e.g. drops, occlusion, CL, frequent clinic visits, etc.).

Equipment

What equipment will help the child function best at home and at school? Reading may require Braille or large print books (usually beneficial if reading vision worse than N10). Normal-sized print may be read by closed circuit television (CCTV) magnification or by a scanner attached to a computer, which has a magnified display facility or which has optical character recognition with a speech synthesizer. The ease of use of standard computer systems has been revolutionized, since accessibility options became a standard feature of computer operating systems (e.g. Windows®).

Schooling

Will the child manage best in a specialist school (for the blind or partially sighted) or in a mainstream school (with specialist teacher support)? This is usually determined by the level of visual impairment, any associated disabilities, and the availability of resources locally. In the UK, the 1981 Education Act signalled the start of a trend to encourage mainstream schooling, where possible.

Resources

How much help (practical and financial) are the family and/or state able to provide? Social workers should ensure that the parents are receiving appropriate financial benefits. Community paediatricians may be invaluable in coordinating local resources. Support organizations often provide help, including advice and emotional support for the parents.

Social

Is the disability accepted by the family/community? The diagnosis may stretch family relationships to breaking point. Siblings may become jealous of the extra attention the child needs. In some communities, blindness is regarded as a stigma. This may adversely affect family dynamics and hinder the child's wider social interactions.

Implications

Are other family members or future siblings at risk of developing the disease or of being carriers? Genetic disease may be emotive, and counselling requires time, patience, and often multiple consultations. The parents may feel guilty about 'passing on' an inherited disease to their child.

Prognosis

Is the visual impairment stationary or progressive? Parents may want to know the probable impact on navigation, education, work, and driving. Where possible, balance the negative (what they will not be able to do) with the positive (what they will be able to do). Stress that our knowledge is limited and that such prognoses are a 'best guess'.

Child abuse

You have a legal duty of care towards any child you see. If you have a concern or suspicion of possible abuse, it is your responsibility to act.

Concern might relate to injuries that are inconsistent with the mobility of the child or with the reported mechanism, histories that are inconsistent with each other or evolve with time, or an unusual relationship between carer and child. All National Health Service (NHS) trust hospitals that deal with children have a named doctor and named nurse with particular expertise in child protection. All suspicions should be discussed with the named doctor and hospital social worker. It is not acceptable to ignore concerns or to assume 'someone else' will act.

On occasion, the ophthalmologist may be asked to examine a child as part of child protection investigations. This should be performed by the most senior ophthalmologist available. It is important to complete as full an examination as possible. Carefully document all findings, including negative ones, and, when describing retinal haemorrhages, include number, size, location, and type (i.e. depth) of haemorrhages with accurate drawings.

Photographs may be helpful; if a digital system is used, an unmodified printout should be made at the time and signed by two witnesses. If a report is required, this should be phrased in terms comprehensible to an educated lay person and include your full name, qualifications, and the situation in which you saw the child.

Retinal haemorrhages and shaken baby syndrome (SBS)

Shaken baby syndrome

Retinal haemorrhages in the absence of bony injury or external eye injury may arise from severe shaking of young children (SBS). They are not diagnostic of abuse and must be taken in the context of the whole child.

Alternative mechanisms

The Child Abuse Working Party of the Royal College of Ophthalmologists[2] have considered other putative mechanisms of retinal and intracranial haemorrhage. They conclude:

- *Normal handling (e.g. vigorous play)*: 'it is highly unlikely that the forces required to produce retinal haemorrhage in a child less than 2 years of age would be generated by a reasonable person during the course of (even rough) play, or in an attempt to rouse a sleeping or unconscious child.'
- *Short-distance falls*: 'in a child with retinal haemorrhages and subdural haemorrhages who has not sustained a high velocity injury and in whom other recognised causes of such haemorrhages have been excluded, child abuse is much the most likely explanation...Rarely accidental trauma may give rise to a similar picture.'

- *High cervical injuries*: cervical injuries alone do not result in retinal bleeding, unless combined with circulatory collapse.
- *Hypoxia*: acute hypoxia from transient apnoea has not been shown to result in the SBS picture, unless combined with circulatory collapse.
- *Intracranial bleeding*: Terson syndrome (retinal haemorrhages 2° to intracranial bleeding) is rare in children, and any haemorrhages tend to be concentrated around the disc.

2. Watts P, Child maltreatment guideline working party of Royal College of Ophthalmologists UK. Abusive head trauma and the eye in infancy. *Eye*. 2013; **27**: 1227–9.

Common clinical presentations: vision and movement

There are a number of common reasons for parents to seek ophthalmic advice. The underlying diseases range from the innocuous to the blinding and/or fatal. A complete ophthalmic (and usually systemic) examination should be performed in all cases. Tables 18.8–18.18 indicate the main causes of these clinical presentations, their key features, and/or a cross reference to further information.

The child who does not see

Unilateral visual loss may not be noticed by parents until picked up at screening or during investigation for an associated abnormality (usually strabismus). Bilateral visual loss will be apparent in the child's visual behaviour. In addition, children who have bilateral poor vision from an early age often have nystagmus or roving eye movements, although this does not occur in patients with retrochiasmal lesions.

- *Examination*: orthoptic, refractive, ophthalmic, neurological ± systemic (as indicated).

Table 18.8 Poor vision: outline of causes

General	Specific
Refractive	Myopia, hypermetropia, astigmatism
Cornea	Opacity, oedema, abnormal curvature, or size
AC	Inflammation
Lens	Cataract, subluxation, lenticonus
Vitreous	Persistent fetal vasculature, inflammation, haemorrhage
Retina	Coloboma, ROP, detachment, dysplasia, dystrophy, albinism
Macula	Hypoplasia, dystrophy, oedema, inflammation, scarring, traction
Optic nerve	Inherited optic atrophy, compression, infiltration, inflammation, hypoplasia
CNS	Hypoxia, inflammation, hydrocephalus, compression, delayed visual maturation
Other	Amblyopia, delayed visual maturation, functional

Abnormal eye alignment

Strabismus is common, affecting about 2% of children. While many cases are detected by parents, significant deviations may be missed due to their size, intermittent nature, or compensatory head posture. Conversely, a number of factors may give the appearance of a squint in a perfectly orthophoric child—'pseudostrabismus'.

- *Examination*: orthoptic, refractive, ophthalmic, neurological ± systemic (as indicated).

Table 18.9 Abnormal ocular alignment: outline of causes and key features

Strabismus	Intermittent or manifest misalignment of eyes that may be horizontal, vertical, or torsional
Pseudostrabismus	Consider epicanthal folds, asymmetry of face, globes (proptosis/enophthalmos), or pupils, abnormal IPD or abnormal angle kappa

Abnormal eye movements

Abnormal supplementary eye movements may occur as an isolated phenomenon or 2° to ocular or systemic disease (usually CNS pathology). They may be broadly divided into nystagmus or saccadic abnormalities.

- *Examination*: orthoptic, refractive, ophthalmic, neurological ± systemic (as indicated).

Table 18.10 Abnormal eye movements: outline of causes and key features

Nystagmus	Slow movement away from fixation, corrected by fast movement (jerk nystagmus) or another slow movement (pendular nystagmus)
Saccadic abnormalities	Fast movement away from fixation, corrected by fast movement immediately (oscillation, e.g. opsoclonus, ocular flutter) or after delay (intrusion)

Common clinical presentations: red eye, watering, and photophobia

Red (see Table 18.11) or watering eyes (see Table 18.12) are among the commonest ocular presentations in primary care. Often these are relatively benign conditions, many of which may be successfully treated by GPs. However, in the presence of atypical features (particularly visual symptoms), more serious diagnoses should be considered. The presence of photophobia (also see Table 18.13) is usually an indication of more severe ocular pathology.

- *Examination*: ophthalmic ± refractive, neurological, systemic (as indicated).

Red eye(s)

Table **18.11** Red eye: causes and key features

Normal VA	
Conjunctivitis (infective, allergic, chemical)	Gritty, often itchy, discharge, diffuse superficial injection ± lid papillae/follicles
FB	FB sensation, FB visible or in fornix/subtarsal, local injection, corneal abrasions (if subtarsal FB)
Episcleritis	Mild local pain, sectoral superficial injection (constricted by phenylephrine)
Scleritis	Severe pain, deep often diffuse injection; complications may lead to ↓VA
Phlyctenulosis	Gritty pain, localized injection, conjunctival/corneal nodule
Vascular malformation	Abnormal conjunctival blood vessels, usually chronic, ± systemic vascular abnormalities
Reduced VA	
Corneal abrasion/erosion	Photophobia, watering, sectoral/circumlimbal injection, epithelial defect
Keratitis	Photophobia watering, circumlimbal injection, corneal infiltrate ± epithelial defect ± AC activity
Glaucoma (acute ↑IOP)	Photophobia, watering, corneal oedema, ↑IOP anterior segment/angle abnormalities
Anterior uveitis (acute)	Photophobia, watering, KPs, AC activity ± PS
Endophthalmitis	Pain, floaters, watering, diffuse deep injection, inflammation (vitreous > AC), hypopyon, chorioretinitis

Watering eyes

Table 18.12 Watering eye: causes and key features

Increased tears	
Blepharitis (posterior)	Chronic gritty, irritable eyes, poor tear film quality, meibomianitis
Conjunctivitis (infective, allergic, chemical)	Gritty, often itchy, discharge may be sticky, diffuse superficial injection ± lid papillae/follicles
FB	FB sensation, FB visible or in fornix/subtarsal, local injection, corneal abrasions (if subtarsal FB)
Corneal abrasion/erosion	Photophobia, sectoral/circumlimbal injection, epithelial defect
Keratitis	Photophobia, sectoral/circumlimbal injection, corneal infiltrate ± epithelial defect ± AC activity
Glaucoma (acute ↑IOP)	Photophobia, injection, corneal oedema, ↑IOP ± anterior segment/angle abnormalities
Anterior uveitis	Photophobia, circumlimbal injection, KPs, AC activity ± PS
Decreased drainage	
Nasolacrimal duct obstruction	Chronic watering (may have sticky discharge) without other ocular signs ± lacrimal sac swelling

Photophobia

Table 18.13 Photophobia: causes and key features

Anterior segment disease	
Corneal abrasion/erosion	Watering, sectoral/circumlimbal injection, epithelial defect
Keratitis	Watering, circumlimbal injection, corneal infiltrate, epithelial defect ± AC activity
Anterior uveitis (acute)	Watering, circumlimbal injection, KPs, AC activity ± PS
Glaucoma (acute ↑IOP)	Watering, injection, corneal oedema, ↑IOP anterior segment/angle abnormalities
Inadequate iris sphincter	Complete/partial absence of tissue (e.g. aniridia, coloboma), mydriasis, or non-pigmentation (albinism)
Posterior segment disease	
Endophthalmitis	Pain, floaters, watering, diffuse deep injection, inflammation (vitreous > AC), chorioretinitis, hypopyon
Retinal dystrophies	Cone deficiencies (achromatopsia, blue cone monochromatism) or later-onset dystrophies
CNS disease	
Meningitis/encephalitis	Fever, headache, neck stiffness, altered mental state, neurological dysfunction, normal ocular examination

Common clinical presentations: proptosis and globe size

Abnormalities of the whole globe are usually congenital and represent developmental abnormalities. Abnormal protrusion of the eye (proptosis; see Table 18.14) usually represents an acquired, progressive disease.

Proptosis

Abnormal protrusion of the eye (proptosis) is uncommon but usually signifies severe orbital pathology. An acute onset in a systemically unwell child may represent orbital cellulitis, an ophthalmic emergency. Orbital tumours usually present with more gradual proptosis, although rhabdomyosarcoma is well known to present acutely, mimicking orbital cellulitis (see Table 18.15).

Table 18.14 Proptosis: causes and key features

Infection	
Orbital cellulitis	Febrile, systemically unwell, with acute pain, lid swelling, restricted eye movements, ↓VA
Inflammation	
Idiopathic orbital inflammatory disease	Acute pain, lid swelling, conjunctival injection, intraocular inflammation, and ↓VA; diffuse orbital disease vs localized (e.g. myositis or dacroadenitis)
TED	Pain, conjunctival injection, lid retraction, restrictive myopathy, ↓VA; usually older children
Vasculitis	Usually present acutely and systemically unwell (e.g. GPA, PAN)
Tumours	
Acquired, e.g. neuroblastoma	Proptosis ± pain, ↓VA, abnormal eye movements; usually gradual onset, but some (e.g. rhabdomyosarcoma) may present acutely
Congenital, e.g. dermoid cysts	Superficial lesions present early as a round lump; deep lesions may cause pain and gradual proptosis
Vascular anomalies	
Congenital orbital varices	Intermittent proptosis exaggerated by Valsalva manoeuvre or forward posture
Carotid–cavernous fistula	Arterialized conjunctival vessels, chemosis ± bruit; usually traumatic in children
Bony anomalies	
Sphenoid dysplasia	Pulsatile proptosis, encephalocele, associated with neurofibromatosis-1
Craniosynostosis	Premature fusion of sutures, resulting in characteristic skull abnormalities
Other	
Pseudoproptosis	Consider ipsilateral large globe or lid retraction, contralateral enophthalmos or ptosis, facial asymmetry, shallow orbits

Table 18.15 Orbital tumours of childhood (selected)

Congenital	
Choristoma	e.g. dermoid cysts, teratoma
Acquired	
Optic nerve	e.g. glioma
Vascular	e.g. capillary haemangioma, lymphangioma
Infiltrative	e.g. myeloid leukaemia, histiocytosis
Other	e.g. rhabdomyosarcoma
Metastases	e.g. neuroblastoma, nephroblastoma (Wilms' tumour), Ewing's sarcoma

Abnormal eye size

Abnormalities of globe size usually result from abnormalities of development, although it may arise 2° to ocular disease (e.g. buphthalmos in glaucoma). While severe forms may be obvious from simple observation, milder isolated aberrations of size may only be obvious as an axial refractive error (see Table 18.16).

Table 18.16 Abnormal eye size: causes and key features

Abnormally large eye	
Axial myopia	Mild (physiological) to severe and progressive (pathological) ↑length; ± other ocular abnormalities
Buphthalmos	Diffusely large eye (with megalocornea) associated with glaucoma
Megalophthalmos	Diffusely large eye (with megalocornea) without glaucoma; ± other ocular abnormalities
'Pseudolarge eye'	Consider proptosis or abnormally small contralateral eye
Abnormally small eye	
Microphthalmos	Diffusely small eye (axial length 2 SD < normal) ± ocular/ systemic anomalies
Nanophthalmos	Microphthalmos with microcornea, normal-sized lens, and abnormally thick sclera
Phthsis bulbi	Acquired shrinkage of the eye due to chronic ocular disease
'Pseudosmall eye'	Consider ipsilateral ptosis or enophthalmos, or abnormally large contralateral eye

Common clinical presentations: cloudy cornea and leucocoria

Opacification of the cornea, lens, or posterior structures is usually associated with poor vision and may indicate serious, even life-threatening, pathology (see Table 18.17).

Cloudy cornea

Corneal opacities may be focal (either central or peripheral) or diffuse. They may be an isolated finding, associated with other ocular abnormalities, or part of an inherited syndrome. In terms of onset, they may be congenital, acquired at birth, or develop during childhood.

Table 18.17 Corneal opacities: causes and key features

Diffuse	
Birth trauma	Forceps injury may induce ruptures in Descemet's membrane (usually unilateral with vertical break)
Glaucoma (acute ↑IOP)	Corneal oedema, ↑IOP, watering, injection ± anterior segment/angle abnormalities, Haab striae
Keratitis (infective, allergic, exposure)	Photophobia, watering, circumlimbal injection, corneal infiltrate ± epithelial defect ± AC activity
Corneal dystrophies	Clinical pattern varies but may be evident from birth (e.g. congenital hereditary endothelial dysfunction)
Metabolic	Bilateral corneal clouding with systemic abnormalities in some mucopolysaccharidoses
Central	
Peter's anomaly	Congenital, usually bilateral central opacities, adhesions to iris or lens
Peripheral	
Sclerocornea	Bilateral (often asymmetric), peripheral / total opacification with vascularization ± other corneal/angle anomalies
Limbal dermoid	Solid white mass that may involve peripheral cornea; rarely bilateral and 360° round limbi
Posterior embryotoxon	Peripheral opacity due to anteriorly displaced Schwalbe's line ± other angle/ocular abnormalities

Leucocoria

All patients with leucocoria must be assessed for the possibility of retinoblastoma. Congenital cataracts are generally easily identified. Other conditions may be less readily differentiated from retinoblastoma, most commonly persistent fetal vasculature syndrome, Coats' disease, toxocara infection, and ROP (see Table 18.18).

Table 18.18 Leucocoria: causes and key features

Lens	
Cataract	Lens opacity: stationary or progressive; isolated, or associated with other ocular/ systemic abnormalities
Vitreous	
Persistent fetal vasculature syndrome	Variable persistence of fetal vasculature/ hyaloid remnants; often microphthalmic; usually unilateral
Inflammatory cyclitic membrane	Fibrous membrane behind the lens arising from the ciliary body due to chronic intraocular inflammation
Retina	
Retinoblastoma	Retinal mass of endophytic, exophytic, or infiltrating type; may spread to anterior segment, orbit, etc.
Coloboma	Developmental defect resulting in variably sized defect involving disc, choroid, and retina
Coats' disease	Retinal telangiectasia with exudation ± ERD
ROP	Early cessation of peripheral retinal vascularization due to prematurity causes fibrovascular proliferation
Familial exudative retinopathy	Avascular peripheral retina, retinal folds and detachment, peripheral retinal exudates
Incontinentia pigmenti	Abnormal peripheral retinal vascularization due to inherited defect causes ROP-like picture
Retinal dysplasia	Grey vascularized mass from extensive gliosis (e.g. Norrie disease, Patau syndrome, etc.)
Toxocara	Unilateral granuloma or endophthalmitis

Intrauterine infections (1)

Congenital infections have a variable effect on morbidity and mortality, dependent on the infecting organism and the stage of gestation of the fetus. Overall, however, ocular morbidity is common. Likely organisms can be remembered by the acronym 'TORCH': toxoplasma, other (e.g. syphilis, lymphocytic choriomeningitis virus, West Nile virus), rubella, CMV, herpes family (HSV and VZV).

Congenital toxoplasmosis

The impact of transplacental infection by toxoplasma is greatest early in pregnancy. The spectrum of disease ranges from an asymptomatic peripheral patch of retinochoroiditis (often an incidental finding years later) to a blinding endophthalmitis. Antenatal screening for toxoplasmosis is no longer used routinely, as there are concerns about the reliability of the test and no clear evidence that treatment reduces mother to fetus transmission. Pregnant women should be informed of 1° prevention measures to avoid toxoplasmosis infection such as not handling cat faeces and not eating undercooked meat or unpasteurized goat's cheese (see Table 18.19).

Table 18.19 Clinical features of congenital toxoplasmosis

Ocular	Retinochoroiditis (more commonly bilateral and affecting the macula than in acquired disease)
	Cataract, microphthalmos, strabismus
Systemic	Hydrocephalus, intracranial calcification, hepatosplenomegaly

Congenital rubella

Rubella has declined since the advent of rubella vaccination in 1969. The virus is well known for its teratogenic effects (especially with early infection). It also has remarkable ongoing pathogenicity, with interstitial pneumonitis and pancreatic inflammation within the first year, virus shedding up to 2y of age, and panencephalitis as late as 12y of age. Virus within the lens may explain the intense uveitis that can follow cataract surgery (see Table 18.20).

Table 18.20 Clinical features of congenital rubella

| Ocular | Pigmentary retinopathy with normal electrodiagnostics (commonest feature), nuclear cataract, microphthalmos, glaucoma (congenital or infantile), corneal clouding (keratitis and/or ↑IOP) |
| Systemic (early/late) | Congenital heart disease, sensorineural deafness, anaemia, thrombocytopenia, bone abnormalities, hepatitis, CNS abnormalities (e.g. encephalitis) |

Congenital syphilis

Having been in decline, syphilis has made a comeback in recent years (see
➲ Syphilis, p. 460). The early stage is characterized by inflammation. Many
of the later manifestations are direct sequelae of this process. Others
(such as interstitial keratitis) may be an immunological phenomenon (see
Table 18.21).

Table 18.21 Clinical features of congenital syphilis

Early disease (<2y of age)	
Ocular	Chorioretinitis and retinal vasculitis (result in the characteristic salt-and-pepper fundus), glaucoma, cataract, anterior uveitis
Systemic	Mucocutaneous rash, periostitis and osteochondritis, jaundice, pneumonia, anaemia
Late disease (>2y of age)	
Ocular	Interstitial keratitis* (usually presents at 5–20y of age), optic atrophy
Systemic	Saddle nose, frontal bossing, sabre shins, Hutchinson's teeth,* scoliosis, hard palate perforation, sensorineural hearing loss*

* The combination of these three signs is known as Hutchinson's triad.

Congenital lymphocytic choriomeningitis virus

Very likely underdiagnosed as congenital cases only recently recognized
(1993). An arena virus with rodents as reservoir causing outbreaks of disease in which pet hamsters may act as vector (see Table 18.22).

Table 18.22 Clinical features of congenital lymphocytic choriomeningitis
virus

Ocular	Retinochoroiditis (similar to toxoplasmosis), optic atrophy, nystagmus, strabismus, cataract, microphthalmos
Systemic	Features at birth rare (meningitis, hepatosplenomegaly), later mental retardation, seizures

Intrauterine infections (2)

Congenital CMV (See Table 18.23)

Although commonly asymptomatic, congenital infection with CMV may cause severe systemic disease. Retinitis tends to be unifocal, more akin to toxoplasmosis than adult CMV retinitis.

Table 18.23 Clinical features of congenital CMV

Ocular	Retinitis (focal), keratitis, cataracts, microphthalmos, optic atrophy
Systemic	Intrauterine growth restriction (IUGR), microcephaly, hydrocephalus, intracranial calcification, hepatosplenomegaly, thrombocytopenia, deafness (which may be progressive)

Congenital HSV (See Table 18.24)

It is rare for HSV to be acquired at the intrauterine stage; more commonly HSV is acquired at birth from maternal genital lesions. HSV2 > HSV1. **NB** Systemic aciclovir for ocular surface disease in neonates limits dissemination. Untreated neonatal infection has a high mortality rate.

Table 18.24 Clinical features of congenital HSV

Ocular	Rash involving lids, conjunctivitis, keratitis, chorioretinitis, cataracts
Systemic	Vesicular rash, mouth sores, jaundice, hepatosplenomegaly, pneumonitis, meningoencephalitis

Congenital VZV (See Table 18.25)

1° varicella infection in the first trimester rarely causes embryopathy. Unusually, the rate of congenital disease is higher if maternal disease is in the second trimester.

Table 18.25 Clinical features of congenital VZV

Ocular	Chorioretinitis (similar to toxoplasmosis), cataracts, microphthalmos, unilateral Horner's syndrome
Systemic	Neuropathic bladder

Ophthalmia neonatorum

Ophthalmia neonatorum is defined as a conjunctivitis occurring within the first month of life. Organisms are commonly acquired from the birth canal. The main risk factor is therefore the presence of sexually transmitted disease in the mother. Ophthalmia neonatorum affects up to 12% of neonates in the Western world and up to 23% in developing countries. It is potentially sight-threatening and may cause systemic complications (see Table 18.26).

Gonococcal neonatal conjunctivitis

Clinical features

- Hyperacute (within 1–3d of birth), with severe purulent discharge, lid oedema, chemosis ± pseudomembrane ± keratitis.

Investigation

- Prewet swab or conjunctival scrapings: immediate Gram stain (Gram-negative diplococci), culture (chocolate agar), and sensitivities.

Treatment

- Cefotaxime 100mg/kg (max 1g) IM as a single dose; frequent saline irrigation of discharge until eliminated.
- After counselling, refer mother (with partner) to GU physician.

Chlamydial neonatal conjunctivitis

This is the commonest cause of neonatal conjunctivitis. A papillary, rather than follicular, reaction is seen due to delayed development of palpebral lymphoid tissue.

Clinical features

- Subacute onset (4–28d after birth), mucopurulent discharge, papillae, may be haemorrhagic ± preseptal cellulitis.
- Systemic (uncommon): rhinitis, otitis, pneumonitis.

Investigation

- Prewet swabs: usually for immunofluorescent staining, but cell culture, PCR, and ELISA may be used.
- Conjunctival scrapings: Giemsa stain.

Treatment

- Erythromycin 12.5mg/kg 4×/d for 2wk.
- After counselling, refer mother (with partner) to GU physician.

Other bacterial neonatal conjunctivitis

Other bacterial causes include *Staphylococcus aureus*, *Streptococcus pneumoniae* (which require topical antibiotics only), and *Haemophilus* and *Pseudomonas* (which require additional systemic antibiotics to prevent systemic complications).

Clinical features

- Subacute onset (4–28d after birth), purulent discharge, lid oedema, chemosis ± keratitis (*Pseudomonas*).

Investigation
- *Prewet swab or conjunctival scrapings*: Gram stain, culture, and sensitivities.

Treatment
- *Gram-positive organisms*: topical (e.g. chloramphenicol Oc 4×/d or erythromycin Oc 4×/d); adjust according to sensitivities.
- *Gram-negative organisms*: topical (e.g. tobramycin Oc 4×/d); adjust according to sensitivities.

HSV neonatal conjunctivitis

Although viral causes of neonatal conjunctivitis are uncommon, they may cause serious ocular morbidity and systemic disease.

Clinical features
- Acute onset (1–14d), vesicular lid lesions, mucoid discharge ± keratitis (e.g. microdendrites), anterior uveitis, cataract, retinitis, optic neuritis (rare).
- *Systemic* (uncommon but may be fatal): jaundice, hepatosplenomegaly, pneumonitis, meningoencephalitis, DIC.

Investigation
- Swab or conjunctival scrapings transported in viral culture medium; PCR.

Treatment
- Aciclovir Oc 5×/d for 1wk ± aciclovir IV 10mg/kg 3×/d for 10d.

Chemical conjunctivitis

Silver nitrate drops are commonly used in some parts of the world as a protective measure against ophthalmia neonatorum. While effective against gonococcal disease, they are of limited use against other bacteria and are of no use against *Chlamydia* or viruses. In the majority of neonates, the drops cause red, watering eyes from 12 to 48h after instillation.

Table 18.26 Timing of onset of ophthalmia neonatorum by cause

Chemical	<2d
Gonococcal	1–3d
Other bacteria	2–5d
HSV	1–14d
Chlamydia	4–28d

Conjunctivitis in the older child

Children are commonly affected by both infective and allergic conjunctivitis. In the older child, it behaves in a more similar manner to adult disease: viral (see ➲ Viral conjunctivitis, p. 186), bacterial (see ➲ Bacterial conjunctivitis (1), p. 182), chlamydial (see ➲ Chlamydial conjunctivitis, p. 188), allergic (see ➲ Allergic conjunctivitis (1), p. 190).

Orbital and preseptal cellulitis

Orbital cellulitis may cause blindness and even death. It requires emergency assessment, imaging, and treatment under the joint care of an ophthalmologist, ENT specialist, and paediatrician. Part of the ophthalmologist's role is to assist in differentiating orbital cellulitis from the much more limited preseptal cellulitis.

Orbital cellulitis

Infective organisms include *Streptococcus pneumoniae, Staphylococcus aureus, Streptococcus pyogenes*, and *Haemophilus influenzae* (previously common in younger children but less likely if Hib-vaccinated).

Risk factors

- *Gender*: ♂:♀ 2:1.[3]
- *Sinus disease*: ethmoidal sinusitis (common), maxillary sinusitis.
- *Infection of other adjacent structures*: preseptal or facial infection, dacrocystitis, dental abscess.
- *Trauma*: septal perforation.
- *Surgical*: orbital, lacrimal, and vitreoretinal surgery.

Clinical features

- Fever, malaise, painful, swollen orbit.
- Inflamed lids (swollen, red, tender, warm), proptosis, painful restricted eye movements ± optic nerve dysfunction (↓VA, ↓colour vision ± RAPD).
- *Complications*: optic nerve compromise is the most important; also orbital or periorbital abscess, exposure keratopathy, ↑IOP, CRAO, CRVO.
- *Systemic*: meningitis, cerebral abscess, cavernous sinus thrombosis.

Differential diagnosis

- Idiopathic orbital inflammatory disease.
- Ruptured dermoid cyst.
- Benign orbital tumours—lymphangioma, haemangioma.
- Malignant tumours—rhabdomyosarcoma, leukaemia, metastatic disease.

Investigation

- Temperature.
- FBC, blood culture (low yield: generally <7% from recent studies).
- CT (orbit, sinuses, brain): diffuse orbital infiltrate, proptosis ± sinus opacity, orbital abscess.

Treatment

- Admit for IV antibiotics (e.g. either flucloxacillin 25mg/kg 4×/d or cefuroxime 50mg/kg 4×/d with metronidazole 7.5mg/kg 3×/d).
- ENT to assess for drainage of sinus ± subperiosteal abscess (subperiosteal abscesses in children under 9y may resolve with medical treatment—if optic nerve compromise or not resolved in 48–72h after starting antibiotics, emergency drainage advised).

Preseptal cellulitis

Preseptal infection is much commoner than orbital cellulitis. The majority of cases are under 5y of age, and 80% of all cases of preseptal cellulitis are under 10y. The main causative organisms are once again staphylococci and streptococci. It is generally a much less severe disease, at least in adults and older children. In younger children, in whom the orbital septum is not fully developed, there is a high risk of progression and so should be treated similarly to orbital cellulitis (see Table 18.27 and Table 18.28).

Clinical features
- Fever, malaise, painful, swollen lid/periorbita.
- Inflamed lids but no proptosis, normal eye movements, normal optic nerve function.

Investigation
- Investigation is not usually necessary, unless there is concern over possible orbital or sinus involvement.

Treatment
- Admit young or unwell children; otherwise daily review until resolution.
- Treat with oral antibiotics (e.g. flucloxacillin).

Table 18.27 Differentiating features of orbital vs preseptal cellulitis

	Orbital	Preseptal
Proptosis	Present	Absent
Ocular motility	Painful + restricted	Normal
VA	↓ (in severe cases)	Normal
Colour vision	↓ (in severe cases)	Normal
RAPD	Present (in severe cases)	Absent (normal)

Table 18.28 Development of paranasal sinuses

Sinus	Onset of development	Onset of adult configuration
Maxillary	In utero	Late childhood (12y)
Sphenoidal	>6mo old	Puberty
Ethmoidal	In utero	Puberty
Frontal	>5y old	Adulthood

3. Nageswaran S et al. Orbital cellulitis in children. *Pediatr Infect Dis J* 2006;25:695–9.

Congenital cataract: assessment

Congenital cataract affects up to 1 in 1,500 live births.[4] Worldwide about 200,000 children are estimated to be blind from cataracts.

As amblyopia is likely to limit final visual outcome, this condition requires urgent expert assessment, with a view to early surgery (see Table 18.29 for causes).

Assessment

- *History*: observed visual function, intrauterine exposure (infections, drugs, toxins, radiation), medical history (e.g. syndromes), FH.
- *Visual function*: clinical tests appropriate to age. Poor fixation, strabismus, and nystagmus suggest severe visual impairment.
- *Cataract density*: indicated by red reflex pre-/post-dilation, and quality of fundal view with a direct/indirect ophthalmoscope. Risk to vision is worse if cataract is posterior, dense, confluent, axial, and >3mm diameter.
- *Cataract morphology*: may suggest underlying cause.
- *Rest of the eye*: visual potential (check pupil reactions, and optic nerve and retina as possible), associated ocular abnormalities (may require treatment, influence surgery, or suggest underlying cause).
- *Rest of the child*: numerous systemic conditions are associated with congenital cataracts (see Table 18.29). Clinical examination will direct appropriate investigation.

Investigation

- Extensive investigations are not always required (e.g. in unilateral cataracts or a known FH).
- Coordinate with a paediatrician, but consider:
  - Urinalysis (reducing substances and amino acids).
  - Serology—'TORCH' screen (toxoplasma, other (e.g. syphilis), rubella, CMV, herpes family (HSV, VZV)).
  - Biochemical profile—including Glu, calcium, phosphate.
  - Erythrocyte enzyme analysis—including galactokinase, G1PUT.
  - Karyotyping and clinical geneticist referral, e.g. if child dysmorphic.

Table 18.29 Causes of congenital/presenile cataracts

Isolated		AD, AR, XR
Chromosomal	Trisomies	Down (21), Edwards (18), Patau (13) syndromes
	Monosomies	Turner syndrome
	Deletions	5p (cri-du-chat syndrome)
	Microdeletion	16p13 (Rubinstein–Taybi syndrome)
	Duplications	3q, 10q
Syndromic	Craniosynostosis	Apert syndrome, Crouzon syndrome
	Craniofacial defects	Smith–Lemli–Opitz syndrome, Hallerman–Streiff–François syndrome
	Dermatological	Cockayne syndrome, incontinentia pigmenti, hypohidrotic ectodermal dysplasia, ichthyosis, naevoid basal cell carcinoma syndrome, Rothmund–Thomson syndrome
	Neuromuscular	Alstrom syndrome, myotonic dystrophy, Marinesco–Sjögren syndrome
	Connective tissue	Marfan syndrome, Alport syndrome, Conradi syndrome, spondyloepiphyseal dysplasia
	AS dysgenesis	Peters anomaly, Rieger syndrome, aniridia
Metabolic	Carbohydrate	Hypoglycaemia, galactokinase deficiency, galactosaemia, mannosidosis
	Lipids	Abetalipoproteinaemia
	Amino acid	Lowe syndrome, homocysteinuria
	Sphingolipidoses	Niemann–Pick disease, Fabry disease
	Minerals	Wilson disease, hypocalcaemia
	Phytanic acid	Refsum disease
Endocrine		Diabetes mellitus, hypoparathyroidism
Infective		Toxoplasma, rubella, herpes group (CMV, HSV1 and 2, VZV), syphilis, measles, poliomyelitis, influenza
Other		Trauma, drugs (steroids), eczema, radiation

4. Haargaard B et al. Incidence and cumulative risk of childhood cataract in a cohort of 2.6 million Danish children. Invest Ophthalmol Vis Sci 2004;45:1316–20.

Congenital cataract: surgery

Timing of surgery

Timely removal of visually significant cataracts (see Table 18.30) is a prerequisite for good outcome.

The two principle factors determining when to intervene are secondary glaucoma risk (which decreases exponentially with each week of life) and amblyopia risk. In the first weeks of life, there is a 'latent period' during which visual deprivation does not result in intractable amblyopia. The aim is to remove the cataract within but at the end of the latent period. A guide is at 6wk for unilateral and 10wk for bilateral cataracts, though opinion varies.

Cataract surgery in children places great demands upon their parents and family. Parents should be carefully counselled. They should understand that the results of surgery depend enormously on their compliance with unpopular treatments, and they must be prepared that functional visual improvement may be fairly modest, particularly in unilateral cases (60% >6/60).[5]

Procedure

Debate continues over the procedure of choice and when to use implantable lenses (see Table 18.30). The current trend is towards implantation at ever younger ages.[6]

A common surgical technique involves a limbal approach with manual anterior and posterior capsulotomies and anterior vitrectomy (anterior or pars plana approach) and primary lens insertion (if appropriate). Suture every incision (absorbable) to close.[6]

Table 18.30 Rationale for post-operative aphakia vs IOL implantation

Advantages of aphakia	Advantages of IOL implantation
Technically easier	Possible reduced post-operative glaucoma
Safer if eye small (corneal diameter <10mm)	Reduced post-operative strabismus
Less visual axis opacification	Better visual outcome in monocular cases*
No IOL long-term safety issues	Reduced refractive error; reduced need for aphakic glasses and/or CL and related problems

* Birch EE *et al.* Visual acuity development after the implantation of unilateral intraocular lenses in infants and young children. *J AAPOS* 2005;9:527–32.

Refractive target for IOL implantation

There is considerable debate over the estimation of IOL power in children undergoing cataract surgery. Problems include: (1) accurately estimating axial length and corneal curvature in children; (2) uncertain reliability of the IOL prediction formulae (such as the SRK I/II, Holladay, etc.), which are based on adult eyes; (3) prediction of how much myopic shift to anticipate with normal eye development; and (4) disagreement as to the optimal post-operative refraction to aim for. Most surgeons target emmetropia in older children (>5y), but, in younger children, there is no consensus; most target hypermetropia (to account for myopic shift), others emmetropia or even mild myopia (to reduce amblyopic risk). In unilateral cataracts, IOL choice may also need to be adjusted to reduce anisometropia to <3D.[7]

Post-operative care

Good post-operative care requires highly motivated parents, coordinated orthoptists/ophthalmologists, and regularly updated refractions.

CL have optical and cosmetic advantages (particularly in aphakia) but may be problematic, particularly in younger children. Increasing implantation of IOLs results in smaller refractive errors that can be easily corrected by spectacles. Older children (≥3y) benefit from bifocal lenses with an 'add' of +3.00 for near.

In unilateral cases, patching of the unaffected eye is essential. Aggressive patching improves the visual outcome in the operated eye but increases disruption and the small risk of induced amblyopia with the normal eye. Close monitoring is a priority, whichever regimen is used.

Parental education pre- and post-surgery is essential.

5. Lambert SR. Treatment of congenital cataract. *Br J Ophthalmol* 2004;**88**:854–5.

6. Solebo AL *et al.* Cataract surgery and intraocular lens implantation in children < or = 2 years old in the UK and Ireland: finding of national surveys. *Br J Ophthalmol* 2009;**93**:1495–8.

7. Eibschitz-Tsimhoni M *et al.* Intraocular lens power calculation in children *Surv Ophthalmol* 2007;**52**:474–82.

Congenital cataract: complications

Post-operative complications

Cataract surgery in children is more challenging and more subject to complications than in adults. A good result is more likely to be achieved with careful case selection, well planned surgery, and meticulous post-operative care (see Table 18.31).

Table 18.31 Post-operative complications and strategies for their management

Complication	Management strategy
Intraocular inflammation (may lead to seclusio pupillae, angle closure, and visual axis opacification)	Steroid (intraoperative periorbital, topical, and sometimes systemic)
	Cycloplegia
	Iridectomy (especially if corneal diameter <10mm), laser iridotomy
	Heparin in irrigation fluid
	Tissue plasminogen activator into AC
Visual axis opacification	1° anterior vitrectomy and posterior capsulotomy
	Acrylic IOL
	Laser capsulotomy
	Surgical capsulotomy (pars plana approach)
	Meticulous post-operative inflammation control (see above)
Glaucoma	1° placement of intracapsular IOL may be protective
	2° surgery: augmented trabeculectomy or tube surgery (where medical treatment fails)
	Cyclodestructive therapies
	NB CCT is often increased in childhood aphakia
Strabismus	Squint surgery
Amblyopia	Penalization
Premature presbyopia	CL/spectacles aiming for +2 to 3
	Bifocals with add of +3 if over 2–3y old
Macula exposure to short wavelength light (clinical significance unproven)	'Yellow' (blue filter) IOL
Retinal detachment (may occur years later)	Vitreoretinal repair
CL problems	See ➜ Contact lenses: complications, p. 844

Uveitis in children

Although uveitis is much less common in children than in adults, it is still a significant cause of ocular morbidity. This is most marked in the context of the 'silent' anterior uveitis of JIA, which accounts for up to 80% of all childhood uveitis. However, it is important to recognize that most other types of uveitis may also affect children (see Table 18.32).

JIA

JIA is the commonest chronic rheumatic disease of childhood. The prevalence of uveitis in JIA overall is ~8–30%, but, in young oligoarticular onset group (i.e. arthritis in which up to four joints are involved), it may be as high as 45–57%. Its classification, screening, and treatment are discussed in more detail elsewhere (see ➋ Uveitis with juvenile idiopathic arthritis, p. 430). A rare cause of uveitis associated with arthritis in children is Blau's syndrome (also known as familial juvenile systemic granulomatosis) due to mutations in the *NOD2* gene (AD). The uveitis seen is most commonly a panuveitis with multifocal choroiditis.

Clinical features
Ophthalmic
- Asymptomatic; rarely floaters; ↓VA from cataract.
- White eye, band keratopathy, small KPs, AC cells/flare, PS, cataract, 2° glaucoma, vitritis, CMO; other complications include hypotony that may lead to phthisis bulbi.

NB In long-standing uveitis, chronic breakdown of the blood–aqueous barrier leads to persistent flare; AC cells are therefore a better guide than flare to disease activity.

Treatment
Refer to a tertiary referral centre for advice about specific immunosuppression if: (1) complications are present at onset, or (2) if the disease is active after 2y of topical treatment. Management of complex cases is optimized in tertiary centres with joint clinics between a paediatric rheumatologist and specialist ophthalmologist.
- *Of uveitis*: treatment options include topical steroid eye drop mydriatics, sub-Tenon injections of steroids, orbital floor injections, occasionally systemic steroids, and increasingly with weekly methotrexate. Ciclosporin, mycophenolate, and anti-TNF agents (infliximab, adalimumab) may also be considered.
- *Of ↑IOP*: initially topical therapy, but up to 2/3 may require surgery (commonly an augmented trabeculectomy or a tube procedure).
- *Of cataract*: aim to defer until the eye has been quiet for a minimum of 3mo, although weigh against the risk of amblyopia in younger children; there is considerable debate over surgery, including whether to implant a lens or leave aphakic.
- *Of band keratopathy*: chelation with EDTA or excimer phototherapeutic keratectomy.

Table **18.32** Uveitis in children

Anterior	JIA	➲ p. 430
	HLA-B27 associated (e.g. psoriasis, ankylosing spondylitis, IBD)	➲ p. 424
	Kawasaki disease	➲ p. 428
	TINU	➲ p. 428
	Idiopathic	➲ p. 422
	Tarantula hairs	
Intermediate	Idiopathic/pars planitis	➲ p. 432
	Toxocariasis	➲ p. 466
	Lyme disease	➲ p. 460
	IBD	➲ p. 425
Posterior	Toxoplasmosis	➲ p. 462
	Toxocariasis	➲ p. 466
	Congenital syphilis	➲ p. 460
	TB	➲ p. 456
	HIV-associated (e.g. CMV retinitis)	➲ p. 454
	Sarcoidosis	➲ p. 436
	Behçet's disease	➲ p. 440
Vasculitis	Leukaemia	➲ p. 434
	Cat-scratch disease	➲ p. 434
	Systemic vasculitis, e.g. SLE	➲ p. 434
	Herpes group, e.g. HSV	➲ p. 448
	HIV-related, e.g. CMV	➲ p. 452

Other causes of uveitis in children

For clinical features, investigation, and treatment of these conditions, see Chapter 11.

Treatment

While there are many similarities to adult disease, it should be noted that:

- *Children are still growing*: systemic steroids reduce growth rate and final height; topical steroids may have systemic side effects.
- *Children are smaller*: all treatments should be appropriately titrated to body size/weight.
- *Children have longer to live*: they are at higher risk of delayed complications, e.g. post-immunosuppression malignancies.

Glaucoma in children: assessment

The childhood glaucomas are a significant cause of blindness in children but may be missed, being both rare and insidious.

Classification

Primary congenital glaucoma (PCG, trabeculodysgenesis)

In this rare syndrome (1/10,000 live births), angle dysgenesis causes reduced aqueous outflow. Presentation is from birth to 10th year of life. It is bilateral in 70% and more common in ♂ (65%).[8] It is usually sporadic, but 10% are familial. Four loci associated with AR PCG are denoted GLC3 A–D, though the genes at these loci are not all known. The gene at GLC3A is *CYP1B1* (Chr 2p).

Primary juvenile glaucoma

The aetiology remains unknown. Presentation is from the 10th to 35th year of life.[8] It may be sporadic or familial. Genes identified include *CYP1B1* (Chr 2p) and *MYOC* (Chr 1q).

Secondary

Anterior segment dysgenesis

(See ➲ Anterior segment dysgenesis, p. 812.)

Developmental abnormalities of the anterior segment result in a spectrum of anterior segment anomalies, including Axenfeld–Rieger syndrome and Peters anomaly, and associated abnormalities of the drainage angle. Glaucoma occurs in about 50%.

Aniridia

In aniridia (*syn* iridotrabeculodysgenesis), the iris tissue is abnormal or absent and is associated with glaucoma in up to 75%.

Lens-/surgery-related

Surgery for congenital cataracts is associated with glaucoma in up to 60%. Risk is highest when surgery is early and in those left aphakic. It is not known whether withholding IOL insertion is causative or merely an association of earlier surgery.

Posterior segment developmental abnormalities

Persistent fetal vasculature syndrome and ROP may cause glaucoma by a 2° angle closure mechanism.

Tumour-related

Tumours may cause ↑IOP by reduced aqueous outflow (mechanical, clogging of trabecular meshwork by cellular debris, 2° haemorrhage, or lead to rubeotic glaucoma). Tumours may be anterior (e.g. juvenile xanthogranuloma, medulloepithelioma), posterior (e.g. retinoblastoma), or systemic (e.g. leukaemia).

Phakomatoses

Sturge–Weber syndrome is associated with ipsilateral glaucoma in up to 50%, being highest where the naevus flammeus involves both upper and lower lid. Neurofibromatosis-1 also carries an increased risk, particularly in the presence of an ipsilateral neurofibroma.

Connective tissue disease
Marfan syndrome, homocystinuria, and Weill–Marchesani are associated with glaucoma. This may arise due to abnormal trabecular meshwork or lens block.

Uveitis
Chronic uveitis of childhood (e.g. associated with JIA) may result in 2° glaucoma. This is usually of relatively late onset.

Clinical features
- Watering eye(s), photophobia, blepharospasm.
- ↑IOP, corneal oedema, enlargement of cornea/globe (buphthalmos, if onset <4y of age), breaks in Descemet's membrane (Haab striae).

Additional features
These may indicate the underlying cause of glaucoma:
- *Ophthalmic*: posterior embryotoxon, leukoma, anterior iris strands, iris hypoplasia, aniridia, iris cyst/tumour, iritis, Lisch nodules (NF-1), cataract, ectopia lentis, aphakia, persistent fetal vasculature, ciliary body tumours, retinal masses.
- *Systemic*: naevus flammeus (Sturge–Weber syndrome), neurofibromas (NF-1 or -2), marfanoid habitus (Marfan syndrome, homocystinuria), brachydactyly (Weill–Marchesani syndrome), abnormal dentition, and umbilical hernia or failure of periumbilical skin involution (Rieger syndrome).

Measuring IOP
The most appropriate technique for measuring IOP will depend on the age and cooperation of the child. Rebound tonometer (iCare) has dramatically reduced the proportion of children who require EUA, because it does not require topical anaesthetic and is much better tolerated than alternatives. A Tonopen or Perkins tonometer can often be used with topical anaesthetic in infants, but GAT remains the gold standard. If IOP measurement is not possible, it may need to be done under general anaesthetic. Inhalational anaesthesia lowers IOP progressively with time and more than ketamine sedation.

IOP and CCT
A higher CCT or thicker cornea (e.g. aphakic glaucoma, aniridia, and microcornea) will lead to overestimating the IOP, i.e. the applanation-measured IOP will be higher than the actual IOP. In contrast a lower CCT or thinner cornea (e.g. keratoconus, keratoglobus) will lead to underestimating the actual IOP.

8. European Glaucoma Society. *Terminology and guidelines for glaucoma, 3rd edition.* Savona: Dogma; 2008.

Glaucoma in children: treatment

Titrate treatment, according to IOP (interpreted in the light of the CCT; see ➲ Ocular hypertension, p. 352), worsening disc appearance, and increasing corneal diameter. In older children, perimetry and OCT of RNFL is also a valuable tool.

Medical treatment

Medical treatment is less effective than in adults but can often temporize and sometimes avoid the need surgery. Topical β-blockers, carbonic anhydrase inhibitors, and prostaglandin analogues are the most commonly used agents. Combination preparations and those which cause less stinging are particularly valuable in order to avoid loss of adherence (a major problem). α2-agonist (brimonidine) causes CNS depression and is contraindicated in children under 2y of age;[9] in younger children, apraclonidine may be safer, though it also can cause drowsiness. Systemic carbonic anhydrase inhibitors can cause lethargy, decreased appetite, and impair growth and should only usually be used for short periods.

Surgical treatment

Preferred surgical technique depends on the type and severity of glaucoma (see Table 18.33). *Options include:*

- *Goniotomy*: incision of the uveal trabecular meshwork under gonioscopic view allows iris root to fall back and presumed to open the drainage angle.
- *Trabeculotomy*: cannulation of Schlemm's canal *ab externo* and disruption of internal wall of canal and trabecular meshwork using trabeculotome.
- *Trabeculectomy*: forms a new drainage channel from AC to subconjunctival space; may be augmented by antimetabolites.
- *Aqueous shunting procedures ('tubes')*: silicone tube flows from AC to episcleral explant.
- *Cycloablation*: Both endoscopic and trans-scleral laser cycloablation may be useful in resistant cases but have limited success rates and often require repeated applications.

Table **18.33** Summary of surgical treatments in paediatric glaucoma

Procedure	Indications	Advantages/*disadvantages*
Goniotomy and/or trabeculotomy	Congenital glaucoma due to trabeculodysgenesis, especially good results (>90% IOP control at 5y) Clear cornea needed for goniotomy (unless endoscopic viewing)	Low rate of serious complications Anatomical route of aqueous maintained Possible in small eyes with difficult access *Less effective for cases other than trabeculodysgenesis*
Trabeculectomy ± augmentation	Refractory glaucoma	*Bleb-related complications (failure, blebitis, leak, hypotony, endophthalmitis)* *Numerous post-operative procedures impractical in children. Increased failure in children due to fibrosis*
Aqueous shunting procedure	Refractory glaucoma Consider especially in aphakic glaucoma	Less post-operative procedures *Explant-related complications (tube migration, plate extrusion, corneal touch, endophthalmitis, strabismus)*
Cyclodestructive laser	Failure of surgical treatment When glaucoma surgery contraindicated due to comorbidities	Minimal post-operative management *Hypotony, phthisis, inflammation, retinal detachment (all rare when titrated procedure)*

9. Coppens G *et al*. The safety and efficacy of glaucoma medications in the pediatric population. *J Pediatr Ophthalmol Strabismus* 2009;**46**:12–18.

Retinopathy of prematurity (1)

ROP was first reported in 1942. By the 1950s, it was the leading cause of childhood blindness. At this point, tight oxygen control was introduced, with a dramatic fall in ROP, but a significant rise in neonatal death and neurological disability. Oxygen delivery is now a compromise between these factors.

Risk factors

- Low gestational age (<32wk).
- Low birthweight (<1,501g).
- High or variable oxygen tension.

Classification

(See Fig. 18.1.)

Stages

These are defined by the International Classification of ROP revisited (ICROP):[10]

- *Stage 1*: demarcation line—flat, white line separating vascular from avascular zones.
- *Stage 2*: ridge—line becomes elevated, thickened, may become pinkish with neovascular tufts ('popcorn') posterior to ridge.
- *Stage 3*: ridge with extraretinal fibrovascular proliferation—vascular tissue grows from posterior margin on to retina or into the vitreous.
- *Stage 4*: subtotal retinal detachment—extrafoveal (4A) or foveal (4B).
- *Stage 5*: total retinal detachment.

Plus and pre-plus disease

- *Plus disease*: there is significant venous dilatation and arteriolar tortuosity (compared with a standard photograph)[10] of the posterior retinal vessels in two or more quadrants.
- *Pre-plus disease*: there is more venous dilatation and arteriolar tortuosity than normal but insufficient to be defined as plus disease.

Location

- *Zone I*: circle centred on the disc, with radius twice the distance from the centre of the disc to the fovea.
- *Zone II*: ring centred on the disc, extending from zone 1 to ora nasally and equator temporally.
- *Zone III*: remaining temporal crescent.

Extent

- Measured in clock-hours.

Threshold disease

- Originally an estimate of when progression and regression were equally likely and so used as the level where treatment is indicated.
- Threshold disease is defined as stage 3 ROP, with plus disease in zones I or II and of 5 continuous or 8 non-continuous clock-hours.

Prethreshold disease

The Early Treatment in ROP (ETROP) trial[11] suggested a benefit in treating some cases of ROP that are not yet at 'threshold'.

Prethreshold disease (type 1)
- Zone I, any stage ROP with plus disease.
- Zone I, stage 3 ROP with or without plus disease.
- Zone II, stage 2 or 3 ROP with plus disease.

Prethreshold disease (type 2)
- Zone I, stage 1 or 2 ROP without plus disease.
- Zone II, stage 3 ROP without plus disease.

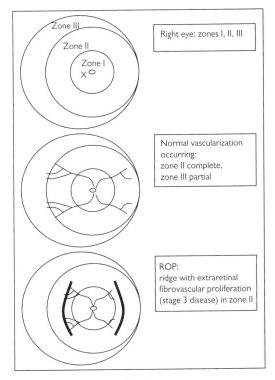

Fig. 18.1 ROP zones and examples of classification.

10. International Committee for the Classification of Retinopathy of Prematurity. The International Classification of Retinopathy of Prematurity revisited. *Arch Ophthalmol* 2005;**123**:991–9.

11. Good WV. Early Treatment for Retinopathy of Prematurity Cooperative Group. Final results of the Early Treatment for Retinopathy of Prematurity (ETROP) randomized trial. *Trans Am Ophthalmol Soc* 2004;**102**:233–48.

Retinopathy of prematurity (2)

Screening (Table 18.34)

Indirect ophthalmoscopy with a 28D lens permits a wide field of view. Dilate in advance (cyclopentolate 0.5% + phenylephrine 2.5%; 2–3 doses; 1h before the examination), consider a sterilized lid speculum and scleral indentation, as needed, and beware of the positions of all tubes/lines that may be vulnerable to a clumsy ophthalmologist.

Table 18.34 Summary of UK ROP screening guidelines[*]

Screening inclusion criteria	
All babies born at <31wk gestational age (i.e. up to 30wk and 6d) or <1,251g birthweight	*Must* be screened
All babies born at <32wk gestational age (i.e. up to 31wk and 6d) or <1,501g birthweight	*Should* be screened (less evidence but considered good practice)
First screening examination[†]	
Babies born <27wk gestational age	First exam to be at 30–31wk post-menstrual age
Babies born between 27 and 32wk gestational age	First exam to be at 4–5wk post-natal age
Babies born >32wk gestational age but <1,501g birthweight	First exam to be at 4–5wk post-natal age
Frequency of screening	
If vessels end in zone I or posterior zone II, *or* any plus or pre-plus disease, *or* any stage 3 disease (any zone)	Screen at least weekly
All other circumstances where termination criteria not reached	Screen at least fortnightly
Termination of screening	
In babies with no ROP	
Vascularization has extended into zone III (usually after 36 completed weeks post-menstrual age)	
In babies with ROP not requiring treatment[‡]	

Two successive examinations showing any of:
- Lack of increase in severity.
- Partial resolution progressing towards complete resolution.
- Change in colour in the ridge from salmon-pink to white.
- Transgression of vessels through the demarcation line.
- Commencement of the process of replacement of active ROP lesions by scar tissue.

[*] RCPCH, RCOphth, BAPN, BLISS. *Guideline for the screening and treatment of retinopathy of prematurity 2008.* (2008). Available at: ⅏ http://www.rcophth.ac.uk

[†] First screening exam should occur prior to discharge.

[‡] Any stage 3 disease may require long-term follow-up as clinically indicated.

Treatment

Treatment has traditionally been recommended for threshold disease and worse; however, recent evidence suggests that 'high-risk' prethreshold disease may also benefit.

Cryotherapy has been used for over 30y but has largely been replaced by laser photocoagulation, which is more portable, better tolerated, and more effective for posterior disease. Photocoagulation should be with a transpupillary diode laser to give nearly confluent burns (half to one burn-width separation) to the whole avascular retina.

Intravitreal anti-VEGF has been shown to be effective in the treatment of ROP, but definitive data are not yet available.

Vitreoretinal surgery aims to repair or prevent progression of ROP-associated retinal detachment (stages 4A, 4B, and 5). Unfortunately, results are generally disappointing (see Table 18.35).

Long-term follow-up and complications

The UK ROP treatment guidelines (see Table 18.35) suggest that all babies with stage 3 ROP which resolved spontaneously and those babies treated for ROP should be reviewed until at least 5y of age.

Common sequelae of ROP include myopia (often severe), retinal folds and dragging of the macula, amblyopia, and strabismus. Eyes that have been treated may develop retinal detachment at the border of the treated and untreated retina.

Table 18.35 Summary of UK ROP treatment guidelines[*]

Treatment criteria	
• Zone I, any ROP with plus disease, *or* • Zone I, stage 3 without plus disease, *or* • Zone II, stage 3 with plus disease	Treat
• Zone II, stage 2 with plus disease	Consider treating
Timing of treatment	
• Aggressive ROP	Treat as soon as possible (<48h)
• All other ROP requiring treatment	Treat within 48–72h
Technique	
Transpupillary diode laser to give near-confluent (0.5–1 burn-width) laser burn spacing to the entire avascular retina[†]	
Post-treatment follow-up	
• First examination	5–7d post-treatment
• Subsequent examination(s)	Initially at least weekly, looking for signs of ↓activity and regression; then as clinically indicated
Retreatment	
• Failure of ROP to regress	10–14d post-initial treatment

[*] RCPCH, RCOphth, BAPN, BLISS (2008) *Guideline for the screening and treatment of retinopathy of prematurity 2008*. Available at: ℘ http://www.rcophth.ac.uk

[†] Where this is not possible, then treatment with cryotherapy or argon laser by an ophthalmologist experienced in these techniques is preferable to a delay in treatment.

Other retinal disorders

ROP-like syndromes

Familial exudative vitreoretinopathy (FEVR)

This rare condition may show AD (Chr 11q) or XR (*NDP* gene) inheritance. The disease is characterized by abrupt cessation of peripheral retinal vessels at the equator (more marked temporally) and vitreous bands in the periphery. The resulting retinal ischaemia leads to fibrovascular proliferation, retinal folds, macular ectopia, retinal detachment (akin to ROP), and subretinal exudation (akin to Coats' disease). The clinical appearance varies markedly, even within families, with severely affected patients being registered blind in infancy, while mildly affected patients may be asymptomatic and just have a small patch of avascularity in the peripheral retina.

Incontinentia pigmenti (Bloch–Sulzberger syndrome)

This rare condition shows XD inheritance which is usually, but not always, lethal *in utero* for ♂ embryos. 80% have a deletion of the *NEMO* gene (Xq28). Clinical features include abnormal peripheral vasculature (akin to ROP), gliosis, TRD, and systemic features such as abnormal teeth, cutaneous pigment whorls, and CNS anomalies. The diagnosis can often be confirmed by the skin changes prior to genetic confirmation.

Retinal dysplasia

A number of conditions are associated with more extensive retinal abnormalities, probably arising as a result of abnormal development involving the inner wall of the optic cup. Clinical features include extensive retinal folds, retinal detachments, retinal haemorrhages, vitreous haemorrhages, retrolental grey mass, and phthisis bulbi. Associated syndromes include Patau syndrome, Edwards syndrome (see ➲ Chromosomal syndromes, p. 816), Norrie disease (retinal dysplasia, deafness, ↓IQ), and Walker–Warburg syndrome (retinal dysplasia, muscular dystrophy, cerebellar malformation).

Other retinochoroidal disorders

Many stationary and progressive disorders of photoreceptors, RPE, choroid, and retinal vasculature present in childhood. They are discussed elsewhere: RP (see ➲ Retinitis pigmentosa (1), p. 572), CSNB (see ➲ Congenital stationary night blindness, p. 576), macular dystrophies (see ➲ Macular dystrophies (1), p. 580), choroidal dystrophies (see ➲ Chorioretinal dystrophies, p. 584), hereditary vitreoretinal degenerations (see ➲ Hereditary vitreoretinal degenerations, p. 494), albinism (see ➲ Albinism, p. 586), and Coats' disease (see ➲ Coats' disease and Leber's miliary aneurysms, p. 568).

Developmental abnormalities: craniofacial and globe

Congenital craniofacial abnormalities

Congenital craniofacial abnormalities may have a profound effect on the developing orbit and globe. They may be divided into craniosynostosis and nonsynostosis abnormalities. They are all rare.

Craniosynostosis

Craniosynostosis arises from premature fusion of the cranial sutures. It occurs in about 1 in 4,000 live births. The clinical appearance and severity depend on the extent of premature suture fusion. Calvarial suture fusion affects cranial shape and orbital development, and the typical appearance is of a tall, broad skull with frontal bossing and proptosis. If severe, compression of the enlarging brain results in ↑ICP. Skull base suture fusion causes midface hypoplasia, characterized by: maxillary hypoplasia, beak-shaped nose, hypertelorism, shallow orbits with proptosis, high arched palate, and mandibular prognathism.

Craniosynostosis may be isolated or part of a syndrome such as Crouzon or Apert syndrome. Crouzon and Apert syndromes are clinically distinct, but both arise from mutations in the gene encoding the fibroblast growth factor receptor-2 (Chr 10q26).

- Apert syndrome: AD or sporadic, occurring in 1 in 100,000 births. Typical features include calvarial bone synostosis, midface hypoplasia, syndactyly, intellectual disability, and low set ears. Ocular associations include keratoconus, ectopia lentis, glaucoma, albinism, exposure keratopathy, papilloedema, and optic atrophy.
- Crouzon syndrome: AD or sporadic, occurring in 1 in 50,000 births. Typical features are similar to Apert syndrome. Other associations include micro-/megalocornea, iris coloboma, cataract, ectopia lentis, glaucoma, and marked retrusion of the orbital floor, leading to prolapse of the globe in front of the lids.

Nonsynostotic craniofacial abnormalities

Branchial arch syndromes are caused by failure of development of the first two branchial arches, which are responsible for the formation of the maxillary and mandibular bones, the ear and facial musculature.

- Treacher Collins syndrome (mandibulofacial dysostosis): AD; mutation in the 'treacle gene' TCOF1 (Chr 5q32). Typical features include bilateral hypoplasia of the mandible and zygoma, downward slanting palpebral fissures, lower lid colobomas, malformed ears, conductive deafness.
- Goldenhar syndrome: part of the same spectrum as hemifacial microsomia. Mostly sporadic mutation in HFM gene (Chr 14q32), occurring in 1 in 5,600 live births; Typical features include unilateral or bilateral hypoplasia of the malar, maxillary, and mandibular regions, microtia, preauricular and facial skin tags, epibulbar dermoid, eyelid coloboma, microphthalmos, vertebral anomaly.

Nasolacrimal duct

Cannulation of the nasolacrimal cord may be delayed distally, resulting in congenital obstruction. More commonly, there is simply an imperforate mucus membrane at the valve of Hasner which disappears within the first year of life. Overall 90% spontaneously resolve by 1y of age. In those that persist, a 'syringe and probe' carries a 90% success rate. If 'syringe and probe' is unsuccessful, it may be repeated or silicone intubation can be used. Where blockage is sufficient to prevent the passage of the probe, a DCR is usually required (see Box 18.1).

> **Box 18.1 Outline of 'syringe and probe' for congenital nasolacrimal obstruction**
>
> - Anaesthesia (usually GA).
> - Dilate punctum, if necessary, with Nettleship dilator.
> - Introduce nasolacrimal cannula into the lower or upper canaliculus.
> - Inject fluorescein-stained saline solution to confirm obstruction.
> - Pull the lower lid laterally, and introduce probe into the inferior punctum and then medially to the sac until a hard stop is felt.
> - Turn the probe 90° so as to direct it inferiorly, aiming slightly posterolaterally down the nasolacrimal duct to perforate membrane.
> - Repeat syringing to confirm patency of nasolacrimal duct with recovery of fluorescein from the nose.

Anophthalmia and microphthalmia

Anophthalmia is the absence of an eye within the orbit. It may be divided into primary anophthalmia (complete failure of any ocular tissue to develop), secondary anophthalmia (partial development which then halts, leaving a very small microphthalmic eye), and degenerative anophthalmia (partially developed eye regresses).

As normal development of the orbit and lids depend on the presence of the globe, early treatment with conformers and expanders is important and continues until the face has fully developed.

Initially, clear conformers are used (until age 2y), as they have to be replaced every few weeks. Subsequently, they may be replaced by painted prostheses. Special conformers are available for microphthalmic eyes in which some limited vision is preserved; these improve cosmesis without obstructing vision. Surgery also has a role in reducing orbital asymmetry. A multidisciplinary approach is needed, including, among others, a paediatric ophthalmologist, orbital surgeon, and orbital prosthesist.

Hamartomas and choristomas

Hamartomas (congenital tumours of tissues normal to that location) include the capillary haemangioma (see ⟳ Capillary haemangioma, p. 618 (for orbital); ⟳ Capillary haemangioma, p. 642 (for retinal)).

Choristomas (congenital tumours of tissues abnormal to that location) include dermoids (see ⟳ Dermoid cyst, p. 614).

Developmental abnormalities: anterior segment

Anterior segment dysgenesis

Anterior segment dysgenesis is the failure of the normal development of the anterior segment of the eye. It includes Axenfeld–Rieger syndrome, Peters anomaly, and aniridia. There is an overlap in the clinical findings of these conditions, and they are thought to be part of a disease spectrum. Glaucoma occurs in 50% of cases (see ➲ Glaucoma in children, pp. 800–2).

Axenfeld–Rieger syndrome

Axenfeld anomaly, Rieger anomaly, Rieger syndrome, iris hypoplasia, and iridogoniodysgenesis have genotypic and phenotypic overlap and are now considered a single entity known as Axenfeld–Rieger syndrome. AD inheritance is most common, with mutations identified in the *PITX2* and *FOXC1* genes.

Clinical features include posterior embryotoxon (an isolated finding in 15% of normal patients), anterior iris strands, and iris hypoplasia. 50% develop glaucoma. Systemic abnormalities include microdontia, oligodontia, maxillary hypoplasia, redundant periumbilical skin, and abnormalities of the cardiovascular outflow tract.[12]

Peters anomaly

This is a congenital corneal opacity (leukoma) associated with a posterior corneal defect (posterior stroma, Descemet's membrane, and endothelium). It may be associated with anterior iris strands, lens–corneal strands, and glaucoma. It is usually sporadic. Early corneal surgery may permit some vision to develop.

Aniridia

Aniridia is characterized by iris hypoplasia. It occurs in up to 1 in 64,000 births, being AD in two-thirds, sporadic in one-third. The disease ranges from mild defects of anterior iris stroma only to almost complete absence of the iris.

Aniridia is often associated with foveal hypoplasia (actually dysgenesis as OCT shows the fovea to be abnormally thick due to preserved inner retinal layers) and nystagmus. It may also be associated with cataract, optic nerve hypoplasia, and glaucoma. Peripheral corneal opacification may develop in childhood due to stem cell deficiency.

Aniridia usually arises from point mutations in the *PAX6* gene (11p13). Sporadic cases may arise from an 11p13 microdeletion which can include the *PAX6* gene and the adjacent *WT1* tumour suppressor gene. Sporadic aniridia is therefore associated with Wilms tumour (nephroblastoma) or the full WAGR syndrome (Wilms tumour, aniridia, GU abnormalities, ↓IQ) Cases of sporadic aniridia should undergo chromosomal deletion analysis to exclude the possibility of Wilms tumour.

Gillespie syndrome is a very rare AR form of aniridia that is not associated with *PAX6* mutations. Aniridia is partial and is associated with ataxia and ↓IQ.

Treatment for aniridia is directed by severity of iris hypoplasia and the extent of associated problems. Interventions include tinted CL, cataract surgery with artificial iris–lens diaphragms, keratoplasty, and medical/surgical therapy for glaucoma.

Iris coloboma

A coloboma is a defect resulting from failure of closure of an embryological fissure. When this occurs at the level of the iris, a typical inferonasal defect is seen. This may be associated with a coloboma of the ciliary body, choroid, retina, and optic nerve.

12. Chang TC et al. Axenfeld-Rieger syndrome: new perspectives. Br J Ophthalmol 2012;**96**:318–22.

Developmental abnormalities: posterior segment

Vitreous

Abnormalities within the vitreal cavity include remnants of the hyaloid vascular system (see Table 18.36) and abnormalities of the vitreous structure, e.g. type II collagen abnormalities resulting in Stickler syndrome.

Table 18.36 Hyaloid remnants

Glial remnant just posterior to lens	Mittendorf's dot
Glial remnant just anterior to disc	Bergmeister's papilla
Vascular remnant arising from disc	Persistent hyaloid artery
Vascular remnant and retrolental mass	Persistent fetal vasculature

Optic fissure

A coloboma is a defect resulting from failure of closure of an embryological fissure. Within the eye, defects may occur anywhere from disc to iris and vary dramatically in size and severity. Colobomas may be blinding and may be associated with more extensive disease.

Optic nerve anomalies

These include optic disc pits, optic disc hypoplasia, coloboma, and morning glory anomaly (see ⟳ Congenital optic disc anomalies, p. 686). Although disc pits are often isolated findings, more severe disc abnormalities are often associated with systemic pathology.

Retina

Premature cessation of peripheral retina vascularization may occur due to an inherited defect (familial exudative vitreoretinopathy, FEVR) or acquired insult (ROP). This results in fibrovascular proliferation, traction, exudation, and retinal detachment.

Retinal dysplasia may occur in isolation but is usually part of a syndrome such as Edwards, Patau, Norrie, Walker–Warburg, or incontinentia pigmenti. Severe forms present with bilateral leucocoria and very poor vision.

Macular hypoplasia may occur in isolation or with syndromes such as albinism or aniridia. There is loss of the normal foveal reflex and, in some cases, loss of the avascular zone.

Chromosomal syndromes

Trisomy syndromes

Down syndrome

Down syndrome (trisomy 21) is the commonest autosomal trisomy, with an incidence of 1 in 650 live births. It is also the commonest genetic cause of learning difficulties. Most cases arise by non-disjunction (94%), some by translocation (5%), and rarely by mosaicism (1%). Mosaic cases usually have a milder phenotype (see Table 18.37).

Table 18.37 Clinical features of Down syndrome

Ocular	Upward slanting palpebral fissures, hypertelorism, epicanthic folds, ectropia, blepharoconjunctivitis
	Myopia, astigmatism
	Strabismus, nystagmus
	Keratoconus, Brushfield spots, cataracts
	Hypoplastic disc
Systemic	Short stature, macroglossia, flat nasal bridge, broad hands, single palmar crease, clinodactyly, 'sandal gap' toes, hypotonia
	Congenital heart disease (ASD, VSD), duodenal atresia, hearing loss, hypothyroidism, diabetes mellitus, ↑risk of leukaemia
	↓IQ and early Alzheimer's dementia

Edwards syndrome

Edwards syndrome (trisomy 18) is the second commonest autosomal trisomy at 1 in 8,000 live births. Life expectancy is <1y (see Table 18.38).

Table 18.38 Clinical features of Edwards syndrome

Ocular	Epicanthic folds, blepharophimosis, ptosis, hypertelorism
	Microphthalmos, corneal opacities, congenital glaucoma, cataracts
	Uveal colobomas
Systemic	Failure to thrive
	Small chin, low set ears, overlapping fingers, 'rocker bottom' feet
	Congenital heart defects, renal malformations

Patau syndrome

Patau syndrome (trisomy 13) is the third commonest autosomal trisomy at 1 in 14,000 live births. Life expectancy is <3mo (see Table 18.39).

Table 18.39 Clinical features of Patau syndrome

Ocular	Cyclopia, microphthalmos, colobomas
	Corneal opacities, cataracts, intraocular cartilage, retinal dysplasia, optic nerve hypoplasia
Systemic	Failure to thrive
	Microcephaly, scalp defects, hernias, polydactyly
	Congenital heart defects, renal malformations, apnoeas

Deletion syndromes

Turner syndrome

Turner syndrome occurs in 1 in 2,000 live ♀ births. Only half are XO (also known as 45,X), with 15% being mosaics and the remainder having partial deletions or other abnormalities. The Turner's phenotype arises from XL genes that escape inactivation (e.g. the *SHOX* short stature homeobox gene) (see Table 18.40).

Other deletion syndromes

Although microdeletions are probably fairly common, macrodeletions, other than Turner's, are rare. Syndromes with ophthalmic features include the cri-du-chat syndrome (5p–), DeGrouchy syndrome (18q–), and the 13q– deletion syndrome. Common features are hypertelorism and epicanthic folds. In addition, in 13q–, there is a significantly increased risk of retinoblastoma.

Table 18.40 Clinical features of Turner syndrome

Ocular	Downward slanting palpebral fissures, epicanthic folds, ptosis, hypertelorism
	Strabismus, convergence insufficiency, ametropia, amblyopia
	Cataracts
	'♂' levels of XR diseases (e.g. red-green colour blindness)
Systemic	Neonatal lymphoedema of hands/feet
	Short stature, webbed neck, low posterior hairline, wide carrying angle, broad chest with apparent wide-spaced nipples
	Congenital heart defects (notably coarctation of the aorta)
	1° gonadal failure
	Normal IQ, sensorineural deafness, delayed motor skills

Metabolic and storage diseases (1)

Although individually these conditions are rare (or very rare) as a group, they feature regularly in the paediatric clinic. The ophthalmologist has an important role both in the diagnostic process and in the ongoing management of affected patients (see Table 18.41, Table 18.42, and Table 18.43).

Table 18.41 Disorders of carbohydrate metabolism

Syndrome	Deficiency	Ocular features	Systemic features
Galactosaemia	Galactose-1-phosphate uridyl transferase	Cataracts (oil droplet)	↓IQ Failure to thrive
Galactokinase deficiency	Galactokinase	Cataracts	Normal
Mannosidosis	α-mannosidase	Cataracts (spoke-like)	↓IQ MPS-like changes but clear corneas

All these conditions are AR. MPS, mucopolysaccharidosis.

Table 18.42 Disorders of amino acid metabolism

Syndrome	Deficiency	Ocular features	Systemic features
Cystinosis	Lysosomal transport protein	Crystalline keratopathy	Renal failure Failure to thrive
Lowe syndrome	Unknown	Cataracts Microphakia Glaucoma Blue sclera AS dysgenesis	↓IQ Failure to thrive Rickets (vitamin D-resistant)
Albinism	See ➔ Albinism, p. 586	See ➔ Albinism, p. 586	See ➔ Albinism, p. 586
Alkaptonuria	Homogentisic acid dioxygenase	Scleral darkening	Ochronosis Arthritis
Sulfite oxidase deficiency	Molybdenum cofactor	Spherophakia Ectopia lentis	Neurodegeneration LE <2y
Tyrosinaemia (II)	Tyrosine transaminase	Herpetiform corneal ulcers	↓IQ (some) Hyperkeratosis of palms/soles
Gyrate atrophy	Ornithine 5-aminotransferase	See ➔ Gyrate atrophy, p. 584	See ➔ Gyrate atrophy, p. 584

All these conditions are AR, other than Lowe syndrome and ocular albinism which are X-linked. LE, life expectancy.

Table 18.43 Disorders of lipid metabolism

Syndrome	Deficiency	Ocular features	Systemic features
Lipoproteins			
Abetalipo-proteinaemia	Triglyceride transfer protein	Pigmentary retinopathy Cataract	Spinocerebellar degeneration Myopathy
Sphingolipids			
G_{M1} gangliosidosis	β-glucosidase	Cloudy corneas Cherry-red spot Optic atrophy	Neurodegeneration (types 1 and 2) Visceromegaly (1)
Tay–Sachs	Hexosaminidase A	Cherry-red spot Optic atrophy	Visceromegaly LE <3y
Sandhoff disease	Hexosaminidase A Hexosaminidase B	Cherry-red spot Optic atrophy	Visceromegaly Neurodegeneration
Gaucher disease (I–III)	β-glucosidase	Supranuclear gaze palsy (type IIIb)	Visceromegaly neurodegeneration LE I (old), II (2), III (15)
Niemann–Pick (type A)	Sphingomyelinase	Cherry-red spot Optic atrophy	Visceromegaly Neurodegeneration LE <3y
Fabry disease	α-galactosidase A	Vortex keratopathy Cataract Tortuous vessels (conjunctival and retinal)	Angiokeratomas Painful episodes Renal failure Vascular disease LE = middle age
Metachromatic leukodystrophy	Arylsulfatase-A	Optic atrophy Nystagmus	Neurodegeneration LE 3–20y from diagnosis
Krabbe disease	Galacto-cerebrosidase	Optic atrophy	Neurodegeneration LE <2y in infants
Farber disease	Ceramidase	Macular pigmentation	Granulomas Arthropathy LE <2y
Other			
Neuronal ceroid lipofuscinosis (Batten's)	Unknown	Macular discoloration RP-like changes Optic atrophy	Neurodegeneration
Zellweger syndrome	Functional peroxisomes	Flat brows ON hypoplasia Pigmentary retinopathy Glaucoma	Dysgenesis of brain, liver, and kidneys Metabolic acidosis LE <1y
Refsum disease	Phytanic acid α-hydrolase	Pigmentary retinopathy	Neuropathy Ataxia Deafness Icthyosis

All these conditions are AR, other than Fabry disease which is X-linked. LE, life expectancy; ON, optic nerve.

Metabolic and storage diseases (2)

See Table 18.44 for disorders of glycosaminoglycan metabolism, Table 18.45 for mineral metabolism, and Table 18.46 for connective tissue.

Table 18.44 Disorders of glycosaminoglycan metabolism (mucopolysaccharidoses)

Syndrome	Deficiency	Ocular features	Systemic features
MPSI (Hurler/ Scheie/ Hurler–Scheie)	α-iduronidase	Cloudy corneas Pigmentary retinopathy Optic atrophy	Skeletal/facial dysmorphism ↓IQ Severity α type: H > H/S > S
MPSII (Hunter)	Iduronate sulfatase	Pigmentary retinopathy Optic atrophy	Variable ↓IQ and dysmorphism
MPSIII (A–D) (Sanfilippo)	Heparan-N-sulfatase (A)	Pigmentary retinopathy Optic atrophy	Neurodegeneration ↓IQ, hyperactivity Mild dysmorphism
MPSIV (A–B) (Morquio)	Galactose-6-sulfatase (A)	Cloudy corneas Pigmentary retinopathy	Skeletal dysplasia Normal facies/IQ
MPSVI (Maroteaux–Lamy)	N-acetyl-galactosamine-4-sulfatase	Cloudy corneas	Skeletal/facial dysmorphism Normal IQ
MPSVII (Sly)	β-glucuronidase	Cloudy corneas Optic atrophy	Skeletal/facial dysmorphism ↓IQ

All these conditions are AR, other than Hunter, which is X-linked.

Table 18.45 Disorders of mineral metabolism

Wilson disease	Cu-binding protein	Kayser–Fleischer ring Cataract	Neurodegeneration Ataxia
Menkes syndrome	Cu transport protein	Optic atrophy	Kinky hair Neurodegeneration Ataxia

These conditions are AR. Cu, copper.

Table 18.46 Disorders of connective tissues

Syndrome	Deficiency	Ocular features	Systemic features
Marfan syndrome	Fibrillin	Ectopia lentis Myopia Retinal detachment Glaucoma Blue sclera Keratoconus	Tall Long-limbed Arachnodactyly High arched palate Aortic dissection Mitral valve disease
Osteogenesis imperfecta	Collagen I	Blue sclera Keratoconus	Brittle bones Hearing loss
Stickler syndrome	Collagen II	Myopia Liquefied vitreous Retinal detachments	Arthropathy Midfacial flattening Cleft palate Hearing loss
Ehlers–Danlos syndrome (six types)	Collagens I and III	Myopia Retinal detachment Ectopia lentis Blue sclera Keratoconus Angioid streaks	Hyperflexible joints Hyperelastic skin Vascular bleeds
PXE	Elastin fragility	Angioid streaks Blue sclera	'Chicken' skin GI bleeds Arterial calcification
Weill–Marchesani syndrome		Ectopia lentis Microspherophakia	Short stature Brachydactyly ↓IQ

Marfan and Stickler are AD; Weill–Marchesani, Ehlers–Danlos, PXE, and osteogenesis imperfecta have dominant and recessive forms.

Phakomatoses

The phakomatoses are a group of conditions with neurological, ocular, and cutaneous features, and a tendency to develop tumours, usually of a hamartomatous type. There is considerable debate about which conditions to include, but neurofibromatosis, tuberous sclerosis, and VHL syndrome are generally considered to be the archetypes.

Neurofibromatosis

Neurofibromatosis-1 (NF-1) is the commonest of all the phakomatoses (prevalence 1/3,000) and arises from mutations in the neurofibromin gene (Chr 17q). Neurofibromatosis-2 (NF-2) is much less common (1/25,000) and arises from mutations in the merlin gene (Chr 22q). Both are AD but with variable expressivity (see Table 18.47 and Table 18.48).

Table 18.47 Features of NF-1

Ocular	Systemic
Optic nerve glioma Lisch nodules (≥2)	Café-au-lait spots (≥6; each >0.5cm pre-puberty or >1.5cm post-puberty) Axillary/inguinal freckling
Lid neurofibroma	Neurofibromas (≥1 plexiform type or ≥2 any type)
Choroidal naevi	Characteristic bony lesion (sphenoid dysplasia, which may cause pulsatile proptosis; long bone cortex thinning/dysplasia)
Retinal astrocytoma	First-degree relative with NF-1

Diagnosis requires two or more of the features in bold.

Table 18.48 Features of NF-2

Ocular	Systemic
Early-onset posterior subcapsular or cortical cataracts	Acoustic neuroma (AN) Meningioma
Combined hamartoma of the RPE and retina	Glioma Schwannoma First-degree relative with NF-2

Definite NF-2: bilateral AN OR first-degree relative with NF-2 AND either unilateral AN (at <30y) or any two of meningioma, glioma, schwannoma, or juvenile cataract.

Probable NF-2: unilateral AN (<30y) AND one of meningioma, glioma, schwannoma, or juvenile cataract; OR multiple meningiomas AND unilateral AN (<30y) or one of meningioma, glioma, schwannoma, or juvenile cataract.

Tuberous sclerosis

Tuberous sclerosis has a prevalence of 1/6,000. It arises from mutations in *TSC1* (Chr 9q) or *TSC2* (Chr 16p), which code for hamartin and tuberin, respectively. It is AD with variable expressivity; however, 50% of cases of tuberous sclerosis are from new mutations (see Table 18.49).

Table 18.49 Features of tuberous sclerosis

Ocular	Systemic
Retinal astrocytoma	Adenoma sebaceum
	Ash leaf spots
	Shagreen patches
	Subungual fibromas
	Cerebral astrocytomas (with epilepsy and ↓IQ)
	Visceral hamartomas (e.g. renal angiomyolipoma, cardiac rhabdomyoma)
	Visceral cysts
	Pulmonary lymphangioleiomyomatosis

VHL syndrome

This rare condition has a prevalence of 1/36,000. It arises from mutations in the *VHL* gene (Chr 3p), which appears to be involved in vascular proliferation. It is AD (see Table 18.50).

Table 18.50 Features of VHL syndrome

Ocular	Systemic
Retinal capillary haemangioma	Haemangioblastoma of cerebellum, spinal cord or brainstem
	Renal cell carcinoma
	Phaeochromocytoma
	Islet cell carcinoma
	Epididymal cysts/adenomas
	Visceral cysts

Sturge–Weber and Wyburn–Mason syndrome

These rare syndromes of vascular abnormalities differ from the 'true' phakomatoses in that they occur sporadically and the tumours (or AVM for Wyburn–Mason) are present from birth (see Table 18.51 and Table 18.52).

Table 18.51 Features of Sturge–Weber syndrome

Ocular	Systemic
Episcleral haemangioma	Naevus flammeus of the face (port-wine stain)
Ciliary body/iris haemangioma	
Choroidal haemangioma (diffuse)	CNS haemangioma
Glaucoma	

Table 18.52 Features of Wyburn–Mason syndrome

Ocular	Systemic
Retinal AVM	Cerebral/brainstem AVM
Orbital/periorbital AVM	

Refractive ophthalmology

Refractive error: introduction

Refractive error is a failure of the eye to focus light from an object onto the retina to form a clear image. It is a frequent cause of reduced visual function. If there is a refractive error when viewing a distant object, the eye is described as ametropic. Ametropia can be divided into myopia (*syn* 'short-sightedness'), hypermetropia (*syn* hyperopia; 'long-sightedness'), and astigmatism (see Table 19.1). If there is no refractive error when viewing a distant object, the eye is said to be emmetropic (see Fig. 19.1).

Epidemiology

It is estimated that refractive error affects around 1–2 billion people worldwide. The prevalence of different types of refractive error varies widely according to the population surveyed, from about 25% in Europe to over 80% in some Asian countries. It also varies according to age.

Definitions

Table 19.1 Summary of definitions

Term	Definition	Optical correction
Emmetropia	No refractive error when looking at a distant object	Nil
Myopia	Light from distant object focuses in front of the retina	Concave lens
Hypermetropia	Light from distant object focuses beyond the retina	Convex lens
Astigmatism	Optical power of eye uneven across different meridians	Toric lens
Presbyopia	Loss of normal accommodation, with failure to focus on near objects	Convex lens addition

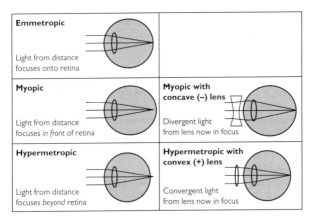

Fig. 19.1 Emmetropia, myopia, and hypermetropia.

Myopia, hypermetropia, and astigmatism

Myopia

Definition

Myopia arises where light from a distance is brought to a focus in front of the retina either because the refracting power of the eye is too great (index myopia) or the anteroposterior diameter is too long (axial myopia).

Classification

Myopia may be classified according to the size of the refractive error; however, there is no universally accepted system. The American Optometric Association (AOA) definitions are: low (<–3D), moderate (–3 to –6D), or high (>–6D). Myopia may physiological or pathological.

Physiological myopia

Physiological myopia is common (20–40% population), is usually <5D, and appears to be associated with increased time spent doing near work (usually reading) through teenage/early adulthood.

Pathological myopia (See ➲ Degenerative myopia, p. 548)

Pathological myopia is much less common (around 2% of the population) and is defined as enlargement of the eyeball with lengthening of the posterior segment. It is usually associated with much higher levels of myopia (>–6D).

Complications of pathological myopia

• Choroidal and retinal degeneration, retinal detachment, staphyloma, open-angle glaucoma. High myopia is also common in many abnormal developmental and genetic conditions.

Treatment

Correction of myopia requires the provision of a concave lens external to the eye (either as spectacles or CL) or a reduction in the refractive power of the eye itself (refractive surgery). Myopia progression can be slowed by orthokeratology and multifocal lens designs or pharmacological treatment.

Hypermetropia

Definition

Hypermetropia arises where light from a distance is brought to a focus behind the retina either because the refracting power of the eye is too weak or the anteroposterior diameter is too short.

Classification

Hypermetropia may be classified according to the size of refractive error. The AOA definitions are: low (≤+2D), moderate (2–5D), and high (>5D). Hypermetropia may be classified as simple, pathological, or functional. In simple hypermetropia, the structures and dimensions of the eye lie within normal limits, whereas, in pathological hypermetropia, the ocular anatomy is abnormal (e.g. developmental abnormality or other ocular pathology). Functional hypermetropia arises from failure of accommodation.

Complications
- Accommodative esotropia, amblyopia (children), early onset of presbyopia, angle-closure glaucoma, retinoschisis.

Treatment
Mild degrees of hypermetropia are often left uncorrected, as a young individual can exert some accommodation to achieve clear distance vision. However, uncorrected hypermetropia may lead to symptoms of ocular fatigue or headaches as a result. Correction of hypermetropia requires the provision of a convex lens external to the eye (spectacles or CL) or refractive surgery to increase in the refractive power of the eye.

Astigmatism

Definition
Astigmatism is where the refracting power of the eye is different in different meridians. It is defined in terms of its magnitude and direction. In the adult population, up to 20% have astigmatism >1D and the majority of the population have some level of detectable astigmatism.

Classification
Astigmatism may be regular (principal meridians 90° apart and so correctable by a toric lens) or irregular. Regular astigmatism may be 'with-the-rule' when the steepest meridian is around 90°, 'against-the-rule' when it is around 180°, or oblique where the principal meridians lie more than 20° from both 90° and 180°. Irregular astigmatism usually arises from an uneven corneal surface (e.g. through scarring or keratoconus).

Treatment
Correction of astigmatism may be achieved with spectacles using toric lenses (i.e. with different power in different meridians), CL, or refractive surgery. RGP CL are particularly suited to the correction of astigmatism (including irregular astigmatism), since their rigidity allows the space between lens and cornea to become filled by the tear film to form a 'lacrimal lens'. This effectively neutralizes corneal astigmatism. In contrast, hydrogel (soft) CLs are less rigid and adopt the same shape as the cornea. Therefore, if a hydrogel CL is to be used to treat astigmatism, a toric design will be necessary. A certain degree of astigmatism may also be corrected as part of refractive surgery procedures.

Spectacles: types

Spectacles (*syn* glasses, eyeglasses) are the oldest and best established of all the refractive options.

Types of spectacles

Single vision

These are single prescription spectacles. Standard single vision spectacles are made up with the 'distance' prescription. 'Reading glasses' are single vision lenses made up with the 'reading' or near prescription and are one option in presbyopia.

- *Advantages*: simple, easily tolerated, economical.
- *Disadvantages*: presbyopes will not be able to perform distance or intermediate tasks with their reading glasses and will require multiple pairs to cope with viewing different tasks/distances.

Bifocals

These are corrective lenses with two distinct regions of differing optical power, enabling refractive correction for two different focal distances in the same set of glasses; usually distance and reading, but may be intermediate, e.g. for VDU use. They have become less popular over the last decade due mainly to the advances in progressive lenses.

- Advantages: more convenient—enables presbyopes to use one set of glasses for tasks at two focal distances.
- Disadvantages: reduces field of vision at each distance (defined by the compromise between the size of each segment); objects may appear to 'jump' when moving between segments; can be poor cosmetically; prismatic effects may be problematic for certain prescriptions.

Types of bifocal

Bifocal lenses are available in a number of designs. These include:

- *Round segment*: near vision region is a distinct small, round segment; advantages: excellent field of vision for distance; better cosmetically; better in terms of prismatic effects, especially for plus powers where segment gives base-down prism. *Disadvantages*: significant 'jump' when moving between segments.
- *D segment (syn half-moon, flat-top)*: near vision region is a 'D' with the flat edge positioned superiorly. *Advantages*: good distance field; well tolerated since little jump; little problem with prismatic effects. *Disadvantages*: relatively poor cosmetically.
- *C segment*: similar to D segment but with the flat edge positioned inferiorly. Advantages: good distance field; well tolerated since little jump; little problem with prismatic effects; reasonable cosmetically.
- Executive (or E line): the lens consists of a straight line segment. *Advantages*: no jump (optical centre of both portions is on dividing line); larger near field of vision. *Disadvantages*: cosmetically poor.
- *Franklin split bifocals*: these consist of two separate lenses mounted together; specially designed to incorporate prisms, especially if different amounts are required for distance and near. *Advantages*: large amounts of prisms can be incorporated and optical centres can be altered. *Disadvantages*: cosmetically poor.

Trifocals

Similar to bifocals but contain three distinct optical regions, enabling three different focal distances (distance, intermediate, and near) in the same set of glasses. Occasionally used in the HES.

Progressive lenses

In progressive lenses (*syn* varifocal lenses), the optical power of the lens changes over the surface of the lens, typically with distance refractive correction in primary gaze, with a corridor of increasing positive power inferiorly to a zone of near refractive correction towards the bottom of the lens.

* *Advantages*: more convenient—enables presbyopes to use one set of glasses for tasks at multiple focal distances with minimal head adjustment; no 'jumping' of images; good cosmetically.
* *Disadvantages*: adaptation period required to adapt to peripheral distortion; more expensive; more distortion away from the optical axis; dependent on careful fitting (needs consideration of vertex distance, pantoscopic angle, and face form angle) to ensure the optics are correctly centred on the pupil.

Types of progressive lenses

There are a number of design features to the optics of progressive lenses such as:

* *'Hard'/'soft' designs*: the 'harder' the progressive lens design, the more the aberrations from blending powers are concentrated into a smaller region on the lens surface, expanding the area of clear vision (wider distance and near zones), but at the expense of increasing unwanted aberrations in the lens periphery.
* *Corridor length*: the corridor length between the distance and near zones can be shortened to improve ergonomic utility (every additional 1mm of corridor length requires roughly 2° of additional ocular rotation to reach the near zone) and smaller frames to be utilized, but this may result in smaller distance and near viewing zones as well as less intermediate vision and a more rapidly increasing level of peripheral aberrations.
* *'Design by prescription' progressive lenses*: vary from hard to soft design within the same lens, according to the different tolerance of hypermetropes and myopes to distortion in the near and distance segments.
* *Bespoke designs*: based on the measurement of aberrations from an individual patient's eyes.

Spectacles: materials

Lens material

Lenses may be made from glass or various plastics (e.g. CR-39 or polycarbonate).

Glass

Glass has the advantage of excellent optical properties, scratch resistance, and has been used in spectacles (or their equivalent) for around 700y.

- The commonest glass is ophthalmic Crown glass (refractive index 1.52), but alternative higher refractive index glasses are also available, e.g. flint glass (refractive index 1.62) may be used with Crown glass in fused bifocals.

Plastics

Plastics have the advantage of a lower density than glass, permitting, lighter lenses. They are also safer if shattered.

- CR-39 is the preferred plastic for most applications, as it has excellent optical properties, is reasonably scratch-resistant, and has low transmission of harmful UV light.
- Polycarbonate or Trivex is mainly used for safety goggles, since it is the most resistant to impact; its main disadvantage is reduced optical quality due to high light dispersion.

Coatings and tints

Surface coatings

Surface coatings may be used to provide scratch resistance, UV inhibition, and anti-reflective properties (for cosmesis and to reduce glare).

Photochromic lenses

Photochromic lenses are lenses which darken on UV/visible light exposure. They may be useful for patients who are very sensitive to glare or are persistently photophobic (e.g. in RP).

Glass photochromic lenses

These depend on a UV-sensitive silver halide (usually silver chloride) which is scattered through the full thickness of the lens.

- *Advantages*: rapid reaction time; photochromic properties long-lasting.
- *Disadvantages*: yellowish tinge when 'clear'; solid tints, so require multiple stock lenses and have uneven transmission and colour across lens according to thickness.

Plastic photochromic lenses

These utilize a surface layer of an organic UV-sensitive compound (usually an oxazine or a naphthopyran).

- *Advantages*: surface layer, so even transmission/colour across lens.
- *Disadvantages*: marginally slower reaction time; do not darken fully in hot weather; photochromic properties wane with time.

Spectacles: prescribing

The principles and practice of refraction are outlined earlier (see ➋ Refraction: outline (1), p. 40). However, when filling in a prescription for spectacles, make sure the following are noted.

General

- Record the prescription carefully and legibly, and double-check that you have transcribed it correctly.
- Ensure that the cylinder and axis are clearly stated and that + and − are clearly distinguishable.
- Ensure that the reading addition is clearly written for each eye (usually the same).
- Record IPD and BVD (especially if the Rx is ± 4.00D in any meridian).

Specific

- If applicable, record eligibility for any vouchers towards expense of glasses (and inform patient) (see ➋ Eligibility for free sight tests and optical vouchers in the NHS (UK), p. 920).
- In young high myopes, state if a high index lens is required.
- Record if a tint is clinically necessary, especially in photophobic patients.
- If applicable, record if a small frame supplement is required for a young child or state any special frame requirements.
- Record if adaptation to the glasses is likely to be required or if the lenses are designed to be used with the reading material at a particular working distance.

Causes of spectacle intolerance

When a patient complains of 'eye strain', they may mean refractive discomfort or asthenopia. It is most commonly seen after a recent moderate change in refractive prescription. However, consider first:

Are the spectacles correct?

- Focimeter them to check that they match the prescription given to the patient.
- Check if the optical centres are correct, especially in high prescriptions with significant induced prismatic effect.
- In the case of progressive lenses. the central fitting crosses of the progressive lens should coincide with the centre of the pupil.
- In the case of reading glasses, ensure that they are being used at the correct working distance.

Was the prescription correct?

- Without necessarily performing a full refraction, it should be possible to quickly test VA and verify whether the prescription given was optimal for distance/near.

Was the prescription a significant change for the patient?

In most cases, asthenopia is simply caused by a recent change in prescription. Look for:

- Significant change in axis or size of cylinder.
- Change of lens form.
- *Anisometropia*: the patient may not be coping with the difference between the two eyes, and optical compromise or further treatment (such as second eye cataract surgery) may need to be reduced.
- Overcorrection, especially of myopes who will end up permanently accommodating.
- Excessive near correction, resulting in an uncomfortably near and narrow reading distance.
- Unsuitable bifocal or progressive lenses—consider occupation, requirements, and general faculties of the patient.

Is there a more serious problem?

Serious ocular pathology may present as a change in refraction (e.g. posterior segment tumour or CMO) or may cause ocular discomfort that the patient misinterprets as 'eye strain'. A full ophthalmic examination may be required.

Contact lenses: outline

Contact lenses (CL) are optical devices that rest on the surface of the cornea. They may be used for correction of refractive error, for a wide range of therapeutic applications, or for cosmesis.

Function

Refractive (or corrective) contact lenses

This is the commonest application of CL. Refractive designs include:

- Simple spherical lenses suitable for hypermetropia, myopia, and low levels of astigmatism; can be used for presbyopia if one eye is prescribed for distance prescription and the other with a near prescription (monovision).
- Toric lenses for more severe astigmatism.
- Bifocal and multifocal lenses for presbyopia.

Therapeutic contact lenses

Commonly called 'bandage' CL, their range of applications is much wider than this implies (see Table 19.2).

Table 19.2 Applications of therapeutic contact lenses

Indication	Examples
Pain relief	Bullous keratopathy, band keratopathy, RCES
Promotion of epithelial wound healing	RCES, persistent epithelial defect
Protection of ocular surface	Entropion, trichiatic lashes
Prevention of ocular dehydration	Dry eye (severe)
Maintain globe integrity	Threatened perforation or early leak
Maintain fornices	SJS, chemical burn
Therapeutic cosmesis	Severely scarred cornea, aniridia, phthisis, leucocoria
Drug delivery	Depot of high drug concentration (seldom used)

Cosmetic contact lenses

In addition to their important 'therapeutic' role in improving cosmesis for a number of pathological conditions, cosmetic CL are widely available for changing eye colour and for 'novelty' or theatrical use (e.g. cat-eyes, national flags, etc).

Material

The ideal CL must not only have excellent optical properties but also be inert, well tolerated by the ocular surface, comfortable to wear, and have good oxygen transmissibility. Oxygen transmissibility (Dk/t) depends on oxygen permeability (Dk) and lens thickness (t). Oxygen permeability itself (Dk) depends on diffusion (D) and solubility (k). The different types of lenses are commonly classified according to their material and are discussed in relevant sections (see ➜ Contact lenses: hard and RGP lenses, p. 838; ➜ Contact lenses: hydrogel lenses, p. 840).

Wearing schedule

Duration of wear: daily wear vs extended wear

In daily wear, there is a regular CL-free period overnight. The lens is cleaned and disinfected (conventional CL) or discarded (disposable CL).

Extended wear has a role in certain patients (e.g. elderly aphakes, young babies) but is generally discouraged for the general population due to the higher risk of infection. The Dk values for soft hydrogels and many RGP materials are sufficient for daily wear but are inadequate for extended wear and result in corneal compromise. For those requiring extended wear, certain silicone hydrogel lenses have been licensed for continuous wear of up to 30d.

Duration of lens: conventional vs disposable

Conventional lenses are usually replaced annually. They are more expensive (per lens); a wider range of parameters are possible but are more vulnerable to damage/loss/deposition due to their long lifespan.

Disposable lenses are commonly replaced either daily, fortnightly, or monthly. They are cheaper, have a narrower range of parameters, but are less likely to be damaged/lost during their lifespan and will attract less lens deposition.

Lens notation

CL parameters are noted as follows: base curves (BC) or back optic zone radii (BOZR), total diameter (TD), and power.

Contact lenses: hard and RGP lenses

'Hard' lenses

Originally made of glass and later of PMMA, these have excellent optical properties but are minimally oxygen-permeable (Dk = 0), so compromising epithelial metabolism with risk of 'overwear'. They are rarely prescribed now.

Rigid gas permeable (RGP) lenses

Made of complex polymers (which may include silicone, fluorene, PMMA, and others). They try to balance oxygen permeability (principally from the silicone molecules) and wettability (contributed to by the fluorene and any coatings) which is important for comfort. For refractive use, they are usually 8.5–11.5mm in size ('corneal'). For therapeutic use, corneal, semi-scleral (14.5–16.5mm), and larger scleral (~23mm) RGP lenses are used (see Box 19.1).

RGP lenses for refractive use

- *Indication*: most types of refractive error, including irregular astigmatism.
- *Design*: due to their rigidity, the space behind the RGP CLs becomes filled in by a 'lacrimal lens'. This effectively neutralizes corneal astigmatism and makes them the treatment of choice for conditions where corneal irregularity is an issue (e.g. keratoconus). Toric lenses may be used for higher degrees of astigmatism; bifocal and multifocal designs for presbyopia.
- *Advantages*: excellent optical quality; good oxygen permeability, particular due to their greater mobility and less corneal coverage than soft CLs; easy to handle (by patient); decreased risk of microbial keratitis.
- *Disadvantages*: moderate initial discomfort/FB sensation; require skilled fitting by CL practitioner (vs hydrogel CL).
- *Use of topical medication*: can safely use fluorescein; preservative-free treatments preferable, but preserved drops can be used with caution.

RGP lenses for therapeutic use

- *Corneal RGP*: indications—severe dry eye, exposure keratopathy, trichiasis; advantages, disadvantages, and use of topical medication—as for RGP lenses for refractive use.
- *Scleral/semi-scleral RGP*: indications—severe dry eye (provide good tear reservoir), exposure keratopathy, trichiasis, maintenance of fornices, more severe keratoconus, severe ocular allergic conditions; advantages—bridge the cornea so can cope with more irregular corneas without causing scarring. Use of topical medication—as for other RGP lenses (see ➲ RGP lenses for refractive use, p. 838). Can be made out of PMMA (more robust) or more oxygen-permeable materials. Scleral impression moulding to make a specialist lens has largely been replaced by simplified fitting sets which are much easier and quicker to fit, although they are usually fitted under the HES or specialist centres.

Box 19.1 Inserting and removing RGP lenses: instructions to patients*

Always wash hands before handling lenses, and inspect lens for any damage/foreign material prior to insertion.

Insertion

- Place lens on tip of index finger of dominant hand, concave side up.
- Place a couple of drops of a suitable wetting and soaking solution onto the lens, and rub them in.
- Look at the lens while you bring it towards the eye.
- Ask the patient to look down and apply pressure to the upper lid margin with your index finger. Ask the patient to look up and apply pressure to the lower lid margin with the index finger of the other hand. Maximize the palpebral aperture.
- Place lens on cornea.
- Look down for a couple of seconds while you release the lids.

Removal

- *Suction method*: a suction holder is applied directly to the lens, allowing it to be directly lifted off the eye. The lens can then be slid off the holder (avoid 'pulling' it off directly). This approach is no longer favoured due to the risk of introducing microbes to the ocular surface.
- *Lid method*: ask the patient to look down and apply pressure to the upper lid margin with your index finger. Ask the patient to look up and apply pressure to the lower lid margin with the index finger of the other hand. Making sure the lens is centred between the fingers, the lids are extracted so the whole lens is exposed, and the lid margins are not turned outwards, bring your fingers together to break the seal between the lens and the ocular surface with the edge curve of the lens.
- *Blink method*: look straight ahead, and open their eyes as wide as possible (so that upper lid is above lens); place a finger at the lateral margin of the lids, and gently pull them laterally; blink firmly to displace the lens (catch it/ensure it will drop onto a suitable clean surface).

* With only minor adjustment, these same techniques can be used by the practitioner (or carer) to insert/remove RGP lenses.

Contact lenses: hydrogel lenses

Hydrogel (soft) lenses

Made of polymers of hydroxethyl methylacrylate, these absorb much more fluid (high water content) than the RGP lenses. In hydrogel lenses, a higher water content results in greater solubility (k) and therefore better permeability (Dk from 10 to around 40) (see Box 19.2).

Hydrogel lenses for refractive use

- *Indication*: most types of refractive error.
- *Design*: hydrogel CLs do not vault over the cornea, and thus there is no significant 'lacrimal lens' to neutralize corneal astigmatism. However, toric CLs can treat astigmatism, provided the lens is stabilized (e.g. prism, thin zones).
- *Advantages*: comfortable, easy to fit, inexpensive.
- *Disadvantages*: less effective vs astigmatism; prone to spoilage if not frequently replaced; oxygen transmissibility not sufficient for overnight wear; optical quality may be less good than RGP lens.
- *Use of topical medication*: avoid fluorescein (will permanently stain); avoid preserved therapies, except for very short-term use.

Hydrogel lenses for therapeutic use

- *Indication*: pain relief, promotion of wound healing, protection of ocular surface, maintenance of globe integrity.
- *Advantages*: wide range of sizes (13.5–20mm for non-frequent replacement lenses); comfortable, easy to fit.
- *Disadvantages*: oxygen transmissibility not sufficient for overnight wear.
- *Use of topical medication*: avoid fluorescein; avoid preserved therapies, except for very short-term use.

Silicone hydrogel lenses

Silicone hydrogel CLs combine some of the advantages of RGP materials with hydrogel lenses. Silicone hydrogel lenses are usually available as 13.5–14.5mm diameter. The silicone is highly permeable to oxygen, so the more silicone (the less water content) the higher the DK (up to ~140). They have a role in both refractive and therapeutic applications.

Silicone hydrogel lenses for refractive use

- *Indication*: most types of refractive error.
- *Advantages*: excellent Dk values (up to 140) which permit longer wearing time.
- *Disadvantages*: generally higher rigidity, high wetting angle.
- *Use of topical medication*: avoid fluorescein (will permanently stain); avoid preserved therapies, except for very short-term use.

Silicone hydrogel lenses for therapeutic use

- *Indication*: promotion of wound healing, pain relief, protection of ocular surface, maintenance of globe integrity.
- *Advantages*: higher Dk leads to ↓risk of vascularization (vs hydrogel CL) (so use in keratoplasty patients).

- *Disadvantages*: less well tolerated in sensitive eyes due to generally higher rigidity and high wetting angle (poorer wetability).
- *Use of topical medication*: avoid fluorescein; avoid preserved therapies, except for very short-term use.

Box 19.2 Inserting and removing hydrogel lenses: instructions to patients*

Always wash hands before handling lenses, and inspect lens for any damage/foreign material prior to insertion. Hold lenses with the tips of the thumb and index finger ; fingernails can cause scratches.

Insertion
- Check that the lens is not 'inside out'; in the correct orientation, the edges should curve slightly inwards, rather than outwards, although not always easy to tell on thin designs.
- Place lens on tip of index finger of dominant hand, concave side up, minimizing contact area.
- Look at the lens while you bring it towards the eye.
- Ask the patient to look down and apply pressure to the upper lid margin with your index finger. Ask the patient to look up and apply pressure to the lower lid margin with the index finger of the other hand. Maximize the palpebral aperture.
- Look up or nasally, and place lens on the sclera.
- Look slowly around to displace air bubbles under the lens and to let the lens settle.
- Look down for a couple of seconds while you gently release the lids.

Removal
- Ask the patient to look down and apply pressure to the upper lid margin with your index finger. Ask the patient to look up and apply pressure to the lower lid margin with the middle finger of the other hand.
- Place index finger of this hand on lens.
- Look up or to your nose, and slide lens down onto inferior or temporal sclera.
- Lift the lens off between the tips of thumb and index finger.

* With only minor adjustment, these same techniques can be used by the practitioner (or carer) to insert/remove hydrogel lenses.

Contact lenses: fitting

Refractive CL

- Measure corneal curvature (keratometry), pupil diameter, vertical palpebral aperture, and corneal/visible iris diameter.
- Either:
  - Predict the lens parameters required (from nomograms incorporating the above measurements and known refractive error), and order the lens on a 'sale-or-return' basis, or
  - Use a trial lens set to determine the best fit.

Rigid gas permeable (RGP)

Estimate CL parameters

The BC is dictated by the type of lens (consult specific manufacturer fitting guide), but is usually the flattest K reading (as the tears fill in the gap between the lens and steeper corneal meridian) or bridging the gap between the meridians (generally corneal astigmatism <2.5D) such as 1/3rd difference steeper than flattest K). If 'on K', for a spherical lens, the lacrimal lens formed by the tear film in the centre of the lens is plano. If steeper or flatter, it confers a plus or minus power of around 0.25D per 0.05mm difference of curvature.

The lens diameter may be influenced by the diameters of the cornea and pupil, and even lid position. A large lens is generally more stable and comfortable and will have less chance of causing flare from the edge of the optic zone impinging on the pupil. Increasing the diameter tightens the fit and vice versa.

The lens power is determined either by calculation (in the form ocular refraction = spectacle refraction / [(1 − BVD) × spectacle refraction] where the spectacle refraction is the spherical component only in negative cylinder form) and can be confirmed together with the alignment of the lens by the 'overrefraction' with a trial lens in place where the ocular prescription = trial lens power + overrefraction + lacrimal lens power.

Assess fit after 20min

The CL should be centred, not crossing the limbus or the optic zone encroaching across the pupil margin, even in dim illumination. The lens should be comfortable after adaptation and should move 1–2mm with blinking, allowing tear flow under the lens. Less movement of a settled lens generally implies too tight/steep; more and a curved movement path implies too loose/flat. However, fluorescein is the key parameter for assessing the lens fit. Good alignment (when the lens is centred) results in shallow clearance (little fluorescence seen) in the centre and mid-periphery, with a bright band of edge clearance around the lens rim. If too steep, there is high central clearance (bright fluorescence) and mid-peripheral touch, along with often a thin edge band; if too flat, there is central touch (black) and clearance in the mid-periphery, extending into the edge curve.

Hydrogel (soft)

Estimate CL parameters

The BC should be in the range of 0.6–1.0mm larger than the average K.

The lens diameter should exceed the corneal diameter covering the limbus by ~1mm. The lens power is calculated as described previously, but using the mean spherical equivalent refraction (ocular refraction = spectacle refraction / [(1 − BVD) × spectacle refraction]).

Assess fit after 20min

The CL should be comfortable, fully cover the cornea, be fairly centred, and should move 0.25–0.50mm with blinking, should displace on ocular excursions (lag) and recover relatively quickly following lens push-up.

Follow-up

Ensure that patients understand how to look after their lenses (including self and case hygiene, together with care solutions). Discuss potential complications (e.g. microbial keratitis), how they present, and the need for lens removal and urgent review in such circumstances. Phrases, such as 'if in doubt, take it out' and the eye should 'look, feel, and see good', can simply impart some key safety concepts.

Follow-up should be fairly frequent initially but, in long-standing uncomplicated CL wear, may be reduced to yearly.

Non-refractive CL

Therapeutic ('bandage') and cosmetic CL are usually plano (or even opaque). Hydrogel and silicone hydrogel CL for therapeutic use generally come in a few standard sizes and are fitted according to diameter/BC. More skilled fitting is required for RGP therapeutic lenses (see RGP lenses for therapeutic use, p. 838). PMMA lenses require a specialist fitting in a dedicated centre.

Contact lenses: complications

The majority of CL complications are associated with poor compliance with recommended CL practice.

Painful red eye in the CL wearer

First rule out microbial keratitis. Then consider alternative diagnoses.

Microbial keratitis (See ➲ Microbial keratitis: assessment, p. 222)
White infiltrate ± epithelial defect, mucopurulent infiltrate, AC inflammation, often large, irregularly shaped, very painful, getting worse with lens removal.
- *Ophthalmic emergency*: treat aggressively (see ➲ Microbial keratitis: treatment, p. 224). Consider *Pseudomonas* and *Acanthamoeba* (more commonly seen in CL wearers).

Sterile keratitis
Small, sometimes multiple, anterior stromal infiltrates, usually non-staining; may be only mildly symptomatic, round, no AC inflammation and watery discharge.
- Differentiate from microbial keratitis. Consider temporarily stopping (if severe) or reducing (if mild) CL wear; improve CL care, using preservative-free solutions or change to alternative CL.

Giant papillary conjunctivitis
Itching + mucoid discharge in the presence of giant papillae under the upper lid.
- Mast cell stabilizer (e.g. sodium cromoglicate 4×/d). Consider temporarily stopping (if severe) or reducing (if mild) CL wear; improve CL care, using preservative-free solutions or change to alternative CL.

CL acute red eye
Lens that has bound to the eye with overnight wear, causing extreme discomfort, red eye, with anterior corneal oedema and AC reaction.
- Remove lens; topical cycloplegic if severe AC reaction; replace with flatter, more mobile lens when recovered, and consider discontinuing extended wear.

Toxic keratopathy
Disinfectant/enzyme inadvertently introduced into eye, resulting in diffuse punctate epithelial erosions ± subepithelial infiltrates.
- Remove lens; preservative-free artificial tears; educate re CL care.

Preservative keratopathy
Preservative (e.g. thiomersal) exposure with punctate epithelial erosions (may be superior limbic pattern) ± subepithelial infiltrates
- Remove lens; preservative-free artificial tears; educate re CL care, and change to preservative-free or differently preserved cleaning solutions.

Tear film disturbance
Poor blink response or ill-fitting RGP lens, resulting in punctate staining at 3 or 9 o'clock with interpalpebral hyperaemia.
- Preservative-free artificial tears; check CL fit.

Painless red eye

Neovascularization

Superficial neovascularization at 3 and 9 o'clock is common or under the thickest toric meridian. It usually does not extend >2–3mm.

- Remove lens; replace with a lens with high oxygen permeability (Dk). Ghost vessels will remain and will refill immediately if hypoxia reintroduced.

Other complications

Other complications include abnormalities of the epithelium, including microcysts, endothelial polymegathism, loss of lens, and superficial corneal abrasion. Optical effects include spectacle blur (their spectacle correction is transiently incorrect after CL wear), flexure (refractive change due to flexing of CL), visual flare (edge effect), accommodative effects (e.g. a myope has to accommodate more when switching from glasses to CL), and aberrations (spherical and chromatic).

Introduction to refractive surgery

Introduction

Refractive surgery reduces or eliminates an individual's dependence on glasses or CL. It is generally safe and produces good results, but it is not risk-free and complications can occur. It should be noted that:

- There is a small risk of permanently damaging vision such that it will not be correctable with glasses/CL.
- Optical correction by refractive surgery may not improve best possible vision. Although vision without glasses/CL is likely to be improved, the patient may still only achieve their best possible VA with glasses/CL.
- Standard photorefractive surgery does not correct for presbyopia, thus myopes may be exchanging dependence on distance glasses for dependence on reading glasses. Surgical options to consider for presbyopia include:
  - Monovision (one eye correct for distance, the other for near) via refractive surgery techniques such as LASIK or conductive keratoplasty (CK).
  - Refractive lens exchange with accommodating/multifocal IOLs.
  - Emerging techniques include presbyopic/multifocal LASIK.
- If developing visually significant cataracts, early cataract surgery with correction by appropriate choice of IOL may be a better alternative.
- In general, lower refractive errors are corrected using laser-based techniques, whereas higher refractive errors are treated with lens-based techniques (see Table 19.3).

General preoperative considerations

The Royal College of Ophthalmologists (UK)[1] have made recommendations on the information that should be provided to the patient considering laser refractive surgery. These include information on the range of refractive options available (whether or not they are available at the particular institution that they are attending), success/complication rates, qualifications of the surgeon, costs of procedures (including refund policies), follow-up arrangements (including emergencies), complaint procedures. In addition, the following factors, which are relevant to their long-term ophthalmic care, must be recorded and a copy provided to the patient:

- Preoperative keratometry.
- Preoperative pachymetry.
- Pre- and post-operative best corrected acuity.
- Pre- and post-operative IOP.
- Preoperative and stabilized post-operative refraction.

---

1. Royal College of Ophthalmologists. *Standards for laser refractive surgery.* (2011). Available at: ⌖ www.rcophth.ac.uk/clinicalguidelines

Table 19.3 Summary of refractive surgery options

Procedure	Abbreviation	Mechanism	Approximate refractive error range
Corneal-based			
Excimer laser			
Photorefractive keratectomy	PRK	Surface ablation technique: epithelium removed, stroma selectively ablated with excimer laser, BCL inserted	−6DS to −12DS 5D cyl
Laser-assisted epithelial keratectomy	LASEK	Surface ablation technique: epithelium removed as sheet using alcohol, stroma selectively ablated with excimer laser, BCL inserted	−6DS to −12DS 5D cyl
Epithelial laser *in situ* keratomileusis	Epi-LASIK	Surface ablation technique: epithelium removed as sheet mechanically with epikeratome, stroma selectively ablated with excimer laser, BCL inserted	−4DS to −12DS 5D cyl
Laser *in situ* keratomileusis	LASIK	Flap-based technique: partial-thickness superficial corneal flap created with microkeratome or FSL, stroma selectively ablated with excimer laser, flap replaced	−4DS to −12DS 5D cyl
Incisional surgery			
Radial keratotomy	RK	Peripheral deep corneal incisions cause central corneal flattening	Myopia up to −6DS
Arcuate keratotomy	AK	Paired arcuate corneal incisions in mid-peripheral cornea cause flattening in that meridian and steepening in opposite meridian	Astigmatism up to 6D cyl
Limbal relaxing incision	LRI	Paired arcuate incisions at limbus cause flattening in that meridian and steepening in opposite meridian	Astigmatism up to 3D cyl

(*Continued*)

Table 19.3 (Cont.)

Procedure	Abbreviation	Mechanism	Approximate refractive error range
Corneal shrinkage surgery			
Laser thermal keratoplasty	LTK	Shrinkage of peripheral corneal stroma in a radial pattern causing flattening and corresponding steepening of the central cornea using Holmium:Nd-YAG laser	Low hypermetropia (and presbyopia) up to 3DS
Conductive keratoplasty	CK	Shrinkage of peripheral corneal stroma in a radial pattern causing flattening and corresponding steepening of the central cornea using high radiofrequency currents	Low hypermetropia (and presbyopia) up to 3DS
Corneal additive surgery			
Intracorneal ring segments	ICRS	Plastic ring segments placed in preformed tunnels in the peripheral cornea causing central flattening	Low myopia (up to −3D) Astigmatism in keratoconus
Lens-based			
Phakic intraocular lens	Phakic IOL	Crystalline lens intact. Synthetic IOL which can be in the AC (iris fixated or angle supported) or in the posterior chamber	−5D to −20D
Refractive lens exchange	RLE	Crystalline lens removed and replaced with PCIOL (monofocal, multifocal, or accommodative)	Any refractive error

Biophysics of refractive lasers (1)

Types of laser-tissue interactions

Photoablation (excimer laser)

Argon fluoride is the main type of excimer (excited-dimer) laser. Electrical energy stimulates argon to form dimers with fluorine, producing 193nm UV light. These high-energy photons have low tissue penetrance, producing high-precision breakage of intermolecular bonds which vaporizes and reshapes the tissue surface. This is used for changing the refractive power of the cornea.

Photodisruption (femtosecond laser)

Infrared light laser of 1,053nm causes photodisruption, the transformation of tissue into plasma, in which very localized high temperature and temperature causes rapid tissue expansion and small microscopic cavities, allowing separation of tissues. This is used for creating flaps in the cornea for LASIK, creating channels in the cornea for intracorneal ring segments (ICRS), and for cutting corneas for lamellar and penetrating keratoplasty.

Photothermal (holmium laser)

Holmium:YAG laser (2.13 microns) is absorbed by water in the cornea, causing thermal shrinkage of collagen used for treating low amounts of hypermetropia.

Types of excimer laser

Broad beam

Large diameter beams (~7mm) with slow repetition rate. High-energy pulses, only small number of pulses needed to treat. Short operating time but uneven ablation more likely.

Scanning slit

Narrow beams that scan across corneal surface, improving smoothness and allowing larger treatment zones than broad beam lasers.

Flying spot

Much smaller diameter beams (0.5–2.0mm) with a high repetition rate. Used in conjunction with a tracking mechanism to ensure precise ablation. This is the main type of laser in use today.

Changes in corneal shape

An understanding of the basic changes that occur to the corneal shape is useful in understanding topographic and pachymetry changes, following different types of treatment, and also the optical zone of treatment required (see Fig. 19.2).

Myopic treatments

Central corneal tissue is removed to make the central cornea *flatter* (see Fig. 19.2a). The amount of tissue removed is more important with higher degrees of myopia, since untreated cornea is thinnest in the centre. The amount of tissue removed in myopic ablations is governed by the Munnerlyn formula:

Depth of ablation (micron) = Diameter (mm) $2 \times$ Power (D) / 3

Thus, depth of ablation for a given refractive correction increases by the square of the treatment diameter. Small ablation zones minimize tissue removal so theoretically would be beneficial in high refractive errors. However, small treatment zones are associated with high degrees of haloes and glare, particularly with large pupil size. They are also associated with greater regression. Large treatment zones reduce visual symptoms and regression but are limited by requiring greater tissue removal. A compromise optical zone size of ~6mm is normally used for removal.

Hypermetropic treatments
A ring-shaped area of mid-peripheral corneal tissue is removed to make the central cornea steeper (see Fig. 19.2b).

Astigmatic treatments
Treatment with an elliptical or cylindrical beam which removes more tissue in the steeper meridian which is then flattened.

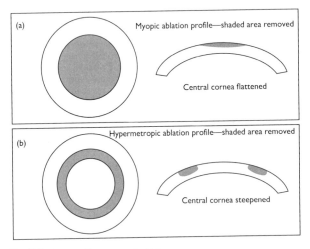

Fig. 19.2 Myopic and hypermetropic ablation.

Biophysics of refractive lasers (2)

Conventional, wavefront-guided, wavefront-optimized, and topography-guided ablations

(See Fig. 19.3.)

Conventional treatment

The only corrected aberrations are low-order aberrations, based on patient's subjective refraction, namely sphere and cylinder. These treatments can increase certain types of higher-order aberrations, particularly spherical aberration which can reduce contrast and cause problems with night vision.

Wavefront-optimized treatment

Treatment based on patient's subjective refraction. Wavefront theory and modelling used to generate additional laser pulses to the periphery of the cornea to negate the spherical aberration induced by conventional treatment.

Wavefront-guided treatment

Higher-order aberrations cause problems with contrast and sharp focus that are not addressed by glasses and CL, e.g. coma, trefoil, spherical aberration. Wavefront technology allows the measurement of these higher-order aberrations with a wavefront aberrometer. Customized excimer laser uses the wavefront scan to drive the ablation, allowing the correction of higher-order aberrations as well as the low-order aberrations. However, there may be an increase in new aberrations that did not exist preoperatively.

Topography-guided treatment

It is not possible to obtain accurate aberrometry in very irregular corneas. Some modern lasers are able to use customized data from corneal topographers to drive the ablation to treat highly irregular corneas.

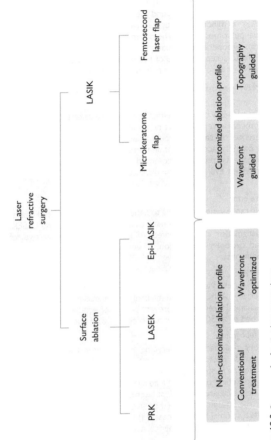

Fig. 19.3 Summary of refractive laser procedures.

Excimer laser refractive surgery: preoperative evaluation

Most patients have excellent results after refractive surgery. Since the introduction of the excimer laser in the 1980s which revolutionized refractive surgery, millions of people around the world have now undergone PRK or LASIK. A small minority of patients have visual complications or unsatisfactory visual outcomes. This can be minimized by careful patient selection and meticulous preoperative evaluation. Patients with unrealistic expectations or unwilling to accept any level of risk should be excluded. Identify patients with relative or absolute contraindications to refractive surgery.

Refractive preoperative assessment

Age

Lower limit 18–21y or when refractive stability reached (no change >0.50D in 2y), otherwise retreatments necessary. No theoretical upper age limit, but presence of cataract would make laser surgery inappropriate. In younger patients (accommodation normal), aim for perfect distance vision. In older patients (reduced accommodation), consider monovision correction (dominant eye perfect for distance, fellow eye low myopia for near vision).

Refractive error

Treatable range varies according to patient corneal thickness and needs. On average, +6D to –12D covers main range for LASIK, PRK, and LASEK. Up to 5D astigmatism can be treated. All patients undergo subjective refraction (and cycloplegic refraction, if deemed necessary, especially young hypermetropes).

Pachymetry

Cornea thickness is a limiting factor for the degree of laser correction possible, especially LASIK. Must be a minimal corneal thickness after laser to provide mechanical strength and prevent post-laser ectasia. A minimal residual stromal bed of >250 microns is an accepted figure but not absolute.

Corneal topography

Mandatory in all patients undergoing excimer laser. Eyes with features of ectatic disease on topography (keratoconus, pellucid marginal degeneration, and forme fruste keratoconus) excluded, since laser ablation can cause further weakening of cornea, leading to further ectasia. Scoring systems exist to help evaluate risk of post-laser ectasia (e.g. the Ectasia Risk Scoring System,[2] risk stratification based on five variables: (1) topography pattern, (2) residual stromal bed thickness, (3) age, (4) preoperative corneal thickness, and (5) preoperative spherical manifest refraction.

Keratometric power

Myopic treatments cause corneal flattening, and hypermetropic treatments cause corneal steepening. Optical quality is significantly degraded beyond certain limits of post-operative keratometry. Accepted values are a minimum of 38D after myopic ablations and a maximum of 50D after hypermetropic ablations.

Pupil size

Pupil size measurement under mesopic conditions is mandatory. In general, large pupils in mesopic conditions (>7.5mm) tend to be associated with increased optical aberrations, and so a larger laser treatment zone may be preferable.

Full ophthalmic examination

Particular attention to ocular surface and evidence of dry eye, tonometry, presence of cataract, and retinal examination.

2. Randleman JB et al. Validation of the Ectasia Risk Score System for preoperative laser in situ keratomileusis screening. Am J Ophthalmol 2008;145:813–18.

Excimer laser refractive surgery: contraindications

Ophthalmic contraindications

(See Table 19.4.)

Table 19.4 Ophthalmic contraindications to refractive laser surgery

Ocular contraindications	Reason
Corneal ectasias: keratoconus, forme fruste keratoconus, pellucid marginal degeneration (absolute CI)	Ablation causes further thinning of ectatic cornea—increases risk of further ectasia
Active or recently active herpes keratitis or HZO (absolute CI)	Increased risk of reactivation due to UV light activation. If inactive >1y, consider treatment with prophylactic aciclovir
Previous herpes keratitis or HZO (relative CI)	
KCS (absolute CI) or dry eye (relative CI)	LASIK causes exacerbation of KCS and increased risk of keratitis
	PRK in KCS increases risk of post-operative haze and delayed epithelialization
Neurotrophic keratopathy (absolute CI)	Ablation associated with delayed epithelialization
Glaucoma (relative CI)	Patients with steroid-induced ↑IOP difficult to manage after PRK due to duration of post-op treatment needed. LASIK requires a high pressure during flap creation which can induce further glaucomatous damage. Changes in corneal thickness means that IOP measurements with applanation tonometry are inaccurate
Previous corneal surgery: radial keratotomy (RK), PK (relative CI)	LASIK unpredictable. Absolutely contraindicated in RK with epithelial plugs at incision site. Consider PRK
Epithelial basement membrane dystrophy (relative CI for LASIK)	Increased likelihood of epithelial defect during flap creation. Surface ablation preferred, may also be therapeutic
Active ophthalmic disease (absolute CI)	For example, diabetic retinopathy, uveitis

CI, contraindication.

Medical contraindications

(See Table 19.5.)

Table 19.5 Medical contraindications to refractive laser surgery

Medical contraindications	Reason
Pregnancy (absolute CI)	Refractive fluctuation. Changes in tear film affecting healing. Unknown risk to fetus of post-operative topical medications
Diabetes mellitus associated with neurotrophic cornea (absolute CI)	Ablation associated with delayed epithelialization
Autoimmune diseases, connective tissue disorders (relative CI)	Altered wound healing
Keloid scars/abnormal wound healing (relative CI)	Increased risk of post-operative haze with PRK. LASIK is preferable
Immunosuppressive medications including oral steroids, isotretinoin, amiodarone (relative CI)	Altered wound healing

Excimer laser refractive surgery: surface treatments

In general, excimer laser treatment is good for spherical refractive errors in the range +6.0D to −12.00D and astigmatism up to 5.00D. Absolute amounts vary according to patient and laser used. Several different techniques are available but can generally be divided into surface treatments (PRK, LASEK, Epi-LASEK) or lamellar/flap-based treatments (LASIK) (see Fig. 19.4).

PRK

Involves the reshaping of the corneal surface following removal of the epithelium. Excimer laser is applied directly to Bowman's layer and removes this layer and anterior stroma.

- *Indications*: previously for low myopia and hypermetropia. Large PRK myopic ablations were associated with increased risk of post-operative corneal haze. With intraoperative MMC, larger ablations are now possible without post-operative haze. Range: myopia from −0.50D to −12.00D; hypermetropia up to +6.00D; astigmatism up to 5.00D.
- PRK is the treatment of choice for:
  - Thin corneas.
  - Corneas with epithelial irregularities, scars, and dystrophies.
  - Very flat or very steep corneas.
  - Eyes with increased risk of trauma such as military personnel and contact sports players.
  - Dry eyes.
  - Patients who had complication from LASIK in fellow eye.
- *Method*: corneal epithelium is removed in area of planned treatment (ablation of epithelium is very uneven with excimer laser). Epithelium removal can be performed: (1) mechanically (blade or rotating brush), (2) chemically (20% ethanol), or (3) laser itself on phototherapeutic keratectomy (PTK) mode. The size of the ablation zone (optical zone) depends on the type of ametropia (larger optical zones necessary for hypermetropic corrections than myopic corrections). Following ablation, CL is inserted until epithelial defect healed. Post-operative topical antibiotics and steroids given.
- *Advantages*: safe, long track record, more ablation possible in thin corneas since no flap required, removal of all complications related to flap creation in LASIK.
- *Disadvantages*: post-operative pain for 2–4d. Slow recovery and slow refractive stability. Wound healing variability and haze formation. Long post-operative drop regimen.

LASEK (laser-assisted subepithelial keratectomy)

A surface ablation related to PRK, but the epithelium is loosened with alcohol and then replaced after laser ablation.

- *Indications*: similar to PRK.
- *Method*: a metal reservoir placed over cornea and filled with 18–20% alcohol to loosen epithelium for ~20s. Loose epithelium is then moved to one side, and the underlying Bowman's layer and stroma are lasered as with PRK. The epithelium is then carefully repositioned, and a bandage lens is placed.

- *Advantages*: theoretically less painful, less haze, and quicker rehabilitation than for PRK.
- *Disadvantages*: more painful, slower visual rehabilitation, and more haze than with LASIK. The use of alcohol means the epithelial sheet is not viable.

Epi-LASIK

A surface ablation related to PRK, but the epithelial flap is made mechanically and lifted before laser applied as for PRK and then flap replaced.

- *Indications*: similar to PRK.
- *Method*: the epithelium is lifted off as a sheet mechanically, using an epikeratome consisting of a blunt plastic blade. The sheet is lifted away intact, and the cornea is sculpted as normal with the excimer laser. The flap is replaced, and a bandage lens is placed over the flap.
- *Advantages*: theoretically less pain, faster healing, and less haze than with PRK and LASEK.
- *Disadvantages*: similar to LASEK. Also risk of stromal penetration by epikeratome.

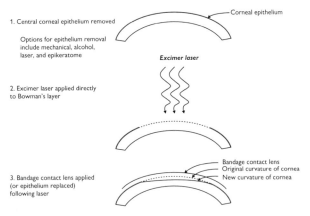

1. Central corneal epithelium removed

   Options for epithelium removal include mechanical, alcohol, laser, and epikeratome

   Corneal epithelium

Excimer laser

2. Excimer laser applied directly to Bowman's layer

3. Bandage contact lens applied (or epithelium replaced) following laser

   Bandage contact lens
   Original curvature of cornea
   New curvature of cornea

Fig. 19.4 Outline of surface-based excimer refractive therapies.

Excimer laser refractive surgery: LASIK

LASIK (laser *in situ* keratomileusis)

Technique involves two stages: firstly creating a thin flap on the surface of the cornea using a microkeratome blade or using FemtoSecond Laser (FSL); secondly, the flap is lifted and the stromal bed is then reshaped with the excimer laser as would occur in surface ablations. It overcomes the pain and slow recovery associated with surface treatments. It is the most popular laser refractive procedure performed today (see Fig. 19.5).

- *Indications*: myopia from −0.50D to −12.00D. Hypermetropia up to +6.00D. Astigmatism up to 5.00D.
- *Method*: a corneal flap is created using a microkeratome or FSL (see Box 19.3). The flap is then lifted (the hinge is usually superior or nasal), and the stroma is ablated with an excimer laser in a similar way to PRK (but Bowman's layer and superficial stroma of flap not lasered). The flap is then replaced and adheres to the bed within a few minutes.
- *Advantages*: less painful than surface ablations. Rapid visual rehabilitation.
- *Disadvantages*: flap-related complications (see Box 19.3), unsuitable for thin corneas, dry eye lasting up to 1y.

> **Box 19.3 LASIK flap creation: options**
>
> **Microkeratome**
>
> Flaps for LASIK were originally created with a microkeratome. A microkeratome consists of an oscillating blade travelling over a suction ring applied to cornea. The suction ring attaches firmly to the globe and raises the IOP to a high level, thereby providing a stable platform across which the cutting head travels. Flap size and thickness are related to size of suction ring and corneal power. Avoid use in steep (>48D) or very flat (<40D) cornea due to increased risk of flap complications.
>
> **FemtoSecond Laser (FSL)**
>
> This is an infrared wavelength laser (1,053nm) which produces very precise lamellar plane dissection and allows very precise ability to control flap size, thickness, and hinge location. No significant difference in visual outcomes between microkeratome and femtosecond LASIK but accepted that FSL associated with fewer flap complications.
>
> **Advantages of FSL over microkeratome**
>
> - Safer and more reliable flap creation with steep and flat cornea.
> - Easier to create thin flaps reliably.
> - Stronger flap adherence.
> - Less epithelial ingrowth.
> - Reduced induction of higher-order aberrations.

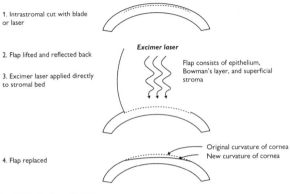

1. Intrastromal cut with blade or laser

2. Flap lifted and reflected back

3. Excimer laser applied directly to stromal bed

Excimer laser

Flap consists of epithelium, Bowman's layer, and superficial stroma

Original curvature of cornea
New curvature of cornea

4. Flap replaced

Fig. 19.5 Outline of LASIK.

Complications of refractive laser: immediate and early

In general, refractive laser is a highly successful procedure with high patient satisfaction and low complication rate. However, due to the high uptake of refractive surgery in the population, it is important that not only refractive surgeons, but also general ophthalmologists, especially those working in primary care and emergency ophthalmology, are able to understand, diagnose, and treat refractive surgery complications.

Microkeratome-related problems (LASIK only)

Incomplete or irregular cut Incidence 0.3–1.2%. Caused by inadequate globe exposure, loss of suction, or mechanical failure. Management depends on how far keratome has advanced. If adequate bed, continue with ablation. If inadequate bed or irregular cut, stop and repeat flap or surface treatment 3–6mo later.

Free cap Incidence 0.1–1%. Amount of cornea protruding above suction ring dictates flap size. Too little protrusion will result in a free flap; can occur with very flat corneas (<40D) or inadequate suction. Ensure cap placed back in correct orientation and allow time for stromal adhesion.

Button hole Incidence 0.1–0.6%. Associated with poorer visual outcome. Risk factors include inadequate suction, poor applanation, slow or non-uniform cutting speeds, steep corneas (>46D), previous ocular surgery, and large flaps. Managed by early recognition and abortion of procedure, and plan surface ablation at later date.

Other complications Include *corneal epithelial defect, corneal bleed* (large flaps in presence of peripheral pannus), *thin/decentred flaps, wound dehiscence* (flap creation after PK), *pizza slicing* (LASIK after RK), and corneal perforation (very rare, seen with old generation microkeratomes lacking prefixed depth plate).

Photoablation-related problems

Treatment decentration (LASIK and surface Rx) Often unrecognized intraoperatively. Leads to irregular astigmatism. Risk factors include high corrections, long treatment duration, poor patient cooperation. Risk minimized by high-speed, real-time eye tracking. Treatment difficult; needs retreatment using a larger, deeper treatment zone or a topography-guided treatment.

Central islands (LASIK and surface Rx) Defined as steep areas (at least 1D with diameter of >1mm) within treatment zone. Common post-operatively but resolve slowly and significantly. Leads to irregular astigmatism, glare, ghosting, monocular diplopia, and reduced VA. Causes include degradation of laser optics (rare with modern flying spot lasers), plume dynamics, acoustic shock waves, water accumulation, varying wound healing. Conservative treatment indicated, as most resolve. If present >6–12mo, repeat laser ablation.

Wrinkles—macro- or microstriae (LASIK only) Present in 0.2–4%. Difficult to see on laser (so all patients examined at slit-lamp post-operatively). Causes include: malposition, excessive irrigation, eye rubbing in early post-operative period, and flap redundancy in high myopia. Treated by gentle repositioning or refloating flap and air-drying; recalcitrant cases are sutured. Early intervention is vital to ensure successful treatment.

Interface debris (LASIK only) From conjunctival or skin epithelial cells, Meibomian secretions, FB (swab fibres, blade fragments). Best avoided by good technique. If present, treat with flap lift and clean.

Early post-operative complications

Undercorrection and overcorrection (LASIK and surface Rx) Undercorrection is most frequent complication and occurs more commonly with treatment of high ametropia. It can be retreated if needed. Overtreatments are less common and usually occur in retreatments and older patients (>50y). Most regress, so observation needed.

Sliding/dislodged flaps (LASIK) Most common in first 24h. Most commonly occurs with large flaps/thin flaps/small-hinged flaps. Treatment is emergency repositioning to prevent fixed folds and epithelial ingrowth.

Flap loss/free cap (LASIK) Can occur intraoperatively or post-operatively (eye rubbing, adhesion to eye patch). If flap found and viable, can be repositioned and secured with or without sutures.

Diffuse lamellar keratitis (DLK) (syn shifting sands of Sahara) (LASIK) Diffuse inflammation at flap interface without microbial cause. Usually seen within first 24h. Aetiology poorly understood; thought to be inflammatory pathway activation by several possible causative agents—toxic or mechanical. Clinical appearance—white sand-like deposits in lamellar cut plane in absence of both epithelial defect and AC activity. Graded I–IV for purpose of treatment and prognosis. Aggressive topical steroid leads to rapid resolution. If any diagnostic doubt, lift flap and culture.

Infectious keratitis (LASIK and surface Rx) Rare but vision-threatening. Incidence 0.1–0.2%. Commonly Gram +ve, *Nocardia, Mycobacterium*, and atypicals. Signs include infiltrate, ciliary injection, hypopyon, and flap melt in severe cases. Adequate and early sampling is key to treatment and consists of flap lift (in LASIK), scrape, and frequent topical antibiotics.

Epithelial ingrowth (LASIK) 3–4 % of cases at 1mo show signs of epithelial ingrowth, severity depending on viability of implanted cells. Sources of cells include implantation from microkeratome, from irrigation, or growth under flap. Risk factors include deficient technique, epithelial defects, and retreatments with flap lift. Treatment depends on extent; if >2mm from edge, progression, flap melting, or reduced VA, then treat. Treatment is by flap lift and scrape. If recurrent, PTK, 50% alcohol, or MMC to stromal bed may be necessary.

Complications of refractive laser: late

Late post-operative complications

Regression (LASIK and surface Rx) Return of refractive error 3–6/12 after treatment. More common in hypermetropic treatments. Occurs as a result of compensatory epithelial hyperplasia. If significant, retreatment required.

Iatrogenic keratectasia (LASIK >> surface Rx) A serious and sight-threatening complication from ectasia due to weakening of corneal mechanical strength following laser. Risk factors include pre-existing ectatic conditions such as forme fruste keratoconus, very large ablations, minimal stromal bed thickness <250 microns, removal of >50% original corneal thickness. Diagnosis confirmed by serial corneal topographies. Treatment difficult—initially with RGP CL but usually require PK. Recently, some benefit shown with corneal cross-linking and ICRS.

Glare and haloes (LASIK and surface Rx) Usually occurs at night and associated with spherical aberration of flattened central cornea after myopic treatments. Associated with large scotopic/mesopic pupil size or small treatment zones. Treatment involves observation. If no improvement with time, consider enlarging optical zone using modern flying spot laser.

Dry eye (LASIK) LASIK may induce or exacerbate pre-existing dry eye. Dry eye is the most frequent complication of LASIK. LASIK flap creation causes corneal nerve disruption which takes 6–12mo to regenerate. Less of a problem with surface treatments. As well as causing symptoms, dry eye can cause poor results due to interference of normal healing. Prevention is best treatment; otherwise treat with intensive lubricants, artificial tears, punctal plugs, and topical ciclosporin.

Corneal haze (surface ablations) Haze is subepithelial and appears a few weeks after surface ablation. Peaks at 1–2mo. Usually resolves over 6–12mo. Persistent haze associated with greater depths of ablation and small treatment zones. If no resolution by 6–12mo, treat with PTK or superficial keratectomy with MMC.

Incisional refractive surgery

Incisional surgery has mostly been replaced by excimer laser techniques and lens-based techniques. A few techniques are still in use, including astigmatic keratotomies. Radial keratotomies (RKs), though now obsolete, were used extensively in the past to treat myopia and may be encountered in clinical practice.

Astigmatic keratotomy

These consist of deep incisions made in the cornea to reduce astigmatism. Two main types in clinical use: arcuate keratotomies (AKs) and LRIs (see Fig. 19.6).

Arcuate keratotomies (AKs)

AKs are paired arc-shaped deep incisions (up to 95% depth) in the mid-peripheral cornea (usually 6–7mm optical zone) centred on the visual axis. Incisions in a particular meridian cause flattening in that meridian and a varying amount of steeping in the opposite meridian (coupling). Performed with guarded blades of variable depth or Femtosecond Laser (FSL). Useful for post-keratoplasty astigmatism. Increased refractive effect with: (1) deeper incision (2) longer incision (3) incision closer to the visual axis. Arcuate cuts are preferred to transverse (straight cuts), because they do not usually change the spherical equivalent (coupling ratio 1:1), compared to transverse cuts that tend to produce a hypermetropic shift (coupling ratio >1).

- *Advantages*: easy to perform; large amounts of astigmatism corrected (up to 10D); reasonably rapid stabilization (4wk).
- *Disadvantages*: unpredictable, even with nomogram use; since increased effect only seen with deep incisions, risk of full-thickness perforation. FSL AK allows increased precision of incision depth, length, and shape.

Limbal relaxing incisions (LRIs)

LRIs are paired arc-shaped deep incisions (600 microns or up to 95%) in the peripheral extent of the clear cornea. They work in the same way as AKs but are less potent in their ability to reduce astigmatism (useful up to 3D) due to their peripheral location. They are used to reduce corneal astigmatism at the time of cataract surgery and tend to have no effect on the spherical equivalent of the eye (coupling ratio 1:1).

- *Advantages*: easy to perform at the same time as cataract surgery; central cornea clear, thus optical quality maintained; rapid healing; cheap, compared to toric IOLs.
- *Disadvantages*: same as for AK.

Radial keratotomies (RKs)

RK was the original incision-based technique for treating myopia (see Fig. 19.6). It consisted of a variable number of deep (85–90% thickness), radial stromal incisions (typically 8) made throughout the peripheral and mid-peripheral cornea, resulting in weakening and bulging of peripheral cornea, with concomitant flattening of the central cornea.

- *Disadvantages*: unpredictable, unstable, progressive flattening leading to hypermetropic shift, visual distortion, permanent corneal weakening leading to rupture following blunt trauma. RK is now an obsolete procedure and has been superceded by excimer laser.

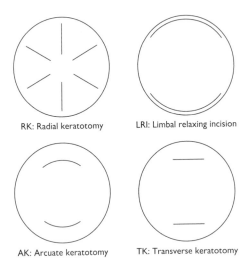

RK: Radial keratotomy

LRI: Limbal relaxing incision

AK: Arcuate keratotomy

TK: Transverse keratotomy

Fig. 19.6 Outline of incisional refractive operations.

Intracorneal ring segments

Intracorneal ring segments (ICRS) (e.g. INTACs, Kerarings, Ferrara rings) consist of thin, arc-shaped segments of PMMA of varying diameters and arc lengths. Mechanism of action is the addition of tissue (ICRS) to the periphery of the cornea causes flattening of the central cornea, leading to myopic correction (see Fig. 19.7). Increased effect with: (1) thicker, (2) longer, and (3) more centrally placed segments. Channels for the rings are made with special trephines or, more precisely, with Femtosecond Laser (FSL). Used to treat myopia with two symmetric ICRS or to treat keratoconus with combinations of different ICRS.

- *Advantages*: reversible; titratable; no corneal tissue removed; potential for surgical treatment of keratoconus other than keratoplasty.
- *Disadvantages*: less predictable than excimer laser techniques; complications from surgery such as AC perforation, infectious keratitis, ICRS extrusion, corneal thinning.

(a)

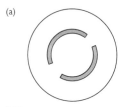

ICRS: intracorneal ring segments
—*central cornea flattened: myopia reduced*

(b)

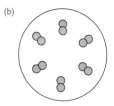

CK: conductive keratoplasty
—*central cornea steepened: hypermetropia reduced*

Fig. 19.7 Outline of ICRS and CK.

Collagen shrinkage procedures

A thermal effect supplied to the peripheral cornea will cause corneal shrinkage that flattens the peripheral cornea and steepens the central cornea, thereby producing a means of treating low hypermetropia (up to 3D). Such an effect can be produced using laser energy (laser thermal keratoplasty) or radiofrequency waves (CK; see Fig. 19.7).

Laser thermokeratoplasty (LTK)

Holmium:YAG laser is used to deliver eight spots of infrared 2.06 microns wavelength in a ring-shaped optical zone of 7mm (corrects ~1.5D hypermetropia) or a double ring of 7mm and 9mm (corrects ~3.0 D hypermetropia).
- *Advantages*: central cornea unscarred; no risk of dry eye; vision improvement immediate.
- *Disadvantages*: small effect; main problem is significant regression. Rarely used now.

Conductive keratoplasty (CK)

Radiofrequency energy delivered through a conductive probe applied directly to peripheral cornea that heats and shrinks the tissue. Increasing effect with increasing numbers of spots and rings (treats up to 3.0D hypermetropia).
- *Advantages*: as for LTK.
- *Disadvantages*: As for LTK, but less regression than LTK.

Lens-based techniques

In general, lens-based techniques are used for high degrees of ammetropia and fall into two categories: phakic IOLs and refractive lens exchange (RLE).

Phakic IOLs

These are lenses that are used in patients who still possess their natural lens. Useful for high myopia (typically >10D) when laser techniques inappropriate due to inadequate corneal thickness/residual stromal bed depth. Useful in younger patients with high ametropia but intact accommodation. In highly ametropic patients older than 50, RLE may be preferred, especially if early cataract is present.

Three current models are approved for clinical use as phakic IOLs:

- *Artisan/Verisyse™ AC iris fixated phakic lens (AMO)*: this lens is clipped to the front of the iris via two claws. Corrects –5.0 to –20.0D.
- *Vision™ (STAAR) ICL (implantable collamer lens)*: this lens sits in the posterior chamber, and so a peripheral iridectomy is performed to prevent pupillary block. Corrects –3.0D to –20.0D.
- *Acrysof CACHET™*: this lens is placed in the AC and is supported by haptics in the angle. It requires an AC depth of ≥3.2mm. Corrects –6.0 to –16.5.
- *Advantages*: larger treatment range, compared to laser treatment.
- *Disadvantages*: intraocular procedure. Phakic IOL removal may need to be removed at later stage when cataract surgery needed. Small anatomic space, so sizing much more critical than for PCIOLs. Not suitable in patients with shallow AC. Sequential one eye surgery recommended, compared to bilateral laser refractive surgery at one sitting.
- *Complications*: increased risk of cataract formation. Potential for endothelial cell loss. Very low risk of endophthalmitis (similar or lower than with cataract surgery).

Refractive lens exchange (RLE)

RLE surgery is identical to modern cataract surgery but carried out in patents with clear lenses for refractive purposes. Any refractive error can be treated, but the procedure is reserved for older patients with reducing accommodation (>50). In addition to treating ametropia, toric IOLs can be used to treat astigmatism, and multifocal/accommodative lenses can be used to reduce dependence on reading spectacles.

- *Advantages*: large range of ametropia can be treated. Combine with toric lenses for astigmatism or multifocal/accommodative lenses for presbyopia. Particularly appropriate for hypermetropia with shallow AC at risk of glaucoma.
- *Disadvantages*: loss of any residual natural accommodation. Slightly higher risk of retina detachment in high myopia, compared to phakic IOLs.
- *Complications*: identical to those of cataract surgery.

Aids to diagnosis

Acute red eye

Normal/near normal vision

Painful/discomfort

Diffuse superficial redness

- *Conjunctivitis*: infective, allergic, or chemical; gritty/itchy; watery, mucoid, mucopurulent, or purulent exudate; papillae or follicles.

Diffuse deep redness

- *Anterior scleritis*: severe pain; diffuse deep injection which does not blanch with vasoconstrictors (e.g. phenylephrine 10%), oedema; globe tender.

Circumlimbal redness

- *Keratitis*: photophobia, watering, circumlimbal injection, corneal infiltrate ± epithelial defect ± AC activity.
- *Anterior uveitis*: photophobia, watering, KPs, AC activity ± PS.
- *Corneal FB*: appropriate history, FB sensation, visible FB.

Sectoral redness

- *Episcleritis*: mild discomfort; may be recurrent; sectoral (occasionally diffuse) redness which blanches with topical vasoconstrictor (e.g. phenylephrine 10%); globe non-tender.
- *Marginal keratitis*: photophobia, watering, marginal corneal infiltrate ± epithelial defect.

Painless

- *Subconjunctival haemorrhage*: well-defined confluent area of haemorrhage.

Reduced vision

Normal IOP

Abnormal corneosclera

- *Corneal abrasion*: photophobia, watering, sectoral/circumlimbal injection, epithelial defect.
- *Keratitis*: photophobia, watering, circumlimbal injection, corneal infiltrate ± epithelial defect ± AC activity ± mucopurulent discharge.

Abnormal uvea

- *Anterior uveitis*: photophobia, watering, KPs, AC activity ± PS.
- *Endophthalmitis*: pain, floaters, watering, diffuse deep injection, inflammation (vitreous > AC), chorioretinitis.

↑IOP

- *Acute glaucoma*: usually due to angle closure; photophobia, watering, corneal oedema ± anterior segment/angle abnormalities such as rubeosis.
- *Hypertensive uveitis*: AC cells and flare ± corneal involvement; often due to herpes group of viruses.

Sudden/recent loss of vision

Few seconds' duration

Unilateral

- *GCA*: usually age >55y, weight loss, fatigue, jaw/tongue claudication, pulseless/tender/thickened temporal artery, ↑ESR/CRP.
- *Papilloedema*: bilateral disc swelling, loss of SVP, peripapillary haemorrhages, features of raised ICP.
- *Impending CRVO*: dilated, tortuous retinal veins, haemorrhages.
- *OIS*: veins dilated and irregular but not tortuous, mid-peripheral haemorrhages; ± NVD, ↑IOP, carotid bruits.

Bilateral

- *Papilloedema*: see described previously.

Few minutes' duration

Unilateral

- *Amaurosis fugax*: curtain across vision ± evidence of emboli, AF, carotid bruits.
- *GCA*: see described previously.

Bilateral

- *Vertebrobasilar artery insufficiency*: recurrent episodes ± ataxia, dysphasia, dysarthria, hemiparesis, hemisensory disturbance.

Up to 1h duration

- *Migraine*: fortification spectra, transient VF defects, unilateral headache, nausea/vomiting, photophobia, aura, FH.

Persistent

Abnormal cornea

- *Hydrops*: acute corneal oedema associated with underlying disease such as keratoconus.

Abnormal vitreous

- *Vitreous haemorrhage*: varies from microscopic level to completely obscuring the fundus.

Abnormal fundus

- *CRAO*: RAPD, attenuated arterioles, pale fundus, cherry-red spot.
- *CRVO*: dilated tortuous veins, haemorrhages in all four quadrants ± CWS, RAPD; BRVO may give symptomatic altitudinal defects, particularly if on temporal arcade.
- *RRD*: flashes/floaters, tobacco dust, convex elevated retina with (multiple) break(s).
- *ERD*: convex elevated retina with shifting fluid, no break.
- *TRD*: concave elevated retina with tractional membranes.
- *Intermediate uveitis*: floaters, vitritis, snow balls/banking ± macular oedema.
- *Posterior uveitis*: floaters, significantly reduced vision; vitritis, retinal/choroidal infiltrates, macular oedema, vascular sheathing/occlusion, haemorrhages.

Abnormal disc
- *AION*: RAPD, pale oedematous disc ± flame-shaped haemorrhages; may have altitudinal field defect; may be arteritic (with signs of GCA) or non-arteritic (usually sectoral).

Abnormal macula
- *Choroidal neovascular membrane*: distortion ± positive scotoma, drusen, subretinal membrane ± haemorrhage, exudate.
- *CSR*: colour desaturation, micropsia, serous detachment of neurosensory retina.

Normal fundus
- *Cortical blindness*: ± denial, small residual field; normal pupil reactions; abnormal CT/MRI head.
- *Functional*: inconsistent acuity between different tests and at different times, normal ophthalmic examination, normal EDTs.

Painful

Abnormal cornea
- *Acute angle-closure glaucoma*: usually hypermetropic, haloes, frontal headache, vomiting; injected, corneal oedema, fixed semi-dilated pupil, shallow AC with closed angle, raised IOP.
- *Bullous keratopathy*: thickened, hazy cornea, stromal/subepithelial oedema, bullae, evidence of underlying pathology, e.g. ACIOL, Fuchs' endothelial dystrophy, etc.
- *Keratitis*: photophobia, watering, circumlimbal injection, corneal infiltrate ± epithelial defect ± AC activity.

Abnormal disc
- *Optic neuritis*: usually age 18–45y, with retro-orbital pain, especially on eye movement, RAPD, reduced colour vision, VF defects, swollen disc ± peripapillary flame-shaped haemorrhages; may also be painless.

Abnormal uvea
- *Anterior uveitis*: anterior pain, photophobia, mildly reduced vision, circumlimbal injection, AC cells and flare, KPs.

Normal fundus
- *Retrobulbar neuritis*: as for optic neuritis but with a normal disc; may also be painless.

Gradual loss of vision

Abnormal cornea

- *Corneal dystrophies*: corneal clouding (deposition/oedema); usually bilateral but may be asymmetric; common types include Fuchs' endothelial dystrophy in the elderly and Reis–Bucklers dystrophy in young adults.
- *Keratoconus*: refractive error from progressive astigmatism; corneal oedema from acute hydrops; usually bilateral but may be asymmetric.

Abnormal lens

- *Cataract*: uni- or bilateral opacification of the lens; cloudy, misty; glare; commonest in the elderly.

Central

Abnormal macula

Macular disease usually leads to distortion ± micropsia and early ↓VA; pupillary responses and colour vision are relatively preserved. Common causes include:

- *AMD*: very common bilateral disease of the elderly; the most common type are 'dry' changes which are associated with gradual, patchy central loss.
- *Macular dystrophies*: group of diseases with specific patterns occurring in younger age group; bilateral disease; may have FH, and genetic testing is sometimes possible.
- *Diabetic maculopathy*: ischaemia may lead to gradual ↓VA; oedema may lead to more acute distortion/↓VA; associated with other diabetic changes.
- *CMO*: oedema resulting in distortion/↓VA; may be associated with surgery, inflammation, or vascular disease.

Abnormal optic disc/nerve

Optic nerve disease usually leads to dimness and darkening of colours; although commonly central, it may lead to peripheral or generalized loss of vision; pupillary responses, colour vision, and brightness testing are all reduced. Important causes include:

- *Compressive optic neuropathy*: progressive ↓VA, disc pallor ± pain, involvement of other local structures.
- *LHON*: severe sequential ↓VA over weeks/months, telangiectatic vessels around disc (acutely); usually young adult ♂; FH.
- *Toxic or nutritional optic neuropathies*: slowly progressive symmetrical ↓VA with central scotomata; relevant nutritional, therapeutic, or toxic history.
- *Inflammatory optic neuropathies*: associated with systemic disease (e.g. sarcoid, vasculitis, and syphilis); often very steroid-sensitive.
- *Chronic papilloedema*: sustained disc swelling due to raised ICP may cause permanent optic nerve dysfunction, including ↓VA and field defects, and optic disc pallor.

Peripheral or patchy

Abnormal choroid/retina

- *Posterior uveitis*: floaters, patchy loss of vision ± central distortion/↓VA from CMO; may include chorioretinitis, vitritis, retinal vasculitis.
- *RP*: bilateral concentric field loss, peripheral 'bone spicule' pigmentation, retinal arteriole attenuation, and optic disc pallor.

Abnormal optic disc

- *Glaucoma*: asymptomatic peripheral field loss; usually bilateral but often asymmetric; characteristic cupping and other disc changes; often associated with ↑IOP.

The watery eye

Increased tear production

Basal increase
- *Increased parasympathetic drive*: from pro-secretory drugs (e.g. pilocarpine) or autonomic disturbance.

Reflex increase
- *Local irritants*, e.g. FB, trichiasis.
- *Chronic ocular disease*, e.g. blepharitis, KCS.
- *Systemic disease*, e.g. TED.

Lacrimal pump failure

Lid tone
- *Lid laxity*: common involutional change in the elderly.
- *Orbicularis weakness*: associated with VIIn palsy.

Lid position
- *Ectropion*: most commonly an involutional change in the elderly but may also be cicatricial, mechanical, or congenital.

Decreased drainage

Punctal obstruction
- *Congenital*: punctal atresia.
- *Acquired*: punctal stenosis is most commonly idiopathic but may arise 2° to punctal eversion, post-HSV infection, or any scarring process (e.g. post-irradiation, trachoma, cicatricial conjunctivitis).

Canalicular obstruction
- *Acquired*: canalicular fibrosis is most commonly idiopathic but may arise 2° to HSV infection, chronic canaliculitis (usually *Actinomycosis*), chronic dacrocystitis, cicatricial conjunctivitis, and 5-FU administration.

Nasolacrimal duct obstruction
- *Congenital*: delayed canalization.
- *Acquired*: stenosis is most commonly idiopathic but may arise 2° to trauma (nasal/orbital fracture), post-irradiation, Granulomatosis with Polyangiitis (GPA), tumours (e.g. nasopharyngeal carcinoma), and other nasal pathology (chronic inflammation/polyps).

Flashes and floaters

Flashes only

Retinal traction

- Vitreoretinal traction, PDR, sickle cell retinopathy, ROP

'Pseudoflashes'

Ocular

- *Photophobia*: discomfort commonly associated with anterior segment inflammation or retinal hypersensitivity.
- *Glare*: dazzle commonly associated with media opacities.
- *Haloes*: ring effect associated with corneal oedema and some media opacities.

CNS

- *Papilloedema*: transient, associated with straining or change in posture.
- *Migraine*: classic enlarging zigzag fortification spectra moving central to peripheral, usually followed by headache.
- *Occipital lobe lesions (tumours, AVMs)*: coloured shapes/blobs.
- *Other visual hallucinations*: bilateral severe visual loss may result in more complex visual hallucinations (Charles Bonnet syndrome).

Floaters only

- *PVD*: partial/complete Weiss ring overlying the optic disc ± visible posterior vitreous face.
- *Vitreous condensations*: degenerative changes within the vitreous lead to translucent opacities.
- *Vitreous haemorrhage*: red cells in the vitreous, varies from minor bleed ('spots' in vision, fundus easily visualized) to severe (severe ↓VA, no fundal view); may be followed by synchysis scintillans (golden particles which settle with gravity).
- *Vitritis*: white cells in the vitreous, may be bilateral and associated with features of intermediate or posterior uveitis.
- *Asteroid hyalosis*: small yellow-white particles that move with the vitreous (rather than settling with gravity), usually innocuous.
- *Amyloidosis*: sheet-like opacities, usually bilateral; most commonly seen with familial systemic amyloidosis.
- *Tumours* (e.g. choroidal melanoma, lymphoma): vitritis of inflammatory and/or tumour cells may be seen.

Flashes and floaters

- *PVD*: partial/complete Weiss ring overlying the optic disc ± visible posterior vitreous face.
- *Retinal tear*: usually U-shaped tear and pigment in the vitreous; may be associated with vitreous haemorrhage or retinal detachment.
- *Retinal detachment*: usually rhegmatogenous (associated with a tear), resulting in elevated retina with SRF.
- *Tumours*: visual phenomena include 'slow-moving ball of light' and floaters 2° to tumour cells/inflammation associated with a choroidal or retinal mass.

Headache

Swollen optic discs

Bilateral

Serious/life-threatening headaches

- *Raised ICP*: worsening headache on lying flat, coughing/sneezing/ Valsalva, visual obscurations, diplopia, disc swelling with loss of SVP, blind spot enlargement, VIn palsy. Causes include:
  - Cerebral tumour, IIH, venous sinus thrombosis, meningitis, encephalitis, brain abscess, congenital ventricular abnormalities, cerebral oedema.
  - Subarachnoid haemorrhage: 'thunderclap headache', meningism, altered consciousness.
- *Accelerated hypertension*: ↑BP, hypertensive retinopathy, including CWS, haemorrhages, exudates.

Unilateral

Serious/life-threatening headaches

- *GCA*: usually age >55y; visual loss, scalp tenderness (± necrosis), jaw/ tongue claudication, limb girdle pain/weakness, fevers, weight loss; non-pulsatile, tender, thickened temporal arteries; AION results in unilateral or, less commonly, bilateral disc swelling.

No optic disc swelling

Serious/life-threatening headaches

- *Raised ICP*: may occur in the presence of non-swollen discs (e.g. myopic discs, atrophic discs, anomalies of the optic nerve sheath).
- *GCA*: endocrine dysfunction (amenorrhoea, galactorrhoea, infertility, acromegaly, Cushing's disease; optic atrophy; bitemporal field loss).
- *Pituitary apoplexy*: recent major hypotensive episode, e.g. surgery, post-partum haemorrhage; acute ↓VA, meningism, ± LOC.

Headache syndrome

- *Tension headache*: very common; tightness, bifrontal/biocciptal/ band-like, may radiate to neck, headache-free intervals, no neurological/ systemic features; this may be associated with cervical spondylosis.
- *Migraine*: common; prodrome, headache (usually hemicranial), nausea, photophobia, phonophobia; visual phenomena include scintillating visual aura (starts paracentral and expands as it moves peripherally), transient visual loss (unilateral or homonymous hemifield), or ophthalmoplegia.
- *Cluster headache*: sudden oculotemporal pain, no prodrome, may have transient lacrimation, rhinorrhoea, and Horner's syndrome.

Facial pain

- *Trigeminal neuralgia*: sudden stabbing pains in trigeminal branch distribution; precipitants include touch, cold, eating.
- *Ophthalmic shingles*: hyperaesthesia in acute phase followed by neuralgic-type pain.

Sinus pain
- *Acute sinusitis*: coryzal/URTI symptoms, tender over paranasal sinuses; proptosis, diplopia, or optic neuropathy warrant urgent exclusion of orbital involvement.

Ocular pain
- *Generalized*: includes AACG, anterior uveitis, keratitis, scleritis, ocular ischaemia.
- *Retrobulbar*: includes optic neuritis, orbital pathology (e.g. infection, infiltration, neoplasm, TED).
- *On eye movement*: includes optic neuritis.

Asthenopia (eye strain)
- Usually worsens with reading/fatigue; ametropia (especially hypermetropia), astigmatism, anisometropia, decompensating phoria, convergence insufficiency, etc.

Diplopia

Monocular

Abnormal refraction
- *High ametropia, astigmatism,* or *edge effect* from corrective lenses: usually correctable with appropriate refraction; CL may be more effective than glasses.

Abnormal cornea
- *Opacity*: associated with scarring (e.g. trauma, infection), oedema (e.g. ↑IOP, decompensation), deposition (e.g. corneal dystrophies).
- *Shape*: peripheral thinning associated with ectasias (e.g. keratoconus), PUK, and other marginal disease.

Abnormal lens
- *Opacity*: cataract.
- *Shape*: lenticonus.
- *Position*: subluxation of lens (ectopia lentis) or implant (especially if complicated surgery).

Abnormal iris
- *Defect*: polycoria due to trauma (e.g. IOFB), peripheral iridotomy (laser or surgical), or disease (e.g. ICE syndrome)

Normal examination
- *Not diplopia*: 'double vision' may be used by the patient to describe other visual anomalies (e.g. ghosting or blurring).
- *Functional*: this is a diagnosis of exclusion.

Binocular

Intermittent or variable
- *Decompensating phoria*: intermittent but usually predictable (e.g. when fatigued) with a constant pattern (e.g. only for distance, only horizontal); underlying phoria with variable/poor recovery.
- *MG*: intermittent diplopia of variable orientation and severity which worsens with fatigue; may be associated with ptosis ± generalized muscular fatigue.
- *Internuclear ophthalmoplegia*: diplopia may only be noticed during saccades when the adducting eye is slower to refixate.
- *GCA*: intermittent diplopia may occur due to ischaemia; may progress to become permanent.

Persistent

Neurogenic

In neurogenic lesions, the diplopia is worst when looking in the direction of the paretic muscle(s); saccades are slowed in this direction; full sequelae will evolve with time. Forced duction test shows normal passive movements.

- *Horizontal only*: typically VIn palsy → underaction of LR → ipsilateral reduced abduction ± convergent.
- *Vertical/torsional only*: typically IVn palsy → underaction of SO, with ipsilateral hypertropia, extorsion, and reduced depression in adducted position.
- *Mixed ± ptosis/pupillary abnormalities*: typically IIIn palsy → underaction of any/all of LPS, SR, MR, IR, IO, sphincter pupillae, resulting in anything from single muscle involvement (rare) to complete ptosis obscuring a hypotropic divergent eye.
- *Complex*: unusual patterns may be due to brainstem lesions, causing nuclear or supranuclear gaze palsies (often associated with other neurological signs), orbital pathology, or disorders of the neuromuscular junction (e.g. MG).

Mechanical

In mechanical lesions, the diplopia is worst when looking away from the restricted muscle(s); signs of restriction may include IOP increase, globe retraction, and pain when looking away from the restricted muscle(s); ductions and versions are equally reduced, but saccades are of normal speed; sequelae are limited to underaction of contralateral synergist. Forced duction test shows restriction of passive movements.

- *Congenital*: these rarely give rise to diplopia unless progressive or decompensating.
- *Acquired*: associated with inflammation (e.g. TED, myositis, idiopathic orbital inflammatory disease), trauma (orbital wall/floor fracture), or infiltration.

Anisocoria

This implies that the larger pupil is the abnormal one.

Abnormal iris appearance (slit-lamp examination)
Vermiform movements
- *Adie's pupil*: pupil initially dilated, later abnormally constricted; response to light is poor, response to near is initially poor, later tonic (exaggerated but slow), i.e. there is light-near dissociation; will constrict with 0.1% pilocarpine due to denervation hypersensitivity.

Structural damage
- *Iris trauma*: dilated pupil (often irregular) due to a torn sphincter with associated anterior segment damage (e.g. transillumination defects).
- *Iris inflammation*: dilated pupil (often irregular) due to sectoral iris atrophy (typically with herpes group of viruses) or stuck down by PS.

Normal iris appearance
Constricts to pilocarpine 1%
- *IIIn palsy*: dilated pupil associated with other features of a IIIn palsy (e.g. ptosis, oculomotor abnormality); will constrict with 1% pilocarpine.

Does not constrict to pilocarpine 1%
- *Pharmacological*: dilated pupil resulting from anticholinergic mydriatics such as atropine (rather than adrenergics).
- *Iris ischaemia*: dilated pupil occurring after angle-closure glaucoma or intraocular surgery (e.g. Urrets–Zavalia syndrome).

This implies that the smaller pupil is the abnormal one.

Abnormal iris appearance (slit-lamp examination)
Structural damage
- *Iris inflammation*: constricted pupil (may be irregular) stuck down by PS.

Normal iris appearance
Dilates at normal speed in dim light
Both pupils dilate equally quickly when ambient light is dimmed.
- *Physiological anisocoria*: anisocoria is usually mild (≤1mm) and only marginally worse in dim, rather than bright, light; responses to light and near are normal; degree of anisocoria varies from day to day and may reverse; will not dilate with 1% apraclonidine (cf. Horner's syndrome).

Dilates in dim light but slowly (i.e. 'dilatation lag')
The smaller pupil is slower to dilate when ambient light is dimmed.
- *Horner's syndrome*: constricted pupil, with mild ptosis; iris hypochromia suggests congenital or very long-standing lesion; confirm with 1% apraclonidine (a Horner's pupil will dilate) or 4% cocaine (a Horner's pupil will not dilate).

Dilates with hydroxyamphetamine 1%
- *Central or preganglionic Horner's syndrome*: constricted pupil, mild ptosis, facial anhydrosis; may have other features related to level of lesion (brainstem, spinal cord, lung apex, neck).

Does not dilate with hydroxyamphetamine 1%
- *Post-ganglionic Horner's syndrome*: constricted pupil, mild ptosis; may have other features related to level of lesion (neck, cavernous sinus, orbit).

Does not dilate in dim light
- *Pharmacological*: constricted pupil may be due to cholinergic miotics such as pilocarpine.

Nystagmus

Early onset

Horizontal jerk

- *Idiopathic congenital*: very early onset (usually by 2mo of age); worsens with fixation; improves within 'null zone' and on convergence; mild ↓VA.
- *Manifest latent*: fast phase towards fixing eye; worsens with occlusion of non-fixing eye, and with gaze towards fast phase; alternates if opposite eye takes up fixation; often associated with infantile esotropia.

Erratic

- *Sensory deprivation*: erratic waveform ± roving eye movements; moderate/severe ↓VA due to ocular or anterior visual pathway disease.

Late onset

Conjugate

Present in primary position

Sustained:
- *Peripheral vestibular*: conjugate horizontal jerk nystagmus, improves with fixation and with time since injury, worsens with gaze towards fast phase (Alexander's law) or change in head position.
- *Cerebellar/central vestibular/brainstem*: conjugate jerk nystagmus which does not improve with fixation; it may be horizontal, vertical, or torsional:
  - *Horizontal type*: e.g. lesions of the vestibular nuclei, cerebellum, or their connections.
  - *Upbeat type*: usually cerebellar/lower brainstem lesions, e.g. demyelination, infarction, tumour, encephalitis, Wernicke's syndrome.
  - *Downbeat type*: usually craniocervical junction lesions, e.g. Arnold–Chiari malformation, spinocerebellar degenerations, infarction, tumour, demyelination.

Periodic:
- *Periodic alternating*: conjugate horizontal jerk nystagmus with waxing–waning nystagmus; 90s in each direction with a 10s 'null' period; usually associated with vestibulocerebellar lesions.

Present only in eccentric gaze
- *Gaze-evoked (GEN)*: conjugate horizontal jerk nystagmus on eccentric gaze, with fast phase towards direction of gaze.
  - *Asymmetric type*: evoked nystagmus usually indicates failure of ipsilateral neural integrator/cerebellar dysfunction.
  - *Symmetric type*: due to CNS depression (e.g. fatigue, alcohol, anticonvulsants, barbiturates) or structural pathology (e.g. brainstem, cerebellum).

Disconjugate

Unilateral

- *Internuclear ophthalmoplegia*: nystagmus of the abducting (and occasionally adducting) eye.
- *SO myokymia*: unilateral high-frequency, low-amplitude torsional nystagmus.

Bilateral

- *See-saw nystagmus*: vertical and torsional components, with one eye elevating and intorting while the other depresses and extorts; slow pendular or jerk waveform.
- *Acquired pendular nystagmus*: usually disconjugate with horizontal, vertical, and torsional components; may be associated with involuntary repetitive movement of palate, pharynx, and face.

Ophthalmic signs: external

The patient

Consider the patient as a whole. Simple observation of the patient provides a vast amount of additional information and should be practised in all cases. Observe that the patient with juvenile cataracts and ↑IOP has severe facial eczema—they may not have thought to mention their topical corticosteroids when you asked about medication. Note the rheumatoid hands of the patient in whom you suspect scleritis. Such information will also help with management (e.g. they need assistance with topical medication). Further 'hands-on' systemic examination is directed according to clinical presentation.

Globe

Ophthalmic signs—the globe

Sign	Causes
Proptosis	• *Infection*: orbital cellulitis
	• *Inflammation*: TED, idiopathic orbital inflammatory disease, systemic vasculitis (e.g. GPA)
	• *Tumours*: capillary haemangioma, lymphangioma, optic nerve glioma, myeloid leukaemia, histiocytosis, dermoid cyst
	• *Vascular anomalies*: orbital varices, carotid–cavernous fistula
	• *Pseudoproptosis*: ipsilateral large globe or lid retraction; contralateral enophthalmos or ptosis; facial asymmetry
Enophthalmos	• *Small globe*: microphthalmos, nanophthalmos, phthisis bulbi, orbital implant
	• *Soft tissue atrophy*: post-irradiation, scleroderma, cicatrizing tumours
	• *Bony defects*: orbital fractures, congenital orbital wall defects

Lymph nodes

Ophthalmic signs—lymph nodes

Sign	Causes
Enlarged preauricular lymph node	• *Infection*: viral conjunctivitis, chlamydial conjunctivitis, gonococcal conjunctivitis, Parinaud's oculoglandular syndrome
	• *Infiltration*: lymphoma

Lids

Ophthalmic signs—lids

Sign	Causes
Madarosis	• *Local*: cicatrizing conjunctivitis, iatrogenic (cryotherapy/radiotherapy/surgery) • *Systemic*: alopecia (patchy/totalis/universalis), psoriasis, hypothyroidism, leprosy
Poliosis	• *Local*: chronic lid margin disease • *Systemic*: sympathetic ophthalmia, VKH syndrome, Waardenburg syndrome
Lid lump	• *Anterior lamella*: external hordeolum, cyst of Moll, cyst of Zeis, xanthelasma, papilloma, seborrhoeic keratosis, keratoacanthoma, naevi, capillary haemangioma, actinic keratosis, BCC, SCC, malignant melanoma, Kaposi's sarcoma • *Posterior lamella*: internal hordeolum, chalazion, pyogenic granuloma, sebaceous gland carcinoma
Ectropion	• Involutional, cicatricial, mechanical, paralytic (VIIn palsy), congenital
Entropion	• Involutional, cicatricial, congenital
Ptosis	• *True ptosis*: involutional, neurogenic (IIIn palsy, Horner's syndrome), myasthenic, myopathic (CPEO group), mechanical, congenital • *Pseudoptosis*: brow ptosis, dermatochalasis, microphthalmos, phthisis, prosthesis, enophthalmos, hypotropia, contralateral lid retraction
Lid retraction	• *Congenital*: Down's syndrome, Duane syndrome • *Acquired*: TED, uraemia, VIIn palsy, IIIn misdirection, Marcus Gunn syndrome, Parinaud syndrome, hydrocephalus, sympathomimetics, cicatrization, lid surgery, large/proptotic globe

Ophthalmic signs: anterior segment (1)

Conjunctiva

Ophthalmic signs—conjunctiva

Sign	Causes
Hyperaemia	*Generalized*, e.g. conjunctivitis, dry eye, drop/preservative allergy, CL wear, scleritis
	Localized, e.g. episcleritis, scleritis, marginal keratitis, superior limbic keratitis, corneal abrasion, FB
	Circumcorneal, e.g. anterior uveitis, keratitis
Discharge	*Purulent*: bacterial conjunctivitis
	Mucopurulent: bacterial or chlamydial conjunctivitis
	Mucoid: vernal conjunctivitis, dry eye syndrome
	Watery: viral or allergic conjunctivitis
Papillae	Bacterial conjunctivitis, allergic conjunctivitis, blepharitis, floppy eyelid syndrome, superior limbic keratoconjunctivitis, CL
Giant papillae	VKC, CL-related giant papillary conjunctivitis, exposed suture, prosthesis, floppy eyelid syndrome
Follicles	Viral conjunctivitis, chlamydial conjunctivitis, drop hypersensitivity, Parinaud oculoglandular syndrome
Pseudomembrane	Infective conjunctivitis (adenovirus, *Streptococcus pyogenes*, *Corynebacterium diphtheriae*, *Neisseria gonorrhoeae*), SJS, GVHD, vernal conjunctivitis, ligneous conjunctivitis
Membrane	Infective conjunctivitis (adenovirus, *Streptococcus pneumoniae*, *Staphylococcus aureus*, *Corynebacterium diphtheriae*), SJS, ligneous conjunctivitis
Cicatrization	Trachoma, atopic keratoconjunctivitis, topical medication, chemical injury, OcMMP, erythema multiforme/SJS/TEN, other bullous disease (e.g. linear IgA disease, epidermolysis bullosa), Sjögren's syndrome, GVHD
Haemorrhagic conjunctivitis	Infective conjunctivitis (adenovirus, enterovirus 70, Coxsackie virus A24, *Streptococcus pneumoniae*, *Haemophilus aegyptius*)

Corneal iron lines (best seen on slit-lamp with cobalt blue light)

Ophthalmic signs—corneal iron lines

Sign	Causes
Ferry	Trabeculectomy
Stocker	Pterygium
Hudson–Stahli	Idiopathic with age (horizontal inferior 1/3 of cornea)
Fleischer	Keratoconus (base of cone)

Cornea (other)

Ophthalmic signs—cornea

Sign	Causes
Shape	
Thinning	*Central*: keratoconus, keratoglobus, posterior keratoconus, microbial keratitis
	Peripheral: PUK, marginal keratitis, microbial keratitis, Mooren's ulcer, pellucid marginal degeneration, Terrien's marginal degeneration
Epithelial	
Punctate epithelial erosions	*Superior*: VKC, superior limbic keratitis, floppy eyelid syndrome, poor CL fit
	Interpalpebral: KCS, UV exposure, corneal anaesthesia
	Inferior: blepharitis, exposure keratopathy, ectropion, poor Bell's phenomenon, rosacea, drop toxicity
Punctate epithelial keratitis	Viral keratitis (adenovirus, HSV, molluscum contagiosum), Thygeson's superficial punctate keratitis
Epithelial oedema	↑IOP, post-operative, aphakic/pseudophakic bullous keratopathy, Fuchs' endothelial dystrophy, trauma, acute hydrops, herpetic keratitis, CL overwear, congenital corneal clouding
Corneal filaments	KCS, recurrent erosion syndrome, corneal anaesthesia, exposure keratopathy, HZO
Stromal	
Pannus	Trachoma, tight CL, phlycten, herpetic keratitis, rosacea keratitis, chemical keratopathy, marginal keratitis, atopic/VKC, superior limbal keratoconjunctivitis, chronic keratoconjunctivitis of any cause
Stromal infiltrate	*Sterile*: marginal keratitis, CL-related
	Infective: bacteria, fungi, viruses, protozoa
Stromal oedema	Post-operative, keratoconus, Fuchs' endothelial dystrophy, disciform keratitis
Stromal deposits	*Corneal dystrophies*: e.g. macular, granular, lattice, Avellino
	Systemic: e.g. mucopolysaccharidoses (some), amyloidosis
Vogt's striae	Keratoconus
Ghost vessels	Interstitial keratitis (e.g. congenital syphilis, Cogan syndrome), other stromal keratitis (e.g. viral, parasitic)
Endothelial	
Descemet's folds	Post-operative, ↓IOP, disciform keratitis, congenital syphilis
Descemet's breaks	Birth trauma, keratoconus/keratoglobus (hydrops), infantile glaucoma (Haab's striae)
Guttata	*Peripheral*: Hassell–Henle bodies (physiological in the elderly)
	Central: Fuchs' endothelial dystrophy
Pigment on endothelium	PDS (Krukenberg spindle), post-operative, trauma
KPs	*Anterior uveitis*: e.g. idiopathic, HLA-B27, FHU, sarcoidosis, associated with keratitis (e.g. herpetic disciform, microbial, marginal)

Ophthalmic signs: anterior segment (2)

Episclera and sclera

Ophthalmic signs—episclera and sclera

Sign	Causes
Injection	*Superficial*: episcleritis *Deep*: scleritis
Pigmentation	*True*: naevus, melanocytoma, bilirubin (chronic liver disease), alkaptonuria, 'pigment spots' (at scleral perforations, e.g. nerve loop of Axenfield) *Pseudo*: blue sclera
Blue sclera	Osteogenesis imperfecta, keratoconus/keratoglobus, acquired scleral thinning (e.g. after necrotizing scleritis), connective tissue disorder (Marfan's, Ehlers–Danlos, PXE), other systemic syndromes (Turner's, Russell–Silver, incontinentia pigmenti)

AC

Ophthalmic signs—AC

Sign	Causes
↑IOP	*Chronic with open angle*: e.g. 1° open angle, normal tension, PXF, pigment dispersion, steroid-induced, angle-recession, intraocular tumour *Chronic with closed angle*: e.g. chronic PAC, neovascular, inflammatory, ICE syndrome, epithelial downgrowth, phacomorphic, aqueous misdirection *Acute with open angle*: e.g. inflammatory, steroid-induced, Posner–Schlossman, pigment dispersion, red cell, ghost cell, phacolytic, lens particle, intraocular tumour *Acute with closed angle*: e.g. PAC, neovascular, inflammatory, ICE syndrome, epithelial downgrowth, phacomorphic, lens dislocation, aqueous misdirection
AC leucocytes	*Corneal*: keratitis, FB, trauma, abrasion, chemical injury *Intraocular*: anterior uveitis, endophthalmitis, tumour necrosis
Hypopyon	*Corneal*: severe microbial keratitis *Intraocular*: severe anterior uveitis, endophthalmitis, tumour necrosis
Hyphaema	*Trauma*: blunt or penetrating *Surgery*: trabeculectomy, iris manipulation procedures *Spontaneous*: NVI/NVA, haematological disease, tumour (e.g. juvenile xanthogranuloma), IOL erosion of iris
Pigment in AC and angle	Idiopathic (↑ with age), PDS, PXF syndrome (Sampaolesi pigment line), intraocular surgery
Blood in Schlemm's canal	Sturge–Weber syndrome, carotid–cavernous fistula, SVC obstruction, hypotony

Iris/ciliary body

Ophthalmic signs—iris and ciliary body

Sign	Causes
Iris mass	*Pigmented*: e.g. iris melanoma, naevus, ICE syndrome, adenoma, ciliary body tumours
	Non-pigmented: e.g. amelanotic iris melanoma, iris cyst, iris granulomata, IOFB, juvenile xanthogranuloma, leiomyoma, ciliary body tumours, iris metastasis
Rubeosis	RVO (usually ischaemic CRVO), PDR, OIS, CRAO, posterior segment tumours, long-standing retinal detachment, sickle cell or other ischaemic retinopathy
Heterochromia	*Hypochromic*: congenital Horner's syndrome, Fuchs' heterochromic cyclitis (the affected eye is bluer), uveitis, trauma/surgery, Waardenberg syndrome
	Hyperchromic: drugs (e.g. latanoprost), siderosis (e.g. IOFB), oculodermal melanocytosis, diffuse iris naevus or melanoma, other intraocular tumours
Transillumination defects	*Diffuse*: albinism, post-angle closure, Fuchs' heterochromic cyclitis
	Peripupillary: PXF syndrome
	Mid-peripheral spoke-like: PDS
	Sectoral: trauma, post-surgery/laser, herpes simplex/zoster, ICE syndrome, iridoschisis
Leucocoria	Cataract, retinoblastoma, persistent fetal vasculature syndrome, inflammatory cyclitic membrane, Coats' disease, ROP, toxocara, incontinentia pigmenti, FEVR, retinal dysplasia (e.g. Norries' disease, Patau's syndrome, Edwards' syndrome)
Corectopia	Iris melanoma, iris naevus, ciliary body tumour, ICE syndrome, PPD, surgery (e.g. complicated cataract surgery, trabeculectomy), anterior segment dysgenesis, coloboma
Ciliary body mass	*Pigmented*: e.g. melanoma, metastasis, adenoma
	Non-pigmented: e.g. cyst, uveal effusion syndrome, medulloepithelioma, leiomyoma, metastases

Ophthalmic signs: anterior segment (3)

Pupil function

Ophthalmic signs—pupil function

Sign	Causes
RAPD	Asymmetric optic nerve disease (e.g. AION, optic neuritis, asymmetric glaucoma, compressive optic neuropathy, etc.) or severe asymmetric retinal disease (e.g. CRAO, CRVO, extensive retinal detachment, etc.)
Anisocoria	*Abnormal mydriasis*: Adie's pupil, iris trauma, iris inflammation, IIIn palsy, pharmacological, ischaemia
	Abnormal miosis: physiological, Horner's, pharmacological, iris inflammation
Light-near dissociation	*Unilateral*: afferent defect (optic nerve pathology), efferent defect (aberrant regeneration of IIIn)
	Bilateral: Parinaud syndrome, Argyll Robertson pupils, diabetes, amyloidosis, alcohol, myotonic dystrophy, encephalitis

Lens

Ophthalmic signs—lens

Sign	Causes
Cataract	*Sutural*: congenital, traumatic, metabolic (Fabry's disease, mannosidosis), depositional (copper, gold, silver, iron, chlorpromazine)
	Nuclear: congenital, age-related
	Lamellar: congenital/infantile (inherited, rubella, diabetes, galactosaemia, hypocalcaemia)
	Coronary: sporadic, inherited
	Cortical: age-related
	Subcapsular: age-related, diabetes, corticosteroids, uveitis, radiation
	Polar: congenital
	Diffuse: congenital, age-related
Abnormal size	*Microphakia*: Lowe syndrome
	Microspherophakia: familial microspherophakia, Peter's anomaly, Marfan's syndrome, Weill–Marchesani syndrome, hyperlysinaemia, Alport's syndrome, congenital rubella
Abnormal shape	Coloboma, anterior lenticonus (Alport's syndrome), posterior lenticonus (sporadic, familial, Lowe syndrome), lentiglobus
Ectopia lentis	*Congenital*: familial ectopia lentis, Marfan's syndrome, Weill–Marchesani syndrome, homocystinuria, familial microspherophakia, hyperlysinaemia, sulfite oxidase deficiency, Stickler syndrome, Sturge–Weber syndrome, Crouzon syndrome, Ehlers–Danlos syndrome, aniridia
	Acquired: PXF, trauma, high myopia, hypermature cataract, buphthalmos, ciliary body tumour
Superficial opacities	PXF, Vossius ring (trauma), glaucomflecken (subcapsular opacities from AACG)

Ophthalmic signs: posterior segment (1)

Fundus (chorioretinal)

Ophthalmic signs—fundus (chorioretinal)

Sign	Causes
Choroid	
Choroidal mass	*Pigmented*: e.g. naevus, CHRPE, melanocytoma, metastasis, BDUMP syndrome
	Non-pigmented: e.g. choroidal granuloma, choroidal detachment, choroidal neovascular membrane, haematoma (subretinal/sub-RPE/suprachoroidal), choroidal osteoma, choroidal haemangioma, posterior scleritis, metastasis
Choroidal folds	Idiopathic, hypermetropia, retrobulbar mass, posterior scleritis, uveitis, idiopathic orbital inflammatory disease, TED, choroidal mass, hypotony, papilloedema
Choroidal detachment	*Effusion*: hypotony, extensive PRP, extensive cryotherapy, posterior uveitis, uveal effusion syndrome
	Haemorrhage: intraoperative, trauma, spontaneous
Retina	
Tractional retinal detachment	ROP, sickle cell retinopathy, PDR, PVR (e.g. trauma/IOFB, intraocular surgery, retinal breaks), vitreomacular traction syndrome, incontinentia pigmenti, retinal dysplasia
Exudative retinal detachment	*Congenital*: nanophthalmos, uveal effusion syndrome, FEVR, disc coloboma/pit
	Vascular: CNV, Coats' disease, CSR, vasculitis, accelerated hypertension, pre-eclampsia
	Choroidal tumours
	Inflammatory: posterior uveitis (e.g. VKH), posterior scleritis, orbital cellulitis, post-operative inflammation, idiopathic orbital inflammatory disease
General	
White dots	*Idiopathic white dot syndromes*: PIC, POHS, MEWDS, APMPPE, serpiginous choroidopathy, birdshot retinochoroidopathy, multifocal choroiditis with panuveitis
	Infective (chorio)retinitis: syphilis, toxoplasma, TB, *Candida*, HSV
	Inflammatory (chorio)retinitis: sarcoidosis, sympathetic ophthalmia, VKH

Fundus (vascular)

Ophthalmic signs—fundus (vascular)

Sign	Causes
Hard exudates	Diabetic retinopathy, choroidal neovascular membrane, macroaneurysm, accelerated hypertension, neuroretinitis, retinal telangiectasias
Cotton wool spots	Diabetic retinopathy, B/CRVO, OIS, hypertension, HIV retinopathy, vasculitis
Retinal telangiectasias	Coats' disease, Leber's miliary aneurysms, idiopathic juxtafoveal telangiectasia, ROP, RP, diabetic retinopathy, sickle retinopathy, radiation retinopathy, hypogammaglobulinaemia, Eales disease, C/BRVO
Arterial emboli	Carotid artery disease, atrial thrombus, atrial myxoma, infective endocarditis, fat embolus (long bone fracture), talc embolus (IV drug abuser), amniotic fluid embolus
Roth's spots	Septic emboli, leukaemia, myeloma, HIV retinopathy
Vasculitis	Idiopathic retinal vasculitis, intermediate or posterior uveitis (idiopathic), sarcoidosis, MS, Behçet's disease, SLE, toxoplasmosis, TB, HSV, VZV, CMV, ARN, GPA, PAN, Takayasu's arteritis, Whipple's disease, Lyme disease
Arteritis	ARN (HSV, VZV); less commonly in other vasculitides

Ophthalmic signs: posterior segment (2)

Macula

Ophthalmic signs—macula

Sign	Causes
CMO	*Post-operative*: cataract/corneal/vitreoretinal surgery
	Post-procedure: cryotherapy, peripheral iridotomy, PRP
	Inflammatory: uveitis (posterior > intermediate > anterior), scleritis
	Vascular: retinal vein obstruction, diabetic maculopathy, ocular ischaemia, choroidal neovascular membrane, retinal telangiectasia, hypertensive retinopathy, radiation retinopathy
	Medication: epinephrine, latanoprost
	Other: vitreomacular traction syndrome, RP, AD CMO, tumours of the choroid/retina
Macular hole	Idiopathic, trauma, CMO, ERM, vitreomacular traction syndrome, retinal detachment (rhegmatogenous), laser injury, myopia, hypertension, PDR
ERM	Idiopathic, retinal detachment surgery, cryotherapy, photocoagulation, trauma (blunt or penetrating), posterior uveitis, persistent vitreous haemorrhage, retinal vascular disease (e.g. BRVO)
Choroidal neovascular membrane	*Degenerative*: AMD, pathological myopia, angioid streaks
	Trauma: choroidal rupture, laser
	Inflammation: sarcoidosis, toxoplasmosis, POHS, PIC, multifocal choroiditis, serpiginous choroidopathy, birdshot retinochoroidopathy, VKH
	Dystrophies: Best's disease
	Other: idiopathic, chorioretinal scar (any cause), tumour
Central serous detachment	CSR, optic disc pit, CNV, posterior uveitis (e.g. VKH), accelerated hypertension; see also ERD
Bull's eye maculopathy	*Drug*: chloroquine group, clofazimine
	Macular dystrophies: cone dystrophy, cone–rod dystrophy, Stargardt's
	Neurological: Batten's disease
Cherry-red spot	*Systemic*: Tay–Sachs disease, Sandhoff disease, GM1 gangliosidoses, Niemann–Pick disease, sialidosis, metachromatic leucodystrophy
	Ocular: CRAO
Foveal schisis	XL juvenile retinoschisis

Optic disc

Ophthalmic signs—optic disc

Sign	Causes
Pallor	*Congenital*: Kjer's, Behr's, or Wolfram's optic atrophy
	Acquired: compression (optic nerve or chiasm), glaucoma, ischaemia, toxins, poor nutrition, inflammation, infection, LHON, trauma, severe retinal disease, post-papilloedema
Apparent swelling	*Pseudo*: drusen, tilted, hypermetropic, myelinated
	True: ↑ICP (usually bilateral) or local causes (may be unilateral), e.g. inflammation, ischaemia, LHON, infiltration, tumour
Pit	*Congenital*
	Acquired: glaucoma

Ophthalmic signs: visual fields

See Fig. 20.1.

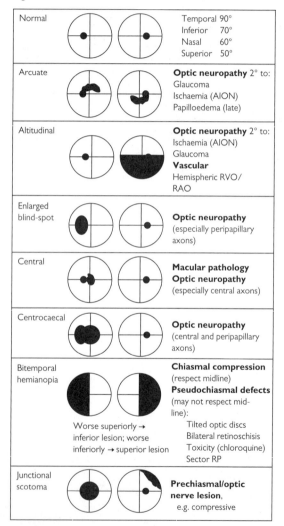

Normal		Temporal 90° Inferior 70° Nasal 60° Superior 50°
Arcuate		**Optic neuropathy** 2° to: Glaucoma Ischaemia (AION) Papilloedema (late)
Altitudinal		**Optic neuropathy** 2° to: Ischaemia (AION) Glaucoma **Vascular** Hemispheric RVO/ RAO
Enlarged blind-spot		**Optic neuropathy** (especially peripapillary axons)
Central		**Macular pathology** **Optic neuropathy** (especially central axons)
Centrocaecal		**Optic neuropathy** (central and peripapillary axons)
Bitemporal hemianopia	Worse superiorly → inferior lesion; worse inferiorly → superior lesion	**Chiasmal compression** (respect midline) **Pseudochiasmal defects** (may not respect midline): Tilted optic discs Bilateral retinoschisis Toxicity (chloroquine) Sector RP
Junctional scotoma		**Prechiasmal/optic nerve lesion**, e.g. compressive

Fig. 20.1 VF defects.

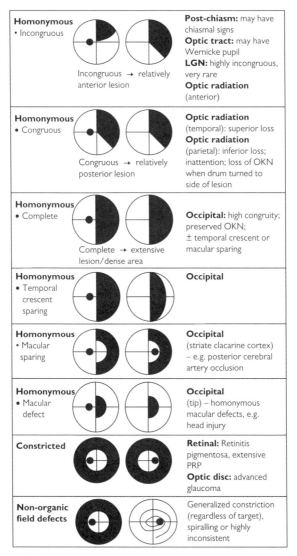

Homonymous • Incongruous	Incongruous → relatively anterior lesion	**Post-chiasm:** may have chiasmal signs **Optic tract:** may have Wernicke pupil **LGN:** highly incongruous, very rare **Optic radiation** (anterior)
Homonymous • Congruous	Congruous → relatively posterior lesion	**Optic radiation** (temporal): superior loss **Optic radiation** (parietal): inferior loss; inattention; loss of OKN when drum turned to side of lesion
Homonymous • Complete	Complete → extensive lesion/dense area	**Occipital:** high congruity; preserved OKN; ± temporal crescent or macular sparing
Homonymous • Temporal crescent sparing		**Occipital**
Homonymous • Macular sparing		**Occipital** (striate clacarine cortex) – e.g. posterior cerebral artery occlusion
Homonymous • Macular defect		**Occipital** (tip) – homonymous macular defects, e.g. head injury
Constricted		**Retinal:** Retinitis pigmentosa, extensive PRP **Optic disc:** advanced glaucoma
Non-organic field defects		Generalized constriction (regardless of target), spiralling or highly inconsistent

Fig. 20.1 (*Cont.*).

Vision in context

Relevant pages
◗ The child who does not see 772

Low vision: taking a history

Around 2.5% of the UK population have some degree of visual impairment which is not correctable by refraction. Of these, up to two-thirds are thought to have sufficiently severe sight loss to qualify for visual impairment registration. However, even amongst those attending ophthalmology units, up to half of those eligible are not actually registered.[1] There is concern that this may reflect a wider problem of access to support and services. It is probable that many of these people never seek help. However, even those who get to an ophthalmologist may only be rewarded with a diagnosis of an incurable eye disease for which 'nothing can be done'.

In these circumstances, those involved in eye care must be aware of 'what *can* be done' to optimize the patient's remaining vision and how best to advise and assist the patient. This is often best coordinated in a dedicated low vision clinic, ideally with access to specialist nurses, optometrists, rehabilitation workers, counsellors, and social services.

Definition

The UK Low Vision Services Consensus Group defines low vision as impairment of visual function which causes restriction to everyday life and which cannot be corrected by conventional spectacles, CL, or medical intervention. This should not be confused with the WHO definition of low vision which is VA <6/18, but ≥3/60 in the better eye with best possible correction; the WHO defines <3/60 as blindness.

History

General—what are their concerns?

People are extremely variable. For some, the priority will be to continue to solve the crossword; others will be afraid of social isolation. Sometimes this will also reveal misunderstandings about their condition.

Specific—consider the following

Reading

Is reading an issue for them? If so, what do they want to read, what size print, and in what context (i.e. at home or out and about)? This will affect the type of optical devices used.

Television

If this is an issue for them, consider size of television, viewing distance, and whether colour or black and white (higher contrast).

Activities of daily living and recreation

Are they managing to look after themselves (± dependants)? What about shopping, cooking, and hygiene? Can they still manage the telephone or do they risk becoming isolated? Can they still do their hobbies?

Medication

Can they manage their tablets, instil drops, and measure their injections?

Mobility

Do they manage to get around? Do they have access to public transport or lifts from family or friends? Mobility training can help them navigate and continue to use public transport with confidence.

Work and financial support

Have they got the help they need to continue working if they wish to? What resources are available to them in terms of equipment or personal assistance? Do they know how to access any benefits that they are entitled to?

Psychosocial

Are they coping emotionally with their visual impairment? Do they have access to local support groups? Would they benefit from talking to a counsellor?

Visual phenomena

Are they troubled by glare? Glare which worsens vision under bright conditions (effectively reducing contrast) is known as disability glare. Glare which is uncomfortable without necessarily affecting vision is known as 'discomfort glare'. Do they find it difficult changing between bright and dark conditions and vice versa? Problems with adaptation to light and dark is common in AMD, RP, and advanced glaucoma.

Visual hallucinations

Ask specifically whether they are being troubled by 'seeing things that are not real'. Charles Bonnet syndrome (visual hallucinations in people with severe sight loss) is relatively common, but patients frequently conceal it for fear of being thought to be mentally ill. Discussing and rationalizing the syndrome (e.g 'your brain is filling in the gaps in your vision') can be very reassuring. The visual hallucinations fall into two broad types: abstract (patterns, lines, etc.) or life-like (people, animals, etc.). The images may be black and white or in colour and may be distorted and of the incorrect size (e.g. images of tiny people). In most cases, it resolves within 12–18mo.[2]

1. Barry RJ et al. Unregistered visual impairment: is registration a failing system. *Br J Ophthalmol* 2005;**89**:995–8.

2. Ffytche DH. Visual hallucinations and the Charles Bonnet syndrome. *Curr Psychiatry Rep* 2005;**7**:168–79.

(Further reading: *Low vision: the essential guide for ophthalmologists* by Anne Sinclair and Barbara Ryan, published by The Guide Dogs for the Blind Association.)

Low vision: assessing visual function

Visual function is more than just distance acuity. Do not overlook the effect of reduced contrast sensitivity or a constricted VF.

VA—distance

Where possible, use a logMAR chart, rather than a Snellen chart. In addition to the usual advantages of logMAR over Snellen (see ➜ Assessment of vision: acuity, p. 4), the fact that there are five letters on every row (including the top row) avoids the 'one chance only' scenario characteristic of the 6/60 line on a Snellen chart and is somewhat less discouraging for the patient. If the top line cannot be read at the test distance, bring the chart nearer—do not just go straight to CF. The jump from 6/60 to CF is a huge difference in functional terms.

VA—near

Previously, most reading charts were aimed at the normally sighted (albeit presbyopic) population with ranges of N5–N48. For low vision assessment, it may be helpful to have a wider range such as the Bailey–Lovie near chart which runs from N2.5 to N80.

Contrast sensitivity

Whilst not commonly used in the general ophthalmic clinic, measuring contrast sensitivity (e.g. with a Pelli–Robson chart) is an important part of assessing visual function in someone with low vision. It can explain an apparent discrepancy between reasonable acuity in the high contrast clinic setting and poor functional vision in a dimly lit home; loss of contrast sensitivity is also associated with increased falls in the elderly.

VF

Day-to-day function is greatly affected by the quality of your VF, even in the presence of 6/6 central vision. Mobility is particularly affected by inferior/central field defects. Reading is also affected by central defects, but also by both right hemianopic defects (they cannot jump to the next word) and left hemianopic defects (they cannot find the next line). Specific reading techniques may be helpful in these cases (see Table 21.1). If a patient is being referred for mobility assessment and training, it is helpful if the rehabilitation officer can be provided with a copy of the VF plot.

Table 21.1 Reading strategies for patients with a hemianopic field defect

Defect	Problem	Strategy
Left hemianopia	Cannot find the start of the line	Keep thumb/marker at the start of the line as a marker to return to
Right hemianopia	Cannot find the next word	Learn to skip beyond the next word so that the target word falls within the field of vision
		Try reading with the text rotated up to 90° so that the whole line falls within the field of vision

The advice depends on the direction of reading—a left-to-right reading direction is assumed here.

Low vision: doing something useful (1)

General

Optimize lighting conditions (e.g. brighter bulbs, more lights around the house, good reading light). Improve contrast where possible.

Make sure information is provided in a suitable format: written (should be in a clear typeface of minimum 14 point font size), audio, or electronic.

Equipment

Refraction (near and distance) should be optimized. In addition, consider:

Optical devices (near)

- *Reading glasses*: these should be optimized, although they are often not sufficient on their own. Up to +4.00D is usually well tolerated, but, beyond this, the reading distance is uncomfortably short. Higher reading additions may require a prism to assist convergence.
- *Hand magnifiers*: these are usually practical and inexpensive but are limited by a small field of view (especially for the higher powers).
- *Stand magnifiers*: these have the advantage of keeping both hands free and keeping the working distance constant but are less transportable.
- *Illuminated magnifiers*: these improve contrast (provided that the batteries are charged) but are generally bulkier.
- *Reading telescopes*: these may be useful for specific near work, since they have a greater working distance than reading glasses of an equivalent magnification. However, they are expensive and are poor cosmetically.
- *CCTV*: excellent magnification with high contrast can be achieved with a TV camera directed down onto a reading plinth and viewed on the adjacent screen. However, it is expensive, not portable, and generally superceded by computer/scanner technology.

Optical devices (distance)

- *Distance telescopes*: can be useful for specific tasks, although generally they are limited by the small field of view. They may be spectacle-mounted (useful for static tasks, e.g. watching TV, theatre, music, sports, etc.) or handheld (used as required, e.g. bus number, signs, etc.).

Computers

Personal computers (either with enlarged text or speech facility) have made a spectacular difference to the lives of many visually impaired people. They provide an easy method of writing, 'reading' (with scanner and optical character recognition), and instant 'letter' communication by email. Web-based facilities also increase access to shopping, entertainment, and support.

Other devices

Other devices include:
- Talking watches/clocks.
- Writing guides.
- Typoscopes (black card with a slit used as a reading window; reduces glare).
- Liquid level indicators (prevent overfilling cups, baths).
- Tactile controls on domestic appliances (either as standard or as 'bump-ons').
- Large button telephones.
- Talking scales.

Entertainment

In addition to the improved accessibility of computers, consider:
- Modified games (e.g. large playing cards).
- Audio description DVDs or videos.
- Talking books/newspapers (available as mp3, audio CD, and other formats).
- Modified sports equipment.

Mobility

Mobility training can help people navigate and continue to use public transport with confidence; a mobility officer will tailor the training to the needs (type of transport/required routes) to that individual. Mobility may be assisted by the use of a cane (see Table 21.2), guide dog (relatively uncommon) or a sighted guide. The use of a cane or a guide dog require training.

Table 21.2 Types of cane (or 'white stick')

Type	Features	Purpose
Symbol cane	Small, lightweight, collapsible	Advises others that the bearer has visual impairment
Guide cane	Longer, more robust	Can be used to detect change in contour, e.g. steps
		Advises others that the bearer has visual impairment
Long cane	Long with a rollerball tip	Used to sweep the path ahead to detect obstacles
		Advises others that the bearer has visual impairment
White walking stick	White, standard walking aid	Used as a walking aid (like a normal walking stick)
		Advises others that the bearer has visual impairment

Support

Ensure that they have access to support from social services and local support groups and that they know how to get help in case of need.

Registration

If they are eligible but are not yet registered, ensure that the purpose of registration is explained and that it is offered to them. (See ➲ Visual impairment registration (1), p. 912.)

Low vision: doing something useful (2)

Benefits

Check that they are aware of what benefits they are entitled to and know where to get help or further information, e.g. social services and local and national support groups (see Box 21.1).

Box 21.1 Benefits available in the UK for those registered visually impaired

Tax relief and allowances

For blind and partially sighted people

- Disability living allowance (DLA, if <16y)/personal independence payment (PIP, if working age, i.e 16–64)/attendance allowance (AA, if ≥65y): for help with personal care and mobility; depends on level of disability.
- Additional income support (if < qualifying age for state pension credit, QASP)/pension credit (if ≥QASP): to top up low income.
- Working tax credit: if disabled and working ≥16h/wk but on low income.
- Employment and support allowance (ESA): for people of working age unable to work.
- Council tax disability reduction scheme.

Additional benefits for those receiving DLA, PIP, or AA

- Additional housing benefit.
- Council tax reduction scheme.
- Exemption from non-dependants deduction from income support, pension credit, housing benefit, and council tax benefit (only applies to those on AA or middle/highest rate DLA or PIP).

Additional benefits for blind people only

- Blind person's income tax allowance.

Other

For blind and partially sighted people

- Community care services and local council assistance: home care, mobility training, counselling, equipment, home modification.
- Free NHS sight test.
- Free NHS prescriptions: depends on age and income.
- Low vision aids.
- Additional equipment/assistance/travel costs to make it possible to work.
- Free postage on 'articles for the blind', e.g. talking books.
- Railcard and other travel concessions.
- Exemption from BT directory enquiries.

Additional benefits for blind people only

- 50% reduction in TV licence fee.
- Car parking concessions (blue badge scheme): also available to partially sighted people if they have mobility problems.
- Free loan of radios, cassette/CD players, and TV sound receivers.
- Help with telephone installation charges and line rental.

The exact benefits change according to governmental initiative; social services are available to provide up-to-the-minute advice for the patient.

Visual impairment registration (1)

Registration of visual impairment has traditionally had three roles: to formally recognize an individual's sight loss, to identify those patients eligible for assistance due to their disability, and to help eye services, social services, and government know the extent and distribution of visual impairment in the community. The National Assistance Act (NAA) 1948 formalized this process and led to the BD8 form which was in use in England and Wales for around 50y before being replaced with the Certificate of Vision Impairment (CVI) forms. Equivalent forms are used in Scotland and in Northern Ireland.

There were a number of reasons that the BD8 registration system was replaced. For many people, the registration process actually excluded or delayed access to services. More than half of those eligible choose not to be registered, and many are unhappy about being registered blind when they have (and are expected to continue to have) residual vision. In response to this, the newer CVI system separates formal registration from the referral for needs assessment. The CVI form is supported by the Referral of Vision Impairment (RVI) and the Low Vision Leaflet (LVL), both of which can be used to notify social services of a person's needs without requiring full registration. Among other changes, the CVI replaced the category 'blind' with 'severely sight-impaired or blind'.

Eligibility

Sight-impaired/partially sighted
This is not legally defined. It is summarized by the Department of Health (UK)[3] (see Table 21.3) as:
- VA 3/60–6/60 with normal VF, *or*
- VA 6/60–6/24 with moderate contraction of the VF, media opacities, or aphakia,
- VA 6/18 or better but with severe field loss. This may be either a large defect, such as hemianopia, or marked contraction of the VF such as in RP or advanced glaucoma.

Severely sight impaired/blind
This is legally defined (NAA 1948) as 'so blind that they cannot do any work for which eyesight is essential'. This is conventionally regarded as:
- VA ≤3/60–6/60 with a very contracted VF, *or*
- VA 6/60 or better with a very contracted VF, especially where there is significant inferior field loss; homonymous or bitemporal hemianopia are specifically excluded, unless the central VA is worse than 6/18.

Table 21.3 Registration for blindness April 1999–March 2000 in England and Wales[*]

Age	Leading causes of blindness
0–15	1st—disorders of the visual cortex (15.9%) 2nd—congenital ocular anomalies (13.4%) 3rd—hereditary retinal disorders (13.1%)
16–64	**1st—diabetic retinopathy (17.7%)** 2nd—hereditary retinal disorders (15.8%) 3rd—degeneration of the macula and posterior pole (7.7%)
All ages	1st—degeneration of the macula and posterior pole (57.2%) 2nd—glaucoma (10.9%) 3rd—diabetic retinopathy (5.9%)

[*] Bunce C *et al.* Causes of blind certifications in England and Wales: April 1999–March 2000. *Eye* 2008;**22**:905–11.

3. Bunce C *et al.* Causes of blind certifications in England and Wales: April 1999–March 2000. *Eye* 2008;**22**:905–11.

Visual impairment registration (2)

See Box 21.2 for relevant documents available.

For the Hospital Eye Service (HES)

Certificate of Vision Impairment (CVI)

This is the declaration of eligibility for registration.

- *Part 1*: contains (1) patient's consent to be registered, (2) consultant ophthalmologist's confirmation of eligibility for registration (sight-impaired vs severely sight-impaired).
- *Part 2*: contains (1) contact details of patient, GP, local social services, (2) visual function (acuity and field), (3) diagnosis (with ICD10 codes).
- *Part 3*: contains (1) relevant social factors (e.g. lives alone, other disability, etc.), (2) urgency of contact required, (3) ethnic origin, and (4) preferred communication format.
- *Explanatory notes*: (1) patient information about the certificate, (2) summary of consent, (3) information about driving.

In signing the form, the patient consents to the information within the form being passed to: (1) their local council, GP, and Primary Care Trust for referral, assessment, and registration purposes and (2) the Royal College of Ophthalmologists on behalf of Moorfields Eye Hospital and the Department of Health for epidemiological research and analysis.

Referral of Vision Impairment (RVI)

This notifies social services of the patient's situation, requests an assessment for them, and states how urgently this is required. It should be completed by ophthalmic clinic staff, with the patient's consent. It does not result in registration.

For optometrists

Low Vision Leaflet (LVL)

These should be provided by optometrists to any person in whom they identify sight impairment. It not only provides the patient with contact details for support and local and national resources, but it also includes a form which can be filled in by the patient, enabling them to 'self-refer' to social services. Social services will then carry out an assessment of their needs and advise them on what resources are available to them. It does not result in registration.

Box 21.2 Relevant documents available from the Department of Health (UK) website*

- CVI.
- RVI.
- LVL.
- Explanatory notes for consultant ophthalmologists and hospital eye clinic staff.
- The identification, referral, and registration of sight loss: action for social services departments and optometrists and explanatory notes.

* Department of Health. *Registering vision impairment as a disability.* (2013). Available at: 🔗 https://www.gov.uk/government/publications/guidance-published-on-registering-a-vision-impairment-as-a-disability

Driving standards

Evidence that visual impairment alone causes accidents is surprisingly scarce. The strictness of driving standards varies internationally, in part affected by the density of traffic and driving conditions. In some parts of the USA, partially sighted people may drive during daylight hours within a specified radius of their home. In the UK, any driver who has a condition which either already affects their fitness to drive or might do so in the future (e.g. glaucoma) must notify the DVLA, unless the visual impairment is anticipated to be of <3mo duration. The following driving standards are enforced by the DVLA.[4]

VA

Group 1 drivers (car and light vehicles)

- Must be able to read in good light either the standard number plate (post-September 2001 format comprising 79mm × 50mm letters) at 20m or the old number plate (pre-September 2001 format comprising 79mm × 57mm letters) at 20.5m, AND
- At least 6/12 with both eyes open (or in the only eye if monocular) with the aid of corrective lenses, if necessary.

Group 2 drivers (large goods vehicles (LGV) and passenger-carrying vehicles (PCV)

- As for group 1 drivers, AND
- At least 6/7.5 in the better eye, AND
- At least 6/60 in the worse eye (with the aid of corrective lenses, if necessary), AND
- Glasses, if required, should be ≤8D in strength.

Some drivers who fail these requirements may be permitted to drive under 'grandfather rights' which take into account the date of licensing. The licence holder needs to contact the DVLA who will require a certificate of recent driving experience and confirmation of no eyesight-related road accidents in the previous 10y.

VF

The preferred method of testing is now the Esterman program on the Humphrey analyser. For those patients who cannot use an automated perimeter, Goldmann testing is acceptable in exceptional circumstances. Bitemporal hemianopia may require monocular Esterman testing to ensure that there is adequate input from both hemifields in at least one eye to prevent dissociation (hemifield slip). A maximum of 20% false positives is allowed.

Group 1 drivers

- At least 120° on the horizontal (target equivalent to a white Goldmann III4e setting), with extension of at least 50° left and right, AND
- No significant defect in the binocular field encroaching within 20° of fixation above or below the horizontal meridian.
- 'Acceptable' central defects comprise:
  - Scattered single missed points.
  - A single cluster of two or three adjoining points.
- 'Acceptable' peripheral defects which are disregarded when assessing the field width comprise:
  - A single cluster of two or three missed points unattached to any other defect on or across the horizontal meridian.

- A vertical defect of only single point width but any length unattached to any other defect on or across the horizontal meridian.

Where a patient has fully adapted to a static, long-standing defect, the DVLA may consider them as an 'exceptional case' and perform a practical driving assessment.

Group 2 drivers

- Horizontal VF should be at least 160°, with extension of 70° to left and right and 30° up and down, AND
- No defects in the central 30°.

Specific cases

All these patients should inform the DVLA of their condition.

Monocularity

Patients may drive group 1 vehicles (but not group 2 vehicles) when clinically advised that they have adapted to the disability and they satisfy the usual VA requirements and have a normal monocular VF.

Diplopia

Patients with uncorrected diplopia must not drive. Driving may be resumed if controlled; patching is acceptable, subject to the above constraints on monocularity for group 1 vehicles; patching is not acceptable for group 2 vehicles. Very rarely, the DVLA may permit someone to drive despite uncorrected diplopia if it is stable (>6mo).

Blepharospasm

Patients with severe blepharospasm must not drive. Patients with mild, treated blepharospasm may drive, subject to consultant approval.

All drivers

If the patient fails to reach these standards, they must not drive and have a legal requirement to notify the DVLA. Failure to comply is a criminal offence and can result in a fine of up to £1,000. Further details are available at ℅ http://www.dvla.gov.uk

Racing licences

For racing in the UK, the Motor Sports Association (MSA) requires a best corrected VA of 6/6 (both eyes together) and a VF of 120° horizontally, with no defects within 20° above or below the horizontal meridian. They must have normal colour vision (specifically red/green discrimination) and no diplopia. Acquired monocularity prevents racing until 5y has elapsed.[5] For racing internationally, the Fédération Internationale de l'Automobile (FIA) requires a best corrected VA of at least 9/10 in each eye or 8/10 in one eye and 10/10 in the other, normal colour vision, normal stereopsis, and a VF of 120° horizontally, without significant defect within 20° above or below the horizontal meridian.[6]

4. Driver and Vehicle Licensing Agency (DVLA). *At a glance guide to the current medical standards of fitness to drive (2013 edition).* Available at: ℅ http://www.dft.gov.uk/dvla/medical/ataglance.aspx

5. Motor Sports Association (UK). *MSA competition licence notes.* Available at: ℅ https://www.msauk.org/uploadedfiles/msa_forms/2013_licence_notes.pdf

6. Fédération Internationale de l'Automobile (FIA). *Appendix L to the International Sporting Code, 2014.* Available at: ℅ http://www.fia.com/sites/default/files/regulation/file/13.12.17_ANNEXE%20L%202014.pdf

Pilot standards

Civil Aviation Authority (CAA)

Class 1 pilots (commercial: aeroplane and helicopter)[7]

VA
- *Distance*: at least 6/9 in each eye and 6/6 with both eyes together (best corrected).
- *Near*: at least N5 at 30–50cm and N14 at 100cm (best corrected).

Refractive error and correction
- Refractive error ≤+5.0D or −6.0D, astigmatism ≤2.0D, and anisometropia ≤2.0D.
- CL may be used if they can be reliably used for >8h/d.
- *Refractive surgery*: stability of refraction must be demonstrated; preoperative refraction must have been ≤+5.0D; glare sensitivity and mesopic contrast must be normal.

Colour
- Satisfactory Ishihara testing; if fails this, then must pass Lantern test.

Other
- Normal VF.
- No diplopia.
- Heterophoria <8Δ exo, 10Δ eso, or 2Δ vertical at 6m and <12Δexo, 6Δeso, or 1Δvertical at 33cm: excess of this will require further assessment by a CAA ophthalmologist.
- No ophthalmic or adnexal disease.

Class 2 pilots (private: aeroplane and helicopter)[8]

VA
- *Distance*: at least 6/12 in each eye and 6/9 with both eyes together (best corrected).
- *Near*: at least N5 at 30–50cm and N14 at 100cm (best corrected).

Substandard VA in one eye may be accepted, subject to a flight test if the other eye has VA of at least 6/6 with N5 and N14.

Refractive error and correction
- Refractive error <+5.0D or −8.0D (in the most ametropic meridian), astigmatism <3D, and anisometropia <3.0D; under some circumstances, stable myopia in the range −5 to −8.0D may be acceptable.
- CL may be used if they can be reliably used for >8h/d.
- *Refractive surgery*: stability of refraction must be demonstrated; usually unable to fly for 3mo post-LASIK and 1y after other procedures; preoperative refractive error may still be a bar to qualification.

Colour
- Satisfactory Ishihara testing; if fails this, then must pass Holmes Wright Lantern test or be restricted to daytime flying.

Other
- Normal VF.
- No diplopia.
- Heterophoria will require further assessment by a CAA ophthalmologist.
- No ophthalmic or adnexal disease.

Further information is available at: ℘ http://www.caa.co.uk

Other occupational visual standards
Numerous occupations have specific occupational standards related to visual requirements which are defined nationally (but may vary from one country to another). The Royal College of Ophthalmologists provide a helpful summary of a number of occupational visual standards within the UK.[8] These should be checked against the latest online resources for each profession (see Table 21.4).

Table 21.4 Selected occupations for which visual standards are required

Organization	Occupation
CAA	Pilots
	Non-pilot flight crew
	Air traffic control officers
	Airfield fire crew
	Airside drivers
London Underground	Train drivers
	Guards
Railway Safety and Standards Board	Train drivers
	Guards
	Shunters
	Conductors
	Signallers
	Railway crossing keepers
Institution of Electrical Engineers	Electrical engineers
Home Office	Police officers
	Prison officers
Fire and Rescue Service	Fire officers
Royal National Lifeboat Institution	Lifeboat crew
Maritime and Coastguard Agency	Merchant navy deck personnel
	Fishing vessel personnel
	Coastguards
Ministry of Defence	Royal Navy
	British Army
	Royal Air Force

7. Civil Aviation Authority. *MED.B.070 Visual System.* Available at: ℘ http://www.caa.co.uk/default. aspx?catid=49&pagetype=90&pageid=13885

8. Bradshaw SE, for the Royal College of Ophthalmologists. *Occupational Visual Standards.* (2009). Available at: ℘ http://www.rcophth.ac.uk/core/core_picker/download.asp?id=123

Eligibility for free sight tests and optical vouchers in the NHS (UK)

Eligibility for support

See Box 21.3 and Box 21.4.

Box 21.3 Eligibility for support with NHS (UK) sight tests

In England, Wales, and Northern Ireland, a patient is eligible for free sight tests if they are:

- <16y old OR ≤18y old and in full-time education OR ≥60y old.
- ≥40y old AND diagnosed with glaucoma or been told by an ophthalmologist that they are at risk of glaucoma or have a parent/sibling/child who has been diagnosed with glaucoma.
- Diagnosed with diabetes.
- Registered as sight-impaired (partially sighted) or severely sight-impaired (blind).
- In need of complex lenses.
- Receiving their sight test through the hospital eye department.
- A prisoner currently on leave.
- Receiving income support, income-based Jobseeker's Allowance, Pension Credit Guarantee Credit, or Universal Credit.
- Entitled to/named on a valid NHS Tax Credit Exemption Certificate.
- Named on a valid HC2 (full) or HC3 (partial) certificate.

In Scotland, everybody is eligible for a free sight test annually.

Box 21.4 Eligibility for NHS (UK) optical vouchers

In England, Wales, and Northern Ireland, a patient is eligible for vouchers towards the costs of glasses or CL if they are:

- <16y old OR ≤18y old and in full-time education.
- Receiving income support, income-based Jobseeker's Allowance, or Pension Credit Guarantee Credit, Universal Credit.
- Entitled to/named on a valid NHS Tax Credit Exemption Certificate.
- Named on a valid HC2 (full) or HC3 (partial) certificate.
- Complex lens prescription.

Up-to-the-minute information is available on the Department of Health (UK) website on ℜ http://www.dh.gov.uk. A useful resource is also available at ℜ http://www.visionmatters.org.uk/sight-tests/eligibility-and-vouchers

---

Chapter 22

Ophthalmic surgery: anaesthetics and perioperative care

Preoperative assessment

Preoperative assessment seeks to identify any factors that may put the patient (or staff) at additional risk. The following are a practical interpretation of the recommendations of the Royal College of Ophthalmologists and the Royal College of Anaesthetists.[1,2]

General

- *Day surgery vs inpatient:* check whether appropriate for day surgery (adequate support) or inpatient care.
- *Casenotes and test results:* ensure medical records and any relevant investigations (including biometry, scans, and blood tests) are available.
- *Alerts:* check for hazards (e.g. known airway problems, allergies, MRSA, blood-borne diseases, e.g. hepatitis, HIV), and ensure that these are communicated appropriately to the rest of the team.
- *Special requirements:* check for special requirements (e.g. patient with learning difficulties, interpreter).

Systemic

History

- Age.
- *PMH:* ask specifically about diabetes, hypertension, IHD (MI, angina), cerebrovascular disease (TIA, CVA), vertigo, and any current problems such as smoking, alcohol intake, incontinence, TB, asthma, claustrophobia, COPD, epilepsy, reflux, hepatic, renal, and thyroid disorders.
- *Past surgical history:* previous surgery ophthalmic and non-ophthalmic, anaesthetics, and adverse reactions. Notes review for presence of intraocular gas, scleral explants, etc.
- *Systemic review:* CVS (e.g. chest pain and precipitating events, palpitations, paroxysmal nocturnal dyspnoea (PND)), RS (recent chest infection, asthma, exercise tolerance, e.g. breathlessness at rest or on exertion, orthopnoea), CNS (pre-existing neurological damage, fits), renal (e.g. dialysis), psychological issues (e.g. alcohol, anxiety), hearing and comprehension, ability to lie still and flat.
- *FH* (including problems with anaesthesia).
- *Medication (both prescription and over-the-counter) and allergies.*
- *SH:* e.g. home care.

NB Any patients with significant anaesthetic risk factors or other concerns (e.g. syndromic patients or those with congenital disorders) should be discussed with the anaesthetist, especially if a general anaesthetic is being considered.

Examination

- *General:* build, weight, height, and BMI.
- *CVS:* anaemia, cyanosis, oedema, pulse (rate + rhythm), BP, heart sounds, any murmurs.
- *RS:* clubbing, respiratory rate and chest expansion, tracheal position, (tracheostomy scars), auscultation (air entry, wheeze, crepitations), pulse oximetry.
- *Musculoskeletal:* neck/jaw/dental/back problems (may affect endotracheal intubation and surgical position).
- *CNS:* comprehension, cooperation, hearing, tremor, neurological deficits, other abnormal movements, and mobility.
- *Miscellaneous:* septic foci, e.g. venous leg ulcers, AV fistulas for haemodialysis, pacemakers, dentures, limb prosthesis, indwelling catheters, etc.
- *Venous thromboembolic (VTE) assessment.*

Ophthalmic examination on the day

The ophthalmic history and examination should identify any new developments since the clinic assessment which may postpone surgery or might modify the planned operation in any way.

Contraindications

Any identified risk factors should be treated preoperatively. This may require postponement of surgery and either coordination with the patient's GP or referral to an appropriate specialist (see Box 22.1).

Box 22.1 Specific systemic contraindications for surgery

- Myocardial ischaemia (unstable angina, coronary stent, or MI in the last 3mo).
- CVA, TIA in the last 3mo.
- Uncontrolled hyperglycaemia.
- Uncontrolled arrhythmias.
- Supratherapeutic INR.
- Acute systemic illness.

1. Royal College of Anaesthetists and Royal College of Ophthalmologists. *Local anaesthesia for ophthalmic surgery. Joint guidelines from the Royal College of Anaesthetists and the Royal College of Ophthalmologists.* (2012). Available at: ℞ http://www.rcophth.ac.uk/page.asp?section=451

2. Royal College of Ophthalmologists. *Cataract surgery guidelines.* (2010). Available at: ℞ http://www.rcophth.ac.uk/page.asp?section=451

Preoperative preparation

Investigations

Operations under local anaesthesia

Routine investigations are usually not required, unless history and systemic examination suggest significant systemic disease which would be worthy of investigation in its own right (e.g. coronary artery disease, diabetes, severe respiratory disease, anticoagulation, renal dialysis).

Operations under GA

It is common practice not to routinely investigate fit ASA I patients (American Society of Anesthesiologists level I; see Table 22.2) under the age of 40y in whom a general history and examination are satisfactory.

Specific investigations

- *Haematological and biochemical profile* (e.g. FBC, U+E, Glu, etc.): tests are indicated for patients in whom abnormalities are likely, e.g. those with renal, hepatic, metabolic, endocrinal dysfunction, or patients on concurrent medication with steroids, bronchodilators, diuretics, cardiac drugs, or those presenting with acute systemic illness.
  - For patients on dialysis, the electrolytes should be checked on the day of surgery.
  - For patients on warfarin, the coagulation screening (INR) should done within 24h preceding surgery.
- *ECG:* is not routinely required for patients under age of 50 unless presenting with history of heavy smoking, diabetes, hypertension, renal disorders, previous cardiac disease, or excessive alcohol intake. Over 50y of age, a baseline ECG is recommended.
- *Sickle cell test:* indicated if African-Caribbean or Mediterranean origin.
- *Pacemaker check:* required in patients with pacemakers.
- *Axial length measurement and B-scan:* to identify staphylomas in high myopes, particularly if contemplating sharp needle blocks.
- *Other investigations:* CXR, echocardiography, LFT, TFT, etc. are indicated, according to patient's history/examination.
- *Infection screening:* for communicable illnesses, dependent on local protocol.

Preoperative topical medication

- *Patients for intraocular surgery*: appropriate preoperative drops (see Table 22.1).

Table 22.1 Common preoperative drop regimes

Cataract surgery	Cyclopentolate 1% + phenylephrine 2.5% + diclofenac 0.1%
Vitreoretinal surgery	Cyclopentolate 1% + phenylephrine 2.5% + diclofenac 0.1%
PK	Pilocarpine 2%

Fasting

Patients receiving GA or moderate/deep sedation

- Patients should be fasted for 6h after a solid meal (includes milk, tea, coffee) and 4h after *clear* fluids and chewing gum.

Table 22.2 ASA classification of fitness for anaesthesia[*]

ASA I	Fit and healthy patient
ASA II	Mild systemic disease; no functional limitation (e.g. mild controlled asthma; smoking)
ASA III	Severe systemic disease; definite functional limitation
ASA IV	Severe systemic disease which is a constant threat to life
ASA V	Moribund patient, not expected to survive for 24h with or without surgical intervention

Suffix E (e.g. ASA IIIE) denotes emergency surgery.

[*] American Society of Anesthesiologists. *ASA physical status classification system*. Available at:
℘ http://www.asahq.org/clinical/physicalstatus.htm

Preoperative management: special patient groups

Patients with diabetes

- Blood sugar should be well controlled prior to surgery. Currently, there is not enough evidence to specify an upper limit of blood sugar above which surgery should be cancelled for local anaesthesia. Normal oral feeding and medication (or near-normal regime) can be continued in most patients having local anaesthesia. Poorly controlled diabetics and those fasting for general anaesthesia will require sliding scale insulin and dextrose infusion (liaise with the anaesthetist) (see Table 22.3).

Table 22.3 Example of insulin sliding scale to be infused along with 5% glucose solution at 100mL/h

Blood sugar (BM)	<2	2.0–4.9	5.0–9.9	10.0–14.9	14.9–19.9	≥20.0
Insulin IV (U/h)	0 Give Glu	0	1.0	2.0	3.0	6.0 Call Dr

This is a guide for use where an alternative locally agreed protocol is not available. It applies to the use of a fast-acting insulin such as Actrapid®. Blood sugar test to be done hourly when on sliding scale. Adjust insulin dose according to blood sugar.

Patients with hypertension

- Continue antihypertensives (including day of surgery); consider postponing elective surgery if BP *consistently* high, e.g. >180/110mmHg. Acute lowering of BP is risky and should be avoided.

Patients with IHD

- Continue usual anti-anginal medication, and ensure their usual *prn* medication (e.g. sublingual glyceryl trinitrate (GTN)) is available in theatre; postpone surgery if unstable angina or within 3mo of MI or coronary angioplasty.

Patients with valvular heart disease

- Antibiotic prophylaxis is not required for intraocular procedures.

Patients on antiplatelet agents and anticoagulants

- Patients on aspirin/clopidogrel/dipyridamole/warfarin:
  - For cataract surgery, these drugs should be continued, as risk of stopping drugs outweighs the risk of haemorrhagic complications.
  - For complex procedures (e.g. glaucoma, vitreoretinal, oculoplastics) and combined procedures where the surgical outcome may be compromised, these drugs may need to be stopped and bridging therapy commenced in consultation with a haematologist and patient's GP/physician. **NB** If the patient has recently had a coronary stent, complex procedures with a risk of bleeding requiring cessation of drug therapy should be postponed where possible (6wk after bare metal stent; 12mo after insertion of drug-eluting stent).

- INR should ideally be checked on the day of surgery.
  - It is advisable (where possible) to have INR <3 for intraocular and strabismus surgery, <2 for orbital and oculoplastic surgery; however, the INR should be kept in the range of the therapeutic values for the original pathology (see Table 22.4). If this is not compatible with their therapeutic target and if it is deemed necessary to stop warfarin, liaise with their haematologist who may consider putting the patient on heparin (either IV or SC) in the perioperative period.
  - Although there is variation in practice, it may be advisable to avoid sharp needle blocks (i.e. peribulbar/retrobulbar) for INR >2.5 and avoid sub-Tenon's for INR >3.5.

Table 22.4 Target INR levels[*]

Prophylaxis of DVT	INR 2.0–2.5
Deep vein thrombosis (DVT) or pulmonary embolism (PE) treatment	INR 2.5
AF	
Cardioversion	
Dilated cardiomyopathy	
Mural thrombus	
Symptomatic inherited thrombophilia	
Paroxysmal nocturnal haemoglobinuria	
Recurrent DVT or PE	INR 3.5
Mechanical heart valve[†]	

[*] See *BNF* and British Society for Haematology recommendations: Guidelines on oral anticoagulation (warfarin): third edition—2005 update. *Br J Haematol* 2005;**132**:277–85.

[†] Some variation in target INR (usually 3–3.5) according to type and location of the valve.

Patients on dialysis

- These patients should have their haematology, blood biochemistry, and haemodynamic status optimized prior to surgery. Protect any AV fistula sites.

Patients with pacemakers or implantable cardioverter-defibrillators (ICDs)

- Will need consultation with cardiologists to identify the model and any specific features. These devices may need to be reprogrammed to prevent perioperative malfunction.

Ocular anaesthesia (1)

Each year, over 250,000 intraocular operations are performed in the UK. During the 1990s, there was a dramatic shift from general to local anaesthesia for the majority of cataract surgery and, more recently, a further shift towards topical anaesthesia. Currently, a similar shift in practice is being seen from general to local anaesthesia for vitreoretinal surgery.

Topical anaesthesia

Indications

If being used for intraocular procedures, topical anaesthesia requires a cooperative patient + experienced surgeon + routine suitable operation (usually cataract surgery).

Method

- Repeated preoperative ± intraoperative anaesthetic drop (e.g. oxybuprocaine 0.4% or proxymetacaine 0.5%)
- For cataract surgery, consider supplementing with intracameral lidocaine (1% isotonic preservative-free) and an anaesthetic-soaked sponge in the inferior fornix (e.g. oxybuprocaine 0.4%).

Complications

Anxiety, pain, eye movement, epithelial toxicity; in an uncooperative patient, surgery may be hazardous, increasing risk of operative complications.

Sub-Tenon's block

Indications

Useful where complete anaesthesia of the globe and akinesia are desired, but the patient is unsuitable for sharp needle blocks (blepharospasm, high myopes, known staphylomas, unknown biometry, deep-set enophthalmic eye, scleral explants, epicanthal folds, INR >2.5, patient unable to maintain 1° gaze). The patient must be sufficiently cooperative to keep head still during block and surgery.

Method

- Establish baseline monitoring (ECG, non-invasive BP (NIBP), SpO$_2$) and venous access.
- Topical anaesthetic to conjunctiva (e.g. oxybuprocaine 0.4% or proxymetacaine 0.5%).
- Observe aseptic precautions.
- Ask patient to look in opposite direction to intended injection site (e.g. superotemporally).
- Open conjunctiva in the inferonasal quadrant around 7–8mm from the limbus; dissect down to bare sclera with blunt curved scissors; insert sub-Tenon's cannula (19G, 25mm, blunt, curved), and slide posteriorly along the globe to reach the equator. Avoid deep posterior placement of the cannula.
- Inject 3–5mL of plain lidocaine 2% for short procedures (or 6–7mL plain levobupivacaine 0.75%) for longer ones. Hyaluronidase 15U/mL improves the quality and speed of onset of the block. Avoid vasopressors in the injectate.
- Apply oculocompression (no more than 30–40mmHg) for 5min (take care in patients with known high IOP/vulnerable optic discs).

Complications

Failure (wide track may lead to backflow; double-perforated conjunctiva may result in leakage), conjunctival chemosis, subconjunctival haemorrhage, vortex vein injury, raised IOP, globe trauma (increased risk with staphyloma, scleral scars, redo retinal surgery, operator's inexperience), EOM damage, retrobulbar haemorrhage. Deep posterior dissection/injections run the risk of central spread of local anaesthetic.

If the inferonasal approach is not accessible, in *experienced hands*, the sub-Tenon's space can be approached from the inferotemporal or super-otemporal quadrant. These approaches carry higher risks of complications.

Ocular anaesthesia (2)

Peribulbar block

Indications

Relatively complete anaesthesia of the globe and akinesia desired; patient sufficiently cooperative to keep the eye and head still during injection and surgery; anaesthetist/surgeon trained in the technique.

Method

The injection is made in the extraconal space. A single medial canthal injection is adequate in experienced hands.

The traditional dual injection technique consisted of making an inferolateral and a medial injection. The disadvantages of this are: (1) the first injection may induce globe shift, increasing the risk of perforation by the second injection; and (2) inferolateral injections are more hazardous, as the technique involves the needle being directed parallel to the floor of the orbit and then posteromedially towards the globe. This poses a risk of penetrating injury, particularly in axial myopes due to globe size and staphylomas (usually posterior pole/posteroinferiorly). Superomedial, superior, superolateral approaches are risky and should not be used.

Medial compartment block

- Establish baseline monitoring (ECG, NIBP, SpO_2) and venous access.
- Topical anaesthetic to conjunctiva (e.g. oxybuprocaine 0.4% or proxymetacaine 0.5%).
- Povidone iodine (5% aqueous solution) preparation of the periorbital skin and the conjunctival sac.
- Ask patient to fix on a target directly ahead in the primary gaze.
- A 25mm, 25G, sharp bevel needle is inserted at the medial canthus, with bevel facing the globe and advanced directly posteriorly in the medial compartment until the hub is at level with the plane of iris. Avoid contact with bones of the medial wall. Apart from being extremely painful there is a risk that delicate lamina papyracea may be perforated.
- Following negative aspiration, inject a total of 6–10mL mixture of 0.75% levobupivacaine and 2% lidocaine with hyaluronidase 15IU/mL. Gentle ptosis of the upper lid is a good sign. Maintain the globe in the primary gaze until needle is withdrawn. Avoid tethering tests which require patients to move eyes whilst the needle is *in situ* (risk of globe/optic nerve injury).
- Following injection, apply ocular compression (30–40mmHg with Honan balloon) for 5min.

NB Globe displacement during needle insertion, excessive pain, chemosis during early phase of injection, trickle of fluid into nasopharynx are warning signs of needle misplacement.

Complications

These can be sight- or life-threatening. Excessive positive pressure (surgery may become hazardous), ptosis, diplopia, globe perforation (<0.1%, but 0.7% if axial length >26mm if using inferolateral routes), oculocardiac reflex (0.03%), expulsive retrobulbar haemorrhage, medial orbital wall puncture, optic nerve injury, systemic neurological complications, acute ischaemic optic neuropathy, amaurosis fugax.

Immediate management of complications

- *Globe puncture*: suspect if loss of red reflex, hypotony, loss of vision, haemorrhage into anterior/posterior chamber. **NB** Avoid oculocompression, defer surgery, and refer to VR surgeons immediately.
- *Retrobulbar haemorrhage*: may require IOP reduction and urgent canthotomy.
- *Systemic neurological complications/anaphylaxis/local anaesthetic toxicity*: require immediate life-supporting treatment (see ➲ Basic and advanced life support, p. 940).

Retrobulbar intraconal block

Retrobulbar intraconal blocks are no longer used in modern practice due to high incidence of local and systemic complications.

Ocular anaesthesia (3)

General anaesthesia

Indications

Complete akinesia and deep anaesthesia required; patient unlikely to keep still (mental impairment, children/young adult, very anxious, uncontrolled tremor) or previous adverse reaction to local anaesthetic; globe trauma contraindicating local anaesthesia; bilateral surgery.

Method

The patient must be adequately fasted (e.g. 6h after solids, 4h after clear fluids; see ➲ Fasting, p. 925) and all appropriate investigations performed (e.g. FBC, U+E, ECG where indicated). GA requires preoperative assessment (to identify and, if possible, minimize anaesthetic risk factors), premedication (sedation, amnesia, anti-emesis), induction, intubation, maintenance, recovery, and post-operative analgesia. Adequate monitoring of the vital signs will be needed throughout.

Effect on IOP (See Box 22.2)

Box 22.2 **General anaesthesia and IOP**

Cause	Effect on IOP
Propofol	↓
Ketamine	Usually ↑ (dose-dependent)
Depolarizing neuromuscular-blocking agents (e.g. suxamethonium)	↑
Non-depolarizing neuromuscular-blocking agents (e.g. vecuronium, rocuronium)	No effect
Volatile anaesthetic agents	↓
Airway manipulation (e.g. laryngoscopy, intubation, laryngeal mask airway (LMA) insertion, extubation)	↑
Coughing/straining, venous congestion/head-down posture	↑
Positive end-expiratory pressure (PEEP) ventilation	↑
Systemic hypotension	↓
Hypoventilation/hypercarbia/hypoxia	↑
Hyperventilation/hypocarbia	↓
Nitrous oxide in presence of intraocular gas (**NB** should be avoided)	↑

Complications

Complications may arise due to patient, drug, equipment, or operator-related factors. The comorbidities of the patients have important bearing on the physiological responses during GA. Emergency surgery carries risk of aspiration of gastric contents. The airway management problems may lead to hypoxia, hypercarbia, and other metabolic disturbances. Anaphylaxis and malignant hyperthermia are noteworthy drug-related issues. Patient awareness during anaesthesia is fortunately a rare phenomenon.

Treatment of anaphylaxis

Anaphylaxis is most commonly encountered by the ophthalmologist during fluorescein angiography (see ➲ Fundus fluorescein angiography (FFA), p. 64). It is an extreme form of type I hypersensitivity reaction. Severe anaphylaxis occurs in 1 out of every 1,900 FFAs. Fatal anaphylaxis occurs in 1 out of every 220,000 FFAs. Although rare, anaphylaxis is not unknown during ophthalmic anaesthesia. Full description is beyond the scope of this chapter; the following is a brief reminder. Local anaesthetics, including topical drops, ocular disinfectants, e.g. chlorhexidine, antibiotics, hyaluronidase, and mydriatic and miotic eye drops may all provoke anaphylaxis.

Clinical features

- Skin and mucocutaneous symptoms include itching, flushing, urticaria, and swelling of conjunctiva, lips, and tongue. Respiratory features consist of hoarseness, stridor, wheeze, cough, severe bronchospasm, and hypoxia. Cardiovascular signs involve arrhythmia, hypotension, and ultimately cardiac arrest.

Management

- *Immediate*: remove allergen; call for help; ensure adequate oxygenation; provide cardiovascular support with IV fluids, vasoactive drugs, and monitoring.
- *Specific therapy involves*:
  - *Drugs*: IM (0.5mL of 1:1,000) or IV (0.5mL of 1:10,000) adrenaline is repeated every 5min until an adequate response is achieved; IV chlorphenamine (10mg); IV hydrocortisone (200mg).
  - *Fluid challenges*: 500mL of crystalloid; repeated, as required.
  - *Tracheal intubation/ventilation*: if required.
- *Late management*: includes referral to a specialist in allergy as well as advice and training in the use of self-injectors. In elderly patient, adrenaline may lead to myocardial ischaemia and other adverse cardiac effects. Caution is required. **NB** Patients on systemic or topical β-blockers may be resistant to treatment.

Hypoglycaemia

Hypoglycaemia is potentially fatal if left untreated. The causes are usually due to excessive utilization or underproduction of glucose. These include hepatic or adrenocortical insufficiency, excessive insulin and sulfonylurea activity, prolonged fasting, and excessive alcohol ingestion.

Clinical features

Clinical features usually appear at blood sugar levels below 2–3mmol/L.
- Range from confusion, restlessness, sweating, pallor, tachycardia, difficulty in speech, diplopia, convulsions, and coma.

NB In the absence of blood sugar levels, hyperglycaemic coma may be indistinguishable from hypoglycaemia. If in doubt, do not delay treatment with dextrose. It will do little harm in hyperglycaemia and be potentially lifesaving in hypoglycaemia.

Treatment (See Fig. 22.1)

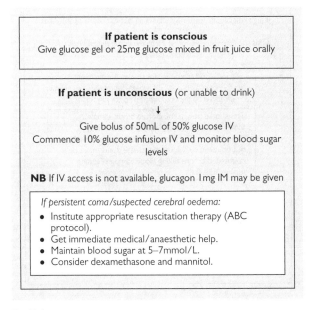

If patient is conscious
Give glucose gel or 25mg glucose mixed in fruit juice orally

If patient is unconscious (or unable to drink)
↓
Give bolus of 50mL of 50% glucose IV
Commence 10% glucose infusion IV and monitor blood sugar levels

NB If IV access is not available, glucagon 1mg IM may be given

If persistent coma/suspected cerebral oedema:
- Institute appropriate resuscitation therapy (ABC protocol).
- Get immediate medical/anaesthetic help.
- Maintain blood sugar at 5–7mmol/L.
- Consider dexamethasone and mannitol.

Fig. 22.1 Management of hypoglycaemia.

Needle-stick injuries

Needle-stick injuries are avoidable. Adopt safe practices for handling sharps, including safe disposal. Needle-stick transmission rates from infected patients are estimated at around 0.5% for HIV, 10–15% for hepatitis C, and 20% for hepatitis B (see Fig. 22.2 and Box 22.3).

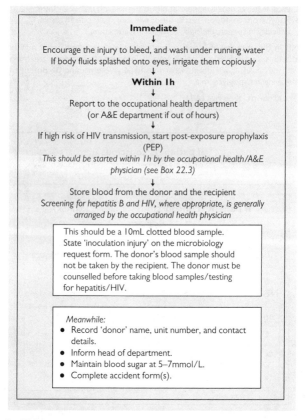

Fig. 22.2 Management of needle-stick injury.

Box 22.3 PEP where exposure to HIV*

The occupational health/A&E physician will assess risk of HIV transmission, based on patient history, nature of body fluid, and route of transmission. The decision of whether to start PEP is made according to risk. The following is common practice but should be confirmed with local occupational health department (for most recent guidelines).

High risk

This includes exposure to blood/high-risk body fluids (from a patient with known/suspected HIV) through sharps injury.
- PEP drugs starting within 1h (e.g. Truvada® (tenofovir disoproxil 245mg/emtricitabine 200mg) one tablet 1×/d; Kaletra® (lopinavir 200mg/ritonavir 50mg) two tablets 2×/d).

If donor is HIV +ve (already known or discovered on testing)
- Continue PEP for 4wk.
- Test recipient for HIV seroconversion at 6wk, 3mo, and 6mo.
- Follow-up with occupational health.

If donor is found to be HIV −ve
- Discontinue PEP.
- Test recipient for HIV seroconversion at 3mo and 6mo.
- Follow-up with occupational health.

Low risk

This applies to non-bloodstained low-risk material.
- PEP is not offered.

* Department of Health. *HIV post-exposure prophylaxis: guidance from the UK Chief Medical Officers' Expert Advisory Group on AIDS (EAGA)*. (2012). Available at: ℞ https://www.gov.uk/government/news/hiv-post-exposure-prophylaxis-guidance-from-the-uk-chief-medical-officers-expert-advisory-group-on-aids

Management of severe local anaesthetic toxicity

Local anaesthesia administration may rarely cause severe toxicity. The warning signs include tinnitus, perioral tingling, muscle twitching, and arrhythmias. This may be followed by loss of consciousness, convulsions, and cardiovascular collapse. Recovery may take up to an hour.

Treatment

See Fig. 22.3 and Fig. 22.4.

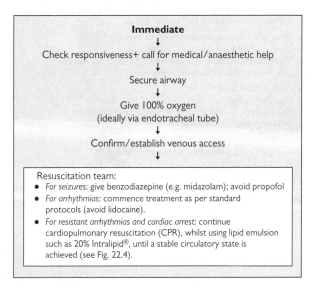

Immediate
↓
Check responsiveness+ call for medical/anaesthetic help
↓
Secure airway
↓
Give 100% oxygen
(ideally via endotracheal tube)
↓
Confirm/establish venous access
↓

Resuscitation team:
- *For seizures*: give benzodiazepine (e.g. midazolam); avoid propofol
- *For arrhythmias*: commence treatment as per standard protocols (avoid lidocaine).
- *For resistant arrhythmias and cardiac arrest*: continue cardiopulmonary resuscitation (CPR), whilst using lipid emulsion such as 20% Intralipid®, until a stable circulatory state is achieved (see Fig. 22.4).

Fig. 22.3 Recommendations for management of severe local anaesthetic toxicity. (See also The Association of Anaesthetists of Great Britain and Ireland Safety Guideline. *Management of severe local anaesthetic toxicity*. (2010). Available at: ℅ http://www.aagbi.org/sites/default/files/la_toxicity_2010_0.pdf)

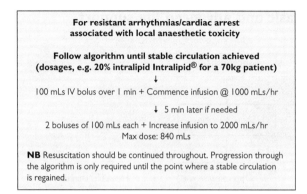

Fig. 22.4 Summary of the use of Intralipid® in severe local anaesthetic toxicity. (The Association of Anaesthetists of Great Britain and Ireland Safety Guideline. *Management of severe local anaesthetic toxicity.* (2010). Available at: ℘ http://www. aagbi.org/sites/default/files/la_toxicity_2010_0.pdf)

Basic and advanced life support

Adult basic life support algorithm

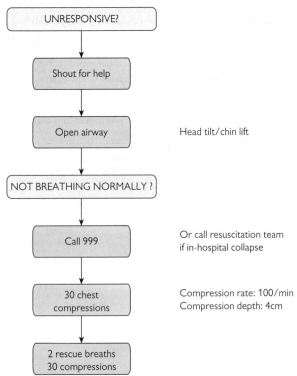

UNRESPONSIVE?

↓

Shout for help

↓

Open airway — Head tilt/chin lift

↓

NOT BREATHING NORMALLY ?

↓

Call 999 — Or call resuscitation team if in-hospital collapse

↓

30 chest compressions — Compression rate: 100/min Compression depth: 4cm

↓

2 rescue breaths 30 compressions

Fig. 22.5 Adult basic life support algorithm. Reproduced from the Resuscitation Guidelines 2010 published by Resuscitation Council (UK); reproduced by kind permission ॐ http://www.resus.org.uk/pages/blsalgo.pdf

Basic life support and in-hospital collapse

The Resuscitation Council (UK) now includes a separate protocol for in-hospital collapse (available at: ॐ http://www.resus.org.uk/pages/inhralgo.pdf) which assumes the rapid availability of resuscitation equipment which is not always immediately available in the ophthalmology setting. The basic life support algorithm (see Fig. 22.5) for out-of-hospital arrest probably more accurately reflects the situation faced by the ophthalmologist when confronted with a collapsed patient in an outlying medical retina clinic, late on a Friday evening (see Fig. 22.5 and Fig. 22.6).

Adult advanced life support algorithm

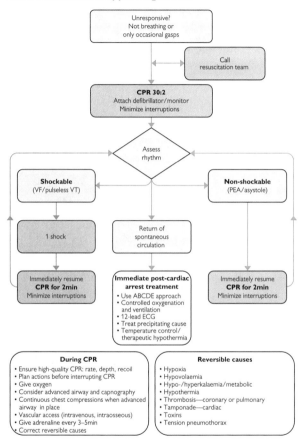

Fig. 22.6 Adult advanced life support algorithm. Reproduced from the Resuscitation Guidelines 2010 published by Resuscitation Council UK, reproduced by kind permission; ℜ http://www.resus.org.uk/pages/alsalgo.pdf

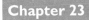

Ophthalmic
surgery: theatre notes

Sterilization services

Sterilization is the process of complete destruction or removal of all microorganisms (bacterial, viral, fungal, spores) from an object or culture medium. No method of sterilization is 100% effective. The sterility assurance level (SAL) is the probability of a single viable organism being present on a unit after sterilization. For an effective sterilization process, the SAL should be very low, e.g. 'one in a million'. Tests to ensure that adequate sterilization has occurred must be carried out routinely. Meticulous cleaning should take place prior to sterilization, as the presence of organic debris reduces its efficacy. The following is a practical interpretation of the recommendations from the Centers for Disease Control and Prevention (CDC)[1] (see Table 23.1 and Box 23.1).

Steam sterilization (autoclave)

This is the most widely used and dependable, as it is non-toxic, inexpensive, rapidly microbicidal, and sporicidal. There are two main operating systems:

- *Gravity displacement autoclave:* steam enters through the top and sides and is lighter than air, which is displaced from the bottom.
- *Pre-vacuum autoclave:* air is removed from the chamber before steam enters; the reduction in trapped air leads to increased efficiency.
- Each object must be exposed to the correct steam *temperature* and *pressure* for the correct amount of *time*. Time at which denaturation occurs is inversely proportional to the amount of water present. At constant temperatures, sterilization times vary, depending on the type of item (wrapped vs unwrapped, metal vs rubber, presence of lumens) and type of sterilizer.

Dry heat sterilization

This can be in the form of either static air or forced air type, which circulates air through the chambers at high velocity, permitting more rapid transfer of heat to instruments. It must only be used for materials that will be damaged by, or are impenetrable to, moist heat, e.g. powders, petroleum, and sharp instruments. Its main disadvantage is that it is slower than steam sterilization.

Ethylene oxide

This colourless gas, which is both inflammable and explosive, is most commonly used for sterilization of temperature- and moisture-sensitive medical devices. Its mechanism of action is through alkylation of DNA and RNA proteins; as such, it both inactivates all microorganisms and is a known human carcinogen. The four essential sterilization parameters are: *gas concentration, temperature, relative humidity*, and *exposure time*.

Ionizing radiation

Low temperature sterilization can be achieved with cobalt-60 γ-rays or electron acceleration. Cost and safety restrictions mean that this technique is generally used industrially, rather than in the health care setting.

Table 23.1 Common parameters for sterilization of surgical instruments

Steam sterilization	Recognized minimum exposure periods for sterilization of wrapped health care supplies are 30min at 121°C (250°F) in a gravity displacement sterilizer or 4min at 132°C (270°F) in a pre-vacuum sterilizer
Heat sterilization	170°C (340°F) for 60min, 160°C (320°F) for 120min, and 150°C (300°F) for 150min
Ethylene oxide	Gas concentration (450–1,200mg/L), temperature (37–63°C), relative humidity (40–80%), and exposure time (1–6h). Within certain limitations, an increase in gas concentration and temperature may shorten sterilization time

Box 23.1 Special considerations for transmissible spongiform encephalitis (TSE)

Prion infectivity is strongly stabilized by drying or fixation with alcohol, formalin, or glutaraldehyde. Contaminated instruments should be kept wet. Boiling, dry heat, radiation, and ethylene oxide are all ineffective in TSE sterilization. Autoclaving at 121°C for 15min may be partially effective.[*] NICE guidelines state that operations involving the vitreous, retina, or optic nerve are high-risk procedures. As such, instrument migration between sets should be eliminated. Supplementary instruments should be either single use or, if reusable, should remain part of the set to which they have been introduced.[†]

[*] World Health Organization. *WHO infection control guidelines for transmissible spongiform encephalopathies. Report of a WHO consultation.* (1999). Geneva: Switzerland. Available at: ℗ http://www.who.int/csr/resources/publications/bse/whocdscsraph2003.pdf

[†] National Institute for Health and Clinical Excellence. *NICE interventional procedure guidance 196. Patient safety and reduction of risk of transmission of Creutzfeldt–Jakob disease (CJD) via interventional procedures.* (2006). Available at: ℗ http://www.nice.org.uk/nicemedia/pdf/ip/IPG196guidance.pdf

Cleaning of tonometer heads

The CDC recommends that tonometer heads should be *wiped clean, disinfected for 5–10min* with either 5,000ppm chlorine or 70% ethyl alcohol, and then *rinsed thoroughly* under tap water before being allowed to *air-dry*. Wiping the tonometer head with 70% isopropyl alcohol does not provide adequate adenoviral disinfection. Disposable tonometer heads may provide a useful alternative.

1. Centers for Disease Control and Prevention. *Guideline for disinfection and sterilization in healthcare facilities.* (2008). Available at: ℗ http://www.cdc.gov/hicpac/pdf/guidelines/Disinfection_Nov_2008.pdf

Hand hygiene

Alcohol-based antiseptics

Alcohols in concentrations of 60–80% are most effective. Higher concentrations are less so, because proteins are not denatured easily in the absence of water. Alcohol-based hand rubs are very effective against Gram-positive and Gram-negative bacteria, *M. tuberculosis*, and a variety of fungi. They have little activity against bacterial spores or protozoal oocysts. They have poor activity against some non-enveloped viruses. HSV, HIV, and influenza are susceptible.

Iodophores

An iodophore is a combination of iodine and a solubilizing agent or carrier, resulting in a complex that releases small amounts of free iodine in aqueous solution (e.g. povidone iodine). Iodine quickly penetrates the cell walls of organisms and disrupts protein and nucleic acid synthesis, leading to cell death. Dilution increases bactericidal activity, possibly through weakening the linkage to the carrier polymer, which increases the concentration of free iodine in solution. Iodophores must therefore be diluted to the manufacturer's recommendation. It is recommended that 5% povidone iodine aqueous solution should be irrigated into the conjunctival sac immediately prior to cataract surgery.[2]

Chlorhexidine

Chlorhexidine is a cationic biguanide developed in the UK. It has good activity against Gram-positive bacteria, less activity against Gram-negatives, and no activity against mycobacteria. It is effective against enveloped viruses (CMV, HSV, HIV) but less so against non-enveloped viruses such as adenovirus. Chlorhexidine 4% hand scrub has been shown to be significantly more effective in reducing bacterial count than povidone iodine (7.5%) scrub agent. It has also been reported to have significantly more residual activity.[3] Chlorhexidine should not be used in the conjunctival sac, as it causes corneal toxicity.

2. Royal College of Ophthalmologists. *Cataract surgery guidelines*. (2010). Available at: ℘ http://www.rcophth.ac.uk/page.asp?section=451&sectionTitle=Clinical+Guidelines

3. World Health Organization. *WHO guidelines on hand yygiene in health care*. (2009). Available at: ℘ http://whqlibdoc.who.int/publications/2009/9789241597906_eng.pdf

Suture materials and needle types

Needle types

Needles vary with respect to wire diameter, wire length, radius of curvature, and type of curvature (half circle, quarter circle). The needle tip determines its tissue-cutting characteristics (Fig. 23.1). Most needles are round at the point of suture attachment and become square more anteriorly. Greatest stability is achieved with the needle holder at the junction between the anterior 2/3 and the posterior 1/3 of the needle.

Needle tip	Design	Use
Spatulate	▽	Flattened cutting profile; cutting edges on the sides so maintains its plane of cleavage and displaces tissue above and below the needle; valuable in suturing sclera
Tapered spatulate	▽	Body of needle is tapered behind the cutting head, allowing easy knot rotation; valuable in suturing cornea
Reverse cutting	▽	Triangular needle with cutting edge on outside of curve. NB: take care as suture track extends deep to path of needle tip
Cutting	△	Triangular needle with cutting edge on inside of curve. Suture track is superficial to needle tip; may be useful in bridal sutures
Round taper point	○	Round taper point. Cuts at tip only, leaving smallest hole of all needles; useful in suturing lacrimal sac, iris repair, bridal sutures under rectus muscles

Fig. 23.1 Suture needles: tips, designs, and usage.

Suture materials

Choice of suture material depends on handling and tying characteristics, desired duration of action, tensile strength, and tolerability to tissue reaction. Suture materials can be divided broadly as follows:

- *Absorbable vs non-absorbable*: absorbable sutures give temporary wound support and are removed by either hydrolysis (synthetic material) or enzymatic degradation (natural material, e.g. silk and catgut); the former causes far less tissue reaction than the latter.
- *Monofilament vs multifilament (braided)*: monofilament sutures are less prone to harbouring microorganisms through capillary action but may weaken if kinked or bent. Multifilaments can be coated to reduce friction generated whilst passing through tissue.
- *Suture size and tensile strength*: sutures are graded according to size and tensile strength. The United States Pharmacopeia (USP) has devised a standard classification system for suture diameter that corresponds to a metric measure (see Table 23.2). Tensile strength and duration of suture survival depend on the suture material, its diameter, and the tissue environment. The duration of effective tensile strength is not the same as the length of time that residual suture material remains in the tissue. Even non-absorbable sutures may degrade over time, reducing their tensile strength (see Table 23.2 and Table 23.3).

Table 23.2 Suture sizes, as defined by USP*

USP size	12-0	11-0	10-0	9-0	8-0	7-0	6-0	5-0	4-0
Average diameter (mm)	0.001–0.009	0.010–0.019	0.020–0.029	0.030–0.039	0.040–0.049	0.050–0.069	0.070–0.099	0.100–0.149	0.150–0.199

* United States Pharmacopeia. Available at: ℅ http://www.usp.org

Table 23.3 Examples of sutures used in ophthalmology

Name	Structure	Other features	Duration	Use
Non-absorbable				
Nylon (polyamide) Ethilon®	Monofilament	High tensile strength, relatively elastic, stiff ends	Loses 10–15% of tensile strength per year	Cornea (10-0) Visual axis (11-0) Sclera (10-0) Limbus (10-0)
Polypropylene Prolene®, Ethicon®	Monofilament	High tensile strength, elastic, stiff ends	Essentially permanent	Iris repair or sutured IOL (10-0)
Polyester Mersiline®, Dacron®, Ethibond®	Braided or monofilament, coated or uncoated	Very high tensile strength. Less elastic than other monofilaments	Essentially permanent	Orbital and plastic surgery procedures
Silk	Twisted or braided, can be coated	Easy handling, soft suture, inelastic	3–6mo (remove at 10d due to tissue reaction)	Sclera (8-0) Skin, greyline, limbal bridal sutures (6-0) Lid traction (4-0)
Absorbable				
Polygalactin 910 Vicryl®	Available as braided and monofilament	High tensile strength	2–3wk	Conjunctiva (10-0) Tarsal plate (5-0) Muscles (6-0) Cornea (10-0)
Polyglycolic acid Dexon®	Braided	High tensile strength	2–3wk	Limbus (8-0) Periosteum (5-0)

Surgical instruments (1)

There are a variety of surgical instruments available, and the list is constantly expanding. Outlined here (see ➲ Surgical instruments, pp. 950, 952, 954) is a brief summary of instruments that can form part of the basic lid and intraocular operating sets, followed by some suggested instrument sets for common ophthalmic emergencies.

Forceps

Forceps can broadly be divided into toothed (for tissue handling) and smooth (for holding and tying sutures). Some have a toothed tip and a suture-tying platform, allowing combined use (see Fig. 23.2).

Instrument	Typical length	Usage	Tip	Design
Pierse	85mm	Fine tissue forceps. Flat surfaces cause less trauma to tissues	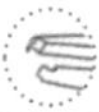	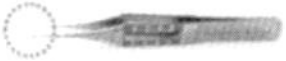
Utrata	85mm	Capsulorrhexis forceps	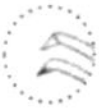	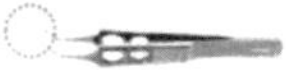
St Martins	85mm	Handling cornea	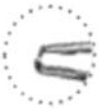	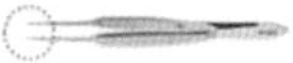
McPherson	85mm	Tying fine sutures. Can incorporate toothed tip	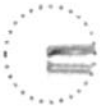	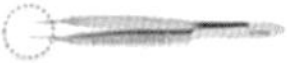
Colibri	90mm	Handling of corneal and scleral edges. May have retro-tip tying platform	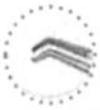	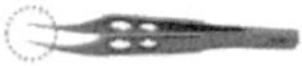
Castroviejo	100mm	Fine tissue forceps for easy grasping. May have retro-tip tying platform	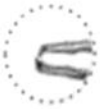	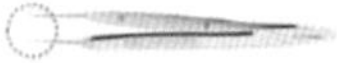
Moorfields	110mm	Serrated tip forceps for handling conjunctiva	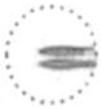	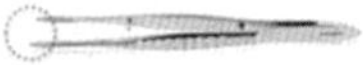
Jayles	115mm	Toothed forceps for easy grasping	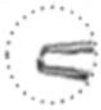	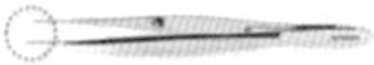
Adsons ½ teeth or serrated tips	125mm	Toothed or serrated tip for handling skin	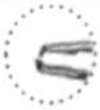 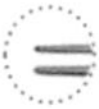	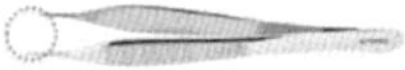

Fig. 23.2 Forceps for ophthalmic surgery.

Blades

There are a variety of blades available for both lid and intraocular surgery. The straight tip of the Bard-Parker™ 11 is ideal for stabbing mucosal incisions in chalazion surgery, whereas the rounded contour of the Bard-Parker™ 15 is more suited to cutting the skin. A keratome is used for the main corneal incision in cataract surgery but may be preceded by a groove made with a 30° (or 15°) blade or a diamond knife. These blades (and the MVR blade) may also be used for creating the smaller paracentesis. The Crescent blade can be used to promote a smooth scleral plane in trabeculectomies or corneal plane in lamellar keratoplasties (see Fig. 23.3).

Instrument	Usage	Tip	Design
Bard-Parker 11	Stabbing incisions	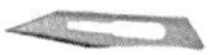	
Bard-Parker 15	Cutaneous incisions	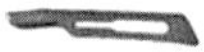	
Keratome	Corneal incision (main section)	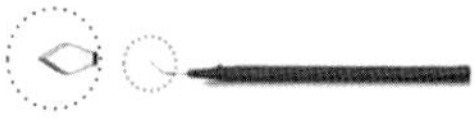	
30° blade	Corneal incision (paracentesis)	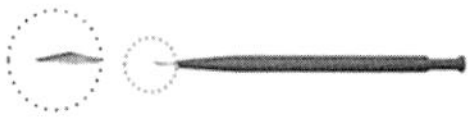	
MVR blade	Corneal or scleral incision (paracentesis, iris hooks, sclerostomies)	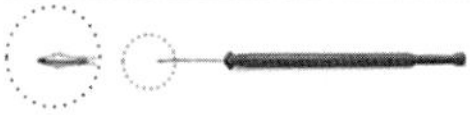	
Crescent knife	Corneal or scleral planar incision/tunnelling	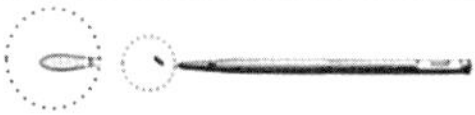	

Fig. 23.3 Blades for ophthalmic surgery.

Surgical instruments (2)

Needle holders

Needle holders are made in various sizes for handling different sutures; they may also be locking or non-locking. In addition, the Castroviejo is a flat-handled suture holder, whereas the Barraquer is round-handled which most surgeons find allows easier rotation during suturing. Locking suture holders can be 'parked', once loaded with the suture; the surgeon is also less likely to inadvertently release the suture prior to addressing the tissue (see Fig. 23.4).

Scissors

Key variables with scissors are: size, curved or straight blades, sharp or blunt/rounded tips, regular or spring-handled. Common examples are Vannas scissors for fine and intraocular use (such as peripheral iridectomy), Westcott scissors which are blunt-tipped, allowing dissection of Tenon's capsule with reduced risk of scleral perforation, and Stevens tenotomy scissors which can have either pointed or round tips (see Fig. 23.5).

Muscle hooks

Muscle hooks ('squint hooks' or 'strabismus hooks') have a number of variations to allow retrieval of muscles/tendons and their safe manipulation. The Stevens tenotomy hook has a short curved hook which gives excellent manoeuvrability; it is often used where accessibility is an issue and to facilitate the introduction of one of the larger muscle hooks. These include the standard Graefe muscle hook, the Jameson which has a kinked end with a bulbous tip to help keep the muscle on the hook, and the Chavasse which has an undulated end to help spread the muscle for manipulation (see Fig. 23.6). Unusual hooks include the Bishop hook which includes a guard to protect the globe during suturing.

Instrument	Typical length	Usage	Design
Barraquer	120mm	Suture holders (round handle, non-locking)	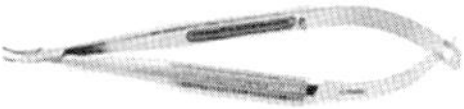
Castroviejo	140mm	Suture holders (flat handle, locking)	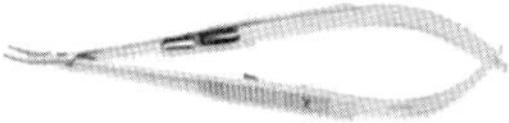

Fig. 23.4 Needle holders for ophthalmic surgery.

Instrument	Typical length	Usage	Design
Vannas	80mm	Fine scissors for intraocular procedures (e.g. iridectomy)	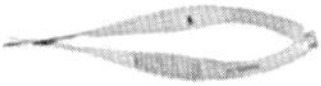
Westcott	115mm	Round-bladed scissors for tenotomy; blunt tips	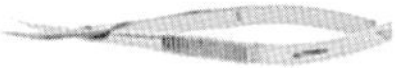
Stevens	115mm	Straight-bladed scissors for tenotomy; with pointed or blunt tips	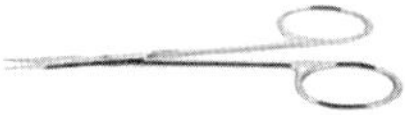

Fig. 23.5 Scissors for ophthalmic surgery.

Instrument	Usage	Design
Stevens	Tenotomy hook	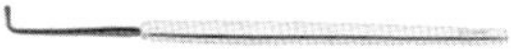
Graefe	Strabismus hook	
Jameson	Strabismus hook	
Chavasse	Strabismus hook	

Fig. 23.6 Forceps for ophthalmic surgery.

Surgical instruments (3)

Retractors and lid specula

Retractors and lid specula are necessary to provide access and good visualization of tissue. Retractors, such as the Desmarres and Blaire, are commonly used in oculoplastic procedures; chalazion clamps facilitate eversion of the lid, with the useful inclusion of a guard to protect the globe. Specula allow the surgeon to gain access to the globe without putting pressure on it. The Barraquer is the most widely used for cataract surgery; variations include adult, paediatric, and neonatal sizes, and standard vs sliding designs. A number of other speculum designs, such as the commonly used Clarke speculum, are more adjustable and provide good fixed control of lid opening; these are commonly used for strabismus surgery (see Fig. 23.7).

Miscellaneous instruments

Calipers, such as the Castroviejo calipers, are useful for taking measurements such as during squint surgery and for 'limbus to limbus' measurement in cases where an ACIOL is required.

A number of specialized instruments are exclusively used in intraocular surgery, such as the cystotome which facilitates capsulorrhexis, and a range of instruments used to manipulate the lens (or sometimes other intraocular structures) such as the Sinskey hook, the mushroom, and various 'phaco choppers'.

Instruments for the assessment and treatment of nasolacrimal problems include lacrimal probes (such as the Bowman or Liebreich lacrimal probes) and punctal dilators (such as the Nettleship dilator) (see Fig. 23.8).

Instrument	Usage	Design
Desmarres retractor	Retractor	
Blaire	Retractor	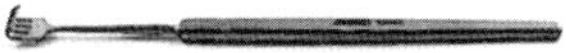
Desmarres chalazion clamp	Clamp	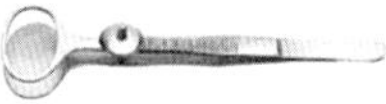
Barraquer speculum	Speculum	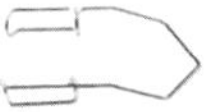
Clarke speculum (right-sided example shown)	Speculum	

Fig. 23.7 Retractors and lid specula for ophthalmic surgery.

Instrument	Usage	Design
Castroviejo Calipers	Calipers	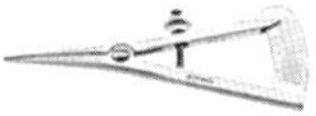
Cystotome	Capsulorrhexis	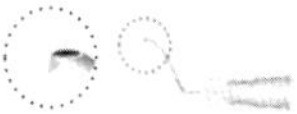
Sinsky hook	Manipulator	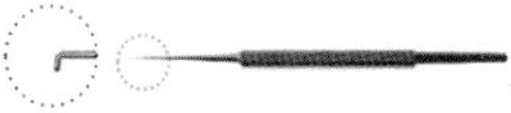
Double-ended mushroom/ phako chopper	Manipulator	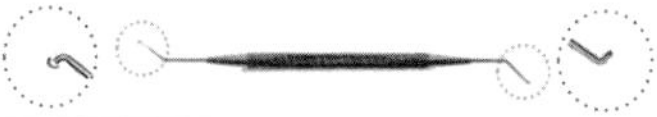
Liebreich lacrimal probe	Lacrimal probe	
Nettleship dilator	Punctal dilation	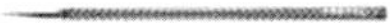

Fig. 23.8 Miscellaneous instruments for ophthalmic surgery.

Laser

Outline

Laser (light amplification of stimulated emission of radiation) is a term that describes the production of a fine beam of light with very specific properties. The properties of any given laser emission are used to produce a certain tissue reaction for a therapeutic effect. The application of this invasive procedure requires compliance with certain health and safety regulations, obtaining informed consent, and compliance with WHO surgical checklist for correct patient, site, and procedure verification. Some of the health and safety regulations will vary slightly between units and more so between countries. Those referred to in this chapter relate to UK regulations at the time of writing.

How lasers work

Subatomic particles in any given medium (in this case, a given gas, liquid, or solid) exist in a 'resting' state. The delivery of energy to the medium excites these particles momentarily to a higher energy state. Their return to the resting state is accompanied by release of energy. Collection of these small 'packets' of energy (usually referred to as photons) results in a coordinated emission that has specific physical properties. The two most important physical properties of this emission are that it is monochromatic (almost the same wavelength throughout) and coherent (its sub-waveforms almost all in the same phase).

There are three generic components required to produce a laser emission: (1) Laser medium; (2) Excitation mechanism; (3) Feedback mechanism.

Laser medium

- *Active medium*: a substance whose atoms or molecules are energized (excited) such that their electrons produce the emission.
- *Medium state*: this can be solid, liquid, or gas and gives the laser its name (e.g. argon laser).

Excitation mechanism (also called the pump)

- External source of energy required to initiate the laser emission process.
- *Types*: electrical (current passes through the active medium); optical (intense light aimed through active medium); chemical (uncommon).

Feedback mechanism

- The process by which the small amounts of released energy are collected and amplified within the machine before the laser beam is emitted.
- This mechanism relies on the use of mirrors with specific reflective properties.
- The process cascades rapidly to a point when the laser beam is finally emitted.
- This process takes place in what is sometimes called the resonance cavity of the laser machine.

Other features

- *Rates of delivery (temporal modes)*: can be continuous or pulsed. This is one of the factors determining tissue reaction and depends on various technical properties of the laser machine.
- *Delivery systems*: slit-lamp (± CL); indirect ophthalmoscope; special probes (endoprobes, cyclodiode probe); others (e.g. LASEK/LASIK).

Laser reactions

Laser emissions passing through tissue will be scattered, reflected, transmitted, or absorbed in varying proportions. Absorption or tissue reaction at a point of focus will depend on the wavelength of the emission, the properties of the different parts comprising the organ involved (the eye in this case), and the properties of the target tissue. The therapeutic effect of the laser can be divided into three broad groups. The reflection back of laser beams is the underlying principle for many of the *diagnostic* equipment that use laser. The following deals with therapeutic laser effects.

Photothermal effect

- Absorption of the laser wavelength causes an effect due to heating up of the target tissue.
- Photocoagulation occurs in retinal tissue, resulting in a scar where the laser is absorbed.
- Photovaporization (photoablation) occurs in corneal tissue during laser corneal refractive procedures.
- Photoshortening occurs in collagen cross-linking procedures.

Photochemical effect

- Here the target tissue is sensitized to a specific laser wavelength using a chemical.
- The commonest ophthalmic use had been PDT of AMD with verteporfin (see ➋ Photodynamic therapy, p. 532).

Photodisruptive effect

- Here the electromagnetic effect of the laser emission at a point of focus alters the stable state of electrons orbiting around their respective nuclei. This produces a chemical breakdown of the material, creating what is called a plasma.
- Once the light emission passes, the electrons and protons reunite, causing this plasma to collapse, creating an acoustic shock wave (audible during the procedure) which destroys the ocular tissue involved (lens capsule or iris tissue).

Clinical applications

Lasers in clinical practice have two broad applications. One is diagnostic (Box 24.1), and the other is therapeutic (Box 24.2). In addition, laser operators should familiarize themselves with the different CL used in laser treatment procedures (see Box 24.1 and Box 24.2). Alternative light-sources to laser include SuperLuminescent Diodes (SLD). A number of OCT machines use an SLD rather than a laser as their light source..

Box 24.1 **Diagnostic applications of laser***

Scanning laser ophthalmoscopy (standard SLO)
- Ophthalmoscopy.
- Fundus camera.
- Angiography (FFA and ICG).
- Psychophysical testing (e.g. microperimetry).

Scanning laser tomography (confocal SLO)
- Retinal tomography.
- Optic nerve head topography.
- Corneal topography.
- Autofluorescence.

OCT
- Anterior segment.
- Posterior segment.

* NB A number of these applications can be performed using non-laser light sources. Most fundus and fluorescein angiography cameras use a standard non-coherent light source and many of the OCT machines in wide-spread usage today use an SLD as their light source.

Box 24.2 Therapeutic applications of laser

Cornea
- Refractive.
- Therapeutic (non-refractive, e.g. Salzmann nodule removal).

Lens
- Capsulotomy.
- Femtosecond-assisted, e.g. capsulorhexis, corneal incision, LRIs, lens fragmentation.

Glaucoma
- Peripheral iridotomy.
- Trabeculoplasty (ALT; SLT).
- Iridoplasty (ALPI).
- Cyclophotocoagulation ('cyclodiode').

Retina
- Photocoagulation.
- Subthreshold macular laser.
- PDT.

Oculoplastics
- Aesthetic laser treatment.
- Therapeutic (e.g. naevus flammeus).

Laser safety in the clinic

In the UK, every hospital has a designated laser protection advisor (LPA). This is usually a medical engineer who is responsible for lasers and other radiation-emitting equipment (mainly in radiology departments) being used in accordance with health and safety laws and regulations. In addition, there are two designated laser safety officers (LSO) at the local departmental level (usually one nurse and one clinician) who are responsible for ensuring that all staff are trained in the use and safety aspects of the laser machines in the unit and that the unit laser procedures and clinics comply with health and safety requirements. The LPA, LSO, and the medical engineering department are jointly responsible for producing and updating the local laser rules.

Laser hazard classification

The commonest classification of lasers is based on power emission (see Table 24.1).

Table 24.1 Laser hazard classification (as per DIN EN 60 825-1/VDE 0837): classification of lasers by potential risks

Class 1	Accessible laser radiation is harmless; very low power (e.g. CD players)
Class 2	Safe by blinking reflex (<0.25s), only for 400–700m; low power (e.g. laser pointers)
Class 3A	Focused laser radiation is harmful when using optical aids; medium power (e.g. aiming laser)
Class 3B	Focused laser radiation is harmful to eyes and partly to skin; medium power (some ophthalmic devices)
Class 4	Also diffusely scattered laser radiation is harmful to eyes and partly to skin, possible fire or explosion hazard; high power (almost all therapeutic lasers)

Practical approaches to laser safety

- *Patient*: check the patient identification (use name, date of birth, and address); consider WHO checklist if assisted by another member of staff; consider marking the eye to be lasered; cross-check the clinical notes; consent the patient, if not already consented; record the procedure accurately and legibly; complete the laser register.
- *Laser room*: ensure the signage outside the room is working; check the machine is working before calling in the first patient; comply with policy of restricted access to laser keys; consider locking the room during laser operation; ensure any windows/reflective surfaces are covered; ensure laser emission is directed away from any doorways.

- *Laser operator*: ensure you have had induction to local safety rules and the locally available machines; report any faults in the room, signage, or equipment; complete all records and checks as previously described; be aware that you are responsible for the patient, attending relatives, and assisting staff.
- *Other factors*: observe infection control; ensure that the correct safety goggles are worn by any attending relatives, assisting staff, or trainees present; ensure the safety goggles are in a safe functional state, and report it if they are not; minimize movement into and out of the room during a given laser session.

Laser procedures in retina

PRP

Indication
- *Diabetic retinopathy*: active proliferative retinopathy, some cases of high-risk preproliferative retinopathy.
- Other ischaemic retinopathies (e.g. CRVO) with either established neovascularization or high-risk features.
- Rubeosis/NVG.

Method
- *Consent.* explain:
  - What the procedure does (aims to stop disease progression; further laser treatment may well be required).
  - What the procedure does not do (does not improve vision; is not an alternative to glycaemic control, etc.).
  - What to expect and possible complications, e.g. pain, loss of peripheral field (with driving implications), scotomas, worsened acuity (e.g. macular decompensation), choroidal or retinal detachment, decreased dark adaptation, and vitreous haemorrhage.
- *Instil topical anaesthetic* (e.g. oxybuprocaine), and position fundus CL (e.g. transequator) with coupling agent.
- *Set argon laser* for 200–500 microns spot size, 0.1s, and adjust power to produce a gently blanching burn.
  - Consider placing a temporal barrier, at least 2–3DD from fovea, to help demarcate a 'no go' zone. Then place ≥1,000 burns outside the vascular arcades, leaving burn-width intervals between them. A second session of ≥1,000 is usually performed a few weeks later.
- *Tips*: the power may need to be adjusted frequently according to variable retinal take-up. If the patient feels pain, consider reducing the duration (e.g. to 0.05s) but increasing the power to maintain burn intensity.
- *Review*: 3-weekly ± fill-in PRP until response.

Complications
- Pain, transient visual loss, permanent loss of peripheral field (with driving implications), decreased dark adaptation (i.e. effect on night vision), permanent scotomas, worsened acuity (e.g. macular decompensation or risk of direct inadvertent macular laser), choroidal or retinal detachment, vitreous haemorrhage.

Macular laser (focal or grid)

Indication

- Clinically significant macular oedema (see Table 13.4).

Method

- *Consent*: explain what the procedure does (aims to reduce sight loss; further laser treatment may well be required), what to expect, and possible complications, e.g. pain, scotomas, worsened acuity, retinal/choroidal detachment.
- *Instil topical anaesthetic* (e.g. oxybuprocaine), and position fundus CL (e.g. area centralis) with coupling agent.
- *Set argon laser* for 50–200 micron spot size, 0.08–0.1s, and adjust power to produce a very gentle blanching burn. Generally, smaller spot sizes and shorter durations are used for more central burns.
- *For focal treatment*: apply burns to leaking microaneurysms between 500 and 3000 microns from the centre of the fovea. Lesions as near as 300 microns to the fovea may be treated, provided this would not be within the foveal avascular zone.
- *For grid treatment*: place similar burns ≥1 burn-width apart in a grid arrangement around the fovea. They must be at least 500 microns from the centre of the fovea and from the disc margin.
- *Review* at 3mo or sooner.

Complications

- Pain, scotomas, worsened acuity (e.g. macular decompensation or scar 'creep'), choroidal or retinal detachment, choroidal neovascular membrane, vitreous haemorrhage.

Laser retinopexy (slit-lamp or indirect delivery systems)

Indication

- Retinal break with risk of progression to rhegmatogenous retinal detachment (usually U-tears) and without excessive subretinal fluid.
- Equatorial and post-equatorial lesions can be reached with slit-lamp delivery system; more anterior lesions require indirect laser with indentation or cryotherapy.

Method

Slit-lamp and indirect retinopexy techniques are discussed alongside Cryopexy in Vitreoretina (see ➲ Laser retinopexy and cryopexy for retinal tears, p. 502).

Laser procedures in glaucoma (1)

Nd-YAG peripheral iridotomy

Indication

- *Treatment*: angle closure with pupil block—may be acute/subacute/chronic, primary/secondary.
- *Prophylaxis*: occludable narrow angles (including fellow eye in angle closure).

Method

- *Consent*: explain what the procedure does, why you are treating both eyes, and possible complications, including failure/need for retreatment, bleeding, inflammation, corneal burns, visual effects (e.g. monocular diplopia).
- *Instil* pilocarpine 2% (tightens the iris) + apraclonidine 1% (prevents IOP spike and may reduce bleeding) + topical anaesthetic (e.g. oxybuprocaine).
- *Set laser* (varies according to model): commonly bursts of two or three pulses of 3–6mJ (greater energy required for irides which are thick and heavily pigmented); the beam should be angled (i.e. not perpendicular).
- *Position CL* (usually the Abraham lens; requires coupling agent).
- *Identify suitable iridotomy sites*: superior (hidden by the normal lid position), peripheral, and ideally in an iris crypt (less energy required).
- *Focus and fire laser*: success is indicated by a forward gush of pigment-loaded aqueous. This usually takes 2–4 shots.

Post-procedure

- Topical steroid (e.g. dexamethasone 0.1% stat, then 6×/d for 1wk).
- Perform an early post-procedure IOP check at about 30–60min post-treatment.
- Review within 10d to recheck IOP and inflammatory response.

Complications

- Bleeding (stops with maintained pressure on lens), inflammation (increase topical steroids), raised IOP, corneal burns (caution with shallow AC), glare, and optical aberrations (avoid interpalpebral iris and particularly the area of iris beneath the marginal tear strip meniscus).

ALT

Indication

- Open-angle glaucoma with pigmented trabeculum—commonly POAG/PXF glaucoma/PDS glaucoma.
- Medical and surgical options undesirable or ineffective.

Method

- *Consent*: explain what the procedure does and possible complications, including failure (short- and long-term), bleeding, and inflammation.
- Instil apraclonidine 1% + topical anaesthetic (e.g. oxybuprocaine).
- *Set laser* (varies according to model): argon—commonly 50 microns spot size, 0.1s duration, 300–1,000mW power (start low, increase, as required); diode—commonly 100 microns spot size, 0.1–0.2s duration, 800–1,200mW power.

- *Position goniolens* (anti-reflective laser lens).
- *Identify trabeculoplasty site*: aim for the anterior border of the pigmented trabecular meshwork.
- *Focus and fire laser*: the ideal reaction is a mild blanching or small bubble; the more pigmented the angle, the less power is usually required. Place 50 equally spaced shots over 180°.

Post-procedure
- All usual glaucoma medications should be continued; topical steroid (e.g. betamethasone 4×/d for 1wk) may be prescribed.
- Perform an early post-procedure IOP check (e.g. at 30–60min).
- *Review in 2–6wk*: if inadequate IOP response, consider ALT on the remaining 180°.
- Failure occurs at a rate of 6–10%/y and is often sudden. Long-term follow-up is necessary.

Complications
- Bleeding (stops with maintained pressure on lens), inflammation (usually mild), PAS, IOP spike, may increase failure rate of subsequent trabeculectomy.

SLT
Indication
- As for ALT, but more targeted and utilizes less energy.

Method
- The usual strategy is to place 50 non-overlapping spots (400 microns spot size, 3ns duration, 0.6mJ initial energy), centred on the trabecular meshwork over the inferior 180°. The power is adjusted to be 0.1mJ below the level that causes bubble formation.
- Pre- and post-procedure management is similar to ALT.

Complications
- Similar to ALT; a transient subclinical reversible corneal endotheliopathy is often seen in the early stages after SLT.

ALPI
Indication
- Plateau iris syndrome (common).
- APAC (rare).

Method
- Place a ring of argon laser burns to the most peripheral iris stroma using a CL (e.g. Abraham or Goldmann); typical applications are 20–50 burns over 360° (with ≥2 spot sizes between burns) of 200–500 microns spot size, 0.2–0.5s duration, and 200–400mW power.

Complications
- Inflammation (usually mild), IOP spike, corneal burns.

Laser procedures in glaucoma (2)

Trans-scleral diode laser cyclophotocoagulation (syn 'cyclodiode')

Indication

- Intractable ↑IOP refractory to other treatments, e.g. in rubeotic or synechial angle closure or where the patient is too systemically unwell to tolerate surgery).
- Less commonly as a temporizing measure prior to trabeculectomy while the ocular surface is being optimized.

Methods

- *Consent*: explain what the procedure does and possible complications, including failure/need for retreatment, hypotony, inflammation, bleeding, and adverse effect on vision; sympathetic ophthalmia has now also been described after diode laser cyclophotocoagulation.
- *Set laser (varies according to model)*: commonly 1,500mW power, 1,500ms duration.
- *Identify ciliary body 0.5–2mm from limbus*: transillumination helps to identify the dark ciliary body. Place the contact probe (of the diode laser) in an anteroposterior manner against the globe, adjusting its position so that the probe is directed at the ciliary body.
- *Fire laser*: 5–10 shots per quadrant; if laser burn is audible ('pop'), decrease power; avoid the 3 and 9 o'clock positions and superior quadrant (in case of possible trabeculectomy in the future).
- *To minimize the risk of overtreatment and hypotony*: reduced number of shots per treatment is recommended, e.g. 10–20 shots (1–2 quadrants). If IOP remains elevated after 6wk, retreat.

Post-procedure

- Topical steroid (e.g. dexamethasone 0.1% 4×/d for 1wk) and all usual glaucoma medication. Review in 1–2wk. Do not be tempted to stop glaucoma treatment in under 6wk.

Complications

- Anterior inflammation (may get hypopyon with NVG), hypotony, haemorrhage, scleral thinning, perforation, cataract, lens subluxation, phthisis, and sympathetic endophthalmitis.

Endodiode laser photocoagulation (syn ECP)

Indication

- As for trans-scleral cyclodiode laser; achieved endoscopically using endolaser cyclophotocoagulation of the ciliary body as an intraocular procedure.

Method

- *Consent*: explain what the procedure does and possible complications, including failure/need for retreatment, hypotony, inflammation, bleeding, endophthalmitis, and adverse effect on vision.
- The ciliary processes can be approached via a limbal or a pars plana entry. The limbal approach avoids anterior vitrectomy and the associated risks. Treatment of at least 180° of ciliary processes is required to achieve significant reductions in IOP. ECP is much easier technically if performed in a pseudophakic eye than a phakic eye. Some surgeons perform ECP as a combined procedure after phacoemulsification of cataract.
- Pupil dilatation with cyclopentolate 1% and phenylephrine 2.5%.
- *Set laser*: 60–90mW power; duration—continuous.
- AC is filled with viscoelastic agent, which is further used to expand the nasal posterior sulcus to allow easier approach to the pars plicata with the ECP probe.
- The probe images the outside of the eye, before being inserted into the AC and the posterior sulcus.
- Apply laser to each process until shrinkage and whitening occur. Only the raised processes are treated, without affecting the 'valleys' between processes.
- If excessive energy is used, the process explodes (or 'pops') with bubble formation, leading to excessive inflammation and breakdown of the blood–aqueous barrier.
- Treat 180–270° of ciliary processes.

Post-procedure

- Topical antibiotics, topical steroid (e.g. dexamethasone 0.1% 4×/d for 1wk) and all usual glaucoma medication. Some surgeons avoid prostaglandin analogues to minimize exacerbation of intraocular inflammation. Stat dose of oral acetazolamide is used to prevent IOP spike. Review next day and 1wk.

Complications

- Inflammation, CMO, cataract (if phakic), endophthalmitis, suprachoroidal haemorrhage, retinal detachment, hypotony, phthisis.

Laser procedures in lens/cataract

Nd-YAG posterior capsulotomy

Indication
- Visually significant PCO.

Method
- *Consent*: explain what the procedure does and possible complications, including failure/need for retreatment, lens damage with visual consequences (pitting, dislocation), floaters, retinal damage (including detachment), ↑IOP, loss of vision.
- *Caution*: check for the presence of coexisting ocular diseases such as uveitis, glaucoma, macular oedema, high-risk retinal degeneration which would make this a higher-risk procedure and might necessitate additional post-procedural therapy/care.
- *Instil mydriatics* (e.g. tropicamide 1% ± phenylephrine 2.5%).
- *Set laser (varies according to model)*: commonly 1–1.5mJ (greater energy required for thicker PCO); the beam should be angled (i.e. not perpendicular).
- *Position CL* (capsulotomy lens; requires coupling agent).
- *Focus and fire laser*: techniques include:
  - Full ring of peripheral shots (effectively a posterior capsulorhexis which leaves the detached capsule free-floating in the vitreous.
  - Partial ring leaving an inferior portion attached (acts as a hinge so that the detached capsule drops out of the visual plane but is not freely mobile).
  - A cross-shaped approach (start in the periphery in each axis).

Post-procedure
- Topical steroid (e.g. dexamethasone 0.1% stat, then 4×/d for 2wk).
- Review in 4–6wk to check visual axis clear and no significant inflammation or other sequelae.

Complications
- Lens damage (pitting, dislocation), inflammation (usually mild but can be severe in uveitic patients), floaters, retinal damage (including tear, detachment), corneal oedema, ↑IOP, CMO, failure/need for retreatment.

Laser-assisted cataract and refractive surgery procedures

Within cataract surgery, FSLs are now being used by some operators to facilitate the following stages: clear corneal incisions, LRIs, capsulorhexis, and lens fragmentation (see ➋ Applications of FSL, p. 320).

Within refractive and other corneal surgery, FSLs can be used for precise separation of tissues such as creating flaps for LASIK, for creating channels in the cornea for ICRS, and for cutting corneas for lamellar and penetrating keratoplasties. The excimer laser is used for ablative reshaping of the cornea which is the basis of PRK, LASIK, and LASEK (see Chapter 19).

Chapter 25

Therapeutics

Principles and delivery of ocular drugs

All doses/frequencies of administration are those for a healthy adult. All medications should be checked against the *BNF*, or equivalent, for licensed indications, side effects, contraindications, interactions, and age- and weight-adjusted dosing.

When considering patients' medication, it is important to check what they are actually taking, rather than what you or anybody else think they are taking. Consider the issue of compliance, particularly when about to treat a suboptimal response with additional medications or more frequent regimens. For more invasive procedures (e.g. injections), formal consent should be taken.

Topical

Only around 1–10% of most topical agents are absorbed into the eye. Absorption is dependent on ocular contact time, drug concentration, and tissue permeability. Small lipophilic drugs pass through the cornea, whereas larger hydrophilic drugs are generally absorbed through conjunctiva and sclera. Topical agents may be in:

- *Aqueous solution* (comfortable, no blurring but very short ocular contact time).
- *Gel preparations* (mild blurring, longer contact time).
- *Suspension* (longer ocular contact time, but bottle must be shaken and may get FB sensation).
- *Ointment* (liquefy at body temperature, longest ocular contact time, but blurs vision).

Technique

- Ensure that patients know how to instil any topical medication and that they can physically manage it.
- If reliable self-administration is not possible, ensure that there is somebody (even a district nurse) who can assist them.
- Consider ways of making it easier, e.g. lying flat, mirror positioning, or eye drop dispensers. Smaller bottles and single use vials tend to be particularly difficult for the frail and elderly.
- Leave at least 5min between instilling topical medications.
- Keep the eye closed, and put pressure over the lacrimal sac for 1–2min to try to increase ocular, and reduce systemic, absorption.

Medications

This includes most ophthalmic medication listed in Tables 25.1–25.6.

Subconjunctival injection

Technique

- Ensure adequate anaesthesia (e.g. a couple of drops of proxymetacaine 0.5%).
- Under direct vision (or slit-lamp or operating microscope), lift an area of conjunctiva to form a small bleb, and slowly inject (sharp needle).

Medications

This route is most commonly used for post-operative injections of corticosteroids and antimicrobials but may be used in acute anterior segment inflammation to deliver mydriatics and corticosteroids (e.g. Mydricaine No. 2 with betamethasone 2–4mg).

Mydricaine No. 1 and No. 2

Mydricaine preparations are used to cause mydriasis and cycloplegia in severe anterior segment inflammation. Mydricaine No. 1 is for children, and Mydricaine No. 2 (which is double strength) is for adults (see Table 25.1).

Table 25.1 Subconjunctival mydriatic preparations

Drug	Dose	Active ingredients
Mydricaine No. 1	0.3mL	3mg procaine hydrochloride, 0.5mg atropine sulfate, and 0.06mL adrenaline solution (1 in 1,000)
Mydricaine No. 2	0.3mL	6mg procaine hydrochloride, 1mg atropine sulfate, and 0.12mL adrenaline solution (1 in 1,000)

These preparations are not commercially available but may be obtained from Special Order Manufacturers (SOM; see *BNF* for list).

Other routes of delivery

Other routes of delivering ophthalmic drugs include: intraocular (see ➲ Intracameral injections, p. 974; ➲ Intravitreal injections, p. 978), periocular (see ➲ Sub-Tenon's and peribulbar injections, p. 976), and systemic (mainly PO, IV, and IM).

Intracameral injections

Intracameral administration of drugs (i.e. into the AC) may be used during an operation, either to facilitate the procedure itself or to reduce post-operative complications. Such drugs may be specifically injected, using a blunt cannula via a paracentesis port, or may be added to the irrigation bottle (e.g. for phacoemulsification surgery; unlicensed use) (see Table 25.2).

Table 25.2 Intracameral preparations

Drug	Dose	Administration	Proprietary
*Anaesthetic**			
Lidocaine 1%	0.3–0.5mL	Intracameral bolus	
Mydriatics†			
Adrenaline	1 in 1,000,000	In irrigation bottle, e.g. 0.5mL of 1 in 1,000 adrenaline added to 500mL of irrigation solution	
Phenylephrine 2.5%†	0.25mL in 1mL BSS	Intracameral bolus	
Miotics			
Acetylcholine 1%	1–2mL	Intracameral bolus	Miochol-E®
Antibiotics			
Cefuroxime	1mg/0.1mL	Intracameral bolus	Aprokam®
Corticosteroids			
Triamcinolone acetonide‡	4mg/0.1mL	Intracameral bolus	Kenalog®

With the exception of Miochol-E® and Aprokam®, these drugs are not licensed for intracameral use.

* Lidocaine also has mydriatic properties.

† Gurbaxani *et al.* (*Eye* 2007;**21**:331–2) describe 0.25mL Minims® phenylephrine in 1mL BSS in cases of idiopathic floppy iris syndrome; however, the presence of sodium metabisulfite disodium edetate in the Minims® preparation is a concern regarding its intracameral use. Intracameral phenylephrine is now available from SOMs.

‡ Triamcinolone acetonide suspension as Kenalog® is preserved with benzyl alcohol and is not licensed for intraocular use. Some surgeons who do use it attempt to remove the triamcinolone from the preservative-containing solution by capturing it in a 5 micron filter before resuspending it in BSS; others simply dilute the neat 40mg/mL solution in BSS.

Sub-Tenon's and peribulbar injections

In addition to their use in ocular anaesthesia (see ➲ Ocular anaesthesia (1), p. 928), the sub-Tenon's and peribulbar routes may be used to deliver drugs, such as corticosteroids, to the posterior aspect of the globe.

Sub-Tenon's injection

Sub-Tenon's cannula technique

Method

See Box 25.1.

- Topical anaesthetic to conjunctiva (e.g. proxymetacaine 0.5%).
- Wash hands, and don sterile gloves.
- Instil 5% povidone iodine onto the ocular surface; drape (optional), and insert lid speculum (optional).
- Ask patient to look in opposite direction to intended injection site (e.g. inferonasally).
- Open conjunctiva around 8mm from the limbus (e.g. superotemporally); dissect down to bare sclera with blunt curved scissors; insert sub-Tenon's cannula (19G, 25mm, blunt, curved), and slide posteriorly along the globe.
- Inject medication.
- Carefully withdraw cannula; forceps or a cotton-tipped applicator can be used to provide countertraction and to hold the conjunctival opening closed (which may help reduce regurgitation).
- Advantage: relatively safe (blunt needle, appropriately curved for the shape of the globe).
- Disadvantage: significant regurgitation of drug along the sub-Tenon's track may result in poor drug delivery.

Sharp needle (Nozik)[1] technique

- Method: insertion and posterior advancement of a 26G, 5/8in needle up to its hub through sub-Tenon's space.
- Advantage: less regurgitation and improved drug delivery.
- Disadvantage: ↑risk of globe perforation.

IV cannula technique[2]

- *Method*: insertion and posterior direction of a 22G or 23G, 0.9/25mm IV cannula (made of polytetrafluoroethylene) through sub-Tenon's space.
- *Advantage*: relatively safe (blunt needle, flexible so moulds to shape of the globe), probably less regurgitation than with sub-Tenon's cannula.
- *Disadvantage*: can be difficult to direct the flexible cannula.

Medications

Although primarily used for ocular anaesthesia (e.g. lidocaine, bupivacaine), these routes may be used for delivering corticosteroids (e.g. triamcinolone, methylprednisolone) in posterior segment inflammation, exudation, or macular oedema.

Box 25.1 Outline of IV cannula technique for sub-Tenon's injection

- Enter the sub-Tenon's space by use of the trocar of a 22G or 23G, 0.9/25mm IV cannula (made of polytetrafluoroethylene).
- Advance the cannula (with the trocar still engaged and in the bevel-up position) for about 3mm within the sub-Tenon's space.
- Slightly withdraw the trocar (so sharp end no longer exposed), and continue to carefully advance the cannula for a further 3mm.
- Completely withdraw the trocar, and direct the cannula posteriorly for a further 12–15mm, using gentle rotatory movements.
- Attach the syringe to the cannula, and inject medication.

Peribulbar injection

Method

Peribulbar injection is a sharp needle technique which is used for delivering medication into the extraconal space. For delivery of local anaesthesia, a medial compartment block via a medial canthal injection is preferred (see ➲ Peribulbar block, p. 930). For delivery of medication, such as corticosteroids, the safer sub-Tenon's route is recommended. However, if the peribulbar route is used, an inferolateral injection is made with a 25G sharp-bevel needle, entering either through the lid or the conjunctiva and directed inferolateral to the globe, just above the orbital floor (see Table 25.3).

Table 25.3 Sub-Tenon's and peribulbar corticosteroids

Drug	Dose	Proprietary
Triamcinolone acetonide	40mg	*Kenalog*® (suspension)
Methylprednisolone	40mg	*Depo-Medrone*® (suspension)*

These are non-licensed uses of the commercial IM/intra-articular preparations of these corticosteroids.

* Contains polyethylene glycol, myristyl-γ-picolinium chloride.

1. Smith RE *et al.* The non-specific treatment of uveitis. In: Smith RE, Nozik RA. Uveitis: a clinical approach to diagnosis and management, 2nd edition. Baltimore: Williams & Wilkins; 1989. pp.51–72.

2. Venkatesh P *et al.* Posterior subtenon injection of corticosteroids using polytetrafluoroethylene (PTFE) intravenous cannula. *Clin Experiment Ophthalmol* 2002;**30**;55–7.

Intravitreal injections

Principle

Intravitreal injections should be isotonic, should have a neutral pH, and must not contain preservatives. Unfortunately, this is not always achievable with commercially available preparations.

Indications

- *Intravitreal antimicrobials for endophthalmitis*: usually performed immediately after a vitreous biopsy or core vitrectomy in theatre.
- *Intravitreal anti-VEGF therapies or corticosteroids for AMD, CMO or various exudative posterior segment diseases*: may be performed in theatre or a dedicated clean room.

Procedure

The following outline summarizes the guidelines of the RCOphth:[3]

Setting

Intravitreal injections may be given in theatre or a dedicated clean room in outpatients which meets stringent conditions such as being enclosed, free from interruptions, good illumination, washable floor, and non-particulate ceiling (i.e. dust-free). In this context, full gowning is not necessary, but hands should be washed and sterile gloves worn. The procedure for an intravitreal injection performed in isolation (i.e. not as part of a vitrectomy/biopsy for endophthalmitis) is:

Preparation

- Confirm consent and correct eye to be injected; measure IOP; ensure adequate dilation; instil topical anaesthesia.
- Set up equipment trolley, and ensure all treatments (including post-injection antibiotics) are available.

Technique

- Wash hands, and don sterile gloves.
- Instil 5% povidone iodine onto the ocular surface, and allow adequate time (3min) prior to injection; clean periocular area with 5–10% povidone iodine; drape, and insert lid speculum.
- Consider whether supplementation of anaesthesia is necessary: subconjunctival or sub-Tenon's (e.g. lidocaine 1%).
- Prepare syringe/needle/drug immediately prior to injection, and ensure any air in the syringe/needle is expelled prior to injection; maintain aseptic technique throughout.
- *Note injection site*: this should be 3.0–3.5mm (aphakic/pseudophakic) or 3.5–4mm (phakic) posterior to limbus, usually in the inferotemporal quadrant. Avoid the horizontal meridians.
- Insert needle (27–30G; 1/2–5/8in long) perpendicularly, aiming towards the centre of the globe.
- Inject appropriate volume of therapeutic agent indicated for intravitreal use (maximum 0.1mL); carefully remove needle; a sterile cotton-tipped applicator can be used as counterpressure and to prevent any reflux.
- Instil topical antibiotic (e.g. chloramphenicol 0.5%). The RCOphth 2013 Guidance advises that routine post-injection antibiotics are not recommended due to a lack of evidence that they reduce endophthalmitis rates, but that they can be used at the discretion of the clinician.

Post-injection
- Test gross VA, and check for central retinal artery patency (may not be necessary if acuity satisfactory).
- If non-perfusion of central retinal artery should occur (often indicated by no perception of light), an AC paracentesis is indicated and should be performed immediately.
- Check injection site (at the slit-lamp) and IOP (not mandatory).
- Topical antibiotics at the discretion of the clinician (e.g. chloramphenicol 0.5% 4×/d) for ≥3d.

Medications (See Tables 25.4–25.6)

Table 25.4 Intravitreal antimicrobials

Drug		Dose	Reconstituted to
Antibacterial	Vancomycin	1–2mg	0.1mL
	Amikacin	400 micrograms	0.1mL
	Ceftazidime	2mg	0.1mL
Antifungal	Amphotericin	5–10 micrograms	0.1mL
Antiviral	Ganciclovir	2–4mg	0.1mL
	Foscarnet	1.2–2.4mg	0.1mL

Table 25.5 Intravitreal corticosteroid

Drug	Dose	Reconstituted to
Dexamethasone*	700 micrograms	Preloaded implant
Fluocinolone acetonide†	190 micrograms	Preloaded implant
Triamcinolone acetate‡	2–4mg	0.05–0.1mL

* Dexamethasone 700 micrograms intravitreal implant (Ozurdex®, Allergan) licensed for macular oedema following retinal vein occlusion (NICE (2011). *Dexamethasone intravitreal implant for the treatment of macular oedema caused by retinal vein occlusion (RVO). Technical appraisals, TA229.* Available at: ℰ http://www.nice.org.uk/guidance/TA229).

† Fluocinolone acetonide 190 microgram intravitreal implant (Iluvien®, Alimera Sciences) licensed for diabetic macular oedema insufficiently responsive to other therapies in pseudophakic patients (NICE (2013). *Fluocinolone acetonide intravitreal implant for treating chronic diabetic macular oedema after an inadequate response to prior therapy. Technology Appraisals, TA301.* Available at: ℰ http://www.nice.org.uk/guidance/TA301)

‡ Non-licensed use of commercial IM/intra-articular preparations of triamcinolone acetate. Triamcinolone acetonide is preserved and not licensed for intraocular use. Some surgeons attempt to remove the triamcinolone from the preservative-containing solution by capturing it in a 5 micron filter before resuspending in BSS; others dilute neat 40mg/mL solution in BSS.

Table 25.6 Intravitreal anti-VEGF therapies (licensed for intraocular use)

Drug	Dose
Ranibizumab	0.5mg/0.05mL
Pegaptanib	0.3mg/0.09mL
Aflibercept	2mg/0.05mL

3. RCOphth. *Guidelines for intravitreal injections procedure.* (2009) and *Age-related Macular Degeneration: Guidelines for Management.* (2013) ℰ http://www.rcophth.ac.uk/clinicalguidelines

Topical antimicrobials

Antibacterials

Generic	Forms	Pres-free	Frequency	Proprietary
Azithromycin dihydrate	g 1.5%	Yes	2×/d	Azyter®
Chloramphenicol	g 0.5%	Minims®	g: see notes	Chloromycetin® Redidrops Minims® chloramphenicol
	Oc 1%	Oc	Oc: 3–4×/d	Chloromycetin® Ophthalmic Ointment
Ciprofloxacin	g 0.3% Oc 0.3%	Oc	See notes*·†	Ciloxan®
Fusidic acid	Gel 1%	No	2×/d	Fucithalmic®
Gentamicin	g 0.3% g 0.3%, 1.4–1.5% (SOM)	Available (SOM)	See notes*	Genticin®
Levofloxacin	g 0.5%	Unit dose	See notes*	Oftaquix® Oftaquix® unit dose
Moxifloxacin	g 0.5%	No	See notes*	Moxivig®
Ofloxacin	g 0.3%	No	See notes*	Exocin®
Propamidine isetionate (dibrompropamidine isetionate in ointment)	g 0.1% Oc 0.15%	Golden Eye® Ointment	g: 4×/d Oc: 1–2×/d	Brolene® Golden Eye®
Tobramycin	g 0.3%	No	See notes‡	Tobravisc®

* Frequency: *BNF* recommends for antibacterial eye drops that they are administered at least every 2h, then reduce frequency as infection is controlled, and continue for 48h after healing; for ointments, *BNF* recommends that they are used at night (with drops used during the day) or 3–4×/d if used alone.

† Ciloxan®: For corneal ulcer, the summary of product characteristics recommend that they are administered throughout day and night, day 1 being applied every 15min for 6h, then every 30min, day 2 being applied every hour, days 3–14 being applied every 4h (max duration of treatment 21d); if ointment used, it should be administered throughout day and night, 1.25cm ointment being applied every 1–2h for 2d, then every 4h for next 12d.

‡ Tobravisc® 2×/d as standard; in severe infections 4x/d for 24h then reduced to 2x/d.

SOM: some preparations may only be available from Special-Order Manufacturers (see *BNF* for list).

Antifungals

Generic	Forms	Frequency
Amphotericin	g 0.15%	≤q 1h initially for fungal keratitis, reducing as infection is controlled (see ❯ Fungal keratitis: treatment, p. 230)
Clotrimazole	g 1%	
Miconazole	g 1%	
Natamycin	g 5%	

SOM: There are no commercially available topical antifungal agents in the UK. These preparations may be available from Special-Order Manufacturers or pharmaceutical importers (see *BNF* for list).

Antivirals

Generic	Forms	Pres-free	Frequency	*Proprietary*
Aciclovir	Oc 3%	Oc	5×/d until healed, then 5×/d for 3d*	*Zovirax*®
Ganciclovir	Gel 0.15%	No	3–5×/d	*Virgan*®
Trifluridine†	g 1%	SOM	9×/d	

* Frequency: *BNF* recommends continuing at 5×/d for at least 3d after healing for aciclovir.

† Trifluridine (*syn* trifluorothymidine) is commonly used in the USA but is not commercially available in the UK. Viroptic®, the brand available in the USA, is not available in pres-free form, but trifluorothymidine eye drops made by SOM are available as pres-free.

Topical anti-inflammatory agents

Corticosteroids

Corticosteroids

Generic	Forms	Pres-free	Frequency	Proprietary
Betamethasone	g 0.1% Oc 0.1%	Oc	See notes*	Betnesol® (g/Oc) Vistamethasone® (g)
Dexamethasone base	g 0.1%	No	See notes*	Maxidex®
Dexamethasone sodium phosphate	g 0.1%	Unit dose	See notes*	Minims® dexamethasone, Dropdex, Dexafree
Fluorometholone	g 0.1%	No	See notes*	FML®
Loteprednol	g 0.5%	No	See notes*	Lotemax®
Prednisolone sodium phosphate	g 0.5% g 0.05%, 0.1%, 0.3% (SOM)†	Minims®	See notes*	Predsol®
Prednisolone acetate	g 1%	No	See notes*	Pred Forte®
Rimexolone	g 1%	No	See notes*	Vexol®

* Frequency: potency and frequency of corticosteroids should be titrated against degree of inflammation in order to achieve control whilst minimizing side effects.

† SOM: some preparations may only be available from Special-Order Manufacturers (see BNF for list).

NB RCOphth/UKOPG guidance discourages use of multiple strengths of low strength prednisolones—suggests 0.1%.

Corticosteroid/antibiotic combinations

Corticosteroid	Antibiotic	Forms	Frequency	Proprietary
Betamethasone 0.1%	Neomycin 0.5%	g	≤6×/d	Betnesol-N®
Dexamethasone base 0.1%	Neomycin 0.35% Polymyxin B sulfate 6,000U/mL	g or Oc*	≤6×/d	Maxitrol®
	Tobramycin 0.3%	g	≤6×/d	Tobradex®
Dexamethasone sodium metasulfobenzoate 0.05%	Framycetin 0.5% Gramicidin 0.005%	g	≤6×/d	Sofradex®

* Unlike most ointments, Maxitrol® Oc is preserved (with parabenzoates).

Antihistamines and other anti-inflammatory agents

Antihistamines and other anti-allergic agents

Generic	Forms	Pres-free	Frequency	Proprietary
Antihistamine[*]				
Antazoline sulfate	g	No	2–3×/d	Otrivine-Antistin®
Azelastine hydrochloride	g	No	2–4×/d up to 6wk	Optilast®
Emedastine	g	No	2×/d	Emadine®
Epinastine hydrochloride	g	No	2×/d up to 8wk	Relestat®
Ketotifen	g	No	2×/d	Zaditen®
Olopatadine	g	No	2×/d up to 4mo	Opatanol®
Mast cell stabilizers				
Lodoxamide	g	No	4×/d	Alomide®
Nedocromil sodium	g	No	2–4×/d	Rapitil®
Sodium cromoglicate	g, unit dose	Unit dose	4×/d	Opticrom® and others Unit dose Catacrom®

[*] Some of these antihistamine preparations also have mast cell-stabilizing properties.

Other anti-inflammatory agents (NSAID type)

Generic	Forms	Pres-free	Frequency[*]	Proprietary
Bromfenac	g 0.09%	No	2×/d	Yellox®
Diclofenac sodium	g 0.1%	Unit dose	1–4×/d	Voltarol® Ophtha unit dose Voltarol® Ophtha Multidose®
Flurbiprofen sodium	g 0.03% (only as SDU)	Unit dose	1–4×/d	Ocufen®
Ketorolac	g 0.5%	No	3×/d	Acular®
Nepafenac	g 0.1%	No	3x/d	Nevenac®

[*] Frequency depends on indication.

A note on ciclosporin: topical ciclosporin is available as eye ointment 0.2% (unlicensed in humans—veterinary medicine) or as drops 0.05% unit dose (Restasis®) available from pharmaceutical importers. 0.06% and 2% forms are available from some SOMs.

Topical glaucoma medications

β-blockers

β-blockers

Generic	Forms	Pres-free	Frequency	Proprietary
Betaxolol hydrochloride	g 0.25%	Unit dose	2×/d	*Betoptic®* suspension *Betoptic®* suspension single dose
	g 0.5%	No	2×/d	*Betoptic®*
Carteolol hydrochloride	g 1 or 2%	No	2×/d	*Teoptic®*
Levobunolol hydrochloride	g 0.5%	Unit dose	1–2×/d	*Betagan®* *Betagan®* unit dose
Timolol maleate	g 0.25% or 0.5%	Unit dose	2×/d	*Timoptol®* *Timoptol®* unit dose
	Gel 0.1%	Unit dose	1×/d	*Tiopex®*
	Gel 0.25% or 0.5%	No	1×/d	*Timoptol-LA®*

Prostaglandin analogues and related drugs

Prostaglandin analogues and related drugs

Generic	Forms	Pres-free	Frequency	Proprietary
Bimatoprost	g 100 and 300 micrograms/mL 0.01% and 0.03%	Unit dose	1×/d (nocte)	*Lumigan®* *Lumigan®* unit dose (0.03%)
Latanoprost	g 50 micrograms/ mL 0.005%	Unit dose	1×/d (nocte)	*Xalatan®* and others *Monopost®*
Travoprost	g 40 micrograms/ mL 0.004%	No	1×/d (nocte)	*Travatan®*
Tafluprost	g 15 micrograms/ mL 0.0015%	Unit dose	1×/d (nocte)	*Saflutan®*

Miotics

Miotics

Generic	Forms	Pres-free	Frequency	Proprietary
Pilocarpine	g 1, 2, or 4%	Minims® (2%)	≤4×/d	Minims® pilocarpine nitrate

Sympathomimetics

Sympathomimetics

Generic	Forms	Pres-free	Frequency	Proprietary
Apraclonidine	g 0.5%	No	3×/d for <1mo	Iopidine® 0.5%
	g 1%	Unit dose	Pre-/post-YAG laser	Iopidine® 1%
Brimonidine tartrate	g 0.2%	No	2×/d	Alphagan®

Carbonic anhydrase inhibitors

(See also Table 25.18.)

Carbonic anhydrase inhibitors

Generic	Forms	Pres-free	Frequency	Proprietary
Brinzolamide	g 1%	No	2–3×/d	Azopt®
Dorzolamide	g 2%	Unit dose	3×/d or 2×/d if with β-blocker	Trusopt® Trusopt® unit dose

Combination drops

Combinations with timolol

Generic	Forms	Pres-free	Frequency	Proprietary
Timolol + bimatoprost	g timolol 0.5%, bimatoprost 0.03%	Unit dose	1×/d	Ganfort® unit dose
Timolol + brimonidine	g timolol 0.5%, brimonidine 0.2%	No	2×/d	Combigan®
Timolol + brinzolamide	g timolol 0.5%, brinzolomide 1%	No	2×/d	Azarga®
Timolol + dorzolamide	g timolol 0.5%, dorzolamide 2%	Unit dose	2×/d	Cosopt® and others Cosopt® and others unit dose
Timolol + latanoprost	g timolol 0.5%, latanoprost 0.005%	No	1×/d	Xalacom® and others
Timolol + travoprost	g timolol 0.5%, travoprost 0.004%	No	1×/d	DuoTrav®

Topical mydriatics

Mydriatics

Mydriatics and cycloplegics[*]

Generic	Forms	Pres-free	Frequency	Proprietary
Antimuscarinic				
Atropine sulfate	g 0.5% or 1% Oc 1%[†]	Minims® (1%) Oc	Single–1×/d	*Minims® atropine sulfate*
Cyclopentolate hydrochloride	g 0.5% or 1%	Minims®	Single–3×/d	*Mydrilate® Minims® cyclopentolate hydrochloride*
Homatropine hydrobromide	g 1%	No	Single–4×/d	
Tropicamide	g 0.5% or 1%	Minims® (0.5% or 1%)	Single	*Mydriacyl® Minims® tropicamide*
Sympathomimetic				
Phenylephrine	g 2.5%, 10%	Minims® (2.5% or 10%)	Single–3×/d	*Minims® phenylephrine hydrochloride*

[*] Mydriasert is a mydratic insert containing 0.28mg tropicamide and 5.4mg of phenylephrine hydrocholoride for insertion into the lower fornix. It is indicated for pre-operative mydriasis or for diagnostic purposes when monotherapy is insufficient.

[†] Oc form may be available from Special-Order Manufacturers (see *BNF* for list) or pharmaceutical importers.

Topical anaesthetics

Anaesthetics

Generic	Forms	Pres-free	Frequency	Proprietary
Oxybuprocaine hydrochloride*	Minims® 0.4%	Yes	Single	Minims® oxybuprocaine hydrochloride
Proxymetacaine hydrochloride	Minims® 0.5%	Yes	Single	Minims® proxymetacaine
Tetracaine hydrochloride	Minims® 0.5% or 1%	Yes	Single	Minims® tetracaine hydrochloride
Combinations with fluorescein				
Lidocaine and fluorescein	Minims® L (4%) + F (0.25%)	Yes	Single	Minims® lidocaine and fluorescein

* Oxybuprocaine hydrochloride was previously known as benoxinate.

Topical tear replacement

Artificial tears and astringents

Artificial tears

Generic	Forms	Pres-free	Frequency	Proprietary
Low viscosity				
Hypromellose	g 0.3%, 0.32%, 0.5%, or 1%	Artelac® unit dose (0.32%) Hydromoor® Tear-Lac® Lumecare® Preservative Free Drops	As required	*Isopto®* plain *Isopto®* alkaline *Tears Naturale®* *Mandanol®* *Artelac®* SDU and others
Hydroxy-ethylcellulose	Minims® 0.44%	Minims®	As required	*Minims®* artificial tears
Polyvinyl alcohol	g 1.4%	Liquifilm® PF, *Refresh®*	As required	*Sno Tears®* *Liquifilm Tears®* *Liquifilm Tears®* PF, *Refresh®*, and others
Sodium chloride	Minims® 0.9%	Minims®	As required	*Minims®* saline
Medium viscosity				
Carbomer 980	Gel 0.2%	Viscotears® PF	≥4×/d	*GelTears®* *Artelac Nighttime gel* *Viscotears®* *Viscotears® PF* *Clinitas®* carbomer gel *Lumecare®* carbomer gel *Xailin®* gel
Carbomer 974P	Gel 0.25%	No		*Liquivisc®*
Carmellose	g 0.5% or 1%	Unit dose and multidose PF	≥4×/d	*Celluvisc®* *Carmize®* *Xailin® Fresh* and others
High viscosity				
Liquid paraffin	Oc 30% or 42.5%	All these ointments are pres-free	Nocte	*Lacri-Lube®* *VitA-POS®** *Xailin Night®*
Yellow soft paraffin	Oc 80%	Simple eye ointment is pres-free	Nocte	Simple eye ointment

* Preservative-free ointment containing vitamin A, liquid paraffin, light liquid paraffin, and soft liquid paraffin.

Mucolytics and astringents

Generic	Forms	Pres-free	Frequency	*Proprietary*
Acetylcysteine	g 5%*	No	3–4×/d	*Ilube®*

* 10% and 20% preparations are available from SOM.

Hyaluronic acid preparations*

Proprietary	Forms	Pres-free	Frequency
Artelac® Splash	g 0.2%	Unit dose	prn
Clinitas®	g 0.4%	Unit dose	2–4×/d or prn
Hyabak®	g 0.15%	Yes	prn
Hylo-Tear®†	g 0.1%	Yes†	prn
Hylo-Care®†	g 0.1%	Yes†	prn
Hylo-Forte®†	g 0.2%	Yes†	prn
Lubristil®	g 0.15%	Unit dose	prn
Lubristil® Gel	Gel 0.15%	Unit dose	prn
Ocusan	g 0.2%	Unit dose	prn
Oxyal®	g 0.1%	Pres-free in the eye‡	prn
Vismed®	g 0.18%	Unit dose	prn
Vismed® Multi§	g 0.18%	Yes§	prn
Vismed® Gel	Gel 0.3%	Unit dose	prn

* A number of other hyaluronic acid preparations are also available.

† Hylo-Tear®, Hylo-Care®, and Hylo-Forte® are preservative-free lubricants available in a multidose bottle. This container utilizes an airless system, thus eliminating all contact of air (and microorganisms) with the solution inside the bottle. It can therefore be used for up to 6mo.

‡ Oxyal® is preserved in the bottle, but this biodegrades on contact with the eye, making it a non-preserved solution in the eye.

§ Vismed® multi is preservative-free; the container is designed to prevent ingress of air (and microorganisms), allowing the preservative-free solution to be used for up to 3mo.

More recent additions to the list of treatments available for treating dry eye include those based on macrogols or soybean oil.

Macrogols are polyethylene glycols. Examples include Systane® (polyethylene glycol 400 0.4%, propylene glycol 0.3%, hydroxypropyl guar) and Systane Ultra® (additional ingredient sorbitol). An example of a soybean oil based preparation is Emustil™ (soybean oil 7%, natural phospholipids 3%).

A note on topical sodium chloride: sodium chloride is available as g. sodium chloride 5% Hypersal® and unit dose NaCl 5% and ointment prescribable medical devices.

Systemic medication: antimicrobials

Table 25.7 is a summary of systemic antimicrobials commonly used in ophthalmology and discussed elsewhere in the text. It is not intended to be exhaustive; consult the *BNF* or other local formulary for details of dosing, contraindications, side effects, and a wider range of alternative therapeutic agents (see also Table 25.8 and Table 25.9).

Table 25.7 Selected systemic antibacterial medications

Drug	Dose	Route
Penicillins		
Flucloxacillin	250–500mg 4×/d	PO/IV/IM
Amoxicillin	250–500mg 4×/d	PO
	500mg–1g 4×/d	IV
Co-amoxiclav	250–500mg amoxicillin 3×/d	PO
	1g 3–4×/d	IV
Cephalosporins		
Cefotaxime	1–2g 2–4×/d	IV/IM
Ceftazidime	2g 3×/d	IV
Cefuroxime	750mg 3–4×/d	IV/IM
Tetracyclines		
Doxycycline	200mg stat, then 100mg 1×/d	PO
Oxytetracycline	250mg 4×/d	PO
Quinolones		
Ciprofloxacin	500–750mg 2×/d	PO
	200–400mg 2×/d	IV
Ofloxacin	200–400mg 2×/d	PO
	200–400mg 2×/d	IV
Macrolides		
Azithromycin	1g stat	PO
Erythromycin	500mg 2×/d	PO
Other		
Metronidazole	200–400mg 3×/d	PO
	500mg 3×/d	IV
Vancomycin	1g 2×/d	IV

Antibiotic prescribing is being modified in the light of challenges such as *Clostridium difficile* and meticillin-resistant *Staphylococcus aureus* (MRSA). In the UK, this has led to a nationwide drive to reduce the use of cephalosporins and quinolones.

Table 25.8 Selected systemic antiviral medications

Drug	Dose	Route
Anti-HSV/VZV		
Aciclovir	800mg 5×/d *(for HZO)*[*]	PO
	5–10mg/kg 3×/d	IV
Valaciclovir	1g 3×/d *(for HZO)*[*]	PO
Famciclovir	250mg 3×/d or 750mg 1×/d	PO
Anti-CMV		
Ganciclovir	5mg/kg 2×/d	IV
Valganciclovir	900mg 2×/d (induction)	PO
	900mg 1×/d (maintenance)	
Cidofovir	5mg/kg every 1wk (induction), every 2wk (maintenance)	IV
Foscarnet	60mg/kg 3×/d (induction)	IV
	60–120mg/kg (maintenance)	

[*] Doses given for aciclovir, valaciclovir, and famciclovir are for treatment of HZO and should be given for 7d. In ARN, aciclovir is usually given IV at 10mg/kg 3×/d 2wk before reverting to the oral dose for 6–12wk.

Table 25.9 Selected systemic antifungal medications

Drug	Dose	Route
Polyene		
Amphotericin	1–3mg/kg/d for liposomal preparations; less for Fungizone®	IV
Fluorinated pyrimidines		
Flucytosine	50mg/kg ×4/d; adjust as per blood level monitoring	IV
Triazoles		
Itraconazole	100–200mg 1×/d	PO
	200mg 2×/d for 2d, then ↓ to 200mg 1×/d	IV
Fluconazole	50–200mg 1×/d	PO
Voriconazole	400mg 2×/d for two doses, then 200mg 2×/d (can ↑ to 300mg 2×/d)	PO
	6mg/kg 2×/d for two doses, then 4mg/kg 2×/d	IV

Systemic medication: glaucoma

Systemic medication may be required to lower IOP in the acute setting (e.g. AACG) or if topical treatment alone has failed. It is also commonly used prophylactically post-procedure (e.g. acetazolamide after cataract surgery). Acetazolamide may also be used in the treatment of raised ICP 2° to IIH, altitude sickness, and epilepsy (see Table 25.10).

Table 25.10 Systemic glaucoma medications

Drug	Dose	Route	Contraindications	Side effects
Acetazolamide	0.25–1g/d in divided doses or 1–2 capsules/d for 250mg SR preparation	IV/PO	Sulfonamide allergy, salt imbalance, renal impairment, hepatic impairment	Nausea Vomiting Diarrhoea Paraesthesiae Rashes Polyuria Hypokalaemia Salt imbalance Mood changes Blood disorders
Mannitol 20%	1–2g/kg over 45min single dose	IV	Cardiac failure	Fluid overload Fever
Glycerol	1g/kg in 50% lemon juice single dose	PO	Diabetes mellitus	Hyperglycaemia

Systemic corticosteroids: general

Indications and mechanism

In severe ophthalmic inflammation, systemic corticosteroids may be required. Corticosteroids are anti-inflammatory but, at higher doses, are immunosuppressive. The immunosuppressive role of corticosteroids is via inhibition of NF-kB transcription factor signalling, so blocking the production of interleukin 2 and other pro-inflammatory cytokines.

Routes of administration (systemic)

- *PO*: the preferred corticosteroid is usually prednisolone. This may be started at 1mg/kg and then titrated down as inflammation is controlled and/or steroid-sparing agents are added. The commonest two forms prescribed are: enteric- and non-enteric-coated, although there is also a soluble form. Absorption of the enteric-coated form may be less predictable. Corticosteroids are best taken in the morning (coincides with physiological morning cortisol peak).
- *IV*: the preferred corticosteroid is usually methylprednisolone. This may be given as a single 500–1000mg dose or 'pulsed', e.g. three doses of 500–1000mg on consecutive or alternate days, given in a 100mL of normal saline over a minimum of 1h.

Efficacy

(See Box 25.2.)

Box 25.2 Corticosteroids: equivalent anti-inflammatory doses

Prednisolone 5mg is equivalent to:
- Dexamethasone, 750 micrograms.
- Betamethasone, 750 micrograms.
- Methylprednisolone, 4mg.
- Triamcinolone, 4mg.
- Hydrocortisone, 20mg.

Contraindications

- Systemic infection (unless covered with appropriate antibiotic(s)).

Monitoring

Pre-treatment

Due to the profound effects of corticosteroids, a short pre-treatment review is advised. This includes selected medical history (varicella status, TB status, pre-existing diabetes/impaired glucose tolerance, hypertension) and examination (weight, BP, Glu). If there is any possibility of TB, a CXR should be performed.

During treatment
- BP, weight, Glu every 3mo.
- Lipids every 1y.
- Bone density (dual X-ray absorptiometry (DXA) scan) if steroid course >3mo; repeated scans may be needed for monitoring bone density in at-risk individuals.

Side effects

(See Table 25.11.)

Table 25.11 Corticosteroid side effects (selected)

Endocrine	Adrenal suppression (risk of Addisonian crisis with withdrawal), Cushing's syndrome, weight gain, moonface
GI	Nausea, indigestion, peptic ulcer, pancreatitis
Musculoskeletal	Myopathy, osteopenia, osteoporosis, avascular necrosis
Skin	Atrophy, bruising, striae, acne, hirsutism
Haematological	Leucocytosis, immunosuppression
Biochemical	Fluid/electrolyte disturbance
Psychiatric	Mood disturbance (high or low), insomnia, psychosis
Neurological	↑ICP, papilloedema, worsening of epilepsy
Cardiovascular	Myocardial rupture after recent MI
Ophthalmic	↑IOP, posterior subcapsular cataracts, worsening of infection (e.g. viral or fungal keratitis)

Systemic corticosteroids: prophylaxis

Avoiding side effects

Prophylaxis of corticosteroid-induced osteoporosis

Consider prophylaxis (e.g. a bisphosphonate such as alendronic acid) if treating with the equivalent of ≥7.5mg prednisolone/d for ≥3mo, as indicated in Table 25.12.

DXA scans compare the bone density of the lower spine and hip against normal (i.e. healthy young adult). The difference is calculated in SD to give the T score, as in Table 25.13.

Table 25.12 Summary of the joint recommendations of the Royal College of Physicians, National Osteoporosis Society, and the Bone and Tooth Society for corticosteroid use of ≥3mo duration[*]

	Fracture Hx	DXA scan	
Age >65y			Investigate[†] + give prophylaxis
Age <65y	Previous fragility fracture		Investigate[†] + give prophylaxis
	No previous fragility fracture	T below −1.5 SD	Give prophylaxis
		T between −1.5 and 0 SD	Repeat DXA in 1–3y
		T above 0 SD	No repeat unless very high dose

[*] Bone and Tooth Society of Great Britain, National Osteoporosis Society, Royal College of Physicians. *Glucocorticoid-induced osteoporosis. Guidelines for prevention and treatment.* (2002). Available at: ⅍ http://www.rcplondon.ac.uk/sites/default/files/documents/glucocorticoid-induced-osteoporosis-guideline.pdf

[†] Investigations advised include: FBC, ESR, bone and LFTs, creatinine, TSH, and other specialist investigations (e.g. isotope bone scan), as indicated.

Table 25.13 Bone densitometry scores

T score	Condition
0 to −1 SD	Normal
−1 to −2.5 SD	Osteopenia
Below −2.5 SD	Osteoporosis

Prophylaxis of GI side effects

Consider prophylaxis (e.g. an H2 antagonist such as ranitidine 150mg 2×/d) if at risk, i.e. higher doses of corticosteroid, history of GI disease, co-administration of NSAIDs (avoid if possible).

Withdrawal of corticosteroids

For most patients having short courses (<10d) of doses ≤40mg/d prednisolone (or equivalent), no tapering is necessary. However, where there is a risk of adrenal suppression (see Box 25.3), tapering is required in which the dose is reduced fairly rapidly to physiological levels (equivalent to 7.5mg prednisolone/d), and thereafter reduced more gradually. One suggested tapering approach is given in Box 25.4.

Box 25.3 Increased risk of adrenal suppression due to corticosteroid administration

- The daily dose has been >40mg/d prednisolone (or equivalent).
- The duration has been >3wk.
- The frequency has been >1×/d.
- There have been other courses recently or long-term steroid administration within the last year.

Box 25.4 Tapering schedule recommended by the Consensus Panel on Immunosuppression for ocular disease*

- Over 40mg/d: reduce by 10mg/d every 1–2wk.
- 40–20mg/d: reduce by 5mg/d every 1–2wk.
- 20–10mg/d: reduce by 2.5mg/d every 1–2wk.
- 10–0mg/d: reduce by 1–2.5mg/d every 1–4wk.

* Jabs DA et al. Guidelines for the use of immunosuppressive drugs in patients with ocular inflammatory disorders: recommendations of an expert panel. *Am J Ophthalmol* 2000;**130**:492–513.

Antimetabolites, calcineurin inhibitors, and cytotoxics

Indications and mechanism

Although corticosteroids are usually the drug of choice in severe systemic or ocular inflammation, other immunosuppressants have an important role, either as second-line agents in unresponsive cases or in permitting reduction/ withdrawal of corticosteroids to minimize their side effects (see Table 25.14).

Table 25.14 Immunosuppressants and their mechanisms[*]

Drug	Dose	Route	Mechanism
Antimetabolites			
Azathioprine	1–3mg/kg	PO	Inhibits purine metabolism
Methotrexate	7.5–20mg/wk	PO/IM/SC	Inhibits dihydrofolate reductase
Mycophenolate mofetil	CellCept® 1g 2×/d	PO	Inhibits purine metabolism
Mycophenolate sodium	Myfortic® 720mg 2×/d	PO	Inhibits purine metabolism
Calcineurin inhibitors			
Ciclosporin	2–5mg/kg/d	PO	Inhibit calcineurin/ NF-AT transcription factor →↓IL-2 + other cytokines
Sirolimus	Adjusted according to blood levels	PO	Inhibit mTOR pathway →↓IL-2 + other cytokines
Tacrolimus[†]	100–200 micrograms/kg/d	PO	Inhibit calcineurin/ NF-AT transcription factor →↓IL-2 + other cytokines
Cytotoxics			
Chlorambucil	100–200 micrograms/kg/d	PO	Alkylating agent: DNA cross-linking blocks cell replication
Cyclophosphamide	2–3mg/kg/d	PO/IV	Alkylating agent: DNA cross-linking blocks cell replication

[*] Many of these immunosuppressants are unlicensed for use in ophthalmology.

[†] Recommended dose for tacrolimus in uveitis is 100–150 micrograms/kg/d, administered in two single doses; however, full dose is not usually tolerated at outset; therefore, start at 50% of the calculated dose, and increase slowly over a few weeks to the full dose. In very resistant cases, an increase to 200 micrograms/kg/d and/or the additional use of another immunosuppressive agent (antimetabolite/alkylating agent) must be considered.

IL-2, interleukin-2.

Cautions

These immunosuppressive agents should only be administered by someone with appropriate experience in their use (normally a GP, rheumatologist, or immunologist) and with adequate monitoring. Patient education is essential. This will include the potential side effects, necessary precautions (e.g. contraception during, and for a period after, taking most of these agents), and warning symptoms which would require urgent medical review (e.g. features suggestive of infection, especially sore throat) (see Table 25.15).

Table 25.15 Immunosuppressants and their side effects

Drug	Side effects (selected)	Suggested monitoring
Antimetabolites		
Azathioprine	Bone marrow suppression GI upset 2° malignancies Alopecia	Pre-treatment: check TPMT levels (low levels increase risk of bone marrow suppression) FBC stat, weekly for 4–8wk, then at least every 3mo
Methotrexate	Hepatotoxicity Bone marrow suppression GI upset	FBC, U+E, LFT stat, weekly until dose stable, then every 2–3mo Commonly folate (1mg/d or 5mg/wk) is given concurrently but not the same day as methotrexate
Mycophenolate mofetil	Bone marrow suppression GI upset 2° malignancies	FBC stat, weekly for 4wk, then fortnightly for 8wk, then monthly for first year
Transcription factor inhibitors		
Ciclosporin	Nephrotoxicity Hypertension Hepatotoxicity Gingival hyperplasia Hypertrichosis	U+E, LFT, BP stat, fortnightly for 4wk, then every 4–6wk
Sirolimus	Hyperlipidaemia Nephrotoxicity Hepatotoxicity	Sirolimus levels, U+E, LFT, lipids weekly for 4wk, then every 2–4wk or as directed
Tacrolimus	Nephrotoxicity Hypertension Neurotoxicity Hepatotoxicity	U+E, LFT, BP stat, fortnightly for 4wk, then every 4–6wk
Cytotoxics		
Chlorambucil	Bone marrow suppression Hepatotoxicity Sterility	Intensive specialist supervision required; includes FBC (+differential), LFT weekly for 4wk, then every 2–4wk
Cyclophosphamide	Bone marrow suppression Haemorrhagic cystitis GI upset Sterility	Intensive specialist supervision required; includes FBC (+ differential), LFT weekly for 4wk, then every 2–4wk

Biologics

The successful use of anti-TNF therapy in RA ushered in the age of biologics. These are monoclonal antibodies or other recombinant proteins which are used in a targeted manner to modulate biological systems.

Nomenclature of monoclonal antibodies

The rationale to naming monoclonal antibodies is as follows:

- Prefix: can be anything but should ensure that the whole name is distinct.
- Infix relating to target: e.g. -lim- for immune system, -tu- for miscellaneous tumour.
- Infix relating to source: e.g. -u- for human, -o- for mouse, -xi- for chimeric, and -zu- for humanized.
- Suffix: the class of medicine, i.e. mab for all monoclonal antibodies.

Examples

- Ada-lim-u-mab is a fully human monoclonal antibody with an immune system target.
- Ri-tu-xi-mab is a chimeric monoclonal antibody with a tumour target (originally developed for use against B-cell non-Hodgkin's lymphoma).

Mechanism

(See Table 25.16.)

Cautions

Biologics should only be administered by someone with appropriate experience in their use (normally a GP, rheumatologist, or immunologist) and with adequate monitoring. Patient education is essential. This will include the potential side effects, necessary precautions (e.g. contraception during, and for a period after, taking most of these agents), and warning symptoms which would require urgent medical review (e.g. features suggestive of infection, especially sore throat) (see Table 25.17).

Table 25.16 Selected biologics and their mechanisms[*]

Drug	Dose	Route	Mechanism
TNFα inhibitors			
Adalimumab	40mg every 2wk	SC	Anti-TNFα: fully human monoclonal antibody against TNFα
Etanercept	25mg twice/wk	SC	Anti-TNFα: Fc fusion protein which binds extracellular TNFαA
Infliximab	3–5mg/kg every 4–8wk	IV	Anti-TNFα: chimeric monoclonal antibody against TNFα
Interleukin receptor antagonists			
Anakinra	100mg/d	SC	Anti-IL-1R: recombinant version of IL-1 receptor antagonist (IL-1RA)
Anti-B-cell			
Rituximab	1g, repeated 2wk later	IV	Anti-CD20: chimeric monoclonal antibody against CD20 (B-cells)
Interferons			
Interferon alfa[†]	Depends on preparation	SC/IV	Antiviral and anti-tumour: decreases NK cell activity

[*] Many of these immunosuppressants are unlicensed for use in ophthalmology.

[†] Interferons: in uveitis, interferon alfa-2a and sometimes interferon alfa-2b are used. In MS, interferon beta may be used.

IL, interleukin.

Table 25.17 Selected biologics and their side effects

Drug	Side effects (selected)	Suggested monitoring
TNFα inhibitors		
Adalimumab	TB and hepatitis B reactivation Severe infections	Pre-treatment: rule out TB infection (may be latent) FBC (+ differential), U+E, LFT stat, fortnightly for 4wk, then every 4–6wk
Etanercept	Hypersensitivity reactions TB and hepatitis B reactivation Severe infections	Pre-treatment: rule out TB infection (may be latent) FBC (+ differential), U+E, LFT stat, fortnightly for 4wk, then every 4–6wk
Infliximab	Human antichimeric antibodies Serum sickness TB and hepatitis B reactivation Anaphylaxis Severe infections	Pre-treatment: rule out TB infection (may be latent) FBC (+ differential), U+E, LFT stat, fortnightly for 4wk, then every 4–6wk
Interleukin receptor antagonists		
Anakinra	Injection site reaction Neutropenia Severe infections (esp. in asthma)	FBC (+ differential) stat, monthly for 6mo, then every 3mo
Daclizumab	Hypersensitivity reactions Hypertension Severe infections	FBC (+ differential), U+E, LFT stat, fortnightly for 4wk, then every 4wk
Anti-B-cell		
Rituximab	Severe infusion reactions (including dyspnoea, hypoxia, bronchospasm) Cytokine release syndrome Cardiac dysfunction (including arrest, hypotension, angina, arrhythmias) TB reactivation Progressive multifocal leukoencephalopathy	Cardiac monitoring during infusion and resuscitation facilities must be available FBC (+ differential), U+E stat, then weekly for 4wk, then every 4–6wk
Interferons		
Interferon alfa	Leukopenia Depression TB reactivation Flu-like symptoms Nephrotoxicity Hepatotoxicity	FBC (+ differential), U+E, LFT stat, fortnightly for 4wk, then every 4–6wk Regular review of mental state

Evidence-based ophthalmology

Study design (1)

More than 2 million research papers are published every year. Faced with an impossible reading list, how should you pick out and critically appraise those that will change your practice and inform future clinical guidelines? The skills of critical appraisal enable you to systematically examine research to assess its validity and usefulness. Apply the same critical thinking to your own work; others will.

Study designs
(See Table 26.1.)

Systematic reviews and meta-analyses

- *Systematic review*: a retrospective review of relevant 1° studies (i.e. original data-gathering studies) meeting pre-specified tests of quality and relevance. Many such reviews have been conducted under the auspices of the Cochrane Collaboration, an organization dedicated to the preparation of such reviews to help better informed decisions about health care (see Box 26.1).
- *Meta-analysis*: a mathematical analysis of the combined results of two or more 1° studies of similar design.

Experimental studies

- *RCT*: a prospective study in which participants are randomly allocated to groups, comparing the intervention(s) with the control (e.g. placebo, standard treatment, or no treatment.). Bias is reduced by masking; in single-masked trials, the participants are unaware of whether they are in the 'treatment' or the 'control' group; in double-masked trials, the participants and the investigators are unaware of who is in which group until after the recording (and sometimes the analysis) of all data. (For obvious reasons, the synonymous term 'blinded' is generally avoided in ophthalmic research.)

Observational studies

- *Cohort study*: a prospective (or sometimes retrospective) study in which a group of individuals are identified at the outset (e.g. by the presence of a disease, exposure to an environmental factor, etc.) and monitored to see outcome over time. This is usually against a control group, although some information on natural history can be obtained without. These studies may be useful in identifying disease risk factors, natural history, and prognosis. For retrospective cohort studies, the group of individuals must be identified as they would have been, had the observer been there at the time (i.e. not with knowledge of the outcome; cf. case control study).
- *Case control study*: a retrospective study in which a group of individuals with outcome of interest (e.g. sympathetic ophthalmia after vitreoretinal surgery) are compared with a suitable control group; this type of study can be useful for rare conditions.
- *Cross-sectional survey*: a single time-point survey in a defined population, observing possible relationships between factors of interest and the disease.
- *Case series*: a description of a series of cases, often describing intervention and outcome, without a control group.

Level of evidence

Table 26.1 Levels of evidence (Scottish Intercollegiate Network (SIGN) classification)

Level	Evidence
1	**Evidence from meta-analyses, systematic reviews of RCTs, or RCTs.** Further classified as:
	1++ (high quality with very low risk of bias)
	1+ (well conducted with low risk of bias)
	1– (high risk of bias)
2	**Evidence from case control or cohort studies** (including systematic reviews of case control or cohort studies). Further classified as:
	2++ (very low risk of confounding, bias, or chance, and high probability that the relationship is causal)
	2+ (low risk of confounding, bias, or chance, and moderate probability that the relationship is causal)
	2– (high risk of confounding, bias, or chance, and significant risk that the relationship is not causal)
3	**Evidence from non-analytic studies (case reports/series)**
4	Evidence from expert opinion

Adapted from Scottish Intercollegiate Network. *SIGN 50: a guideline developer's handbook, Edinburgh 2008.* (Revised 2011). Available at: ℜ http://www.sign.ac.uk

Also see: Harbour R *et al.* A new system for grading recommendations in evidence based guidelines. *BMJ* 2001;**323**:334–6.

Study design (2)

Most studies are not simply descriptive but seek to detect clinically important associations between variables (e.g. IOP and progression of glaucoma) or the effects of interventions (e.g. differences between treatments A and B in their reduction of IOP). Integral to the design of such studies is a clear definition of the hypothesis and a calculation of the statistical power of the study (see Box 26.1).

The null and the alternative hypotheses

The null hypothesis is the default. It states that there is no effect or association of interest. For example, in a study of a new treatment for AMD, the null hypothesis might be that there is no difference between treatment vs placebo in the extent of visual loss at 6mo. The alternative hypothesis is that the null hypothesis is false, i.e. that there is an effect or association of interest. In the example shown, this might be that the extent of visual loss from AMD is significantly less in the group receiving treatment.

Power calculations

Study design should include a calculation of the statistical power of the study. This is its ability to detect an effect of a specified size. Technically, this can be defined as the probability that the appropriate statistical test will reject a false null hypothesis (known as a type II error; see Box 26.2). Generally, a power of ≥80% is considered acceptable in study design. Statistical power depends on:

- Statistical significance level required (i.e. p value; conventionally $p < 0.05$).
- Size of the effect (difference) being looked for.
- *Sensitivity of the data*: this includes sample size and data reliability.

It should be noted that, as most of these variables will already be determined, the main role of power calculations is to estimate how many participants will need to be recruited to have ≥80% chance of finding an effect.

Power calculations are also sometimes used retrospectively in studies where no effect has been found to see whether this is likely to be due to inadequate powering of the study (i.e. a type II error).

Box 26.1 The Cochrane Collaboration

Since its foundation in 1993, the Cochrane Collaboration has been at the forefront of the movement to an evidence-based approach to medicine. It is named after Archie Cochrane, a pioneering clinical trialist, who conducted his first controlled study whilst he was a prisoner of war and who later became the head of the Medical Research Council (MRC) Epidemiology Unit in the UK. His thesis was that 'resources, however limited, should be used to provide forms of health care that have been shown to be effective by properly controlled research'.

THE COCHRANE
COLLABORATION

The Cochrane logo symbolizes two reflected Cs for Cochrane Collaboration and contains a forest plot of the results of one of the earliest systematic reviews, containing a meta-analysis of the effect of prenatal corticosteroid treatment vs placebo on neonatal mortality of preterm infants. Seven studies are shown as horizontal lines, with the vertical line representing the point of no effect. The shorter the line, the more certain the result (narrower confidence intervals).

More recent Forest plots may also include a square (or 'blob'), indicative of the weight attributed to the study. The calculated summary measure of the meta-analysis is presented as a diamond, with the lateral points indicating the confidence intervals.

The Cochrane Collaboration and links to resources may be found at ℘ http://www.cochrane.org. The UK Cochrane Centre is at ℘ http://www.ukcc.cochrane.org

Box 26.2 Hypotheses and type I and type II errors

- *Null hypothesis*: there is no effect or association of interest.
- *Alternative hypothesis*: the null hypothesis is false, i.e. there exists an effect or association.
- *Type I error*: false positive, i.e. the null hypothesis is incorrectly rejected (statistical significance falsely claimed).
- *Type II error*: false negative, i.e. the null hypothesis is incorrectly accepted (statistical insignificance falsely accepted).

Critical appraisal

Questions to ask of a research paper

Question 1: is it worth reading at all?
• Does it ask a clear question?
• Was an appropriate method used to answer the question?

Unless the answer is 'yes' to both these points, it is probably not worth carrying on.

Question 2: what type of study is it?
Your appraisal of the validity of a paper will depend on the study design (see ➲ Study design (1), p. 1004). Specific questions to ask are:

Systematic review and meta-analysis
Would the search strategy have identified all relevant papers? Were studies assessed for quality? If data are combined, was this appropriate?

Randomized controlled study
Were patients satisfactorily allocated/randomized between groups? What was the level of masking/blinding (participants ± investigators ± data analysts)? Were both groups treated in the same way (apart from the intervention)? Was there a high 'loss-to-follow-up rate', and could this have affected the results? Was the study sufficiently powered (i.e. did it recruit enough patients to reduce the likelihood of a type II error (see Box 26.2)?

Cohort study
Was there a control group, and was it appropriate? How were patients selected, and would they be typical of the defined cohort? Has the 'exposure' under consideration and the outcomes been accurately measured? Have any important confounding factors been overlooked? Was there a high 'loss-to-follow-up rate', and could the lost participants be atypical of the group (e.g. important to know about 'loss to follow-up' due to death)? Was the study sufficiently powered and of long enough duration to pick up important events which are uncommon or have a long lag-time?

Case control study
Were the 'controls' appropriate matches for the cases? Is the assessment of the 'exposure' under consideration based on recall or records, and how reliable is this likely to be? Have any important confounding factors been overlooked?

Question 3: what are the main results, and are they statistically and clinically significant?
A statistically significant difference is of little interest, unless it reflects a change that is meaningful in clinical terms. In a comparison of ocular hypotensives, a difference in mean IOP reduction of 0.3mmHg at one particular time-point may be statistically significant but most unlikely to translate into clinical benefit.

Question 4: are there other factors that need to be considered?
What other outcomes were reported or should be estimated? This is likely to include side effects, quality of life, costs, etc.

Question 5: are the conclusions of this study locally applicable?
Is the study scenario similar enough to your local situation (e.g. population demographics, potential availability of intervention) to make these results applicable to the patients you see?

Question 6: should we change our practice?
In the final analysis, will the intervention overall benefit your patients (consider side effects, quality of life, etc.)? You may also have to consider the cost–benefit profile in terms of its affordability to either the patient or the health service, depending on local/national health economics.

Clinical guidelines

Aims

Clinical guidelines usually aim to achieve the following:
- Summarize the available evidence for the management of a particular clinical scenario.
- Provide evidence-based recommendations for best management.
- Provide expert consensus recommendations for good practice where evidence is lacking.

Process

The process of guideline development includes:
- The identification of the clinical questions.
- A systematic literature search directed towards answering these questions.
- Selection of evidence according to previously determined inclusion criteria.
- Critical appraisal of the included papers (see ➔ Critical appraisal, p. 1008).
- Formulation of recommendations (graded according to strength of evidence).
- And, if necessary, consensus process to agree 'good practice' in those areas where there is insufficient evidence.

Strength of recommendations

This is based on critical appraisal of the available evidence (see ➔ Critical appraisal, p. 1008). There are a number of grading systems that help identify the level of evidence on which any recommendation is based (Table 26.2).

Table 26.2 Strength of recommendations (SIGN grading system)

Recommendation	Evidence
A	At least one meta-analysis, systematic review, or RCT rated as 1++ and directly applicable to the target population; or
	A systematic review of RCTs or a body of evidence consisting principally of studies rated as 1+, directly applicable to the target population and demonstrating overall consistency of results
B	A body of evidence, including studies rated as 2++, directly applicable to the target population and demonstrating overall consistency of results; or
	Extrapolated evidence from studies rated as 1++ or 1+
C	A body of evidence, including studies rated as 2+, directly applicable to the target population and demonstrating overall consistency of results; or
	Extrapolated evidence from studies rated as 2++
D	Evidence level 3 or 4; or
	Extrapolated evidence from studies rated as 2+

This table should be read in conjunction with Table 26.1. Adapted from Scottish Intercollegiate Network. *SIGN 50: a guideline developer's handbook*, Edinburgh 2008. (Revised 2011). Available at: ✍ http://www.sign.ac.uk. Also see: Harbour R *et al.* A new system for grading recommendations in evidence based guidelines. *BMJ* 2001;323:334–6.

NICE guidelines

In the UK, NICE aims to provide evidence-based guidance to identify which drugs, procedures, and devices provide the best quality care and which offer the best value for money for the NHS. Since its inception in 1999, its remit has expanded to include health promotion and, since April 2013, social care under the provisions of the Health and Social Care Act 2012.

The procedure by which NICE develops its clinical guidelines is as follows:

1. *Guideline topic is referred* to NICE by the Department of Health.
2. *Stakeholders register their interest*, ensuring that patients, carers, health professionals are consulted throughout the process.
3. *The scope of the guideline is prepared* by the appropriate National Collaborating Centre (usually in ophthalmology, this will be the National Clinical Guideline Centre).
4. *The guideline development group is established*, comprising health professionals, representatives of patients/carers groups, and technical experts.
5. *Draft guideline produced*, based on the available evidence and including recommendations.
6. *Consultation*, allowing registered stakeholders to comment on the draft guideline.
7. *Final guideline produced*, by the National Collaborating Centre, based on the recommendations of the guideline development group.
8. *Guidance issued to the NHS*, with formal approval by NICE of the final guideline.

Health care economics

The economic analysis of evidence base is vital in a world where resources within most health care systems are limited. Sometimes termed 'value-based medicine', the application of these analytical tools seeks to quantify the value of an intervention in terms of its benefit in relation to its cost.

Aims

Puts a value on each intervention in relation to its cost; may help to direct allocation of resources.

Tools

Cost minimization analysis

This simply considers which option costs less. It makes the assumption that there is no significant difference in benefit between the two interventions (or that any such difference does not matter). It is therefore very limited.

Cost–benefit analysis

This considers an intervention in terms of economic cost vs 'money saved', e.g. the cost of a cataract operation vs the saving of preventing blindness (work productivity, avoidance of disability costs/social care/health care).

Cost effectiveness analysis

(**NB** Some health economists do not distinguish between cost effectiveness analysis and cost–utility analysis.) This considers an intervention in terms of the cost to achieve a particular end-point, e.g. to attain a VA of ≥6/12.

Cost–utility analysis

(**NB** Some health economists do not distinguish between cost effectiveness analysis and cost–utility analysis.) This considers an intervention in terms of its benefit on length and quality of life. The benefit in terms of length of life is estimated from the literature. Quality of life can either be estimated from questionnaires, such as the National Eye Institute Visual Functioning Questionnaire-25 (NEI VFQ-25), or by utility analysis (see Box 26.3). This provides an estimate of the number of quality-adjusted life years (QALYs) gained by the intervention. This is then compared with the cost associated with the intervention to give the cost–utility analysis, measured in cost/QALY gained (e.g. £/QALY).

Based on these techniques, it has been estimated that:

- Laser therapy for threshold ROP costs about $781/QALY gained.
- Initial cataract surgery costs about $2141/QALY gained.
- PDT for neovascular AMD (6/60 initial VA) costs about $184,423/QALY gained.[1]
- Intravitreal ranibizumab for neovascular AMD (non-classic; based on MARINA with 22 injections over 2y) costs about $50,691/QALY gained in a second eye model (i.e. where vision already lost in the first eye) or $123,887/QALY gained in a first eye model (i.e. normal vision in the other eye).[2]

Box 26.3 **Utility analysis**

If a year of life lived in perfect health = 1 QALY, what is the value of a year of life with impaired vision? Utility analysis tries to put numbers on this by a variety of methods.

Time trade-off technique

Ask the patient:

1. How many more years do you expect to live?
2. How many of your remaining years of your life would you trade to have perfect health (or perfect vision)?

Utility value = 1 − (years traded / years of life expected)

Examples

Using this technique, utility scores for vision have been estimated as follows:[*]

- VA 6/6 (permanent and bilateral) 1.0.
- VA 6/12 (in the better eye) 0.8.
- VA 6/60 (in the better eye) 0.66.
- VA CF (in the better eye) 0.52.
- VA HM (in the better eye) 0.35.
- VA NPL (bilateral) 0.26.

Thus, according to these estimates, 1y of life with bilateral NPL has a value of 0.26 QALYs. Note that this value is derived from judgements made by the patient, rather than by their ophthalmologist.

Other utility estimation techniques

Other methods include the standard gamble and the willingness-to-pay techniques.

[*] Brown MM *et al.* Healthcare economic analyses and value-based medicine. *Surv Ophthalmol* 2003;**48**:204–23.

1. Brown MM *et al.* Healthcare economic analyses and value-based medicine. *Surv Ophthalmol* 2003;**48**:204–23.

2. Brown MM *et al.* A value-based medicine analysis of ranibizumab for the treatment of subfoveal neovascular macular degeneration. *Ophthalmology* 2008;**115**:1039–45.

Patient-reported outcomes (PROs)

Who defines whether a clinical intervention is successful? It is increasingly recognized that the clinical outcome measures that health professionals value so highly (such as VA, VF) fail to capture the full impact of ophthalmic disease on a patient's life. PROs and the tools that measure them (patient-reported outcome measures, PROMs) describe any report or measure of the patient's health that comes directly from the patient without interpretation by a clinician, a researcher, or anyone else. PROMs are an integral part of most modern clinical trials, either as a 1° or 2° outcome. They may measure outcome in absolute terms (e.g. severity of a symptom) or may measure change (e.g. the extent to which a symptom has improved/worsened). PROMs may cover a range of factors such as patients' ability to carry out activities of daily living, psychological welfare, social functioning, perception of health status, sense of stigma, and satisfaction with life. The most appropriate PROM for a study will depend on the study objectives and the target population.

Vision status measures

Visual impairment

These measures relate to the function of vision.

- *Example from the NEI VFQ-25:* 'At the present time, would you say your eyesight using both eyes (with glasses or contact lenses if you wear them) is excellent, good, fair, poor or very poor, or are you completely blind?'[3]

Visual disability

These measures relate to limitations in activities of daily living and social participation.

- *Example from the NEI VFQ-25:* 'Because of your eyesight, how much difficulty do you have finding something on a crowded shelf? No difficulty at all, a little difficulty, moderate difficulty, extreme difficulty, stopped doing this because of your eyesight, stopped doing this for other reasons, or not interested in doing this'

Vision satisfaction measures

Vision-related quality of life

These measures relate to the extent to which these effects bother the individual.

- *Example from the Vision Core Module 1 (VCM1):* 'In the past month, how often has your eyesight stopped you doing the things you want to do? Not at all, very rarely, a little of the time, a fair amount of the time, a lot of the time, or all of the time.'[4]

Generic vs disease-specific tools

Generic tools cover broad aspects of health status and have been designed for use in general populations or across a wide range of disease conditions. They can therefore be used to compare outcomes across conditions. More specific instruments may focus on a key function (such as vision) or disease (such as glaucoma). Advantages include their ability to record issues of importance to a specific population, can be more sensitive to detecting changes over time, and can provide highly specific data to inform and improve clinical practice.

Examples of generic measures include:

- *EuroQoL-5D (EQ-5D)*: five questions covering mobility, self-care, usual activities, pain/discomfort, and anxiety/depression, followed by a global health scale on which the patient marks their own assessment of health state between 0 and 100.[5]
- *Short Form-36 (SF-36)*: 11 questions covering physical functioning, physical health impact on role, bodily pain, general health, vitality, social functioning, emotional health impact on role, and mental health.[6]

Examples of vision-specific measures include:

- *NEI VFQ-25*: 25 questions divided into: (1) general health and vision, (2) difficulty with activities (including items such as close-up work, reading, noticing objects in the peripheral vision, driving a car, matching clothes), and (3) responses to vision problems (including items such as do they feel that they achieve less, do they stay at home, are they embarrassed by their eyesight).
- *VCM1*: ten questions concerning whether visual impairment induces negative feelings (embarrassment, frustration, loneliness, sadness), worry about deterioration, concern about safety or ability to cope, and extent of interference with daily life.

Examples of disease-specific measures

Some conditions, such as glaucoma and cataract, have multiple validated disease-specific PROMs. Most ophthalmic conditions do not yet have robust disease-specific PROMs but may have data supporting the use of more generic tools in these populations.

- *Glaucoma quality of life (Glau-QoL)*: 36 questions assessing sense of well-being, self-image, daily life, burden of treatment, driving, anxiety, and confidence in care.[7]
- *Treatment satisfaction survey for intraocular pressure (TSS-IOP)*: assesses patient's satisfaction with various factors associated with topical medications to control IOP.[7]
- *Catquest-9SF*: nine questions assessing visual impact on specific activities, on daily life, and on satisfaction validated in 10,886 patients.[8]

3. Mangione CM *et al.* Development of the 25-item National Eye Institute Visual Function Questionnaire. *Arch Ophthal* 2001;**119**:1050–8.

4. Frost NA *et al.* Development of a questionnaire for measurement of vision-related quality of life. *Ophthalmic Epidemiol* 1998;**5**:185–210.

5. EuroQol Group. EuroQol--a new facility for the measurement of health-related quality of life. *Health Policy* 1990;**16**:199–208.

6. Brazier JE *et al.* Validating the SF-36 health survey questionnaire: new outcome measure for primary care. *BMJ* 1992;**305**:160–4.

7. Che Hamzah J *et al.* Choosing appropriate patient-reported outcomes instrument for glaucoma research: a systematic review of vision instruments. *Qual Life Res* 2011;**20**:1141–58.

8. Lundström M *et al.* Catquest-9SF patient outcomes questionnaire: nine-item short-form Rasch-scaled revision of the Catquest questionnaire. *J Cataract Refract Surg.* 2009;**35**:504–13.

Statistical terms

Populations and samples
- *Population*: the defined group of interest.
- *Sample*: a selected number of that population who are studied.

Types of statistics

Descriptive statistics
Technique of describing the sample by the use of a typical value (e.g. the median) and its distribution (e.g. the interquartile range).

Inferential statistics
Technique of using statistical analysis of the sample to make inferences about a particular parameter in the population. This includes hypothesis testing and estimation.

Hypothesis testing
Considers whether there is an effect or association of interest. For example, consider the clinical question 'Which of two treatments A or B is more effective at lowering IOP?' The null hypothesis would state that there is no difference in IOP reduction in the two groups, whereas the alternative hypothesis would state that the null hypothesis was false, i.e. that there was a statistically significant difference. Conventionally, a difference is considered significant if the probability of it arising by chance is <5% (i.e. p <0.05).

Estimation
What magnitude of effect would be expected in the actual population? Estimation predicts, from statistical analysis of the sample, the size of the effect to be expected in the population, usually expressed as a 95% confidence interval. This is the range within which there is a 95% probability that the actual effect observed in the population will lie.

Types of variables
The main division is between categorical and numerical variables. The type of variable will dictate which statistical tests are appropriate to the data set.
- *Categorical variables*: variables that have values that can be distinguished from each other but that are qualitative, rather than quantitative. Examples include gender and race.
- *Numerical variables*: quantitative variables that can be measured numerically or to which numbers can be meaningfully assigned. They can be further divided into:
  - *Discrete*: variable can only take certain values (e.g. number of patients).
  - *Continuous*: variable can be measured on a continuous scale (e.g. IOP, duration of operation).

Frequency distribution

Frequency distributions may be normal or skewed. The type of distribution will dictate which statistical tests are appropriate to the data set (see Fig. 26.1).

Normal distribution

Many biological variables (e.g. height) have a 'bell-shaped' or normal (*syn* Gaussian) distribution. These can be described in terms of a mean and SD. If uncertain as to whether a data set is normally distributed, this can be tested, e.g. with the Kolmogorov–Smirnoff test.

Skewed distribution

Some variables (e.g. IOP) have an asymmetric distribution, in which a few very high or very low values result in the distribution being skewed positively or negatively (respectively). Distributions that are not normally distributed are better described in terms of median and interquartile range, rather than in terms of mean and SD.

Independent vs dependent data

If samples are unrelated to each other, they are said to be independent. If samples are related to each other (e.g. VA pre- and post-intervention), then they are described as being dependent. If only two groups of samples are being considered, independent and dependent data are commonly described as 'unpaired' and 'paired', respectively. The independence of the samples will dictate which statistical tests are appropriate for a given data set.

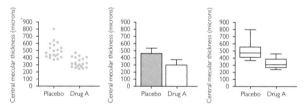

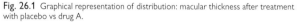

Fig. 26.1 Graphical representation of distribution: macular thickness after treatment with placebo vs drug A.

Graphs of single grouped variables vary in the amount of information they convey. The same data set is illustrated in Fig. 26.1 by three different plots:

A scatter plot retains all information regarding distribution, as it presents all the raw data; it usually lacks any summary statistics, i.e. central tendency (e.g. median) or variability (e.g. interquartile range).

A traditional column or bar chart provides the central tendency (median shown here) and may provide a measure of variability (interquartile range shown here).

Box and whisker plots retain more information, as they contain five summary statistics. The classic box and whisker plot shows the minimum sample value (lower whisker), the lower quartile (base of the box), the median (line within the box), the upper quartile (top of the box), and the maximum sample value (higher whisker). One of the advantages of the box and whisker plot is that it is easy to visualize the degree to which data are skewed. Variations of the box and whisker plot include variations in the values of the whiskers (e.g. may represent SD or alternative centiles) and variable width boxes to represent the size of the sample population.

Statistical tests

The types of statistical tests undertaken will be dictated by the nature of the data: type of variable (categorical, numerical), its distribution (normal or skewed), and whether the samples are independent or dependent.

Statistical tests for categorical data

Categorical data can be conveniently described by a contingency table (see Table 26.3). Hypothesis testing is with either chi-squared (χ^2) or Fisher's Exact test.

Chi-squared test

Commonly used test for categorical data, it compares observed and expected frequencies of mutually exclusive events. Actual numbers, not percentages, should be used; all expected values should be >1, and 80% should be >5.

Yates' correction helps adjust for smaller sample sizes and should generally be used for all chi-squared tests.

Fisher's Exact test

Similar to the chi-squared test but more robust for small sample sizes. It should be used when the above conditions cannot be met.

Table 26.3 Example of categorical data that can be described in a 2 × 2 contingency table

		Outcome	
		Anatomical closure of macular hole	
		Success	Failure
Intervention	Vitrectomy with platelets	a	b
	Vitrectomy alone	c	d

Having constructed a 2 × 2 contingency table, the possible association of the use of platelets with improved surgical success can be tested by the chi-squared or Fisher's Exact tests.

Statistical tests for continuous data

Test selection will depend on the distribution of the data, whether values in the two data sets are paired, and whether testing for a difference (or lack of) between groups or testing for correlation between the groups.

- *Parametric tests*: assume that the data are normally distributed (see ➔ Statistical terms, p. 1016).
- *Non-parametric tests*: make no assumptions about the distribution of the data, sometimes termed 'distribution-free'.

It is important to use a test appropriate to the number of groups being considered. For example, one cannot sequentially apply the *t*-test to multiple groups to look for 'any' significant difference; applying such a test in this way greatly increases the chance of erroneously finding a 'statistically significant' difference (i.e. a type I error) (see Table 26.4).

Table 26.4 Common statistical tests used for continuous data

	Parametric	Non-parametric
Tests on two groups		
Paired data	Paired *t*-test	Wilcoxon test
Unpaired data	Unpaired *t*-test	Mann–Whitney *U* test
Correlation	Pearson's test	Spearman's rank test
Tests on >2 groups		
Dependent data	Repeated measures ANOVA	Friedman test
Independent data	One-way ANOVA	Kruskal–Wallis test

Linear and logistic regression

Linear regression

Linear regression builds a model that describes the relationship between one or more independent (or predictor) variables and a single continuous dependent (or outcome) variable. At its simplest, it describes the relationship between the dependent variable (y) and the independent variable (x) as a linear equation:

$$y = a + bx$$

(where a and b are constants.)

- Simple linear regression determines the best equation to predict Y from a single variable X; both variables must be continuous.
- Multiple linear regression finds the equation that best predicts Y from multiple independent variables. You would consider this approach when there are several independent (predictor) variables (e.g. X_1, X_2, X_3) and a single continuous dependent variable (e.g. Y); predictor variables may be continuous or categorical.

Logistic regression

Logistic regression quantifies the association between a risk factor (or treatment) and a disease (or any event), after adjusting for other variables. Whereas, in multiple linear regression, it is the value of the continuous variable (e.g. IOP) that can be predicted from two or more predictor variables (e.g. age, gender, time of day), in logistic regression, it is the probability of obtaining one of the outcomes (e.g. the chance of being alive 1y after phacoemulsification) that can be predicted.

Risks, odds, and number needed to treat (NNT)

Absolute and relative risk

Absolute risk describes the likelihood of an event occurring in one particular group. Relative risk (or risk ratio) compares the likelihood of an event occurring in two groups. A relative risk of 1 means that there is no difference between the two groups. Relative risk is the preferred method of expressing likelihood in RCTs and cohort studies (see Table 26.5).

Relative risk = Risk of event on treatment / Risk of event in control group
$$= (a / [a + b]) / (c / [c + d])$$

Table 26.5 Risk table

		Outcome	
		Event occurs	No event
Intervention	Treatment group	a	b
	Control group	c	d

NB The 'event' may be beneficial (e.g. surgical success) or harmful (e.g. drug side effect).

Odds ratio

The odds ratio compares the odds of an event occurring in two groups. An odds ratio of 1 means that there is no difference between the two groups. Odds ratios are the preferred method of expressing likelihood in case-control studies and retrospective studies.

Odds ratio = Odds of event on treatment / Odds of event in control group
$$= (a / b) / (c / d)$$

NNT

NNT or number needed to harm (NNH) describes the number of people that must be treated in order for one beneficial (or harmful) event to occur. It is derived from the absolute risk reduction (ARR).

ARR = Risk of event in control group – Risk of event on treatment
$$= (c / [c + d]) - (a / [a + b])$$

NNT = 1/ARR

Statistical issues relating to two eyes

The 'two-eye' problem

The classical 'two-eye' problem is that observations from left and right eyes will tend to be correlated. If data from both eyes are pooled, this will violate an important assumption of hypothesis testing, namely, that these are independent observations. However, dealing with this issue is problematic. For conditions that are equally likely to affect either eye, analyses based on either right or left eyes, or on a randomly selected eye, are statistically equivalent. If information has been collected on both eyes, then half of the data will be unused. In addition, bias may be introduced if there is non-random selection of the eye for inclusion in the analysis. This would also apply to the choice of the first eye with disease, better/worse eye, or operated eye.

Averaging results from right and left eyes also results in a loss of information and would not be appropriate for studies that operate at the ocular level, e.g. the impact of topical treatment or ocular surgery.

Solutions to the 'two-eye' problem

In dealing with the 'two-eye' problem, it is important to take account of between-eye correlation. In statistical terms, the 'two-eye' problem is an example of clustered data where the maximum cluster size is always 2 (at least in humans). Many different univariate and multivariate approaches to this problem have been suggested. The degree of between-eye correlation can be assessed by calculating the kappa statistic. If there is little or no correlation between eyes, the kappa statistic will be close to zero. If the kappa statistic is greater than about 0.3, then between-eye correlation is likely to be an important problem. In one recent survey, it was noted that over 40% of relevant ophthalmic research papers failed to address this issue.[9] Statistical techniques exist that can utilize all available data while allowing for the correlation.[9,10]

There are of course occasions where the 'two-eye' problem can be useful, such as where the second eye can be used as a control in a paired comparison of unilateral treatment such as in the Diabetic Retinopathy Study.[11]

9. Karakosta A et al. Choice of analytic approach for eye-specific outcomes: one eye or two? Am J Ophthalmol 2012;**153**:571–9.

10. Murdoch I et al. People and eyes: statistical approaches in ophthalmology. Br J Ophthalmol 1998;**82**:971–3.

11. The Diabetic Retinopathy Study Research Group. Photocoagulation treatment of proliferative diabetic retinopathy: the second report from the Diabetic Retinopathy Study. Arch Ophthalmol 1978;**85**:82–106.

Investigations

The process of clinical assessment—comprising history, examination, and investigation—is directed towards reaching a diagnosis. During this process, we acquire a wealth of clinical data that we process, often subconsciously, to narrow down the diagnosis. The usefulness of each symptom, sign, and investigation in predicting a particular diagnosis can be described statistically by its sensitivity, specificity, positive predictive value (PPV), and negative predictive value (NPV).

Sensitivity and specificity are performance measures of a particular test, whereas PPV and NPV give the post-test probabilities of disease/health and so are affected by disease prevalence (i.e. the proportion of the population with that condition).

Sensitivity and specificity

Sensitivity

This is the 'pick-up' or how good a test is at being positive in disease (true positive; see Table 26.6). This is the number of people in whom the test correctly predicts disease as a proportion of the number of people who do have the disease, i.e.

Sensitivity = True positive / (True positive + False negative)

Specificity

This is how good the test is at being negative in the healthy (true negative; see Table 26.6). This is the number of people in whom the test correctly predicts no disease as a proportion of the number of people who do not have the disease, i.e.

Specificity = True negative / (False positive + True negative)

PPV and NPV

PPV

This indicates what proportion of people with a positive test do in fact have the disease. It is helpful in interpreting the significance of a positive test result. It is, however, affected by the prevalence of a particular condition. A test with a high PPV will be useful for confirming a particular condition.

PPV = True positive / (True positive + False positive)

NPV

This indicates what proportion of people with a negative test are in fact free from the disease. Like the PPV, it will be affected by disease prevalence. A test with a high NPV will be useful for ruling out a particular condition.

NPV = True negative / (True negative + False negative)

Table 26.6 Sensitivity and specificity depend on the rate of true positives and true negatives in their respective populations

Test result	Patients have disease	Patients do not have disease
Test is positive	True +ve	False +ve
Test is negative	False −ve	True −ve

Bayesian vs frequentist approaches

Our usual approach to trial design is based on the null hypothesis: 'there is no difference between A and B'(see ➲ The null and the alternative hypotheses, p. 1006). The difference is considered significant (i.e. the null hypothesis is rejected) if the probability of it arising by chance is <5% (i.e. p <0.05). This is based on a 'frequentist' approach to probability, in which one considers the experiment (such as a clinical trial) to be one of an infinite number of repetitions of the same experiment and defines an event's probability, based on its relative frequency in those hypothetical repetitions of the experiment.

A Bayesian approach to experiments actively utilizes prior knowledge and allows the outcome of earlier experiments to inform subsequent ones. Specifically, Bayes' theorem relates the probabilities from previous knowledge (the prior distribution) to the probabilities recalculated after the experiment (posterior distribution). The 'posterior' probability is the estimate of the probability of the hypothesis being true, based on the result of the experiment (the data) but taking the prior knowledge into account. A key tenet of a Bayesian approach to clinical trials is that the prior information (e.g. from earlier studies) and the trial results are part of a continuous stream of data and that inferences may be continually revised as new data emerge.

In their Guidance for the Use of Bayesian Statistics in Medical Device Clinical Trials,[12] the FDA points out the following potential advantages and disadvantages of a Bayesian approach to trial design (see Box 26.4).

Advantages

More information for decision making

The use of relevant prior data may inform the process and increase the precision of the Bayesian estimate.

Sample size reduction via prior information

The use of prior information may reduce the estimated sample size required.

Sample size reduction via adaptive trial design

A Bayesian approach provides greater flexibility during the trial, permitting an 'adaptive' design. The cumulative data are continually assessed and can be used, according to pre-specified determinants, to direct aspects of the trial. For example, the trial may be stopped early if certain conditions are met (either success or failure).

Mid-course changes via adaptive trial design

A Bayesian approach can also offer the flexibility of changes midway through a trial, notably dropping an unfavourable treatment arm or altering the randomization scheme (i.e. the treatment to control ratio). The latter is particularly relevant for an ethically sensitive study, since it 'adapts' to promote recruitment to the superior arm(s) of the study.

Other potential benefits

Other potential advantages include the possibility of an exact Bayesian analysis (vs an approximate frequentist analysis), greater flexibility in dealing with missing data and in dealing with multiplicity (end-points and/or subgroups).

Disadvantages

Extensive preplanning

In addition to the critical elements of standard trial design (protocol, conduct, and analysis), a Bayesian approach requires the following additional elements to be defined:

- The prior information,
- The data to be collected from the trial, and
- The mathematical model used to combine the two.

The prior information is critical to the final result, so advance agreement of its validity (e.g. with regulatory authorities) is recommended.

Extensive model building

Extensive mathematical modelling may be recommended to support the trial design, including aspects relating to prior information, patient outcomes, missing data, and sensitivity analyses on the model choices. Again, advance agreement of the validity of these models is recommended.

Specific statistical and computational expertise

Although Bayesian theory has been around for several centuries, it is only with the support of computers that the statistical aspects of a Bayesian trial analysis have been possible. A Bayesian approach does require more highly skilled statistical and computational support than the standard frequentist design.

Box 26.4 I-SPY-2: a case study of an adaptive trial*

One of the most dramatic examples of an adaptive trial design is I-SPY-2, a phase II rolling drug-screening programme to test new therapies for breast cancer. The trial has six treatment arms, including an arm for standard therapy. Randomization is adaptive so that the probability of being assigned to a particular treatment arm increases if the outcome of the prior patients in the group is good. As the trial progresses, the treatment arms are replaced either because (1) they show sufficient success to graduate to a smaller, focused phase III study or (2) they show lack of benefit and are terminated. The more successful a drug, the faster it will move through the screening process. It also means that trial participants will tend to receive the more effective treatments. Fewer patients are required (per drug outcome), and it is predicted to be significantly cheaper than standard single drug non-adaptive designs. Up to 12 drugs will be tested through the I-SPY-2 programme. If successful, I-SPY-2 could head a major new chapter in our approach to clinical trials.

* Berry DA. Adaptive clinical trials in oncology. *Nat Rev Clin Oncol* 2012;9:199–207.

12. US Food and Drug Administration. *Guidance for the use of Bayesian statistics in medical device clinical trials.* (2010). Available at: ℜ http://www.fda.gov/medicaldevices/deviceregulationandguidance/guidancedocuments/ucm071072.htm

Resources

Eponymous syndromes

Aarskog syndrome XL; megalocornea, hypertelorism, antimongoloid palpebral fissures; short stature, syndactyly.

Aicardi syndrome Probably XL; lethal to ♂; corpus callosal agenesis and other CNS abnormalities, infantile spasms, mental retardation, vertebral and rib malformations; chorioretinal lacunar defects, colobomas.

Albright syndrome Disorder of G-proteins resulting in polyostotic fibrous dysplasia (of bone), endocrine abnormalities (including precocious puberty) and café-au-lait spots; orbital involvement may cause proptosis, sinus mucoceles, and compressive optic neuropathy.

Alagille syndrome AD (Chr 20); posterior embryotoxon, optic disc drusen, pale fundi, hypertelorism; intrahepatic bile duct hypoplasia, butterfly vertebrae, congenital heart disease.

Alport syndrome Disorder of type IV collagen; XD but autosomal inheritance described; anterior lenticonus, anterior polar, and cortical cataracts, fleck retina; sensorineural deafness, nephritis.

Alström–Olsen syndrome AR; cone–rod dystrophy with features of RP, posterior subcapsular cataracts; diabetes mellitus, sensorineural deafness, nephropathy, obesity, acanthosis nigricans.

Anderson–Fabry disease See Fabry's disease.

Apert syndrome AD or sporadic; gene encoding the fibroblast growth factor receptor 2 (Chr 10q26); craniosynostosis, syndactyly, broad distal phalanx of great thumb/toe, mental handicap; hypertelorism, proptosis, strabismus, keratoconus, ectopia lentis, congenital glaucoma, optic atrophy.

Arnold–Chiari malformation Congenital herniation of the cerebellum/brainstem through the foramen magnum may cause hydrocephalus, cerebellar signs (e.g. nystagmus, ataxia)., and may be associated with syringomyelia.

Bardet–Biedl and Laurence–Moon syndromes AR overlapping conditions; RP with early macular involvement; polydactyly, hypogonadism, obesity, microcephaly, nephropathy, ↓IQ.

Batten disease (neuronal ceroid lipofuscinosis) AR metabolic disorder resulting in neurodegeneration. Juvenile form: bull's eye maculopathy, pigmentary retinopathy, optic atrophy, epilepsy, life expectancy <25y.

Bassen–Kornzweig (abetalipoproteinaemia) AR deficiency of triglyceride transfer protein; RP, cataract; spinocerebellar degeneration, steatorrhoea, acanthosis (of erythrocytes).

Bloch–Sulzberger syndrome (incontinentia pigmenti) XD, lethal to ♂; abnormal peripheral retinal vasculature, gliosis, TRD; abnormal teeth, cutaneous pigment whorls, and CNS anomalies.

Bourneville disease (tuberous sclerosis) AD (Chr 9q TSC1 and Chr 16p TSC2), phakomatosis with neurocutaneous features and retinal astrocytomas.

Brown syndrome Mechanical restriction syndrome attributed to the SO tendon sheath.

Caffrey disease Hyperplasia of subperiosteal bone and proptosis.

Cogan syndrome Idiopathic, probably autoimmune; interstitial keratitis, sensorineural deafness, tinnitus, vertigo, systemic vasculitis (including life-threatening aortitis).

Crouzon syndrome AD or sporadic; gene encoding the fibroblast growth factor receptor 2 (Chr 10q26); craniosynostosis, maxillary hypoplasia, prognathism, hooked nose; proptosis, strabismus, micro-/megalo-cornea, iris coloboma, cataract, ectopia lentis, glaucoma.

De Morsier syndrome Optic nerve hypoplasia; midline brain abnormalities, including absent septum pellucidum and corpus callosal hypo-/aplasia.

Down's syndrome Trisomy 21; 1 in 650 live births; blepharitis, keratoconus, cataracts; musculoskeletal abnormalities, congenital heart disease, ↓IQ.

Duane syndrome Aberrant coinnervation of LR and MR, resulting in horizontal gaze anomalies.

Edwards' syndrome Trisomy 18; 1 in 8,000 live births; microphthalmos, glaucoma, cataracts; failure to thrive, congenital heart disease; life expectancy <1y.

Fabry's disease XL; α-galactosidase A deficiency results in glycosphingolipid accumulation; vortex keratopathy, cataracts (posterior cortical and granular), conjunctival and retinal telangiectasia; peripheral neuropathy with painful 'Fabry crises', renal failure, angiokeratoma corporis diffusum, lymphoedema.

Foster–Kennedy syndrome Ipsilateral optic atrophy due to compressive optic neuropathy, with contralateral disc swelling from ↑ICP.

Foville syndrome Lesion of lateral pons, resulting in ipsilateral facial paresis, horizontal gaze palsy (towards side of lesion), and a contralateral hemiparesis.

Friedreich's ataxia AR; triplet repeat expansion (GAA) of non-coding region of the frataxin gene (Chr 9); degeneration of spinocerebellar tracts (ataxia, dysarthria, nystagmus), corticospinal tracts (weakness, extensor plantars), posterior columns (proprioception), and peripheral neuropathy (with absent tendon reflexes), pes cavus.

Gardner's syndrome Variant of familial adenomatous polyposis (AD) with bone cysts, hamartomas, and soft tissue tumours; atypical CHRPE.

Gaucher's disease AR; β-glucosidase deficiency; visceromegaly (type I) or neurodegeneration (type II or III); supranuclear palsy (type IIIb).

Gerstmann's syndrome Dominant parietal lobe lesion, resulting in finger agnosia, right/left confusion, dysgraphia, acalculia; may be associated with failure of ipsilateral pursuit movements.

Gillespie syndrome Variant of aniridia (*PAX-6* mutation) with mental retardation and cerebellar ataxia.

Goldenhar syndrome Part of the spectrum of hemifacial microsomia; accessory auricle, limbal dermoid, hypoplasia of face, vertebral anomaly. corneal hyposthesia. Duane syndrome, iris and upper eyelid coloboma.

Goldman–Favre disease AR; optically empty vitreous, retinoschisis, macular changes, peripheral pigmentary retinopathy.

Gorlin syndrome AD (tumour suppressor gene *PATCHED*; Chr 9q); multiple BCCs, jaw cysts, skeletal abnormalities, ectopic calcification (e.g. falx cerebri); hypertelorism, prominent supraorbital ridges.

Gradenigo syndrome VIn palsy and pain in Vn distribution due to lesion at the apex of the petrous temporal bone; this may be related to chronic middle ear infection.

Gronblad–Strandberg syndrome Angioid streaks with PXE.

Hallermann–Streiff–François syndrome Microphthalmos, cataract, hypotrichosis, blue sclera; dyscephaly, short stature.

Heerfordt syndrome (uveoparotid fever) Presentation of sarcoidosis with fever, parotid enlargement, uveitis.

Hermansky–Pudlak syndrome Type II oculocutaneous albinism with platelet dysfunction, pulmonary fibrosis, granulomatous colitis.

Kasabach–Merritt syndrome Giant haemangioma with localized intravascular coagulation causing low platelets and fibrinogen.

Kearns–Sayre syndrome Mitochondrial inheritance; CPEO, pigmentary retinopathy (granular pigmentation, PPA) and heart block; usually presents before 20y.

Laurence–Moon syndrome Grouped with Bardet–Biedl syndrome but no obesity or polydactyly.

Leber's congenital amaurosis AR; blind from birth, eye poking (oculodigital sign), hypermetropia, sluggish or paradoxical pupillary reflexes, macular dysplasia but fairly normal fundal appearance.

Leber's hereditary optic neuropathy Mitochondrial inheritance; rapid sequential visual loss in 20–30s due to optic neuropathy.

Löfgren syndrome Presentation of sarcoidosis with fever, erythema nodosum, bihilar lymphadenopathy.

Louis–Bar syndrome (ataxia telangiectasia) AR (Chr 11q, *ATM* gene); conjunctival telangiectasia, progressive oculomotor apraxia; cerebellar ataxia, ↓IQ, immunodeficiency.

Lowe syndrome (oculocerebrorenal syndrome) XL disorder of amino acid metabolism; congenital cataract, microspherophakia, blue sclera, anterior segment dysgenesis, glaucoma; ↓IQ, hypotonia, vitamin D-resistant rickets.

Maffuci syndrome Multiple haemangiomas and enchondromas (which may cause limb deformities), with risk of malignant transformation.

Marfan's syndrome AD (Chr 15, fibrillin); ectopia lentis, retinal detachment, glaucoma, axial myopia; arachnodactyly, long-limbed, aortic dissection.

Meckel–Gruber syndrome AR; coloboma; microcephaly, occipital encephalocele, cleft lip/palate, polydactyly, polycystic kidney disease.

Menke disease XR deficiency of copper transport protein; optic atrophy, retinal dystrophy; wiry hair, ataxia, neurodegeneration.

Mikulicz syndrome Infiltrative swelling of salivary and lacrimal glands.

Millard–Gubler syndrome Lesion of the facial colliculus (dorsal pons), resulting in ipsilateral VIn and VIIn palsies ± contralateral hemiparesis.

Miller–Fisher syndrome Variant of Guillain–Barré syndrome characterized by acute external ophthalmoplegia, ataxia, and areflexia.

Moebius syndrome Congenital facial paresis with ipsilateral abducens palsy. Other cranial nerves may be affected.

Niemann–Pick disease AR; deficiency of sphingomyelinase; type A is infantile onset with visceromegaly, neurodegeneration and cherry-red spot; type B juvenile onset with visceromegaly, rarely cherry red spot; type C has variable onset, vertical supranuclear gaze palsy, ataxia, and neurodegeneration.

Norrie disease XL; retinal dysplasia, retinal detachment, leucocoria, vitreous haemorrhage, cataract, phthisis; ↓IQ, deafness.

Oguchi disease AR; non-progressive nyctalopia (CSNB), pseudotapetal reflex which normalizes with dark adaptation (Mizuo phenomenon).

Parinaud syndrome Lesion of dorsal midbrain, resulting in light-near dissociation, supranuclear upgaze palsy, convergence retraction nystagmus, and failure of convergence and accommodation.

Patau syndrome Trisomy 13; 1 in 14,000 live births; cyclopia, colobomas, retinal dysplasia; microcephaly; life expectancy <3mo.

Raymond syndrome Lesion of the corticospinal tract in the ventral pons, resulting in VIn palsy and contralateral hemiparesis.

Refsum disease AR; deficiency of phytanic acid α-hydrolase results in accumulation of phytanic acid; pigmentary retinopathy, optic atrophy; ichthyosis, deafness, cardiomyopathy, ataxia.

Riley–Day syndrome (familial dysautonomia) AR; commoner in Ashkenazi Jews; tear deficiency → KCS, commonly with ulceration, reduced corneal sensation; sensory neuropathy, autonomic dysfunction/crises.

Rubinstein–Taybi syndrome (otopalatodigital syndrome) Developmental abnormality; hypertelorism, colobomas; broad thumbs/big toes, maxillary/mandibular hypoplasia, hypertrichosis, ↓IQ.

Sandhoff disease AR (Chr 5q, *HEXB*); GM2 gangliosidosis with deficiency of hexosaminadase A and B; cherry red spot, optic atrophy; splenomegaly, neurodegeneration.

Sjögren's syndrome Autoimmune condition affecting up to 4% of population; inflammation of lacrimal and salivary glands → dry eyes (may be severe and lead to cicatrization) and dry mouth; can be 1° or 2° to conditions such as RA and SLE; diagnosis supported by anti-Ro (SS-A), anti-La (SS-B), and parotid gland US; labial gland biopsy; ↑risk of B-cell lymphoma.

Stargardt disease (and fundus flavimaculatus) AR (usually Chr 1p, ABCA4); commonest of the macular dystrophies with two clinical presentations: Stargardt's ('beaten-bronze' atrophy, yellowish flecks of the posterior pole, significant dVA) and fundus flavimaculatus (widespread pisciform flecks with relative preservation of vision).

Steele–Richardson–Olszewski (progressive supranuclear palsy) Neurodegenerative disease of the elderly; supranuclear vertical gaze; postural instability, parkinsonism, pseudobulbar palsy, and dementia.

Stickler syndrome (hereditary arthro-ophthalmopathy) AD (Chr 12q, *COL2A1*); abnormality of type II collagen; high myopia, optically empty vitreous, retinal detachments, cataract, ectopia lentis, glaucoma; arthropathy, Pierre–Robin sequence (micrognathia, high arched/cleft palate), sensorineural deafness, mitral valve prolapse.

Sturge–Weber syndrome Phakomatosis with port-wine stain of the face, with ocular and CNS haemangiomas.

Tay–Sachs disease AR (Chr 15q, *HEXA*); GM2 gangliosidosis with deficiency of hexosaminadase A; cherry red spot, optic atrophy; neurodegeneration.

Treacher Collins syndrome (mandibulofacial dysostosis) AD; 'treacle gene' *TCOF1* (Chr 5q32); clefting syndrome; antimongoloid palpebral fissures, lower lid colobomas, dermoids; mandibular hypoplasia, zygoma hypoplasia, choanal atresia.

Turcot syndrome Variant of familial adenomatous polyposis (AD) with CNS neuroepithelial tumours, especially medulloblastoma and glioma; atypical CHRPE.

Turner's syndrome XO; 1 in 2,000 live ♀ births; antimongoloid palpebral fissures, cataracts, convergence insufficiency; short stature, wide carrying angle, low hair line, webbed neck, 1° gonadal failure, congenital heart defects.

Vogt–Koyanagi–Harada syndrome Multisystem inflammatory disease; bilateral granulomatous panuveitis; vitiligo, alopecia, deafness, tinnitus, sterile meningoencephalitis, and cranial neuropathies.

von Hippel–Lindau AD (Chr 3p, *VHL* gene); phakomatosis with retinal capillary haemangiomas, CNS haemangioblastomas, renal cell carcinomas, and other tumours.

Waardenburg syndrome AD (*PAX3*); heterochromia, hypertelorism; white forelock, deafness.

Wallenberg syndrome (lateral medullary syndrome) Lesion of the lateral medulla (typically posterior inferior cerebellar artery occlusion), resulting in ipsilateral Horner's syndrome, ipsilateral cerebellar signs, ipsilateral palatal paralysis, ipsilateral decreased facial sensation (pain and temperature), contralateral decreased somatic sensation (pain and temperature).

Walker–Warburg syndrome AR; retinal dysplasia; muscular dystrophy, Dandy–Walker malformation.

Weber syndrome Upper midbrain lesion, causing ipsilateral oculomotor paralysis (with loss of reaction to light and accommodation) with contralateral hemiparesis.

Weill–Marchesani syndrome AR; ectopia lentis, microspherophakia, retinal detachment, anomalous angles; short stature, brachydactyly, ↓IQ.

Wildervanck syndrome Klippel–Feil malformation (short neck due to cervical vertebrae anomalies) with deafness and Duane syndrome.

Wyburn–Mason syndrome Phakomatosis with AVMs of retina, orbit, and CNS.

Zellweger syndrome (cerebrohepatorenal syndrome) AR; severe end of a spectrum of peroxisomal disorders which includes neonatal adrenoleukodystrophy and infantile Refsum disease; cataract, optic nerve hypoplasia, pigmentary retinopathy, corneal clouding; high forehead, flat brows; life expectancy <1y.

Web resources for ophthalmologists (1)

Ophthalmic and related associations
(See Box 27.1.)

Box 27.1 Ophthalmic and related associations

American Academy of Ophthalmology
↪ http://www.aao.org

Association for Research in Vision and Ophthalmology
↪ http://www.arvo.org

American Association for Pediatric Ophthalmology and Strabismus
↪ http://www.aapos.org

American Society of Cataract and Refractive Surgery
↪ http://www.ascrs.org

British Association of Retinal Screening
↪ http://www.eyescreening.org.uk

British Contact Lens Association
↪ http://www.bcla.org.uk

British and Eire Association of Vitreoretinal Surgeons
↪ http://www.beavrs.org

British Oculoplastic Surgery Society
↪ http://www.bopss.co.uk

British Ophthalmic Anaesthesia Society
↪ http://www.boas.org

British and Irish Orthoptic Society
↪ http://www.orthoptics.org.uk

British Society for Refractive Surgery
↪ http://www.bsrs.co.uk

Club Jules Gonin
↪ http://www.clubjulesgonin.com

College of Optometrists
↪ http://www.college-optometrists.org

European Association for Vision and Eye Research
↪ http://www.ever.be

European University Professors of Ophthalmology
↪ http://www.eupo.eu

European Neuro-Ophthalmological Society
↪ http://www.eunosweb.org

European Society of Cataract and Refractive Surgeons
↪ http://www.escrs.org

European Society of Ophthalmic Plastic and Reconstructive Surgery
 http://www.esoprs.eu

European Society of Ophthalmology
 http://www.soevision.org

European Society of Retina Specialists
 http://www.euretina.org

Institute of Ophthalmology
 http://www.ucl.ac.uk/ioo

International Council of Ophthalmology
 http://www.icoph.org

International Ocular Inflammation Society
 http://www.iois.memberlodge.org

International Society for Clinical Electrophysiology of Vision
 http://www.iscev.org

International Society of Refractive Surgery
 http://www.aao.org/isrs

International Uveitis Study Group
 http://www.iusg.net

Medical Contact Lens and Ocular Surface Association
 http://www.mclosa.org.uk

Moorfields Eye Hospital
 http://www.moorfields.nhs.uk

Ocular Immunology and Uveitis Foundation
 http://www.uveitis.org

Ophthalmic Imaging Association
 http://www.oia.org.uk

ORBIS International
 http://www.orbis.org

Oxford Ophthalmological Congress
 http://www.oxford-ophthalmological-congress.org.uk

Royal Society of Medicine—Ophthalmology Section
 http://www.rsm.ac.uk/academ/smtophth.php

Scottish Ophthalmological Club
 http://www.s-o-c.org.uk

United Kingdom and Ireland Society of Cataract and Refractive Surgeons
 http://www.ukiscrs.org.uk

Medical Colleges (UK)
(See Box 27.2.)

Box 27.2 Medical Colleges (UK)

The College of Emergency Medicine
🕮 http://www.collemergencymed.ac.uk

The Royal College of Anaesthetists
🕮 http://www.rcoa.ac.uk

The Royal College of General Practitioners
🕮 http://www.rcgp.org.uk

The Royal College of Obstetricians and Gynaecologists
🕮 http://www.rcog.org.uk

The Royal College of Ophthalmologists
🕮 http://www.rcophth.ac.uk

The Royal College of Paediatrics and Child Health
🕮 http://www.rcpch.ac.uk

The Royal College of Pathologists
🕮 http://www.rcpath.org

The Royal College of Physicians
🕮 http://www.rcplondon.ac.uk

The Royal College of Physicians of Edinburgh
🕮 http://www.rcpe.ac.uk

The Royal College of Physicians and Surgeons of Glasgow
🕮 http://www.rcpsg.ac.uk

The Royal College of Psychiatrists
🕮 http://www.rcpsych.ac.uk

The Royal College of Radiologists
🕮 http://www.rcr.ac.uk

The Royal College of Surgeons of Edinburgh
🕮 http://www.rcsed.ac.uk

The Royal College of Surgeons of England
🕮 http://www.rcseng.ac.uk

The Royal College of Surgeons in Ireland
🕮 http://www.rcsi.ie

Other professional bodies and defence organizations
(See Box 27.3.)

Box 27.3 Other professional bodies and defence organizations

Academy of Medical Royal Colleges
  🖱 http://www.aomrc.org.uk

Association of Surgeons in Training
  🖱 http://www.asit.org

British Medical Association
  🖱 http://www.bma.org.uk

General Medical Council
  🖱 http://www.gmc-uk.org

Medical Defence Union
  🖱 http://www.themdu.com

Medical and Dental Defence Union of Scotland
  🖱 http://www.mddus.com

Medical Protection Society
  🖱 http://www.medicalprotection.org

Neither the authors nor Oxford University Press are responsible for the content of any the websites listed.

Web resources for ophthalmologists (2)

Training and career issues
(See Box 27.4.)

Box 27.4 Training and career issues

BMJ Careers
   🔗 http://careers.bmj.com

NHS Jobs
   🔗 http://www.jobs.nhs.uk

British Medical Association
   🔗 http://www.bma.org.uk

General Medical Council
   🔗 http://www.gmc-uk.org

Royal College of Ophthalmologists
   🔗 http://www.rcophth.ac.uk

ePortfolio for the Royal College of Ophthalmologists
   🔗 http:portfolio.rcophth.ac.uk

Curriculum for Ophthalmic Specialist Training (OSTs)
   🔗 http:curriculum.rcophth.ac.uk

Web resources for ophthalmologists (3)

Journals
(See Box 27.5.)

Box 27.5 Journals

Ophthalmic

Acta Ophthalmologica
 http://www.onlinelibrary.wiley.com/journal/10.1111/
(ISSN)1755-3768

American Journal of Ophthalmology
 http://www.ajo.com

BMC Ophthalmology
 http://www.biomedcentral.com/bmcophthalmol

British Journal of Ophthalmology
 http://bjo.bmj.com

Clinical and Experimental Ophthalmology
 http://www.onlinelibrary.wiley.com/journal/10.1111/
(ISSN)1442-9071

Cornea
 http://www.corneajrnl.com

Current Opinion In Ophthalmology
 http://www.co-ophthalmology.com

Experimental Eye Research
 http://www.journals.elsevier.com/experimental-eye-research

Eye
 http://www.nature.com/eye

Eye News
 http://www.eyenews.uk.com

Graefe's Archive for Clinical and Experimental Ophthalmology
 http://http://link.springer.com/journal/417

Investigative Ophthalmology & Visual Science
 http://www.iovs.org

JAMA Ophthalmology
 http://archopht.jamanetwork.com/journal.aspx

Journal of Cataract & Refractive Surgery
 http://www.jcrsjournal.org

Journal of Glaucoma
 http://www.glaucomajournal.com

Journal of Neuro-Ophthalmology
 http://www.jneuro-ophthalmology.com

Box 27.5 (*Cont.*)

Ophthalmic (contd.)

Journal of Vision
   🖑 http://www.journalofvision.org/*Molecular Vision*
   🖑 http://www.molvis.org/molvis/about.html

The Ocular Surface
   🖑 http://www.journals.elsevier.com/the-ocular-surface

Ophthalmic Epidemiology
   🖑 http://informahealthcare.com/loi/ope

Ophthalmic and Physiological Optics
   🖑 http://www.onlinelibrary.wiley.com/journal/10.1111/
(ISSN)1475-1313

Ophthalmology
   🖑 http://www.aaojournal.org

Optometry and Vision Science
   🖑 http://journals.lww.com/optvissci/pages/default.aspx

Progress in Retinal and Eye Research
   🖑 http://www.journals.elsevier.com/
progress-in-retinal-and-eye-research

Retina
   🖑 http://www.retinajournal.com

Survey of Ophthalmology
   🖑 http://www.surveyophthalmol.com

Vision Research
   🖑 http://www.journals.elsevier.com/vision-research

General

British Medical Journal
   🖑 http://www.bmj.com

Nature
   🖑 http://www.nature.com

New England Journal of Medicine
   🖑 http://www.nejm.org

The Lancet
   🖑 http://www.thelancet.com

Other medical resources
(See Box 27.6.)

Box 27.6 Other medical resources

PubMed and MEDLINE
 ⌖ http://www.pubmed.com

Cochrane Eyes and Vision Group
 ⌖ http://www.cochraneeyes.org

ClinicalEvidence
 ⌖ http://www.clinicalevidence.com

Doctors net
 ⌖ http://www.doctors.net.uk

Medscape
 ⌖ http://www.emedicine.medscape.com

EMBASE
 ⌖ http://www.embase.com

Ovid
 ⌖ http://www.ovid.com

Web of Knowledge
 ⌖ http://wokinfo.com

Google Scholar
 ⌖ http://scholar.google.com

Internet Ophthalmology
 ⌖ http://www.ophthal.org

National Audit Office
 ⌖ http://www.nao.org.uk

Evidence Search Health and Social Care
 ⌖ http://www.evidence.nhs.uk

The Knowledge Network
 ⌖ http://www.knowledge.scot.nhs.uk/home.aspx

Department of Health
 ⌖ http://www.dh.gov.uk

UK National Statistics
 ⌖ http://www.statistics.gov.uk

National Institute for Health and Clinical Excellence
 ⌖ http://www.nice.org.uk

Scottish Intercollegiate Guideline Network
 ⌖ http://www.sign.ac.uk

Scottish Medicines Consortium
 ⌖ http://www.scottishmedicines.org.uk

Centers for Disease Control and Prevention
 ⌖ http://www.cdc.gov

World Health Organization
 ⌖ http://www.who.int

Charities/institutions supporting ophthalmic research (selected)
(See Box 27.7.)

Box 27.7 Charities/institutions supporting ophthalmic research (selected)

Action Medical Research
   🕮 http://www.action.org.uk

British Council for Prevention of Blindness
   🕮 http://www.bcpb.org

Fight for Sight
   🕮 http://www.fightforsight.org.uk

Guide Dogs for the Blind Association
   🕮 http://www.guidedogs.org.uk

International Agency for the Prevention of Blindness
   🕮 http://www.iapb.org

Medical Research Council
   🕮 http://www.mrc.ac.uk

National Eye Research Centre
   🕮 http://www.nerc.co.uk

Royal National Institute of Blind People
   🕮 http://www.rnib.org.uk

Sightsavers
   🕮 http://www.sightsavers.org

Vision 2020 UK
   🕮 http://www.vision2020uk.org.uk

Wellcome Trust
   🕮 http://www.wellcome.ac.uk

Neither the authors nor Oxford University Press are responsible for the content of any of the websites listed.

Web resources for patients

Accessibility and information for patients
(See Box 27.8.)

Box 27.8 Accessibility and information for patients

Action for Blind People
 ⇽ http://www.actionforblindpeople.org.uk

BBC Disability Site
 ⇽ http://www.bbc.co.uk/ouch/messageboards

Benefits of Blind Registration
 ⇽ http://www.rnib.org.uk/livingwithsightloss/registeringsightloss/
Pages/registration_benefits.aspx

Blind Business Association Charitable Trust
 ⇽ http://www.bbact.org.uk

British Blind Sport
 ⇽ http://www.britishblindsport.org.uk

British Computer Association of the Blind
 ⇽ http://www.bcab.org.uk

British Wireless for the Blind Fund
 ⇽ http://www.blind.org.uk

Calibre Audio Library
 ⇽ http://www.calibre.org.uk

Disability Rights UK
 ⇽ http://www.disabilityrightsuk.org

DIAL Network
 ⇽ http://www.scope.org.uk/dial

Driver & Vehicle Licensing Agency (DVLA)
 ⇽ http://www.dvla.gov.uk

iNFOsound
 ⇽ http://www.infosound.org.uk

Jobability (job site for disabled people)
 ⇽ http://www.jobability.org

The Royal National College for the Blind
 ⇽ http://www.rncb.ac.uk

Vitalise
 ⇽ http://www.vitalise.org.uk

WellChild Trust
 ⇽ http://www.wellchild.org.uk

The Royal Blind Society
 ⇽ http://www.royalblindsociety.org

Specialist holidays for the visually impaired

Action for Blind People
  🖰 http://www.actionforblindpeople.org.uk/holidays

The Royal Blind Society
  🖰 http://www.royalblindsociety.org/holidays.htm

Traveleyes
  🖰 http://www.traveleyes-international.com

Vitalise
  🖰 http://www.vitalise.org.uk/centre_breaks

Support groups for patients and their families
(See Box 27.9.)

Box 27.9 **Support groups for patients and their families**

Albinism Fellowship
   🕮 http://www.albinism.org.uk

Aniridia Network
   🕮 http://aniridia.org

Behçet's Syndrome Society
   🕮 http://www.behcets.org.uk

Birdshot Uveitis Society
   🕮 http://www.birdshot.org.uk

British Retinitis Pigmentosa Society
   🕮 http://www.brps.org.uk

British Sjögren's Syndrome Association
   🕮 http://www.bssa.uk.net

British Thyroid Association
   🕮 http://www.british-thyroid-association.org

Childrens Chronic Arthritis Association
   🕮 http://www.ccaa.org.uk

Childhood Eye Cancer Trust (retinoblastoma)
   🕮 http://www.chect.org.uk

deafblind UK
   🕮 http://www.deafblind.org.uk

International Glaucoma Association
   🕮 http://www.iga.org.uk

UK Keratoconus Self Help and Support Association
   🕮 http://www.keratoconus-group.org.uk

Look UK (families with visually impaired children)
   🕮 http://www.look-uk.org

Macular Society
   🕮 http://www.macularsociety.org

Micro and Anophthalmic Children's Society (MACS)
   🕮 http://www.macs.org.uk

National Association of Local Societies for Visually Impaired People
   🕮 http://www.nalsvi.org

National Blind Childrens Society
   🕮 http://www.nbcs.org.uk

National Ankylosing Spondylitis Society
   🕮 http://www.nass.co.uk

National Rheumatoid Arthritis Society
  ✍ http://www.nras.org.uk

nystagmus network information and research
  ✍ http://www.nystagmusnet.org

olivia's vision
  ✍ http://www.oliviasvision.org

sense (The National Deaf Blind and Rubella Association)
  ✍ http://www.sense.org.uk

Thyroid Eye Disease Charitable Trust
  ✍ http://www.tedct.co.uk

Uveitis Information Group (Scotland)
  ✍ http://www.uveitis.net

See also RNIB website
  ✍ http://www.rnib.org.uk

Reference intervals

See Tables 27.1–27.4 for reference intervals.

Table 27.1 Haematology

FBC	
Hb	130–180g/L ♂
	115–165g/L ♀
Hct	0.40–0.52 ♂
	0.36–0.47 ♀
RCC	4.5–6.5 × 10^{12}/L ♂
	3.8–5.8 × 10^{12}/L ♀
MCV	77–95fL
MCH	27.0–32.0pg
Reticulocytes	50–100 × 10^9/L (0.5–2.5%)
WCC	4.0–11.0 × 10^9/L
Neutrophils	2.0–7.5 × 10^9/L
Lymphocytes	1.5–4.5 × 10^9/L
Eosinophils	0.04–0.4 × 10^9/L
Basophils	0.0–0.2 × 10^9/L
Monocytes	0.2–0.8 × 10^9/L
Platelets	150–400 × 10^9/L
Clotting	
INR	0.8–1.2
PT	12–14s
APTT ratio	0.8–1.2
APTT	26.0–33.5s
Protein C	80–135U/dL
Protein S	80–135U/dL
Antithrombin III	80–120U/dL
APCR	2.12–4.0
Haematinics	
Serum B12	150–700ng/L
Serum folate	2.0–11.0 micrograms/L
Red cell folate	160–640 micrograms/L
Serum ferritin	15–300 micrograms/L
Others	
HbA1c	20–40 mmol/mol (4–5.9%)
ESR	Variable: some suggest an upper limit based on age and gender: age/2 for ♂ and (age + 10) / 2 for ♀

Table 27.2 Biochemistry

U+E and glucose	
Sodium (Na)	135–145mmol/L
Potassium (K)	3.5–5.0mmol/L
Urea	3.0–6.5mmol/L
Creatinine	60–125 micromoles/L
Glucose (fasting)	3.5–5.5mmol/L
Glucose (random)	3.5–11.0mmol/L (normal/IGT)
LFTs and protein	
Total protein	63–80g/L
Albumin	32–50g/L
Bilirubin	<17 micromoles/L
Alkaline phosphatase	100–300IU/L
ALT	5–42IU/L
AST	5–42IU/L
γGT	10–46IU/L
Bone	
Calcium (total)	2.15–2.55mmol/L
Phosphate	0.7–1.5mmol/L
Lipids	
Cholesterol	3.9–6.0mmol/L
Triglycerides	0.55–1.90mmol/L
Iron studies	
Iron	14–33 micromoles/L
	11–28 micromoles/L
TIBC	45–75 micromoles/L
Hormones	
TSH	0.35–5.5mU/L
Free T4	9–24pmol/L
Cortisol (morning)	450–700nmol/L
FSH	2–8U/L (luteal ♀); >25u/L (menopausal ♀)
LH	3–16U/L (luteal ♀)
Prolactin	<325U/L ♂
	<500U/L (non-pregnant ♀)
Other	
CRP	<8mg/L
ACE	12–71 (age ≥20); 5–87 (age <20)
Arterial blood gases	
pH	7.35–7.45
PaO₂	>10.6kPa
PaCO₂	4.7–6.0kPa
BE	± 2.0mmol/L

Table 27.3 Immunology

IgG	5.3–16.5g/L
IgA	0.8–4.0g/L
IgM	0.5–2.0g/L
C3	0.9–2.1g/L
C4	0.12–0.53g/L
C1 esterase	0.11–0.36g/L
CH50	80–120%

Table 27.4 CSF analysis

Lymphocytes	<4/mL
Neutrophils	0/mL
Glucose	≥2/3 plasma level
Protein	<0.4g/L
Opening pressure	<20cmH$_2$O or <25cmH$_2$O in the obese

For some tests (such as ACE level), there may be significant variation between labs as to what constitutes the 'normal' range. It is therefore important to check values against local standards.

Index

Adult basic life support algorithm

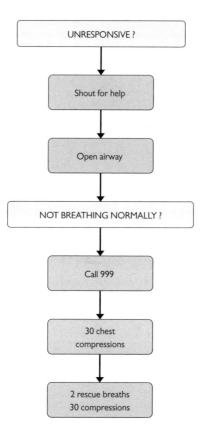